Basic Electrical and Electronics Engineering

Basic Electrical and Electronics Engineering

Shikha Shrivastava
M Tech (Electrical Engineering)
Associate Professor
Department of Electronics Engineering
Shah & Anchor Kutchhi Engineering College
Chembur, Mumbai
India
E-mail: shikha.12ap@gmail.com

CBS

CBS Publishers & Distributors Pvt Ltd

New Delhi • Bengaluru • Chennai • Kochi • Kolkata • Mumbai
Bhopal • Bhubaneswar • Hyderabad • Jharkhand • Nagpur • Patna • Pune • Uttarakhand • Dhaka (Bangladesh)

Basic Electrical
and
Electronics Engineering

ISBN: 978-93-88327-50-3

CBS Edition: 2019
First Edition: 2014

Published by Satish Kumar Jain and produced by Varun Jain for
CBS Publishers & Distributors Pvt Ltd
4819/XI Prahlad Street, 24 Ansari Road, Daryaganj, New Delhi 110 002, India.
Ph: 23289259, 23266861, 23266867 Fax: 011-23243014 Website: www.cbspd.com
e-mail: delhi@cbspd.com; cbspubs@airtelmail.in.
Corporate Office: 204 FIE, Industrial Area, Patparganj, Delhi 110 092
Ph: 4934 4934 Fax: 4934 4935 e-mail: publishing@cbspd.com; publicity@cbspd.com

Branches

- **Bengaluru:** Seema House 2975, 17th Cross, K.R. Road, Banasankari 2nd Stage, Bengaluru 560 070, Karnataka
  Ph: +91-80-26771678/79 Fax: +91-80-26771680 e-mail: bangalore@cbspd.com
- **Chennai:** 7, Subbaraya Street, Shenoy Nagar, Chennai 600 030, Tamil Nadu
  Ph: +91-44-26680620, 26681266 Fax: +91-44-42032115 e-mail: chennai@cbspd.com
- **Kochi:** 42/1325, 1326, Power House Road, Opp KSEB Power House, Ernakulam 682 018, Kochi, Kerala
  Ph: +91-484-4059061-65 Fax: +91-484-4059065 e-mail: kochi@cbspd.com
- **Kolkata:** 6/B, Ground Floor, Rameswar Shaw Road, Kolkata-700 014, West Bengal
  Ph: +91-33-22891126, 22891127, 22891128 e-mail: kolkata@cbspd.com
- **Mumbai:** 83-C, Dr E Moses Road, Worli, Mumbai-400018, Maharashtra
  Ph: +91-22-24902340/41 Fax: +91-22-24902342 e-mail: mumbai@cbspd.com

Representatives

• **Bhopal**	0-8319310552	• **Bhubaneswar**	0-9911037372	• **Hyderabad**	0-9885175004
• **Jharkhand**	0-9811541605	• **Nagpur**	0-9021734563	• **Patna**	0-9334159340
• **Pune**	0-9623451994	• **Uttarakhand**	0-9716462459	• **Dhaka (Bangladesh)**	01912-003485

Printed by Rashtriya printers, Delhi

to

My Husband

Vinod Srivastav and

Children

Vishesh and Kriti

Preface

This book has been written with two main objectives in view: *First* to cover the ground of the important examination syllabi of basic electrical and electronics, for undergraduate first year engineering students of all branches; *second* to configure the book in a manner suitable for self-study.

This book gives a good number of solved problems in order to get ease over the subject. Students who work through these problems should not experience difficulty with the chapter problems, which are chosen to aid understanding of the text. The solutions of these problems are also given at the end of the book for reference. Looking at the need of the hour, multiple-choice questions are also given with answers at the end of the book.

Chapter 1 deals with the simple methods to solve circuits with steady state DC supply. It also help students get acquainted with various theorems used for solving the circuits. More number of problems which are self explanatory, are given for self help. Some of the numericals are repeated purposely for different theorems so as to make students aware with the fundamental aspect that irrespective of methods used, the electrical quantities do not change and also for a comparative analysis of various methods.

Chapter 2 describes the basics of electromagnetic induction with suitable examples.

Chapter 3 presents the basic principles of generation of AC supply and definitions associated with AC supply and its vector representation.

Chapter 4 presents various components and their behaviour with steady state AC supply. A good number of problems, varying from simple to complex are given for students so that these methods may be implemented for various practical circuits. Students are encouraged to make proper use of modern day calculators for ease of calculations in complex algebra.

Chapter 5 enumerates three-phase supply system, and the basic analysis of supply system is given with the help of numericals.

Chapter 6 introduces the first static machine, the transformer. After reading and practicing AC circuits and their vector representation, its applications in this chapter would help students understand the operation and behaviour of the transformer.

Chapter 7 presents students to the various basic rotating electrical machines which are commonly used. It only introduces the concept and constructions of the motors to a very small extent, just to make students familiar with them.

Chapter 8 introduces students to the semiconductor world. The basic device being the diode and its application as a rectifier.

Chapter 9 deals with the transistor to the introductory level only. A great majority of diagrams have been specially drawn and steps for doing so are explained with details for ease of students.

Constructive criticism and suggestions from the readers of the book will be gratefully accepted to enable further improvement of the book.

Your feedback is welcome at shikha.12ap@gmail.com

Shikha Shrivastava

Acknowledgements

I would like to acknowledge all the students who have come in contact with my teaching experience and have given a greater insight into the subject from their point of view. This edition is the outcome of the tremandous response to the first edition. I am thankful to them for their constant encouragement.

I am also thankful to Mrs Sushma Srivastava, for her help in getting a better understanding on the electronic devices. I acknowledge Mrs Manjusha Kulkarni's effort for her critical analysis of the content from time to time. I am thankful to all my friends and colleagues for their constant help.

This work would not have been possible without the constant support and encouragement from my husband Mr Vinod Shrivastav and children Vishesh and Kriti, to whom I wish to express my deep gratitude.

I am grateful to Sh Satish Kumar Jain (Mataji), CMD, and Sh Varun Jain, Director, CBS Publishers & Distributors, New Delhi, for their patience, goodwill and cooperation. I express my gratitude to Mr YN Arjuna (Senior Vice President Publishing, Editorial and Publicity); Mrs Ritu Chawla (AGM Production); Mrs Sanjubala Tripathy and Mr Parmod Kumar, for their skillful service and immense help.

Shikha Shrivastava

Contents

Preface *vii*

1. D.C. CIRCUITS **1.1–1.88**

1.1 Basic Definitions 1.1
1.2 Ohm's Law 1.3
1.3 Resistances in Series 1.4
1.4 Resistances in Parallel 1.4
1.5 Kirchhoff's Laws 1.5
1.5.1 Kirchhoff's Current Law or Point Law 1.5
1.5.2 Kirchhoff's Voltage Law (KVL) or Mesh Law 1.6
1.6 Star-Delta Transformation 1.12
1.7 Mesh Analysis or Maxwell's Loop Current Method 1.23
1.7.1 Concept of Supermesh 1.28
1.8 Nodal Analysis 1.30
1.8.1 Concept of Super Node 1.36
1.9 Source Transformation 1.39
1.10 Superposition Theorem 1.45
1.11 Thevenin's Theorem 1.57
1.13 Norton's Theorem 1.70
1.14 Maximum Power Transfer Theorem 1.77
Unsolved Problems 1.84

2. ELECTROMAGNETIC INDUCTION **2.1–2.10**

2.1 Direction of Induced emf and Current 2.1
2.1.1 Dynamically Induced emf 2.1
2.1.2 Statistically Induced emf 2.2
2.2 Magnetomotive Force (mmf) 2.3
2.3 Magnetic Field Strength 2.3
2.4 Reluctance 2.4
2.5 Co-efficients of Self Inductance 2.4
2.6 Co-efficient of Mutual Inductance 2.5
2.7 Coupling Co-efficient 2.6
2.8 Rise of Current in Inductive Circuits 2.7
2.9 Decay (Fall) of Current in Inductive Circuit 2.1

3. A.C. FUNDAMENTALS **3.1–3.28**

3.1 Introduction 3.1
3.2 Generation of Alternating Voltages and Currents 3.3

3.3 Terminologies of Sinusoidal Functions 3.5
3.4 Important Value of Alternating Voltage and Current 3.8
3.4.1 Average Value 3.8
3.4.2 Effective or RMS Value 3.9
3.4.3 Form Factor and Peak Factor 3.10
3.5 Vector Representation of Sinusoidal A.C. 3.21
3.6 Vector Representation Using RMS Values 3.22
3.7 Mathematical Operation of Vectors 3.22
Unsolved Examples 3.26

4. A.C. CIRCUITS **4.1–4.58**

4.1 A.C. Through Pure Resistance 4.1
4.2 A.C. Through Pure Inductance 4.3
4.3 A.C. Through Pure Capacitance 4.5
4.4 Resistance and Inductance in Series 4.7
4.5 Resistance and Capacitance in Series 4.9
4.6 R-L-C Series Circuit 4.11
4.7 A.C. Parallel Circuits 4.27
4.8 Resonance in A.C. Circuits 4.38
4.8.1 Series Resonant Circuit 4.39
4.8.2 Parallel Resonant Circuit 4.48
4.8.3 Comparison of Resonance in Series and Parallel Circuits 4.52
Unsolved Examples 4.55

5. THREE PHASE CIRCUITS **5.1–5.29**

5.1 Generation of 3-Phase A.C. System 5.1
5.2 Inter Connection of Three Phases 5.2
5.3 Star or Y Connection 5.3
5.3.1 Relation Between Phase and Line Voltages (Star Connection) 5.4
5.3.2 Relation Between Line and Phase Currents (Star Connection) 5.5
5.5.3 Power Consumed in Star Connected Load 5.5
5.3.4 Volt-Ampere and Reactive Volt-Ampere Relation in Star Connected Load 5.5
5.4 Delta or D Connection 5.6
5.4.1 Relation Between Phase and Line Voltages in Delta Connected Load 5.6
5.4.2 Relation Between Line and Phase Currents 5.7
5.4.3 Power Consumed in Delta Connected Load 5.8
5.4.4 Volt-Ampere and Reactive Volt-Ampere Relation in Delta Connected Load 5.8
5.5 Comparisons 5.15
5.5.1 Comparison Between Star and Delta Connected Loads 5.15
5.5.2 Comparison Between the Power Consumed in Star Connected Load and Delta Connected Load 5.16
5.6 Measurement of Power in 3-Phase Circuits 5.16
5.6.1 One Wattmeter Method 5.17
5.6.2 Three Wattmeter Method 5.18

5.6.3 Two Wattmeter Method 5.18
5.6.3.1 Star Connected Load 5.19
5.6.3.2 Delta Connected Load 5.21
5.6.3.3 Effect of Power Factor on Wattmeter Readings 5.22
Unsolved Examples 5.27

6. TRANSFORMER **6.1–6.39**

6.1 Need of Transformer 6.1
6.2 Transformer Construction 6.1
6.3 Principle of Transformer 6.3
6.4 Ideal Two Winding Transformer 6.3
6.5 Phasor Diagram of Ideal Transformer on No-Load 6.7
6.6 Phasor Diagram of Ideal Transformer on Load 6.7
6.7 Ratings of Transformer 6.8
6.8 Practical Transformer 6.11
6.9 No Load Vector Diagram of Practical Transformer 6.11
6.10 Transformer Vector Diagram Under Load Conditions 6.12
6.11 Equivalent Circuit of a Transformer 6.14
6.11.1 Approximate Equivalent Circuit of Transformer 6.16
6.12 Open Circuit and Short Circuit Test on Transformer 6.17
6.13 Losses and Efficiency of a Transformer 6.21
6.14 Efficiency Calculation Using O.C/S.C. Test Results 6.23
6.15 Regulation 6.23
6.16 All Day Efficiency 6.31
Unsolved Examples 6.37

7. ROTATING ELECTRICAL MACHINE **7.1–7.22**

7.1 D.C. Machines 7.1
7.1.1 D.C. Generator Principle 7.2
7.1.2 Parts of D.C. Machines 7.3
7.1.2.1 Stator 7.3
7.1.2.2 Rotor 7.4
7.1.3 emf Equation of a D.C. Generator 7.6
7.1.4 Representation of a D.C. Machine 7.7
7.1.5 Types of D.C. Machines 7.8
7.1.5.1 Separately Excited D.C. Machine 7.8
7.1.5.2 Self Excited D.C. Machines 7.8
7.1.6 D.C. Motors 7.10
7.1.7 Comparison of Generator and Motor 7.10
7.1.8 Back emf 7.11
7.2 3-Phase Induction Motors 7.12
7.2.1 Construction of 3-Phase Induction Motors 7.12
7.2.2 Production of Rotating Magnetic Field 7.13
7.2.3 Principle of Operation 7.15

7.2.4 Slip and Rotor Speed 7.16
7.3 Single-Phase Induction Motors 7.16
7.3.1 Constructional Features of Single-Phase Induction Motors 7.16
7.3.2 Double Field Revolving Theory 7.16
7.4 Split-Phase Induction Motors 7.18
7.5 Shaded Pole Induction Motor 7.21

8. SEMICONDUCTOR DIODES AND THEIR APPLICATIONS **8.1–8.12**

8.1 Classification of Materials 8.1
8.2 Semiconductors 8.1
8.3 Donor and Acceptor Impurities 8.2
8.4 Semiconductor Diode 8.2
8.5 Half-Wave Rectifier 8.5
8.6 Full-Wave Rectifier Circuit (with Centre Tap Transformer) 8.7
8.7 Full-Wave Bridge Rectifier 8.8
8.8 Filter Circuit (Capacitor Filter) 8.10
8.9 Zener Diode 8.11

9. TRANSISTORS **9.1–9.8**

9.1 Naming the Terminals of Transistor 9.1
9.2 Operation of N-P-N Transistor 9.2
9.3 Transistor Symbol 9.3
9.4 Transistor Connection 9.4
9.5 Common Base Connection 9.4
9.6 Common Emitter Configuration 9.6

Appendix A: Multiple Choice Questions A.1–A.14
Appendix B: Solution To Unsolved Examples B.1–B.72
Appendix C: Some Useful Formulae C.1

CHAPTER

1

D.C. CIRCUITS

There are certain theorems which can be applied to electric networks for their simplification or for analyzing their solutions. These theorems can be applied to d.c. circuits as well as steady state analysis of a.c. circuits with a difference, that in d.c. circuits the resistances (scalar quantities) are replaced by impedances (vector quantities) and in a.c., the analysis is in vector form, where as in d.c. all these analysis are done in scalar quantities. Different types of circuits are defined below according to their properties.

1.1 Basic Definitions

(a) **Circuit :** A circuit is a conducting part through which either an electric current flows or is intended to flow.

(b) **Linear Circuit :** A linear circuit is one in which circuit parameters do not change with change in voltage or current.

(c) **Parameters :** The various elements of a circuit that is resistance, inductances and capacitance are called parameters.

(d) **Bilateral Circuits :** A bilateral circuit is one whose properties or characteristics are same in both the directions Resistance, inductance and capacitance etc. are bilateral circuit elements.

(e) **Unilateral Circuit :** If the properties or characteristics of a circuit or element change with the direction of its operation it is said be unilateral circuit. Diode is a good example of unilateral circuit.

(f) **Electric Network :** A combination of various electric elements, connected to one another is called electric network.

(g) **Passive Network :** A circuit which does not contain any source of emf in it is called passive network.

(h) **Active Network :** A circuit or a network which contains one or more sources of emf is called active network.

(i) **D.C. Voltage Source (Ideal) :** A d.c. voltage source is one whose output voltage does not change with time and has no internal resistance. The voltage of a d.c. source does not depend upon the resistance connected across it. [Fig. 1.1.(a)]

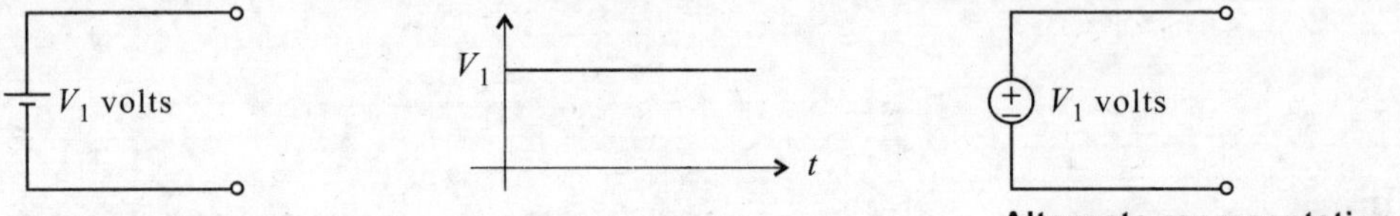

Alternate representation

Fig. 1.1(a) : Ideal voltage source.

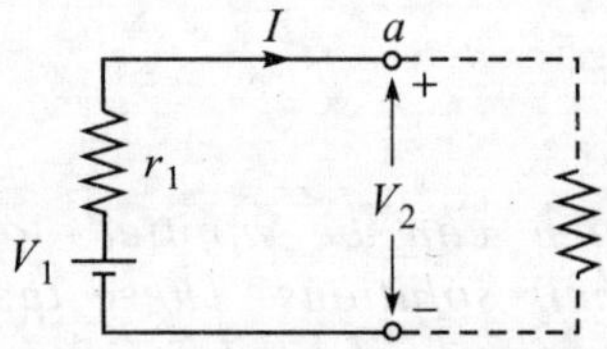

Fig. 1.1 (b) : Practical voltage source.

(j) **Practical D.C. Voltage Source :** Practically, no source can be ideal i.e. Every source has some internal resistance r_1 [Fig. 1.1(b)]. Because of presence of this internal resistance the voltage available across the external terminals *ab* of the source is lesser than V_1. Depending upon the current I drawn from the source the terminal voltage V_2 will be given by

$$V_2 = V_1 - Ir_1 \qquad \text{..... (1.1)}$$

e.g. If a resistance R is connected across *ab* then,

$$I = \frac{V_1}{R + r_1}$$

$$\text{and } V_2 = V_1 - Ir_1$$

Usually, value of r_1 is very small (negligible or zero in case of ideal voltage source)

(k) **Ideal Current Source :** A d.c. source whose output current remains constant irrespective of the circuit connected across its terminals is called an *ideal current source* [Fig. 1.2(a)].

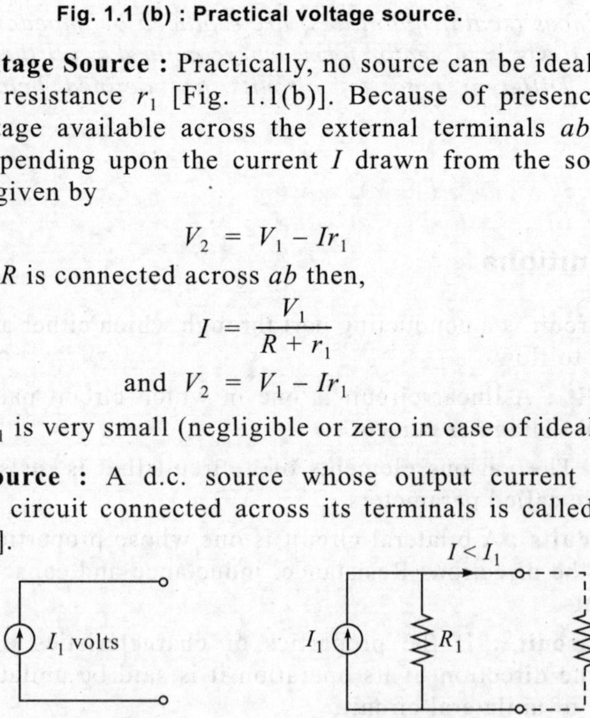

(a) Ideal source. **(b) Practical source.**

Fig. 1.2 : D.c. current source.

(l) Practical Current Source : Fig. 1.2(b) shows the representation for a practical current source. Here, the output current I is not the same as I_1, but is less than I_1. Usually the internal resistance of a current source R_1 is very large (Ideally infinity for an ideal current source).

(m) Resistance : It may be defined as the property of a substance due to which it opposes the flow of current through it. Its unit is ohms (Ω). It is represented as in Fig. 1.3.

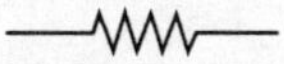

R

Fig. 1.3 : Representation of resistance.

(n) Laws of Resistance : The resistance R offered by a conductor depends upon the following factors.

(i) It varies directly as its length l.

(ii) It varies inversely as its cross-section area A, of the conductor.

(iii) It depends upon the nature of material.

(iv) It also depends upon the temperature of the conductor.

At a constant temperature,

$$R \propto \frac{l}{A} \qquad \text{..... (1.2)}$$

$$\text{or } R = \rho \frac{l}{A} \qquad \text{..... (1.3)}$$

ρ is a constant that depends upon the nature of material of the conductor. It is called *resistivity* or *specific resistance*.

We will now discuss various theorems and techniques which will help us in solving complicated networks.

1.2 Ohm's Law

Ohm's law states that "*the ratio of potential difference (V) between any two points on a conductor to the current flowing between them is constant, provided the temperature of the conductor remains constant.*"

$$\text{i.e. } \frac{V}{I} = \text{constant}$$

$$\text{or } \frac{V}{I} = R \qquad \text{..... (1.4)}$$

where, R is the resistance of the conductor between those points. In other words, "*if resistance R remains constant the current through a conductor is directly proportional to the potential difference across the ends of the conductor.*"

1.3 Resistances in Series

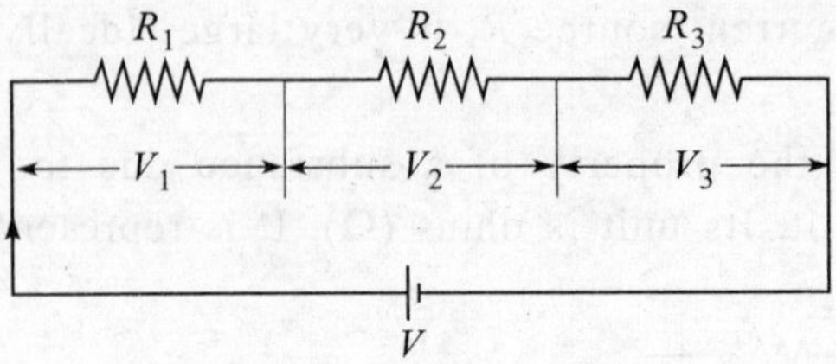

Fig. 1.4(a) : Series resistances.

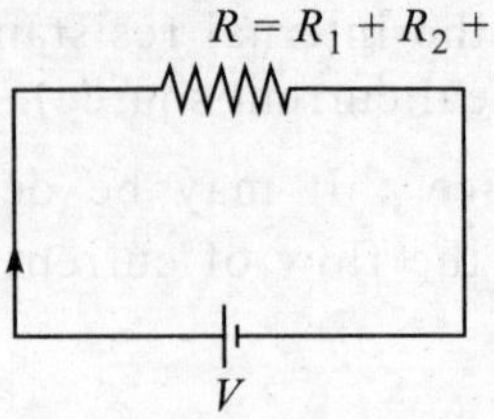

Fig. 1.4(b) : Equivalent resistance.

The resistance R_1, R_2 and R_3 are joined end on end in Fig. 1.4(a), are said to be connected in series. The equivalent resistance is R, as shown in Fig. 1.4(b), where

$$R = R_1 + R_2 + R_3$$

Important observations here are

(i) All the three resistance carry the same current.

(ii) The voltage across each resistance is given using Ohm's law and these voltages will be different if R_1, R_2 and R_3 are different.

$$V_1 = IR_1 \; ; \; V_2 = IR_2 \; ; \; V_3 = IR_3$$

(iii) Sum of the three voltages is equal to the supply voltage.

$$\text{i.e. } V = V_1 + V_2 + V_3 \quad \text{..... (1.5)}$$

but $V = IR$ from Fig. 1.4(b)

$$\therefore \; IR = IR_1 + IR_2 + IR_3$$

$$\text{or } R = R_1 + R_2 + R_3 \quad \text{..... (1.6)}$$

1.4 Resistances in Parallel

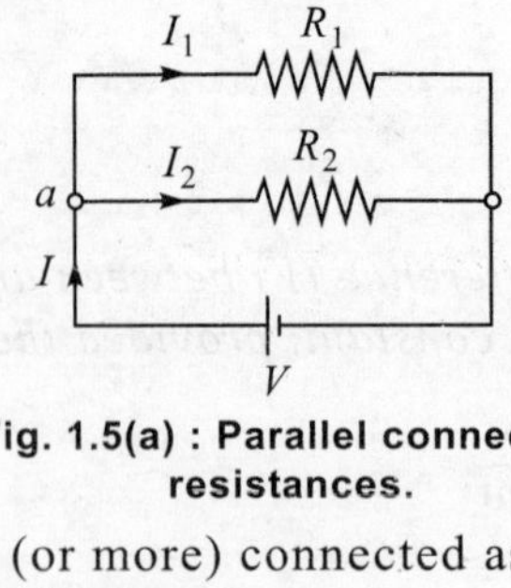

Fig. 1.5(a) : Parallel connected resistances.

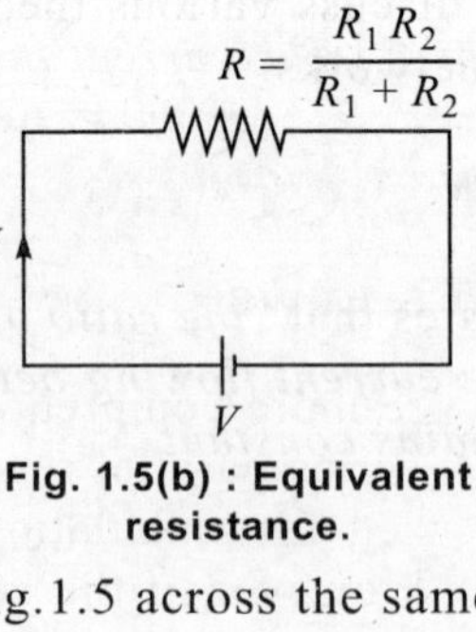

Fig. 1.5(b) : Equivalent resistance.

Two resistances (or more) connected as shown in Fig.1.5 across the same terminals ab are called parallel resistances.

(i) They share the same voltage V.

(ii) They carry different currents if the resistances are of different values given by Ohm's law.

$$\therefore \; I_1 = \frac{V}{R_1} \text{ and } I_2 = \frac{V}{R_2}$$

(iii) The total current I is the sum of the currents I_1 and I_2.

If R is the equivalent resistance in Fig. 1.5(b) then both the circuits the current drawn from supply I would be same.

$$I = \frac{V}{R} \quad \text{and} \quad I = I_1 + I_2$$

$$\therefore \quad \frac{V}{R} = \frac{V}{R_1} + \frac{V}{R_2}$$

$$\text{or} \quad \frac{1}{R} = \frac{1}{R_1} + \frac{1}{R_2} \qquad \text{..... (1.7)}$$

$$\text{or} \quad R = \frac{R_1 R_2}{R_1 + R_2} \qquad \text{..... (1.8)}$$

Note : Current Division Rule in Parallel Resistance

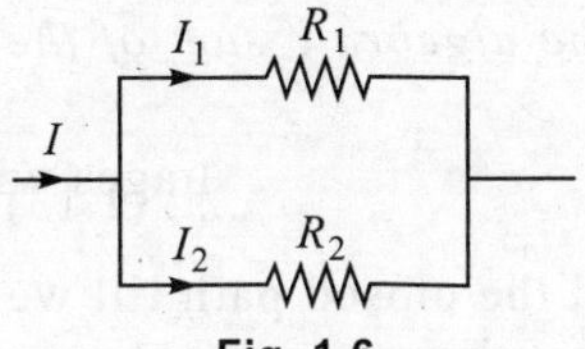

Fig. 1.6

If there are two resistance connected in parallel (Fig. 1.6) and total current entering is I then

$$I = I_1 + I_2 \qquad \text{..... (1.9)}$$

and for parallel resistance as they share same voltage

$$I_1 R_1 = I_2 R_2$$

From equation (1.9)

$$I_2 = I - I_1$$

$$\therefore \quad I_1 R_1 = (I - I_1) R_2$$

$$I_1 R_1 = I R_2 - I_1 R_2$$

$$I_1 (R_1 + R_2) = I R_2$$

$$\therefore \quad I_1 = I \frac{R_2}{R_1 + R_2} \qquad \text{..... (1.10)}$$

How to Remember : *The current through a resistance R_1 when connected in parallel with another resistance R_2, knowing total current entering I is given by the neighbour's resistance R_2 divided by total resistance ($R_1 + R_2$) multiplied by the total current I.*

1.5 Kirchhoff's Laws

These laws are more comprehensive than Ohm's law. The circuits which can not be readily solved by series-parallel resistances and Ohm's laws can be solved by Kirchhoff's laws. It can be used for calculating currents and voltages in various components of a complex circuits. However, if the complexity of the circuits increase than other methods described later are more useful.

1.5.1 Kirchhoff's Current Law or Point Law

It states that "*in any electrical network, the algebric sum of currents meeting at a junction (called node) is zero.*"

It simply means that total current entering a node is equal to total current leaving that node. Obviously, as there is no accumulation of current at any junction.

From Fig. 1.7 thus we can write KCL equation as

$$I_1 + I_3 = I_2 + I_4 + I_5 \quad ..... (1.11)$$

From this we can derive the following equation.

$$I_2 + I_4 + I_5 - I_1 - I_3 = 0 \quad ..... (1.12)$$

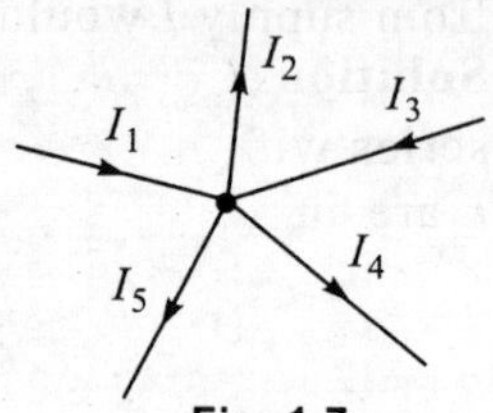

Fig. 1.7

Note : *We will hence forth take outgoing currents as positive and incoming currents at the node as negative.*

1.5.2 Kirchhoff's Voltage Law (KVL) or Mesh Law

It states that "*the algebraic sum of the products of current and resistance in each of the conductors in any closed mesh (or path) in a network plus the algebraic sum of the emfs in that path is zero.*"

$$\text{i.e. } \Sigma\, IR + \Sigma\, emf = 0 \quad ..... (1.13)$$

This means that if we start from particular junction and go around the closed path till we reach the starting point, without repeating a node then we must be at the same potential at which we started. Hence, all the emf sources must necessarily be equal to the voltage drops in the resistances, every voltage being given its proper sign (positive or negative).

The proper signs for emfs and drops will be as under from now onwards. Refer Fig.1.8.

Here *ABCD* is a part of a circuit, where currents I_1, I_2 and I_3 are assumed to flow in the marked directions. To assign proper signs to the various drops and emfs, when we travel the loop from *A-B-C-D-A*, if we are going in the direction of current we will take the drop as positive, if the direction of current is opposite to the direction of travel then take that drop as negative. For emf source if while going in the direction of travel we get positive terminal of source, we will take it positive and if we get negative terminal first then we will take it negative. Refer Fig. 1.8 and its equation (1.14) while going from *A-B-C-D-A*.

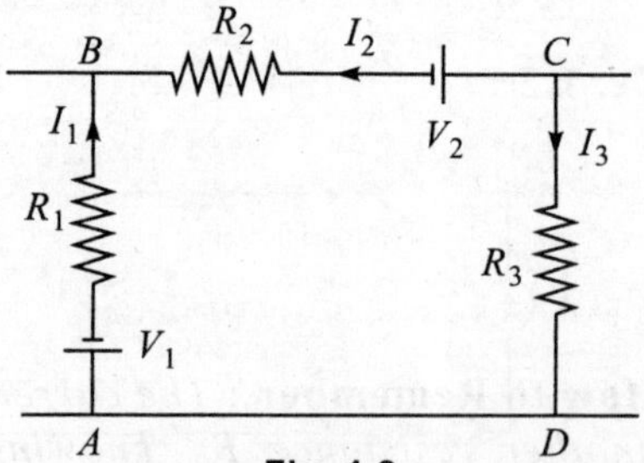

Fig. 1.8

$$+ V_1 + I_1 R_1 - I_2 R_2 - V_2 + I_3 R_3 = 0 \quad ..... (1.14)$$

Important : *In applying Kirchhoff's laws to circuits, we assume certain direction of currents. However, the important point here is that once a particular direction has been assumed, the same should be used through out the solution of the question. If the value of current we calculate comes out to be positive, it indicates that the assumed current is in the same direction as actual current and if the calculated value of current is negative than the actual current is opposite to the assumed current.*

Ex. 1.1 : Using KCL, KVL find I_1, I_2 and r in the following circuit. (Fig. 1.9)

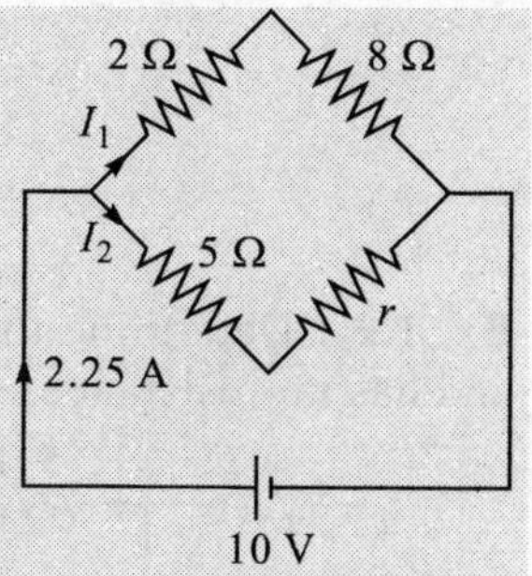

Fig. 1.9

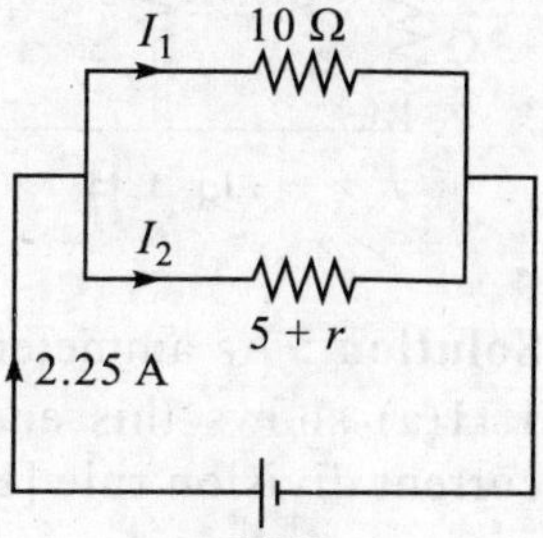

Fig. 1.9(a)

Solution : From Fig. 1.9. Resistance 2 Ω and 8 Ω are in series with equivalent resistance 8 + 2 = 10 Ω and 5 Ω and r are in series with equivalent resistance of $(5 + r)$ ohms.

$$I_1 = \frac{10\text{ V}}{10\ \Omega}$$

$$\therefore \boxed{I_1 = 1\text{ A}}$$

But $I_1 + I_2 = 2.25$ ... (KCL)

$$\therefore I_2 = 2.25 - 1$$

$$\therefore \boxed{I_2 = 1.25\text{ A}}$$

From the circuit

$$I_2 = \frac{10}{5 + r}$$

$$\therefore 1.25 = \frac{10}{5 + r} \quad \text{or } 5 + r = \frac{10}{1.25}$$

$$\therefore \boxed{r = 3\ \Omega}$$

Ex. 1.2 : Find I in Fig. 1.10.

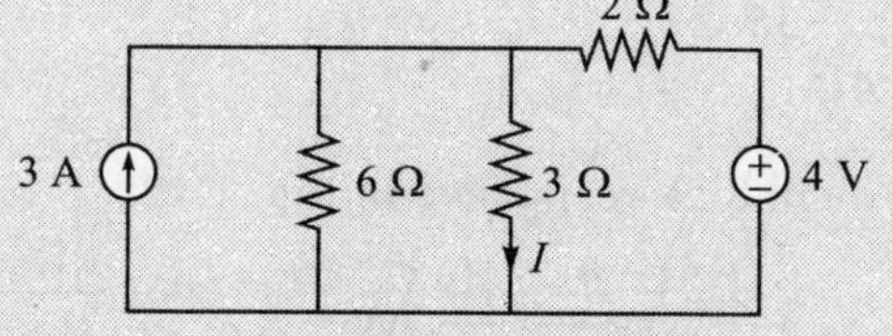

Fig. 1.10

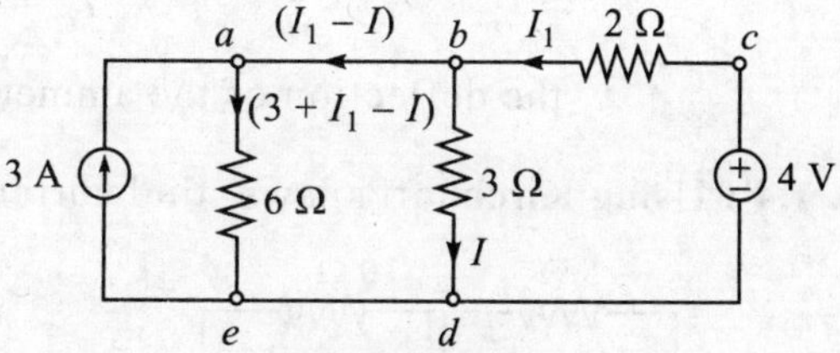

Fig. 1.10(a)

Solution : Assuming branch current and using KCL finding various other currents we will write KVL equations. As there are two variables I and I_1, we need two equations from the circuit in Fig. 1.10(a).

Apply KVL in *abdea*

$$3I - 6(3 + I_1 - I) = 0$$

$$9I - 6I_1 = 18 \quad \text{.... (i)}$$

Apply KVL in *bdcb*

$$3I - 4 + 2I_1 = 0$$

$$3I + 2I_1 = 4 \quad \text{.... (ii)}$$

Thus,

$$\begin{bmatrix} 9 & -6 \\ 3 & 2 \end{bmatrix} \begin{bmatrix} I \\ I_1 \end{bmatrix} = \begin{bmatrix} 18 \\ 4 \end{bmatrix}$$

$$\therefore I = \boxed{1.67 \text{ A}}$$

Ex. 1.3 : Determine the deflection of the ammeter in Fig. 1.11. Assume ammeter is ideal and has no resistance.

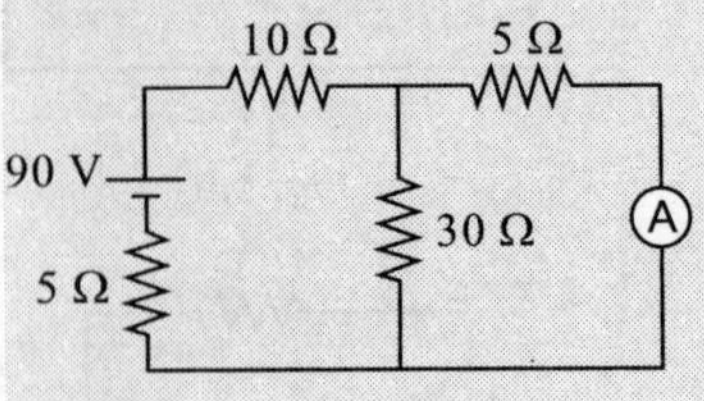

Fig. 1.11

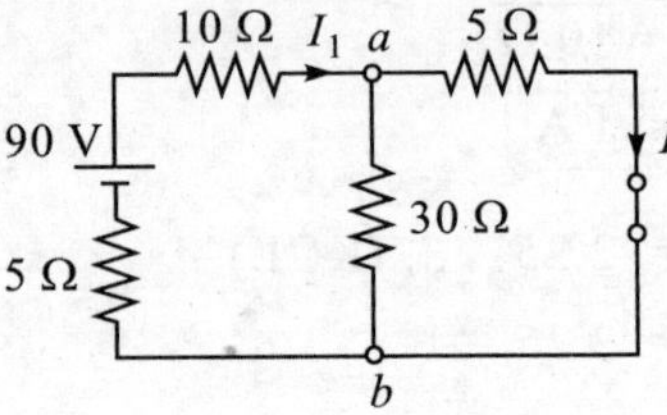

Fig. 1.11(a)

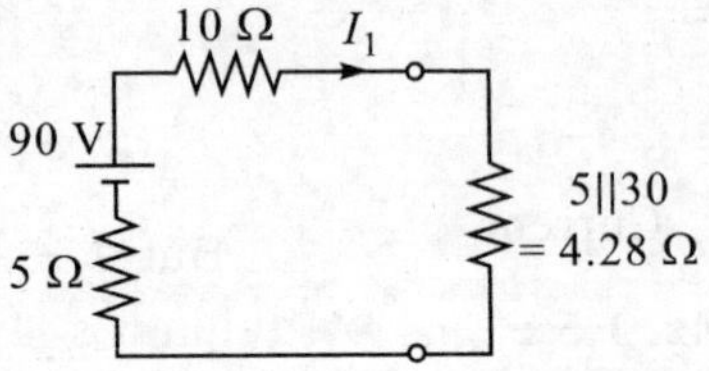

Fig. 1.11(b)

Solution : As ammeter is ideal it can be replaced by a short circuit (zero resistance) Fig. 1.11(a) shows this and let the current here be I_2. 30 Ω and 5 Ω are in parallel using current division rule [equation (1.10)]

$$\therefore I_2 = I_1 \times \frac{30}{30+5} \qquad \text{... (i)}$$

From Fig. 1.11(b)

$$I_1 = \frac{90}{10 + 4.28 + 5} = 4.67 \text{ A}$$

∴ From (i) we get

$$I_2 = 4.67 \times \frac{30}{35} = \boxed{4 \text{ A}}$$

∴ the deflection of the ammeter is 4 A.

Ex. 1.4 : Using Kirchhoff's laws, find current through 8 Ω resistance in Fig. 1.12.

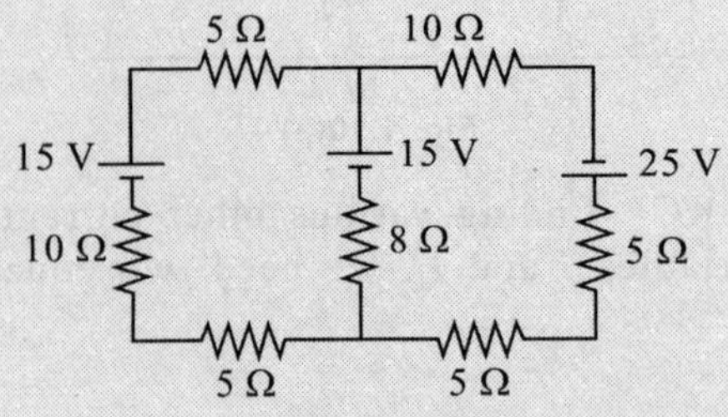

Fig. 1.12

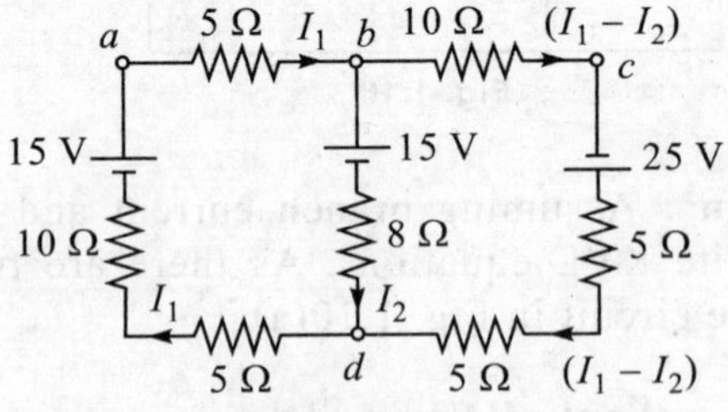

Fig. 1.12(a)

Solution : Let us redraw the circuit and assume currents I_1 and I_2, thus applying KCL find other currents. Name the junctions *abcd*. Fig. 1.12(a).

Apply KVL in mesh *abda*

$$5I_1 + 15 + 8I_2 + 5I_1 + 10I_1 - 15 = 0$$

$$\therefore 20\, I_1 + 8I_2 = 0 \qquad \text{.... (i)}$$

Apply KVL in mesh *bcdb*

$$10(I_1 - I_2) - 25 + 5(I_1 - I_2) + 5(I_1 - I_2) - 8I_2 - 15 = 0$$

$$\therefore 20I_1 - 28I_2 = 40 \qquad \text{.... (ii)}$$

Solving equations (i) and (ii) by Cramer's Rule

$$\begin{bmatrix} 20 & 8 \\ 20 & -28 \end{bmatrix} \begin{bmatrix} I_1 \\ I_2 \end{bmatrix} = \begin{bmatrix} 0 \\ 40 \end{bmatrix}$$

$$\therefore I_1 = \boxed{0.44 \text{ A}}$$

$$\text{and } I_2 = \boxed{-1.11 \text{ A}}$$

$\therefore$ Current through 8 Ω is –1.11 A i.e. 1.11 A opposite to the marked direction.

Ex. 1.5 : Using Kirchhoff's laws find V_{bc} in Fig. 1.13.

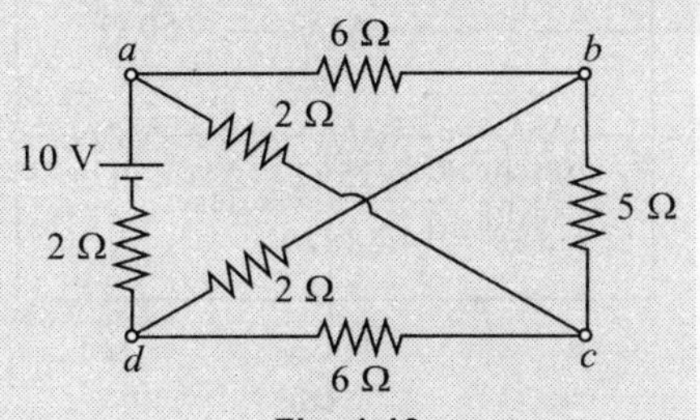

Fig. 1.13

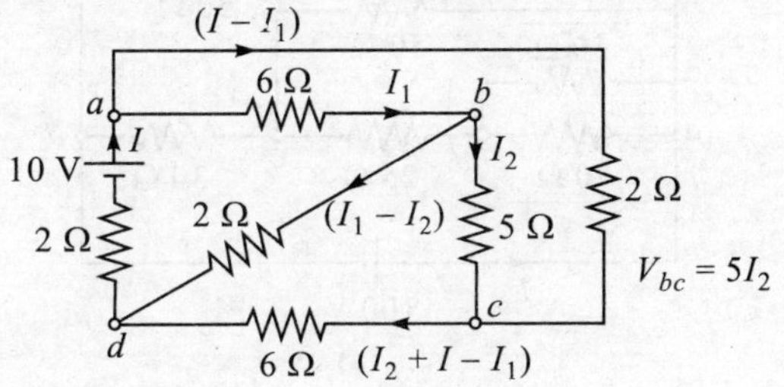

Fig. 1.13(a)

Solution : Redraw the circuit and assume various current as in Fig. 1.13(a).

Applying KVL in *abda*

$$6I_1 + 2(I_1 - I_2) + 2I - 10 = 0$$

$$\therefore 8I_1 - 2I_2 + 2I = 10 \qquad \text{.... (i)}$$

Applying KVL in *bcdb*

$$5I_2 + 6(I_2 + I - I_1) - 2(I_1 - I_2) = 0$$

$$\therefore -8I_1 + 13I_2 + 6I = 0 \qquad \text{.... (ii)}$$

Applying KVL in outer mesh *abca*

$$6I_1 + 5I_2 - 2(I - I_1) = 0$$

$$\therefore 8I_1 + 5I_2 - 2I = 0 \qquad \text{.... (iii)}$$

From (i), (ii) and (iii)

$$\begin{bmatrix} 8 & -2 & 2 \\ -8 & 13 & 6 \\ 8 & 5 & -2 \end{bmatrix} \begin{bmatrix} I_1 \\ I_2 \\ I \end{bmatrix} = \begin{bmatrix} 10 \\ 0 \\ 0 \end{bmatrix}$$

$$\therefore I_2 = \boxed{-0.4 \text{ A}}$$

$$\text{and } V_{bc} = 5I_2$$

$$\therefore V_{bc} = \boxed{-2 \text{ volts}}$$

Ex. 1.6 : Find I in the Fig.1.14.

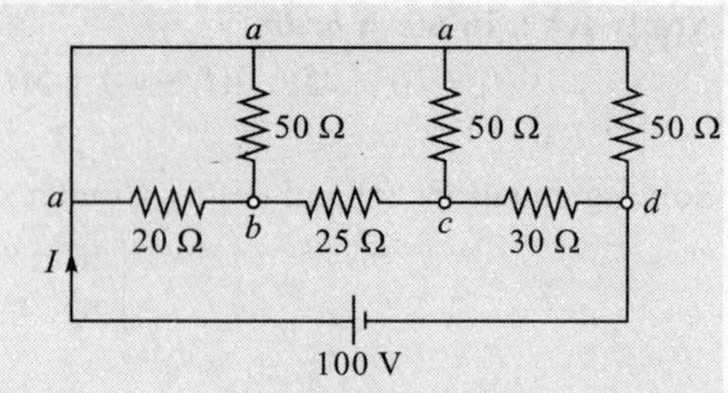

Fig. 1.14

Solution : I here is the source current. Hence we find the equivalent resistance between ad.

Note : *Let us name all junction, keeping in mind that if there is no element connected between two junctions, than those will be equipotential, hence they will be given the same name.*

Now let us redraw, the same circuit with a different layout [Fig. 1.15] and follow steps (a) to (f).

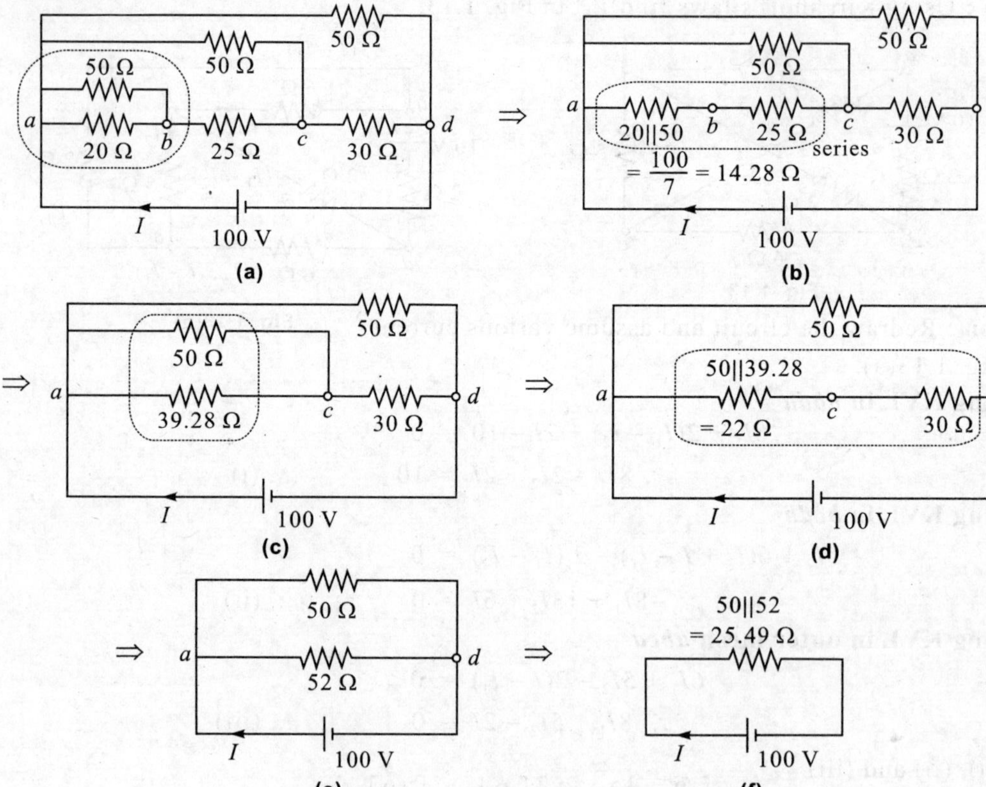

Fig. 1.15

$$\therefore\ I = \frac{100}{25.49} = \boxed{3.92\text{ A}}$$

Remember $R_{eq} = \dfrac{R_1 R_2}{R_1 + R_2}$ for two parallel resistances R_1 and R_2

and for two series resistances R_a and R_b

$$R_{eq} = R_a + R_b$$

Ex. 1.7 : Find I_1, I_2 and I_3 in Fig. 1.16. Also find power loss in the three resistances.

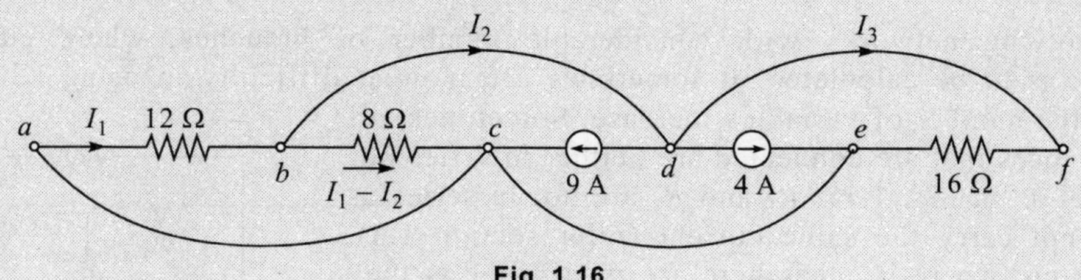

Fig. 1.16

Solution : Apply KCL at *d* [refer equation (1.22)]

$$-I_2 + 9 + 4 + I_3 = 0$$

$$\therefore I_3 = I_2 - 13 \qquad \text{.... (i)}$$

Now, as there are two unknowns i.e. I_1 and I_2 we require two equations.

KVL in *abca*

$$12I_1 + 8(I_1 - I_2) = 0$$

$$20I_1 - 8I_2 = 0 \qquad \text{.... (ii)}$$

KVL in *abdfeca*

$$12I_1 + 16I_3 = 0$$

Substituting for I_3 from equation (i)

$$\text{or } 12I_1 + 16(I_2 - 13) = 0$$

$$12I_1 + 16I_2 = 208 \qquad \text{.... (iii)}$$

From (ii) and (iii) we get

$$\begin{bmatrix} 20 & -8 \\ 12 & 16 \end{bmatrix} \begin{bmatrix} I_1 \\ I_2 \end{bmatrix} = \begin{bmatrix} 0 \\ 208 \end{bmatrix}$$

$$I_1 = \boxed{4\text{ A}}$$

$$I_2 = \boxed{10\text{ A}}$$

From (i) we have $I_3 = I_2 - 13$

$$\therefore I_3 = \boxed{-3\text{ A}}$$

$$\therefore \text{Power loss in } 12\ \Omega = I_1^2 \times 12 = 4^2 \times 12$$

$$= \boxed{192\text{ watts}}$$

$$\text{Power loss in } 8\ \Omega = (I_1 - I_2)^2 \times 8 = (4 - 10)^2 \times 8 \text{ watts}$$

$$= \boxed{288\text{ watts}}$$

$$\text{Power loss in } 16\ \Omega = I_3^2 \times 16 = (-3)^2 \times 16$$

$$= \boxed{144\text{ watts}}$$

1.6 Star-Delta Transformation

In solving networks with considerable number of branches, where equivalent resistance is to be calculated, it sometimes offers great difficulty in using Kirchhoff's laws, as the number of variables increase. Sometimes, all the resistances that are connected are neither in series nor in parallel as in Fig. 1.17. R_1 and R_3 are not in series as they do not carry the same current (refer section 1.3). Similarly no two resistances here are in parallel as they do not share the same voltage.

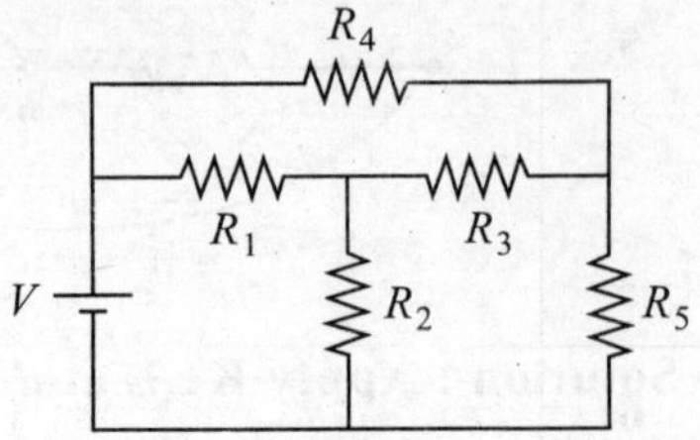

Fig. 1.17

Thus, here we identify two different types of connections.

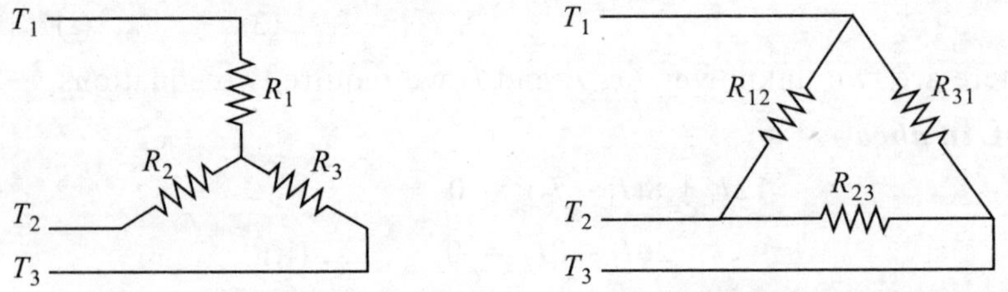

Fig. 1.18

(i) If three resistances are connected to a common point N [Fig. 1.18(a)] with three other terminals T_1, T_2 and T_3 it is called *star connected resistances*.

(ii) If three resistances are connected in cyclic order [as in Fig. 1.18(b)] across three terminals T_1, T_2 and T_3 they are said to be *delta connected resistances*.

So far as the respective terminals are connected a star connected network can be replaced by a delta connected network and vice-versa. The two arrangements will be equivalent electrically, only if the resistance measured between any pair of terminals is the same in both the arrangements, keeping the third terminals open. Let us find this condition in tabular form.

S.No.	Step	Star Connection	Equivalent Delta Connection
1.	Resistance between T_1-T_2 with T_3 open	$R_1 + R_2$ $\therefore\ R_1 + R_2$	$= R_{12} \parallel (R_{23} + R_{31})$ $= \dfrac{R_{12}(R_{23} + R_{31})}{R_{12} + R_{23} + R_{31}}$ ..... (1.15)
2.	Resistance between T_2-T_3 with T_1 open	$R_2 + R_3$ $\therefore\ R_2 + R_3$	$= R_{23} \parallel (R_{12} + R_{31})$ $= \dfrac{R_{23}(R_{12} + R_{31})}{R_{23} + R_{12} + R_{31}}$ ..... (1.16)
3.	Resistance between T_3-T_1 with T_2 open	$R_1 + R_3$	$= \dfrac{R_{31}(R_{12} + R_{23})}{R_{12} + R_{23} + R_{31}}$ ..... (1.17)

4.	Equation (1.15) – (1.16)	$R_1 - R_3$	$= \dfrac{R_{12} R_{31} - R_{23} R_{31}}{R_{12} + R_{23} + R_{31}}$ ..... (1.18)
5.	Equation (1.17) + (1.18)	$2R_1$ $\therefore\ R_1$	$= \dfrac{2R_{12} R_{31}}{R_{12} + R_{23} + R_{31}}$ $= \dfrac{R_{12} R_{31}}{R_{12} + R_{23} + R_{31}}$ ..... (1.19)
6.	Similarly, observe Fig. 1.18 and equation (1.19)	R_2	$= \dfrac{R_{12} R_{23}}{R_{12} + R_{23} + R_{31}}$ ..... (1.20)
7.	Similarly,	R_3	$= \dfrac{R_{31} R_{23}}{R_{12} + R_{23} + R_{31}}$ ..... (1.21)
8.	Equation (1.19) ÷ (1.20)	$\dfrac{R_1}{R_2}$ $\therefore\ R_{31}$	$= \dfrac{R_{31}}{R_{23}}$ $= \dfrac{R_1}{R_2} R_{23}$ ..... (1.22)
9.	Equation (1.19) ÷ (1.21)	$\dfrac{R_1}{R_3}$ $\therefore\ R_{12}$	$= \dfrac{R_{12}}{R_{23}}$ $= \dfrac{R_1}{R_3} R_{23}$ ..... (1.23)
10.	Substituting R_{31} and R_{12} from equations (1.22) and (1.23) in (1.19)	R_1	$= \dfrac{\dfrac{R_1}{R_3} R_{23} \cdot \dfrac{R_1}{R_2} R_{23}}{\dfrac{R_1}{R_3} R_{23} + R_{23} + \dfrac{R_1}{R_2} R_{23}}$ ..... (1.24)
11.	Simplifying equation (1.24), we get	R_{23}	$= \dfrac{R_1 R_2 + R_2 R_3 + R_3 R_1}{R_1}$ ..... (1.25)
	Observe this equation (1.25) and the circuit of Fig. 1.18.		
12.	Similarly,	R_{12}	$= \dfrac{R_1 R_2 + R_2 R_3 + R_3 R_1}{R_3}$ ..... (1.26)
13.	And	R_{31}	$= \dfrac{R_1 R_2 + R_2 R_3 + R_3 R_1}{R_2}$ ..... (1.27)

How to Remember : Look at Fig. 1.19 where star and delta are drawn together.

Observe equation (1.19) i.e. delta values being known the star value is

$$R_1 = \frac{R_{12}\,R_{31}}{R_{12} + R_{23} + R_{31}}$$

Resistance R_1 is placed between R_{12} and R_{31} whereas, above equation (1.25). Star values being known, the delta value is

$$R_{23} = \frac{R_1\,R_2 + R_2\,R_3 + R_3\,R_1}{R_1}$$

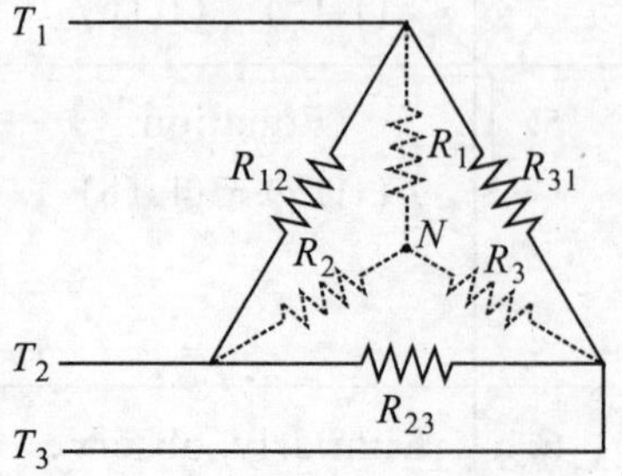

Fig. 1.19

Delta resistance R_{23} is placed opposite R_1. In both the conversions numerator is product term or sum of product and denominator is single term or addition of single terms.

Ex. 1.8 : Find equivalent resistance between *ab* in Fig. 1.20.

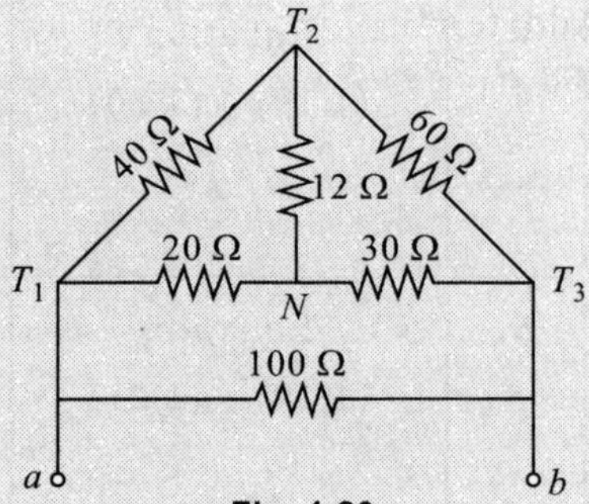

Fig. 1.20

Solution :

Step 1: Identify the three star connected resistances i.e. 20 Ω, 12 Ω and 30 Ω across T_1, T_2 and T_3 with N as the middle terminal.

Step 2: Formula for star to delta

$$R_{12} = \frac{R_1\,R_2 + R_2\,R_3 + R_3\,R_1}{R_3}$$

$$R_{12} = \frac{20 \times 12 + 12 \times 30 + 20 \times 30}{30}$$

$$R_{12} = \frac{1200}{30} = 40\ \Omega$$

$$R_{23} = \frac{1200}{12} = 100\ \Omega$$

$$R_{31} = \frac{1200}{20} = 60\ \Omega$$

Step 3: Combine marked parallel resistances [Fig. 1.20(b)]

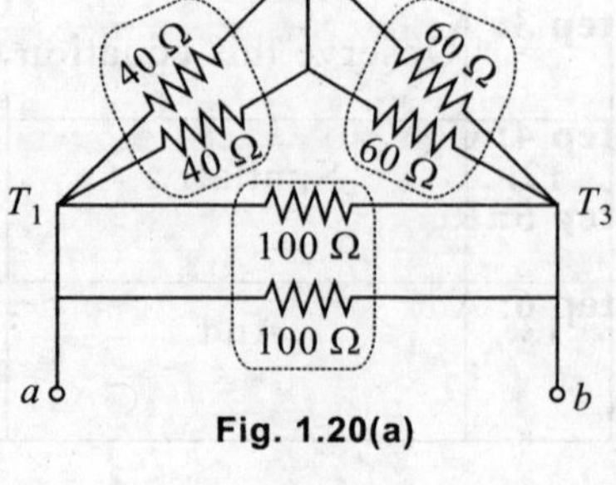

Fig. 1.20(a)

Step 4: Add series resistance [Fig. 1.20(c)]

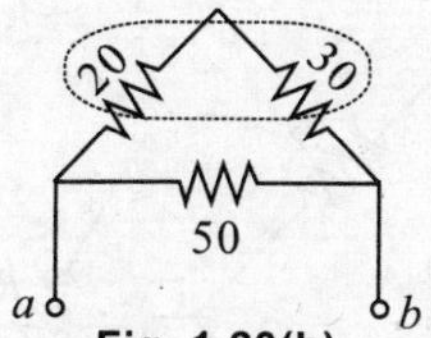

Fig. 1.20(b)

⇒

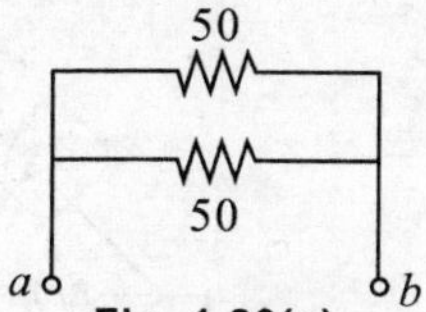

Fig. 1.20(c)

⇒

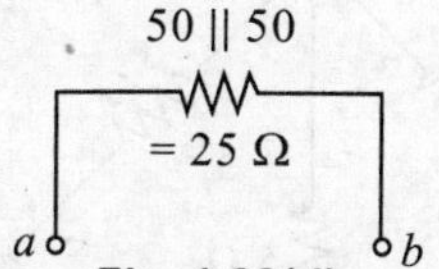

Fig. 1.20(d)

$$\boxed{R_{ab} = 25\ \Omega}$$

Ex. 1.9 : Find R_{ab} in Fig. 1.21.

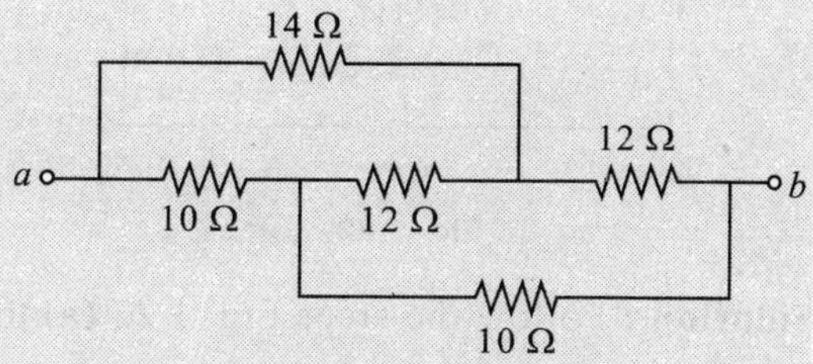

Fig. 1.21

Solution :

Step 1: Identify the delta connected resistances (14, 10, 12) and their junctions *a,c,d*. [Fig. 1.21(a)]

Step 2: As delta is to be converted to star. Add terminal N_1 and replace the delta by star R_1, R_2 and R_3. [Fig. 1.21(b)]

$$R_1 = \frac{10 \times 14}{10 + 12 + 14} = 3.89$$

$$R_2 = \frac{10 \times 12}{10 + 12 + 14} = 3.33$$

$$R_3 = \frac{12 \times 14}{10 + 12 + 14} = 4.67$$

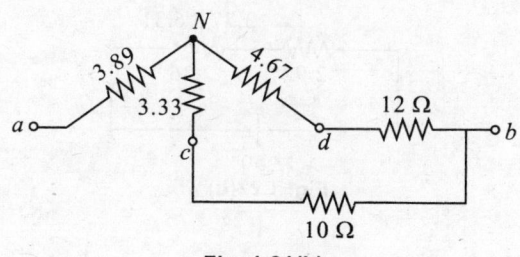

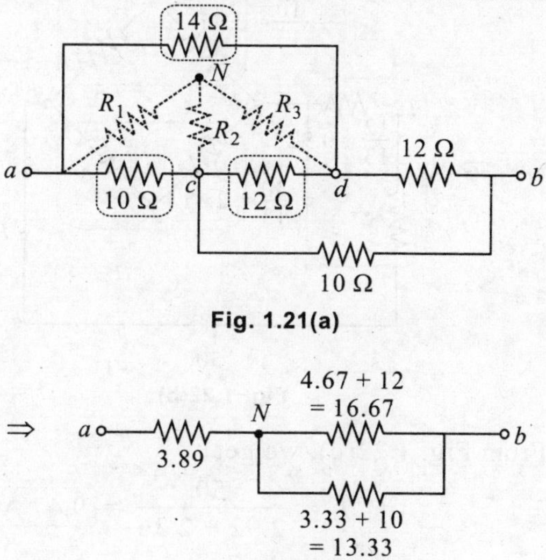

Fig. 1.21(a)

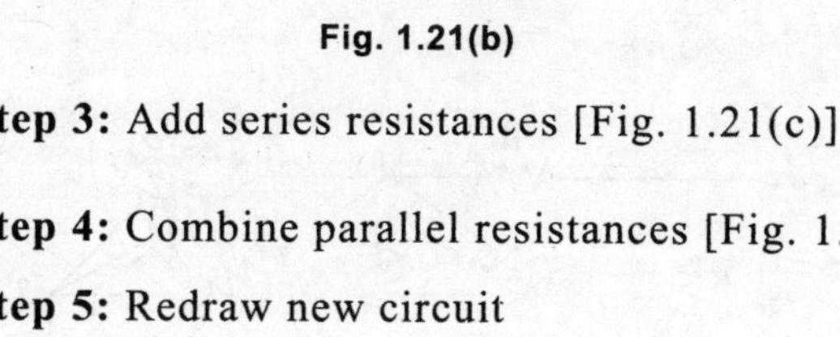

Fig. 1.21(b)

⇒

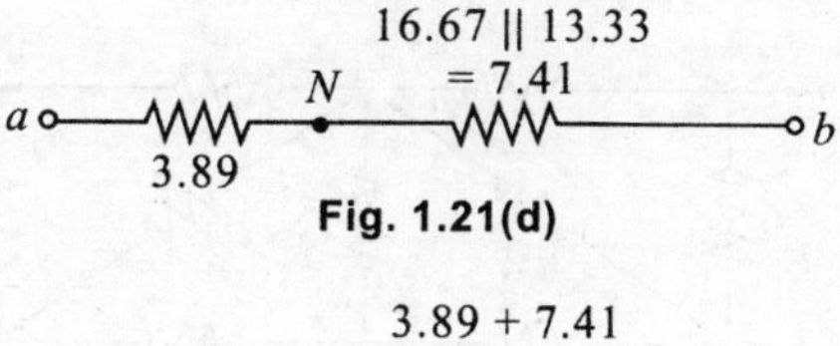

Fig. 1.21(c)

Step 3: Add series resistances [Fig. 1.21(c)].

Step 4: Combine parallel resistances [Fig. 1.21(d)]

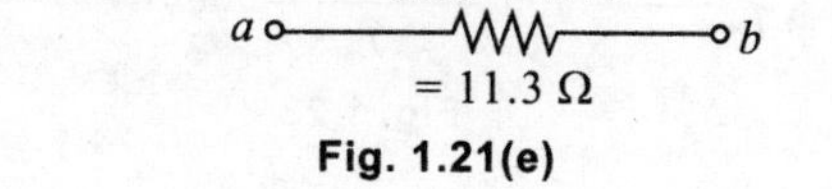

Fig. 1.21(d)

Step 5: Redraw new circuit

Step 6: Add series resistances

Fig. 1.21(e)

$$\boxed{R_{ab} = 11.3\ \Omega}$$

Ex. 1.10 : Find I in Fig. 1.22.

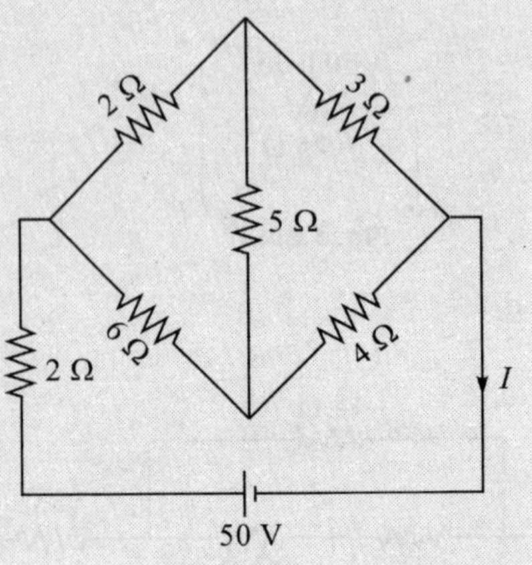

Fig. 1.22

⇒

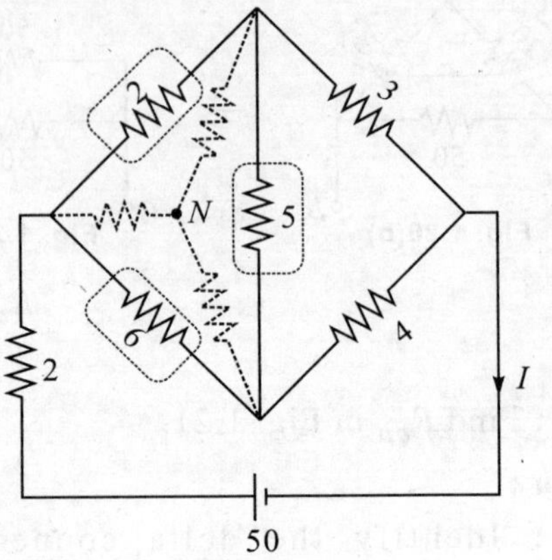

Fig. 1.22(a)

Solution : Follow the steps Fig. 1.22 (a) to (d)

⇒

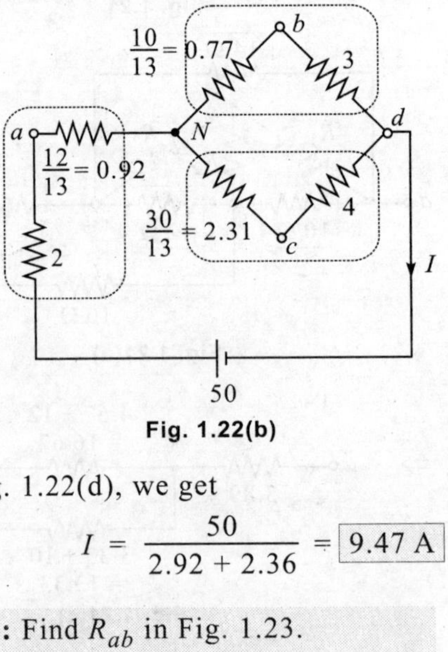

Fig. 1.22(b)

⇗

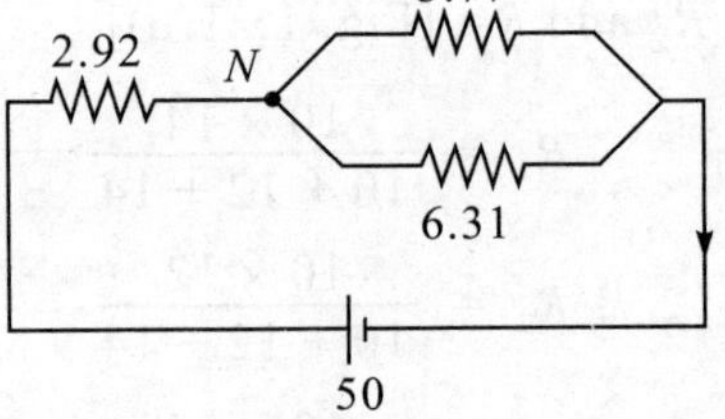

Fig. 1.22(c)

⇓

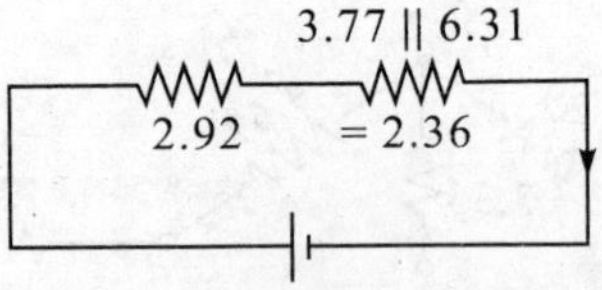

Fig. 1.22(d)

From Fig. 1.22(d), we get

$$I = \frac{50}{2.92 + 2.36} = \boxed{9.47 \text{ A}}$$

Ex. 1.11 : Find R_{ab} in Fig. 1.23.

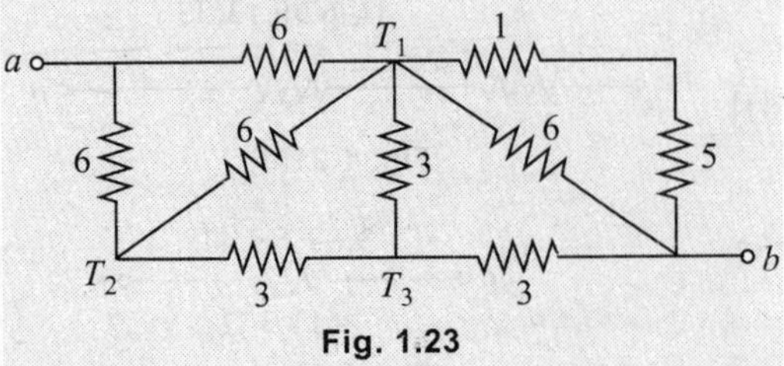

Fig. 1.23

⇒

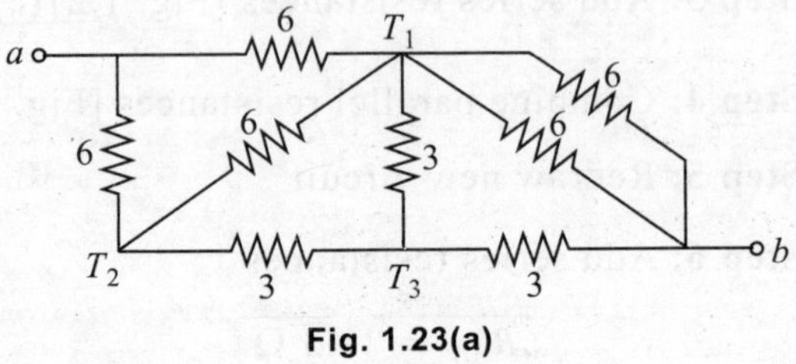

Fig. 1.23(a)

Solution : [Hint : Always identify series-parallel resistances before star-delta connections] follow steps (a) to (f) i.e. Figs. 1.23(a) to 1.23(f).

⇒ 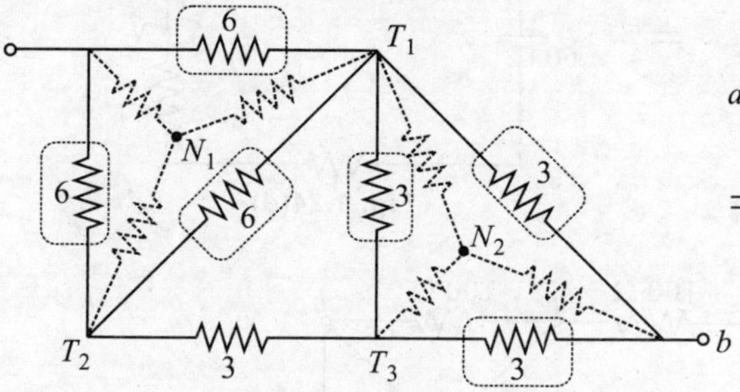

Fig. 1.23(b)

⇒ 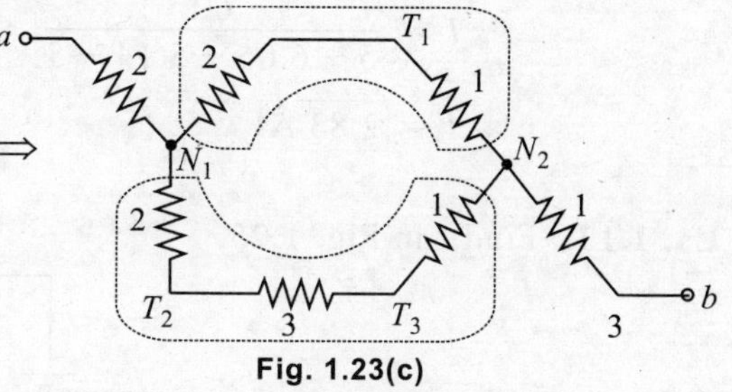

Fig. 1.23(c)

⇒ 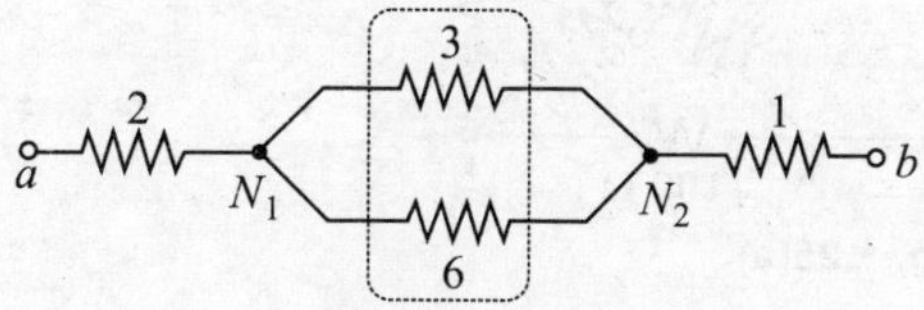

Fig. 1.23(d)

⇒ 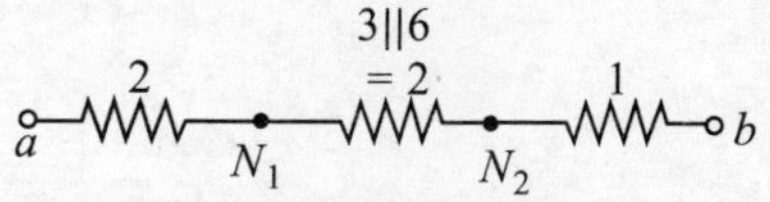

Fig. 1.23(e)

⇒ 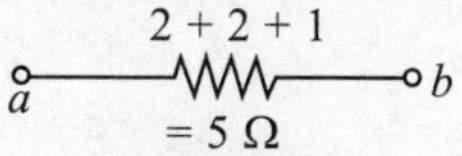

Fig. 1.23(f)

$$R_{ab} = 5\ \Omega$$

Ex. 1.12 : Find *I* in Fig. 1.24.

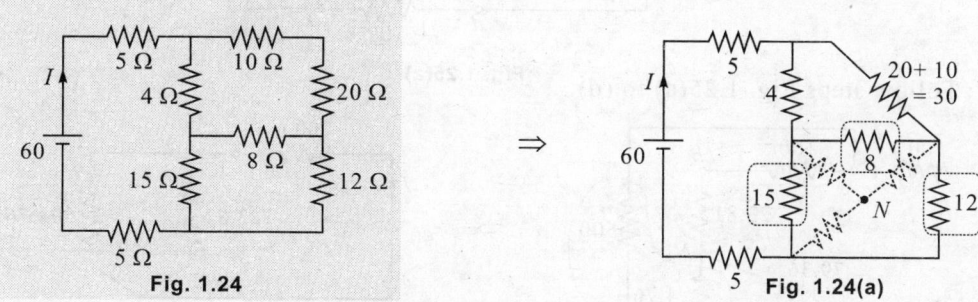

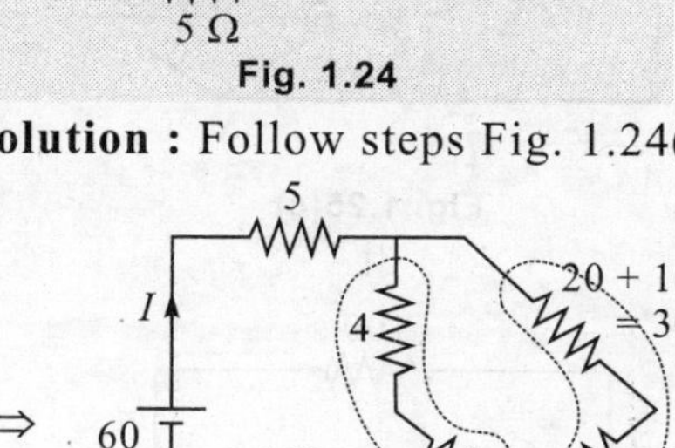

Fig. 1.24

⇒ 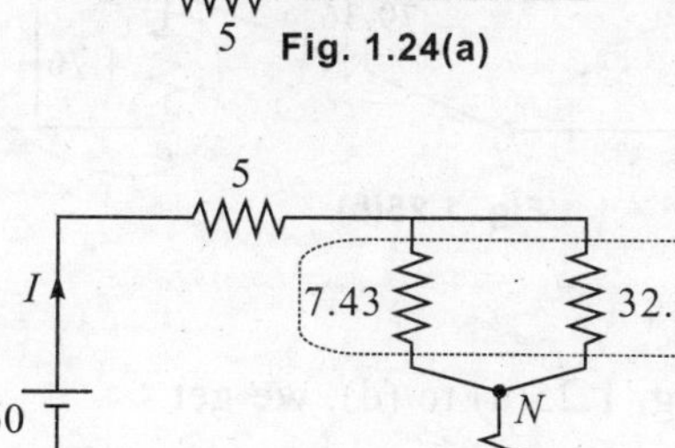

Fig. 1.24(a)

Solution : Follow steps Fig. 1.24(a) to (d)

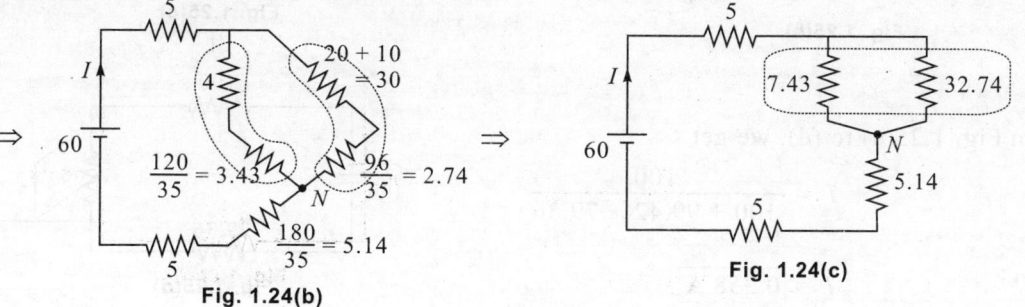

⇒ 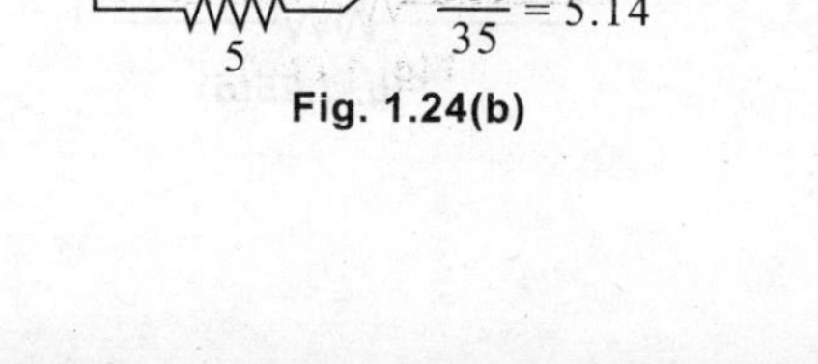

Fig. 1.24(b)

⇒ 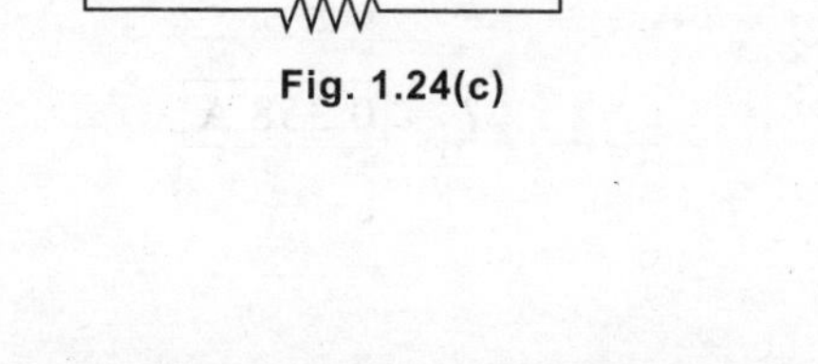

Fig. 1.24(c)

From Fig. 1.24(a) to (d), we get

$$I = \frac{60}{5 + 6.05 + 5.14 + 5}$$

$$\therefore\ I = \boxed{2.83\ \text{A}}$$

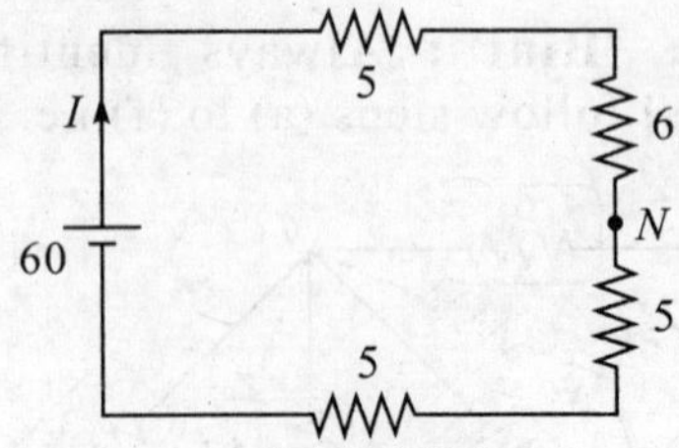

Fig. 1.24(d)

Ex. 1.13 : Find *I* in Fig. 1.25.

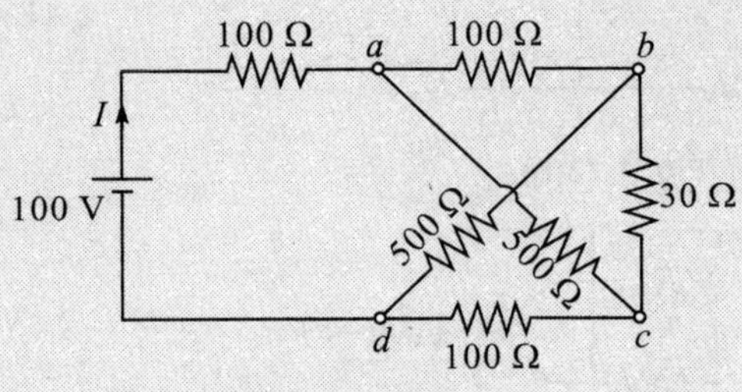

Fig. 1.25(a)

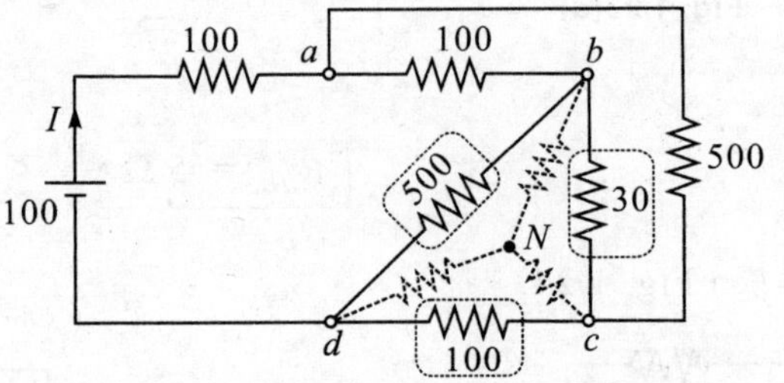

Fig. 1.25(a)

Solution : Follow steps Fig. 1.25(a) to (d)

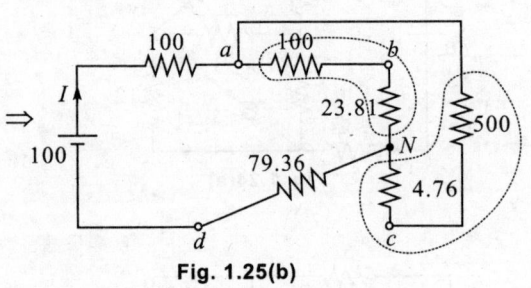

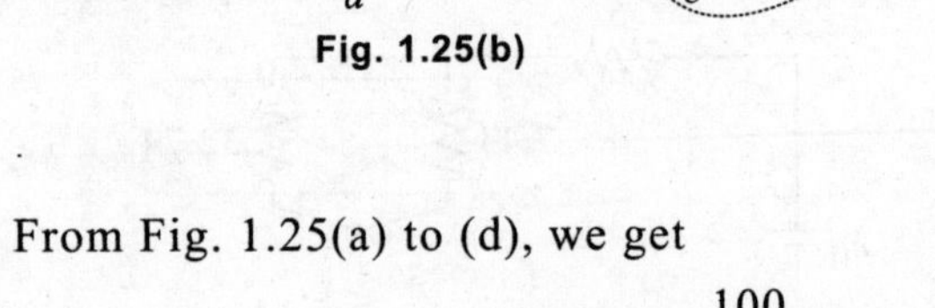

Fig. 1.25(b)

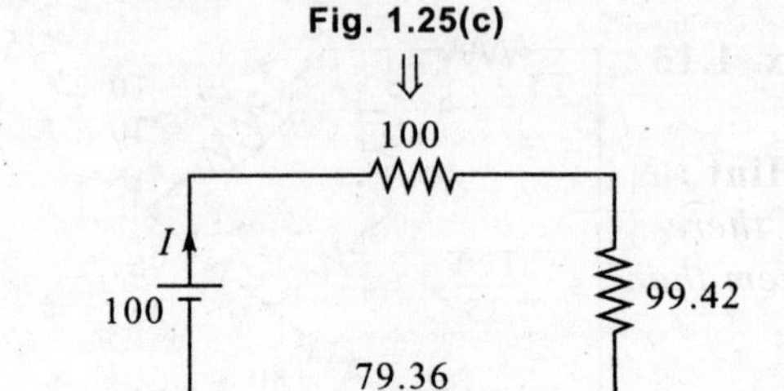

Fig. 1.25(c)

⇓

Fig. 1.25(d)

From Fig. 1.25(a) to (d), we get

$$I = \frac{100}{100 + 99.42 + 79.36}$$

$$\therefore\ I = \boxed{0.358\ \text{A}}$$

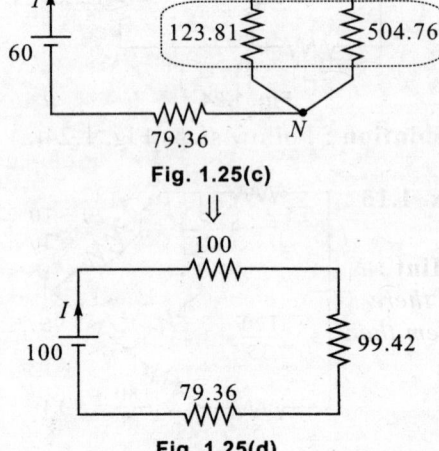

Ex. 1.14 : Find I in Fig. 1.26.

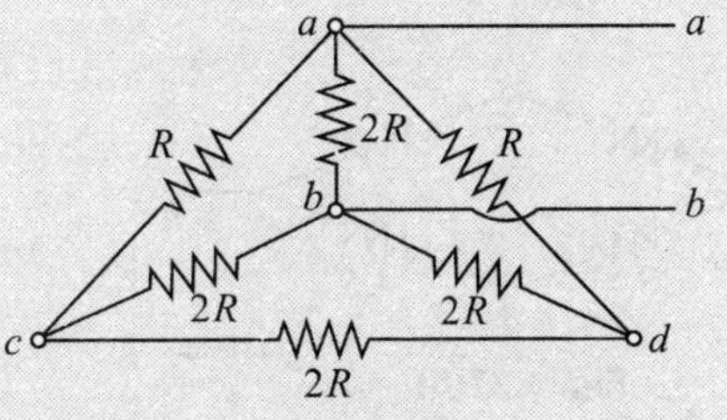

Fig. 1.26

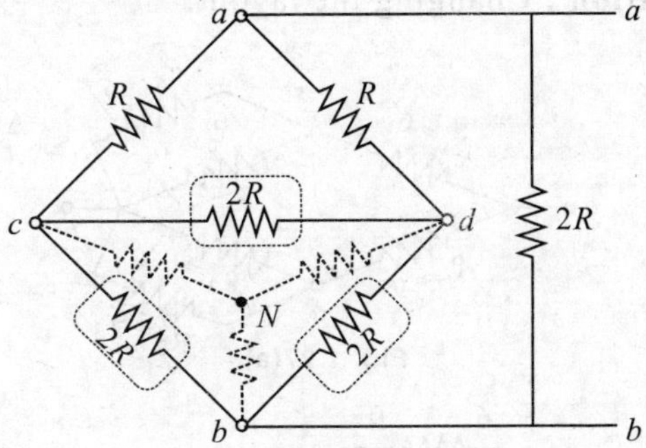

Fig. 1.26(a)

Solution : Redraw the circuit by bringing terminal b out as in Fig. 1.26(a).

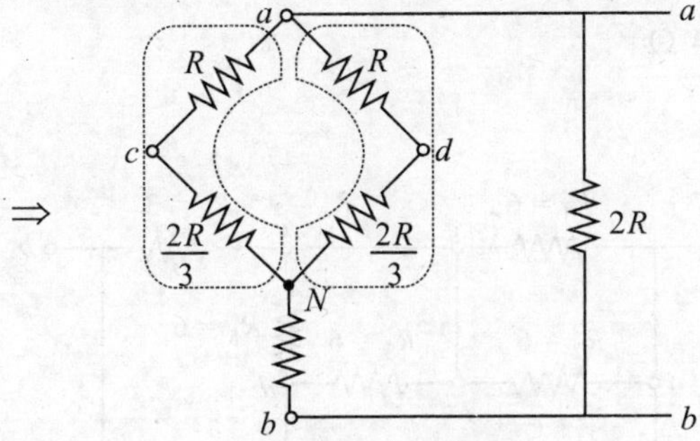

Fig. 1.26(b)

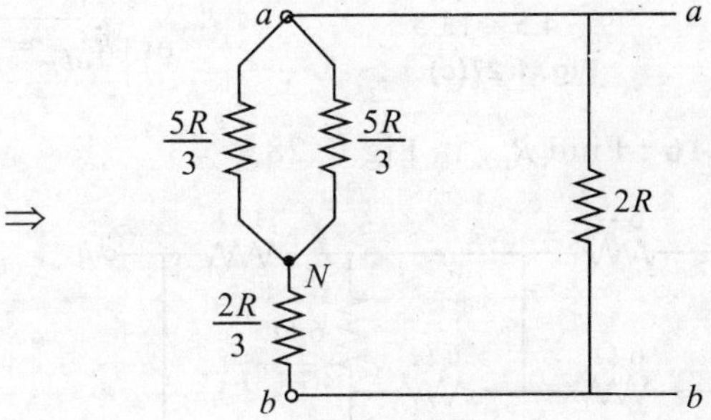

Fig. 1.26(c)

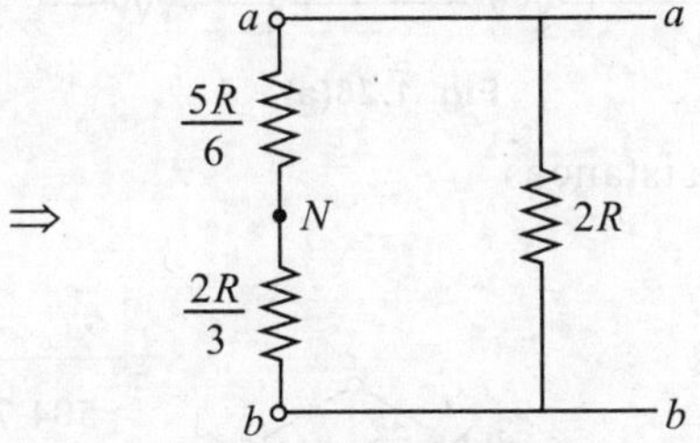

Fig. 1.26(c)

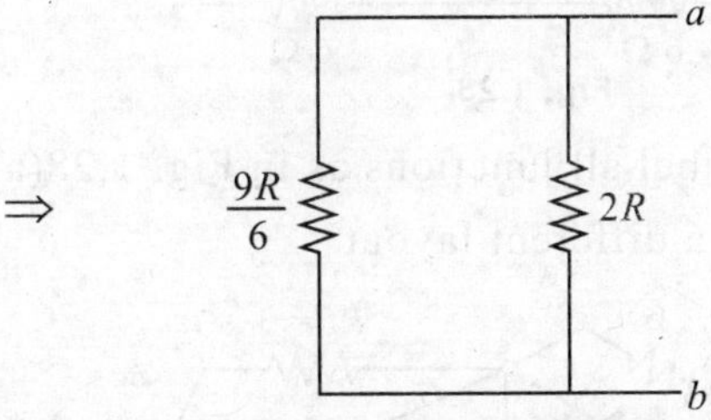

Fig. 1.26(d)

$$\therefore \; R_{ab} = \frac{9R}{6} \,||\, 2R = \boxed{\frac{6}{7}R}$$

Ex. 1.15 : Find R_{ab} in Fig. 1.27.

[Hint : *Name all junctions keeping in mind if there is no element connected between them then name will be same.***]**

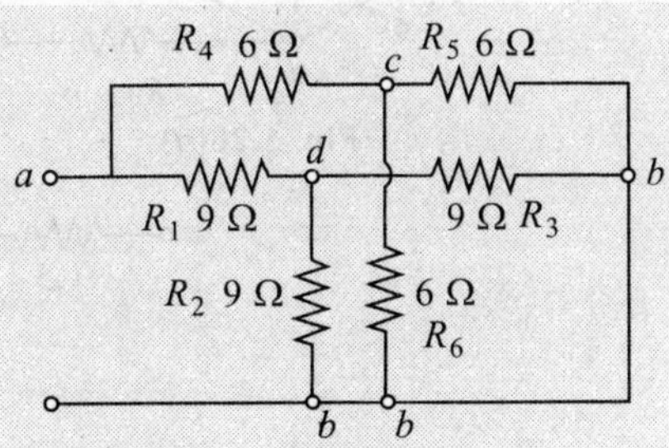

Fig. 1.27

Solution : Changing the layout.

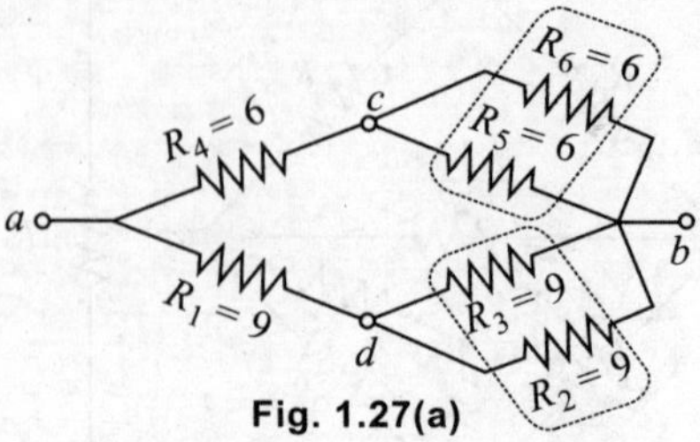

Fig. 1.27(a)

$\Rightarrow$

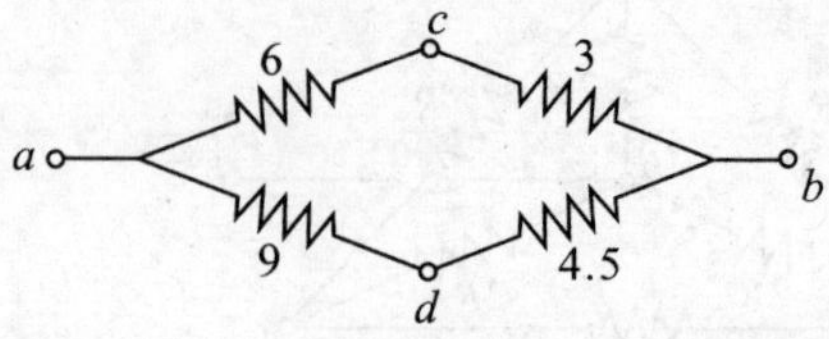

Fig. 1.27(b)

$\Rightarrow$

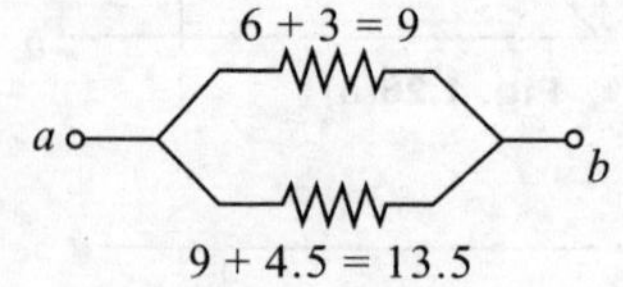

Fig. 1.27(c)

$$\therefore \; R_{ab} = 9 \,||\, 13.5 = \frac{9 \times 13.5}{9 + 13.5}$$

$$\text{or } \boxed{R_{ab} = 5.4\ \Omega}$$

Ex. 1.16 : Find R_{ab} in Fig. 1.28.

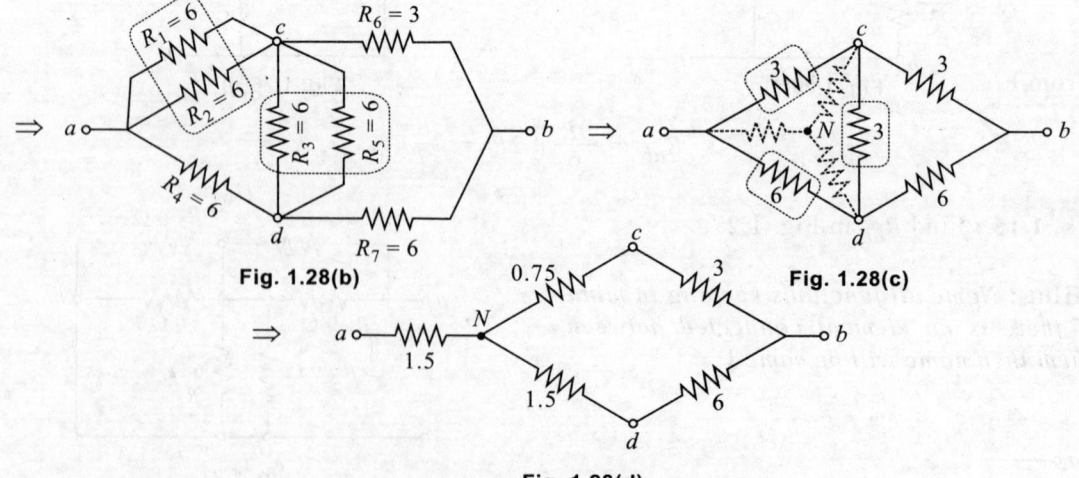

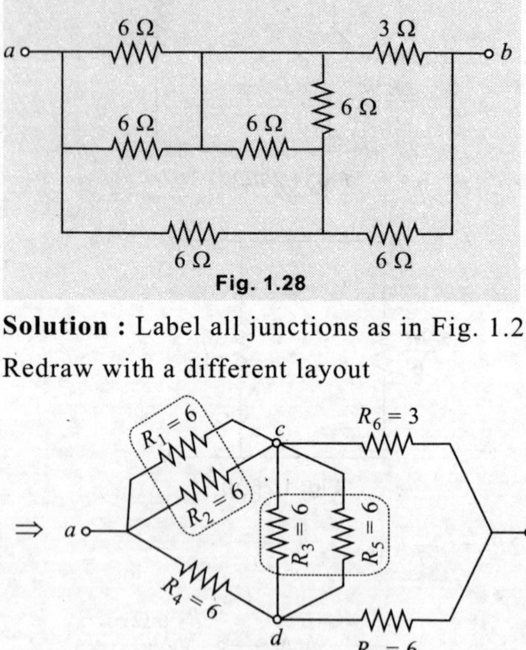

Fig. 1.28

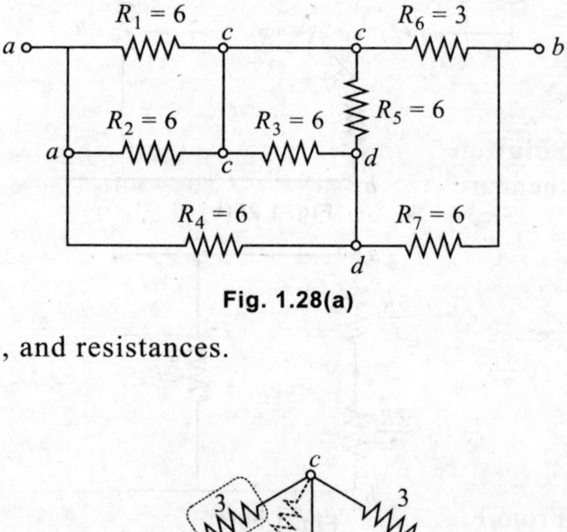

Fig. 1.28(a)

Solution : Label all junctions as in Fig. 1.28(a), and resistances.

Redraw with a different layout

$\Rightarrow$

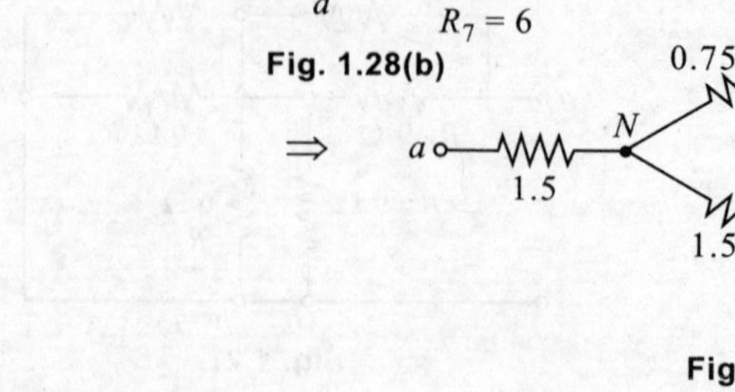

Fig. 1.28(b)

$\Rightarrow$

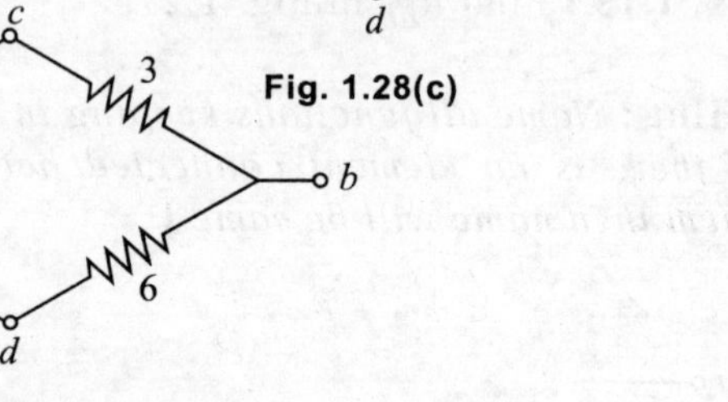

Fig. 1.28(c)

$\Rightarrow$

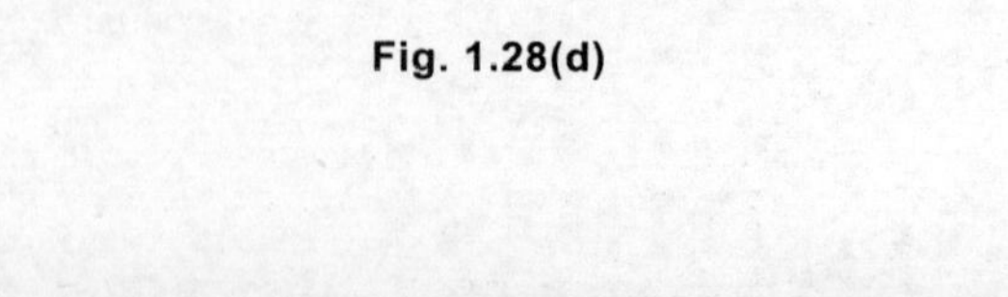

Fig. 1.28(d)

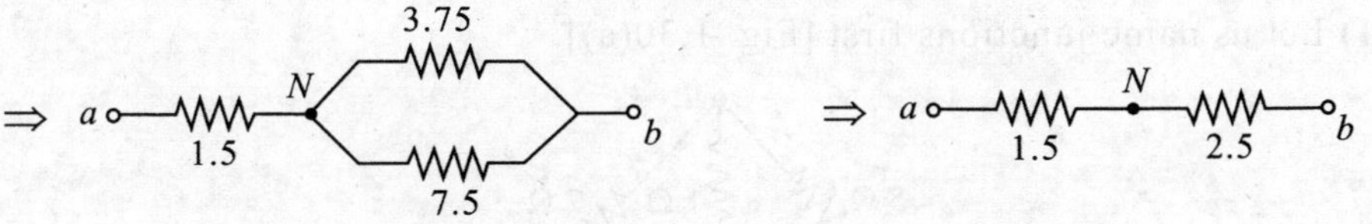

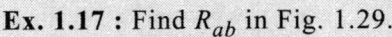

From Fig. 1.28(a) to (f)

$$\therefore R_{ab} = 1.5 + 2.5$$

$$\text{or } \boxed{R_{ab} = 4\ \Omega}$$

Ex. 1.17 : Find R_{ab} in Fig. 1.29.

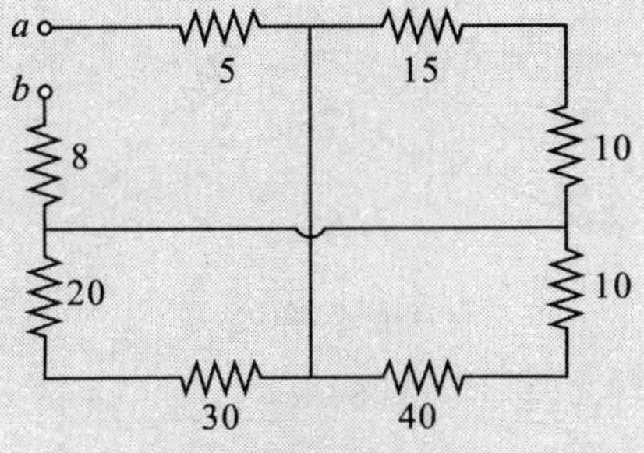

Fig. 1.29

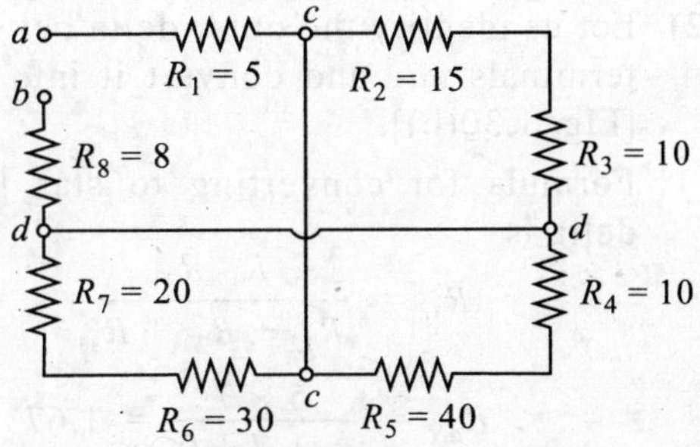

Fig. 1.29(a)

Solution : First label the junctions (remember junctions without any element between them are equipotential) as shown in Fig 1.29(a). Redraw as in Fig 1.29(b).

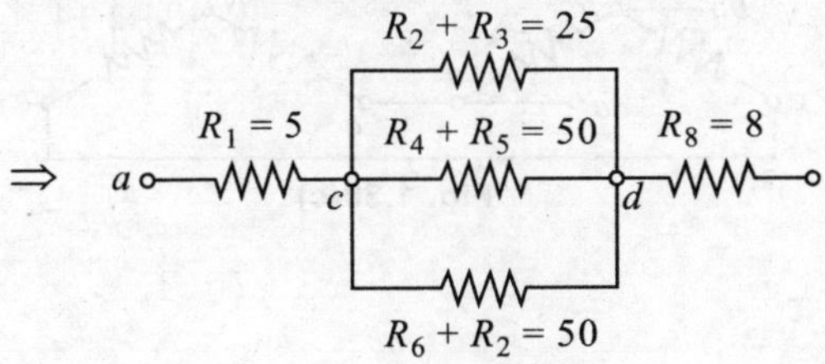

Fig. 1.29(b)

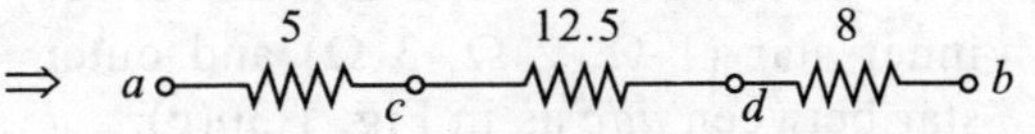

Fig. 1.29(c)

From Fig. 1.29(a), (b) and (c)

$$\therefore R_{ab} = 5 + 12.5 + 8$$

$$\text{or } \boxed{R_{ab} = 25.5\ \Omega}$$

Ex. 1.18 : Find R_{ab} by converting the outer delta to star in Fig. 1.30.

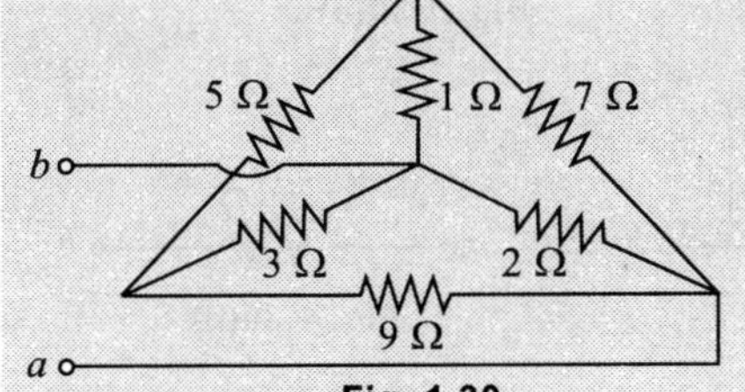

Fig. 1.30

Solution : (1) Let us name junctions first [Fig. 1.30(a)].

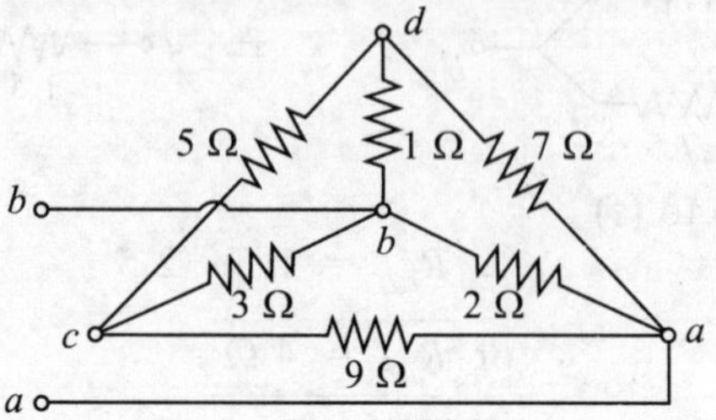

Fig. 1.30(a)

(2) Let us identify the outer delta between terminals *adc* and convert it into star [Fig. 1.30(b)].

Formula for converting to star from delta is

$$R_1 = \frac{R_{12} R_{31}}{R_{12} + R_{23} + R_{31}}$$

$$\therefore \; R_{dN} = \frac{5 \times 7}{5 + 7 + 9} = 1.67$$

$$R_{cN} = \frac{5 \times 9}{5 + 7 + 9} = 2.14$$

$$R_{aN} = \frac{9 \times 7}{5 + 7 + 9} = 3$$

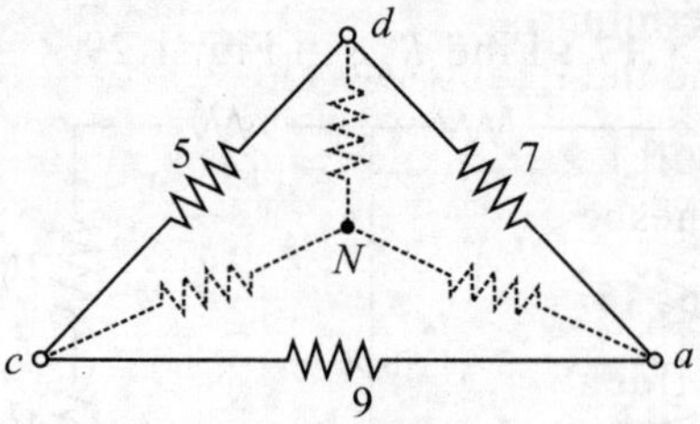

Fig. 1.30(b)

(3) Now mark *abcd* and *N* and connect the inner star (1 Ω, 2 Ω, 3 Ω) and outer star between *adc* as in Fig. 1.30(c).

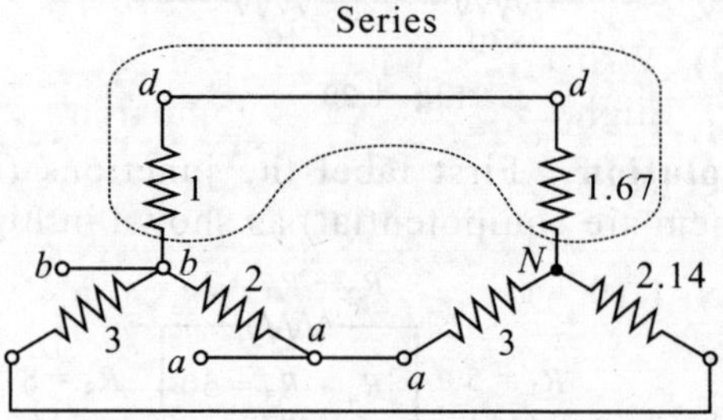

Fig. 1.30(c)

(4) Change the layout as in Fig. 1.30(d).

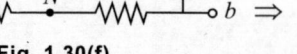

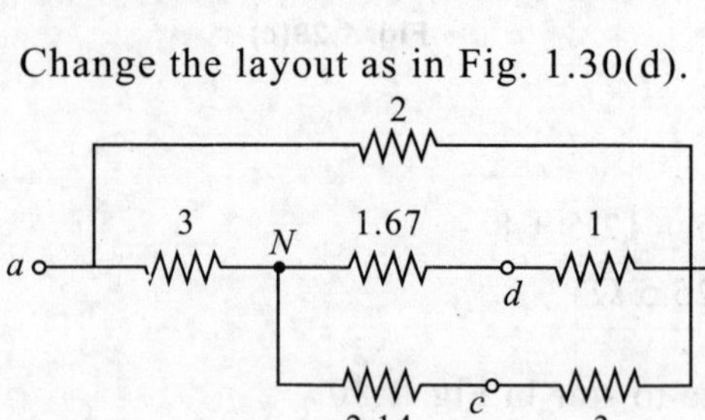

Fig. 1.30(d)

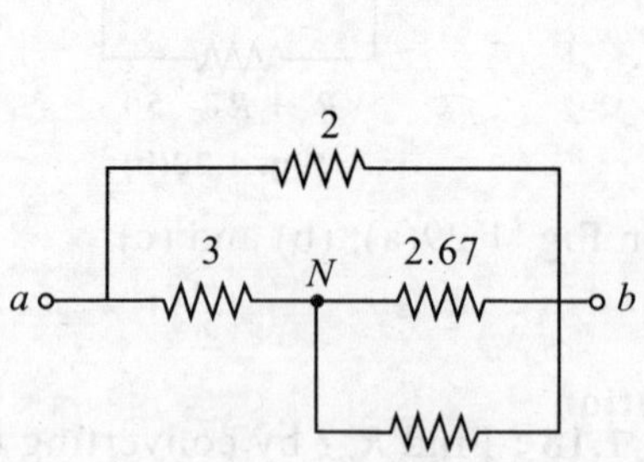

Fig. 1.30(e)

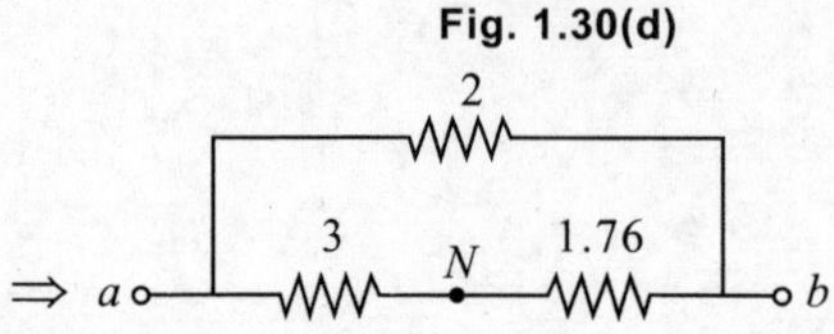

Fig. 1.30(f)

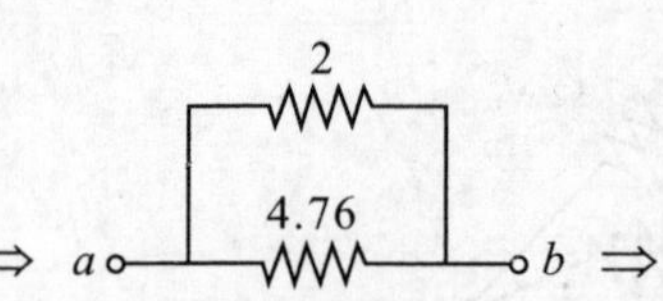

Fig. 1.30(g)

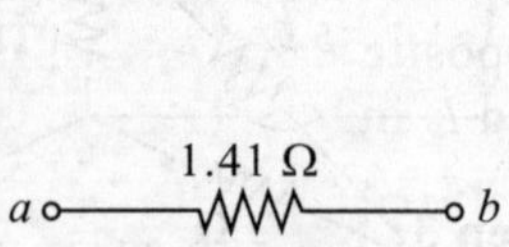

Fig. 1.30(h)

$$R_{ab} = 1.41 \; \Omega$$

1.7 Mesh Analysis or Maxwell's Loop Current Method

This method is more suitable than Kirchhoff's laws. In Kirchhoff's laws each branch current was specified where as in "*Mesh Analysis*" currents in different meshes are assigned continuous paths so that they do not split at junctions into branch currents.

Basically this method uses KVL equations in terms of different mesh currents. Rather, here the mesh under consideration while writing the KVL equation is assumed to have current higher than any other mesh currents, i.e. direction of voltages in a given mesh are determined by that particular mesh current which is under consideration (as it is assumed to be the largest current).

It will be seen later that the number of independent equations here is equal to the number of meshes.

Steps for Mesh Analysis :

(1) Identify closed loops (meshes) in the circuit, which do not contain any other closed loop inside it.

(2) Assume currents in each mesh.

(3) Write KVL equations for each mesh assuming which ever mesh you consider has a higher magnitude as compared to other currents.

Let us consider the following example.

Ex. 1.19 : Using mesh analysis find I. Fig 1.31.

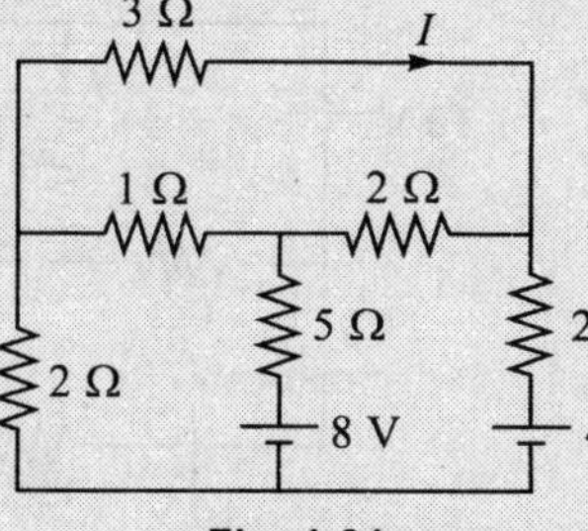

Fig. 1.31

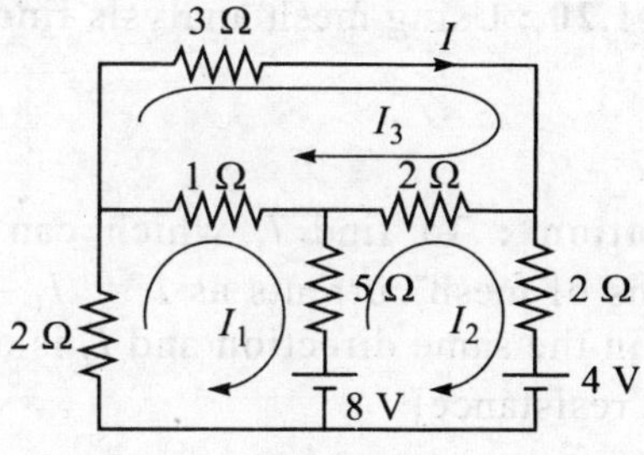

Fig. 1.31

Solution : Step 1: Identify meshes [Fig 1.31(a)]

Step 2: Assume currents I_1, I_2 and I_3 as shown.

Observe : In the middle 5 Ω resistance two currents I_1 and I_2 are flowing and they are in opposite directions. Similarly, in 1 Ω (I_1 and I_3 in opposite directions flow) and 2 Ω (I_3 and I_2 in opposite directions.

Step 3: KVL in mesh I : According to section 1.5.2.

$$2I_1 + (I_1 - I_3) + 5(I_1 - I_2) + 8 = 0$$

$$\therefore 8I_1 - 5I_2 - I_3 = 8 \quad .... \text{(i)}$$

KVL in mesh I_2

$$2I_2 + 4 - 8 + 5(I_2 - I_1) + 2(I_2 - I_3) = 0$$

$$\therefore -5I_1 + 9I_2 - 2I_3 = 4 \quad .... \text{(ii)}$$

KVL in mesh I_3

$$3I_3 + 2(I_3 - I_2) + 1(I_3 - I_1) = 0$$

$$\therefore -I_1 - 2I_2 + 6I_3 = 0 \quad .... \text{(iii)}$$

From equation (i), (ii), (iii), we get

$$\begin{bmatrix} 8 & -5 & -1 \\ -5 & 9 & -2 \\ -1 & -2 & 6 \end{bmatrix} \begin{bmatrix} I_1 \\ I_2 \\ I_3 \end{bmatrix} = \begin{bmatrix} -8 \\ 4 \\ 0 \end{bmatrix}$$

$$\therefore I_1 = -1.23 \text{ A}$$

$$I_2 = -0.307 \text{ A}$$

$$I_3 = -0.307 \text{ A}$$

But observe Fig. 1.30(i) carefully, desired current I is same as I_3 [as I_3 is the only mesh current flowing through 3 Ω resistance where I is defined, and has same direction as I]

$$\therefore I = I_3 = \boxed{-0.307 \text{ Amp}}$$

–ve sign indicates that actual current is 0.307 in opposite direction to marked polarity.

Ex. 1.20 : Using mesh analysis find I (Fig. 1.32).

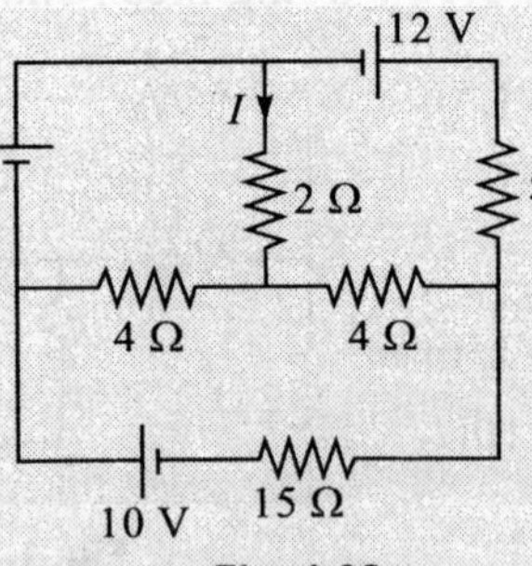

Fig. 1.32

Solution : To find I, which can be defined in terms of mesh currents as $I = I_1 - I_2$ [as I_1 and I are in the same direction and I_2 is opposite to I_1 in 2 Ω resistance]

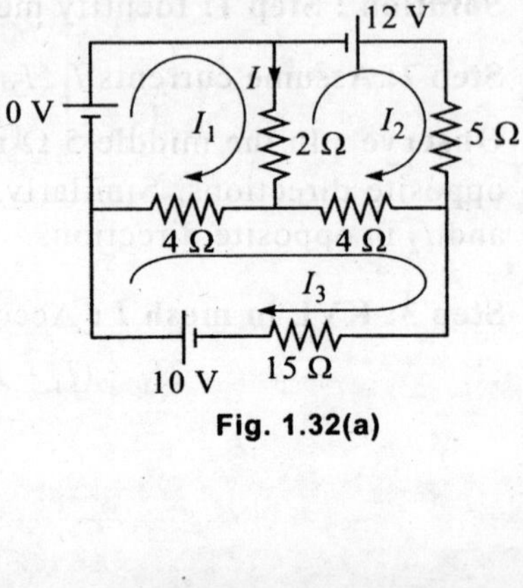

Fig. 1.32(a)

KVL in mesh I_1

$$-10 + 2(I_1 - I_2) + 4(I_1 - I_3) = 0$$

$$\therefore 6I_1 - 2I_2 - 4I_3 = 10 \quad .... \text{(i)}$$

KVL in mesh I_2

$$-12 + 5I_2 + 4(I_2 - I_3) + 2(I_2 - I_1) = 0$$

$$\therefore -2I_1 + 11I_2 - 4I_3 = 12 \quad .... \text{(ii)}$$

KVL in mesh I_3

$$4(I_3 - I_1) + 4(I_3 - I_2) + 15I_3 - 10 = 0$$

$$\therefore -4I_1 - 4I_2 + 23I_3 = 10 \quad .... \text{(iii)}$$

Using equaiton (i) (ii) and (iii), we get

$$\begin{bmatrix} 6 & -2 & -4 \\ -2 & 11 & -4 \\ -4 & -4 & 23 \end{bmatrix} \begin{bmatrix} I_1 \\ I_2 \\ I_3 \end{bmatrix} = \begin{bmatrix} 10 \\ 12 \\ 10 \end{bmatrix}$$

$$\therefore I_1 = 3.33 \text{ A}$$

$$I_2 = 2.20 \text{ A}$$

$$\therefore I = I_1 - I_2 = 3.33 - 2.20$$

$$\therefore I = \boxed{1.13 \text{ A}}$$

Ex. 1.21 : Find V_{ab} in Fig. 1.33.

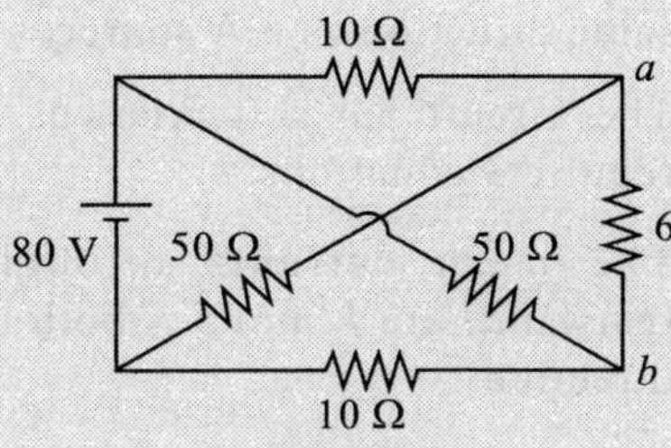

Fig. 1.33

Solution : Redraw the circuit as in Fig. 1.33(a).

$$V_{ab} = 60(I_2 - I_3) \quad .... \text{(i)}$$

[as a is at a higher potential current I_2 will be taken as higher current]

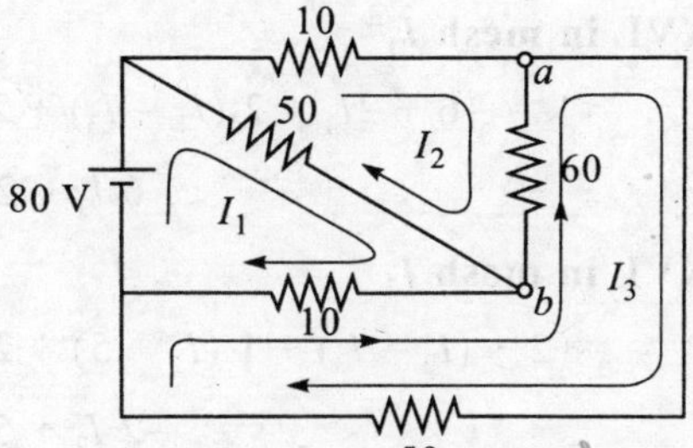

Fig. 1.33(a)

KVL in mesh *I*

$$-80 + 50(I_1 - I_2) + 10\,(I_1 - I_3) = 0$$

$$\therefore 60\,I_1 - 50\,I_2 - 10\,I_3 = 80 \quad .... \text{(ii)}$$

KVL in mesh I_2

$$10\,I_2 + 60(I_2 - I_3) + 50\,(I_2 - I_1) = 0$$

$$\therefore -50\,I_1 + 120\,I_2 - 60\,I_3 = 0 \quad .... \text{(iii)}$$

KVL in mesh I_3

$$10(I_3 - I_1) + 60(I_3 - I_2) + 50\,I_3 = 0$$

$$\therefore -10\,I_1 - 60\,I_2 + 120\,I_3 = 0 \quad .... \text{(iv)}$$

Thus,

$$\begin{bmatrix} 60 & -50 & -10 \\ -50 & 120 & -60 \\ -10 & -60 & 120 \end{bmatrix} \begin{bmatrix} I_1 \\ I_2 \\ I_3 \end{bmatrix} = \begin{bmatrix} 80 \\ 0 \\ 0 \end{bmatrix}$$

$$\therefore I_2 = 1.91 \text{ A}$$

$$I_3 = 1.22$$

$$V_{ab} = 60(I_2 - I_3) = 60(1.91 - 1.22)$$

$$V_{ab} = \boxed{41.4 \text{ volts}}$$

Ex. 1.22 : Find I in Fig. 1.34.

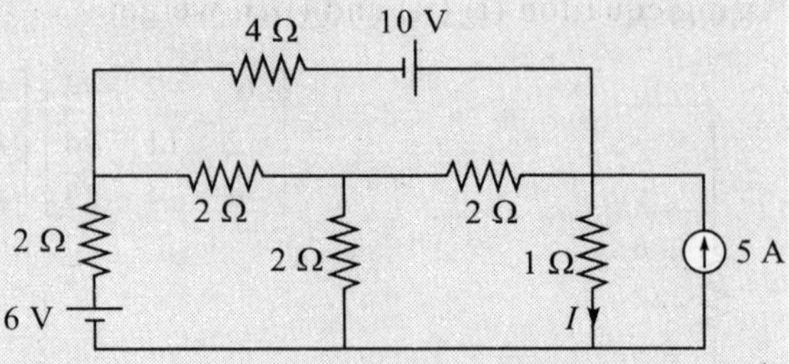

Fig. 1.34

Solution : Redraw the circuit as in Fig. 1.34(a).

Note :

(i) In this circuit there are 4 meshes.

(ii) There is a current source of 5 A in the outer most mesh.

(iii) As there is only one mesh current defined through the current source, the mesh current is also 5 A in the same direction as 5 A source.

(iv) The circuit has 3 unknowns, so we require 3 equations.

(v) The mesh currents through 1 Ω resistance are I_2 and 5 A both in same direction.

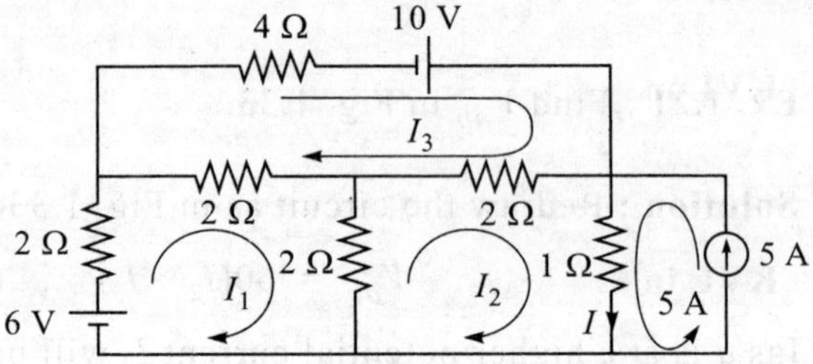

Fig. 1.34(a)

$$\therefore I = I_2 + 5 \quad .... \text{(i)}$$

KVL in mesh I_1

$$-6 + 2I_1 + 2(I_1 - I_3) + 2(I_1 - I_2) = 0$$

$$\therefore 6I_1 - 2I_2 - 2I_3 = 6 \quad .... \text{(ii)}$$

KVL in mesh I_2

$$+2 + (I_2 - I_3) + 1(I_2 + 5) + 2(I_2 - I_1) = 0$$

$$\therefore -2I_1 + 5I_2 - 2I_3 = -5 \quad .... \text{(iii)}$$

KVL in mesh I_3

$$4I_3 - 10 + 2(I_3 - I_2) + 2(I_3 - I_1) = 0$$

$$\therefore -2I_1 - 2I_2 + 8I_3 = 10 \quad .... \text{(iv)}$$

$$\begin{bmatrix} 6 & -2 & -2 \\ -2 & 5 & -2 \\ -2 & -2 & 8 \end{bmatrix} \begin{bmatrix} I_1 \\ I_2 \\ I_3 \end{bmatrix} = \begin{bmatrix} 6 \\ -5 \\ 10 \end{bmatrix}$$

$$\therefore I_2 = 0.4$$

From (i), we have $I = I_2 + 5$

$$\therefore I = \boxed{5.4 \text{ Amp}}$$

Ex. 1.23 : Find I using mesh analysis in Fig. 1.35.

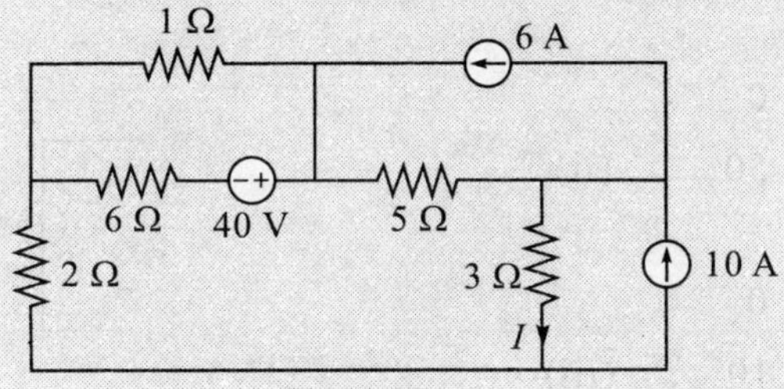

Fig. 1.35

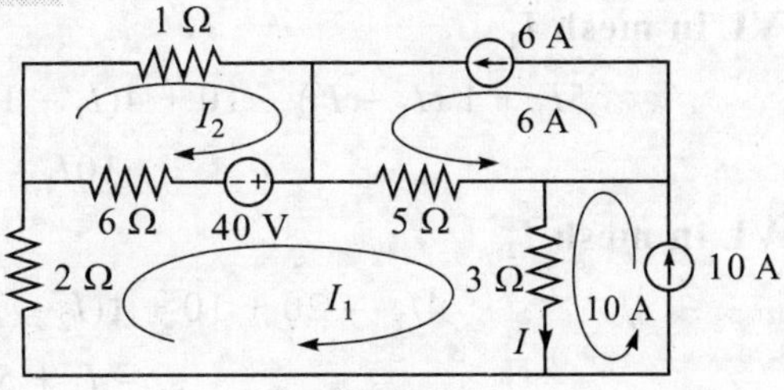

Fig. 1.35(a)

Solution : Refer Fig. 1.35(a).

$$I = I_1 + 10 \quad .... \text{(i)}$$

KVL in mesh I_1

$$2I_1 + 6(I_1 - I_2) - 40 + 5(I_1 + 6) + 3(I_1 + 10) = 0$$

$$\therefore 16I_1 - 6I_2 = -20 \quad .... \text{(ii)}$$

KVL in mesh I_2

$$1I_2 + 40 + 6(I_2 - I_1) = 0$$

$$\therefore -6I_1 + 7I_2 = -40 \quad .... \text{(iii)}$$

$$\therefore \begin{bmatrix} 16 & -6 \\ -6 & 7 \end{bmatrix} \begin{bmatrix} I_1 \\ I_2 \end{bmatrix} = \begin{bmatrix} -20 \\ -40 \end{bmatrix}$$

$$I_1 = \boxed{-5 \text{ A}}$$

From (i), we have $I = I_1 + 10 = -5 + 10$

$$\therefore I = \boxed{5 \text{ A}}$$

Ex. 1.24 : Using mesh analysis find V_{AB} in Fig. 1.36.

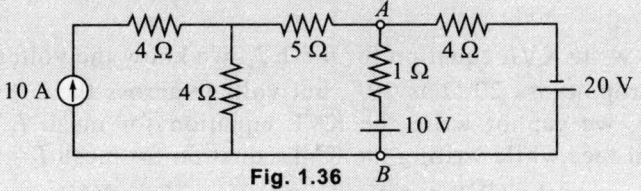

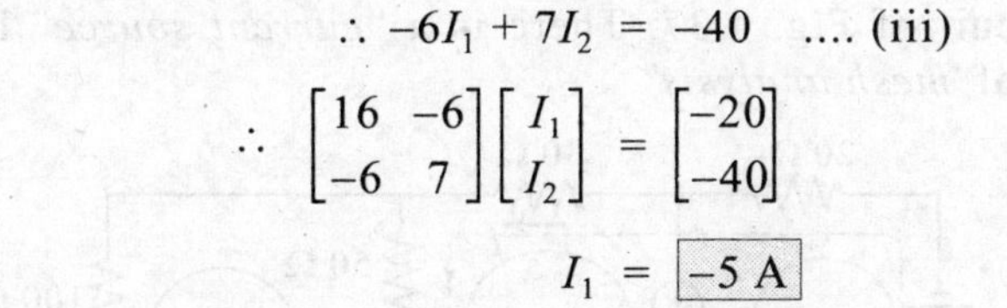

Fig. 1.36

Solution :

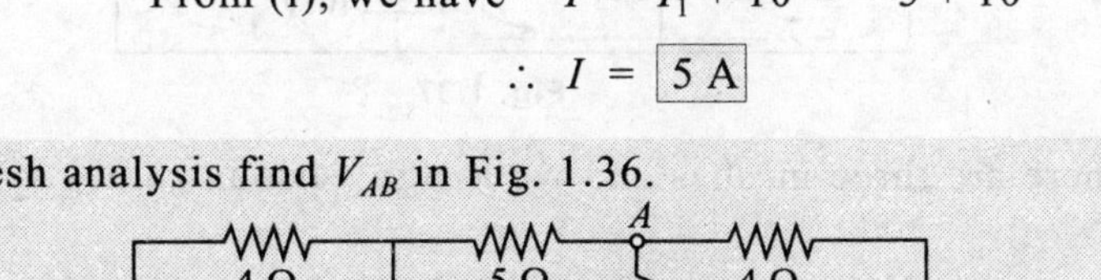

Fig. 1.36(a)

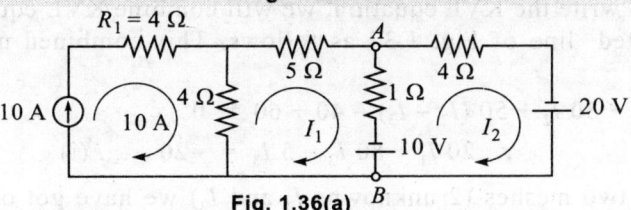

[Hint : Resistance $R_1 = 4\ \Omega$ in series with 10 A source is "redundant" i.e. has no meaning and should not be considered as current through 10 A source remains 10 A for any value of R_1**]**

$$V_{AB} = 1(I_1 - I_2) - 10 \quad \text{.... (i)}$$

KVL in mesh I_1

$$5I_1 + 1\,(I_1 - I_2) - 10 + 4(I_1 - 10) = 0$$

$$\therefore 10I_1 - I_2 = 50 \quad \text{.... (ii)}$$

KVL in mesh I_2

$$4I_2 - 20 + 10 + 1(I_2 - I_1) = 0$$

$$\therefore -I_1 + 5I_2 = 10 \quad \text{.... (iii)}$$

$$\therefore \begin{bmatrix} 10 & -1 \\ -1 & 5 \end{bmatrix} \begin{bmatrix} I_1 \\ I_2 \end{bmatrix} = \begin{bmatrix} 50 \\ 10 \end{bmatrix}$$

$$\therefore I_1 = 5.31 \text{ and } I_2 = 3.06$$

$$\therefore V_{AB} = (5.31 - 3.06) - 10 \quad \text{.... from (i)}$$

$$V_{AB} = \boxed{-7.75 \text{ volts}}$$

1.7.1 Concept of Supermesh

Look at the circuit of Fig. 1.37. There is a "*current source*" between two meshes. Following the steps of '*mesh analysis*'.

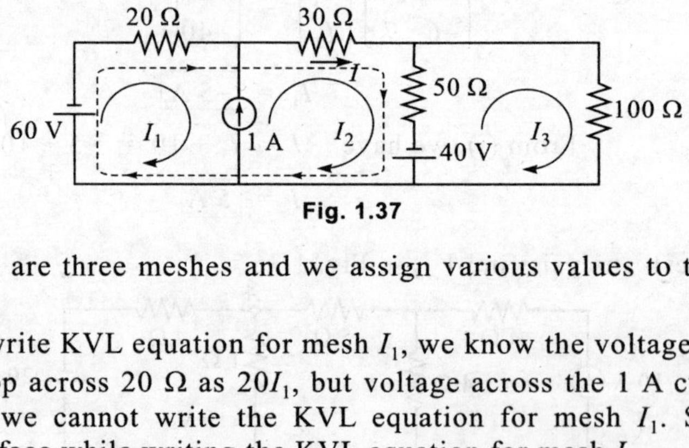

Fig. 1.37

We find that there are three meshes and we assign various values to these meshes i.e. I_1, I_2 and I_3.

Now, in order to write KVL equation for mesh I_1, we know the voltage of 60 V source, we can define the drop across 20 Ω as $20I_1$, but voltage across the 1 A current source is not defined!! Hence, we cannot write the KVL equation for mesh I_1. Similarly, the same difficulty we will face while writing the KVL equation for mesh I_2.

Thus, in order to write the KVL equation, we will combine KVL equations of mesh I_1 and I_2 along the dotted line of Fig. 1.37 as follows. This combined mesh is called "*Super mesh*".

$$20\,I_1 + 30\,I_2 + 50\,(I_2 - I_3) - 40 + 60 = 0$$

$$\therefore 20\,I_1 + 80\,I_2 - 5\,I_3 = -20 \quad \text{.... (i)}$$

Note : Here for two meshes (2 unknowns I_1 and I_2) we have got only one equation. We have actually lost one equation, which can be found as follows: the mesh currents through 1 A source are I_1 and I_2 and direction of I_2 is same as that of 1 A source.

$$\therefore I_2 - I_1 = 1 \text{ A} \quad .... \text{(ii)}$$

Now writing the KVL equation for mesh I_3, we get

$$100\, I_3 + 40 + 50(I_3 - I_2) = 0$$

$$-50\, I_2 + 150\, I_3 = -40 \quad .... \text{(iii)}$$

Thus, the three equations (i), (ii) and (iii) can be simplified as

$$\begin{bmatrix} 20 & 80 & -50 \\ -1 & 1 & 0 \\ 0 & -50 & 150 \end{bmatrix} \begin{bmatrix} I_1 \\ I_2 \\ I_3 \end{bmatrix} = \begin{bmatrix} -20 \\ 1 \\ -40 \end{bmatrix}$$

$$I_1 = -1.16 \text{ A} ;\ I_2 = -0.16 \text{ A} ;\ I_3 = -0.32 \text{ A}$$

If I was to be calculated (from Fig. 1.37) then $I = I_2$

$$\therefore I = \boxed{-0.16 \text{ A}}$$

Ex. 1.25 : Using mesh analysis find I in Fig. 1.38.

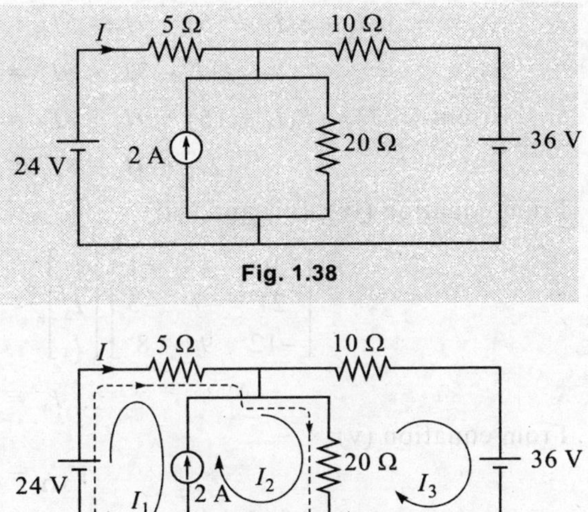

Fig. 1.38

Solution : As there is a current source of 2 A between two meshes I_1 and I_2 it is a case of super mesh.

KVL in super mesh I_1 and I_2

$$-24 + 5I_1 + 20(I_2 - I_3) = 0$$

$$\therefore 5I_1 + 20I_2 - 20I_3 = 24 \quad .... \text{(i)}$$

and

$$I_2 - I_1 = 2 \quad .... \text{(ii)}$$

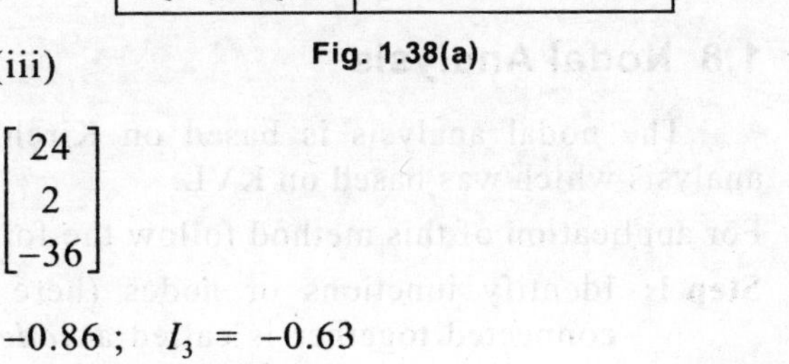

Fig. 1.38(a)

KVL in mesh I_3

$$10I_3 + 36 + 20(I_3 - I_2) = 0$$

$$\therefore -20I_2 + 30I_3 = -36 \quad .... \text{(iii)}$$

$$\begin{bmatrix} 5 & 20 & -20 \\ -1 & 1 & 0 \\ 0 & -20 & 30 \end{bmatrix} \begin{bmatrix} I_1 \\ I_2 \\ I_3 \end{bmatrix} = \begin{bmatrix} 24 \\ 2 \\ -36 \end{bmatrix}$$

$$I_1 = -1.14 ;\ I_2 = -0.86 ;\ I_3 = -0.63$$

But $I = I_1$

$$\therefore I = \boxed{-1.14 \text{ A}}$$

Ex. 1.26 : Using mesh analysis find voltage across 3 Ω resistance in Fig. 1.39.

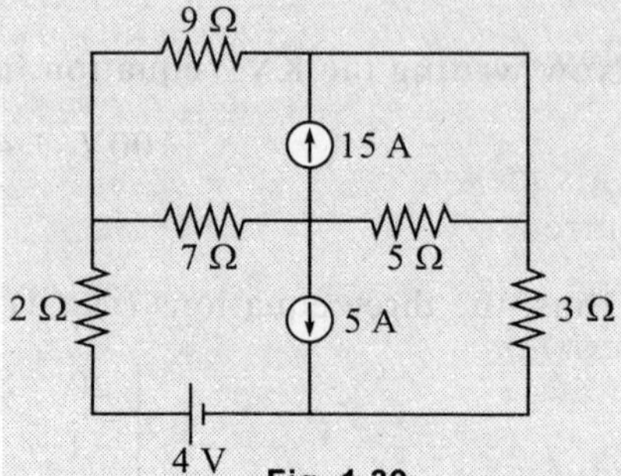

Fig. 1.39

Solution : KVL in super mesh I_1, I_2

$$9I_1 + 5(I_2 - I_4) + 7(I_1 - I_3) = 0$$

$$16I_1 + 5I_2 - 7I_3 - 5I_4 = 0 \quad .... \text{(i)}$$

$$\text{and } I_2 - I_1 = 15 \quad .... \text{(ii)}$$

KVL in super mesh I_3, I_4

$$7(I_3 - I_1) + 5(I_4 - I_2) + 3I_4 - 4 + 2I_3 = 0$$

$$-7I_1 - 5I_2 + 9I_3 + 8I_4 = 4 \quad .... \text{(iii)}$$

$$\text{and } I_3 - I_4 = 5 \quad .... \text{(iv)}$$

$$V_{3\,\Omega} = 3I_4 \text{ from Fig. 1.39(a)} \quad .... \text{(v)}$$

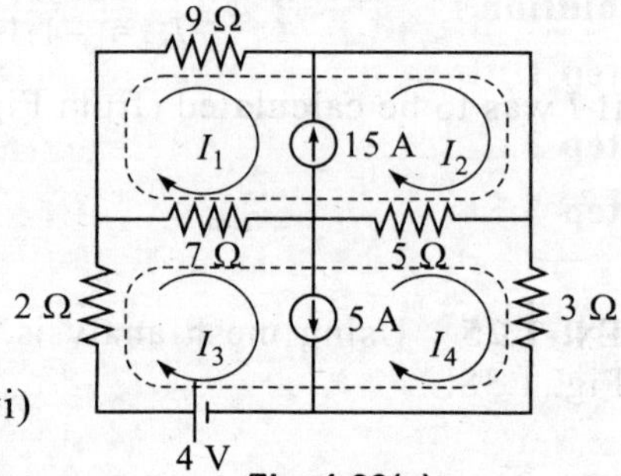

Fig. 1.39(a)

From equation (ii) $I_2 = I_1 + 15$

Substituting I_2 in equations (i) and (iii) we get

$$16I_1 + 5(I_1 + 15) - 7I_3 - 5I_4 = 0$$

$$21I_1 - 7I_3 - 5I_4 = -75 \quad .... \text{(vi)}$$

$$\text{and } -7I_1 - 5(I_1 + 15) + 9I_3 + 8I_4 = 4$$

$$-12I_1 + 9I_3 + 8I_4 = 79 \quad .... \text{(vii)}$$

From equation (iv), (vi) and (vii)

$$\begin{bmatrix} 0 & 1 & -1 \\ 21 & -7 & -5 \\ -12 & 9 & 8 \end{bmatrix} \begin{bmatrix} I_1 \\ I_3 \\ I_4 \end{bmatrix} = \begin{bmatrix} 5 \\ -75 \\ 79 \end{bmatrix}$$

$$\therefore I_4 = 1.098$$

From equation (v)

$$V_{3\,\Omega} = 3I_4$$

$$V_{3\,\Omega} = \boxed{3.294 \text{ volts}}$$

1.8 Nodal Analysis

The nodal analysis is based on Kirchhoff's Current Law (KCL) unlike the mesh analysis which was based on KVL.

For application of this method follow the following steps:

Step 1: Identify junctions or nodes (here terminal where more than 2 elements are connected together is called a *node*). Be careful that "nodes which do not have any element connected between them are considered as one node."

Step 2: Consider any one node (normally the lowest where all the elements or branches are connected) as the reference or datum node.

Step 3: Assume voltages at each node with respect to the reference.

Step 4: Write KCL equation at each node assuming which ever you consider is at a higher potential than any other potential in the circuit.

This means that all the assumed currents will be away from the node, unless there is a current source in a branch whose direction of current is known.

The currents in each branch is defined by *difference of potentials divided by the resistance in a particular branch.*

Ex. 1.27 : Using nodal analysis find V in Fig. 1.40.

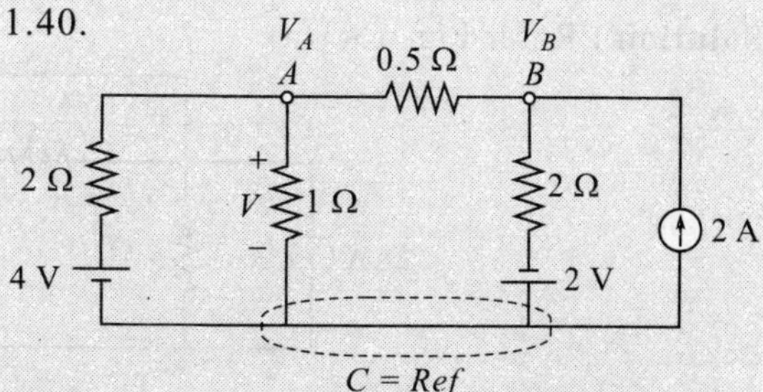

Fig. 1.40

Solution :

Step 1 : Identify junctions, A, B, C.

Step 2 : Take C as the reference node.

Step 3 : Assume voltages V_A and V_B with reference to C.

Step 4 : Write KCL equation at each node.

$$V = V_A$$

KCL at A

$$\frac{V_A - 4}{2} + \frac{V_A}{1} + \frac{V_A - V_B}{0.5} = 0$$

Multiply this equation by 2 we get

$$(V_A - 4) + 2V_A + 4(V_A - V_B) = 0$$

$$\therefore \; 7V_A - 4V_B = 4 \quad .... \text{(i)}$$

KCL at B

$$\frac{V_B - V_A}{0.5} + \frac{V_B - (-2)}{2} - 2 = 0$$

Multiply this equation by 2 we get

$$4(V_B - V_A) + V_B + 2 - 4 = 0$$

$$\therefore \; -4V_A + 5V_B = 2 \quad .... \text{(ii)}$$

$$\therefore \; \begin{bmatrix} 7 & -4 \\ -4 & 5 \end{bmatrix} \begin{bmatrix} V_A \\ V_B \end{bmatrix} = \begin{bmatrix} 4 \\ 2 \end{bmatrix}$$

From Fig.1.40,

$$\therefore \; V_A = 1.47 \text{ volts and } V_B = 1.58 \text{ volts}$$

$$\therefore \; V = \boxed{1.47 \text{ volts}}$$

Ex. 1.28 : Using nodal analysis find I in Fig. 1.41.

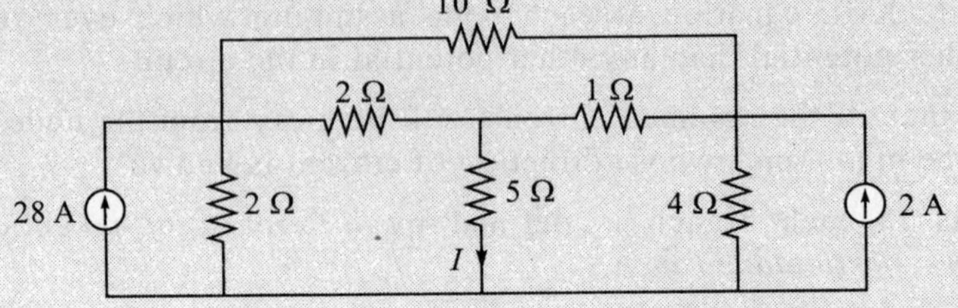

Fig. 1.41

Solution : Refer Fig. 1.41(a).

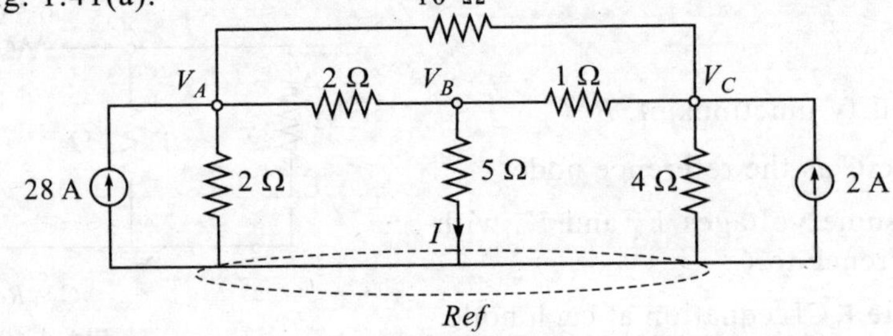

Fig. 1.41(a)

KCL at ***A***

$$-28 + \frac{V_A}{2} + \frac{V_A - V_B}{2} + \frac{V_A - V_C}{10} = 0$$

Multiply this equation by 10, we get

$$-280 + 5V_A + 5V_A - 5V_B + V_A - V_C = 0$$

$$11V_A - 5V_B - V_C = 280 \quad .... \text{(i)}$$

KCL at ***B***

$$\frac{V_B - V_A}{2} + \frac{V_B}{5} + \frac{V_B - V_C}{1} = 0$$

Multiply this equation by 10, we get

$$5V_B - 5V_A + 2V_B + 10V_B - 10V_C = 0$$

$$5V_A + 17V_B - 10V_C = 0 \quad .... \text{(ii)}$$

KCL at ***C***

$$\frac{V_C - V_B}{1} + \frac{V_C}{4} + \frac{V_C - V_A}{10} - 2 = 0$$

Multiply this equation by 20, we get

$$20V_C - 20V_B + 5V_C + 2V_C - 2V_A - 40 = 0$$

$$-2V_A - 20V_B + 27V_C = 40 \quad .... \text{(iii)}$$

$$\therefore \begin{bmatrix} 11 & -5 & -1 \\ -5 & 17 & -10 \\ -2 & -20 & 27 \end{bmatrix} \begin{bmatrix} V_A \\ V_B \\ V_C \end{bmatrix} = \begin{bmatrix} 280 \\ 0 \\ 40 \end{bmatrix}$$

From Fig. 1.41(a), $I = \frac{V_B}{5}$

$$\therefore \; V_B = 24.74 \text{ volts}$$

$$\text{and } I = \frac{24.74}{5}$$

$$\therefore \; I = \boxed{4.95 \text{ amp}}$$

Ex. 1.29 : Using nodal analysis, find V in Fig. 1.42.

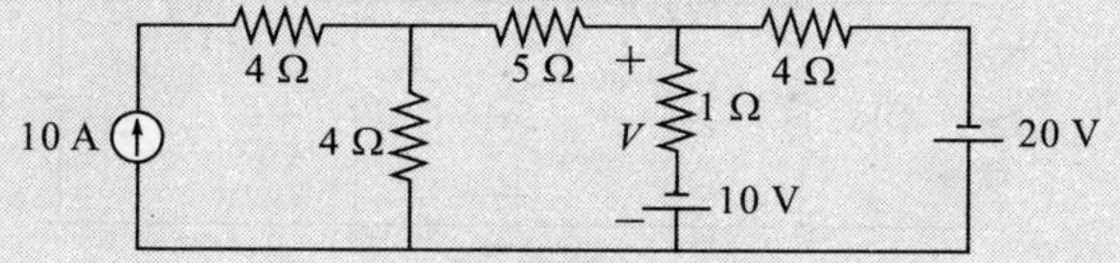

Fig. 1.42

Solution : Refer Fig. 1.42(a).

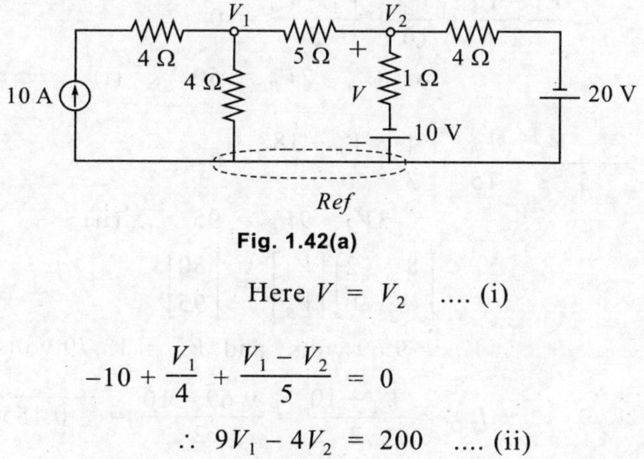

Fig. 1.42(a)

$$\text{Here } V = V_2 \quad \text{.... (i)}$$

KCL at V_1

$$-10 + \frac{V_1}{4} + \frac{V_1 - V_2}{5} = 0$$

$$\therefore \; 9V_1 - 4V_2 = 200 \quad \text{.... (ii)}$$

KCL at V_2

$$\frac{V_2 - V_1}{5} + \frac{V_2 - (-10)}{1} + \frac{V_2 - (-20)}{4} = 0$$

$$\therefore \; -4V_1 + 29V_2 = -300 \quad \text{.... (iii)}$$

$$\therefore \begin{bmatrix} 9 & -4 \\ -4 & 29 \end{bmatrix} \begin{bmatrix} V_1 \\ V_2 \end{bmatrix} = \begin{bmatrix} 200 \\ -300 \end{bmatrix}$$

$$\therefore \; V_2 = -7.75 \text{ volts}$$

$$\text{From (i) } V = \boxed{-7.75 \text{ volts}}$$

Ex. 1.30 : Find current through 2 Ω and 3 Ω resistances using nodal analysis in Fig. 1.43..

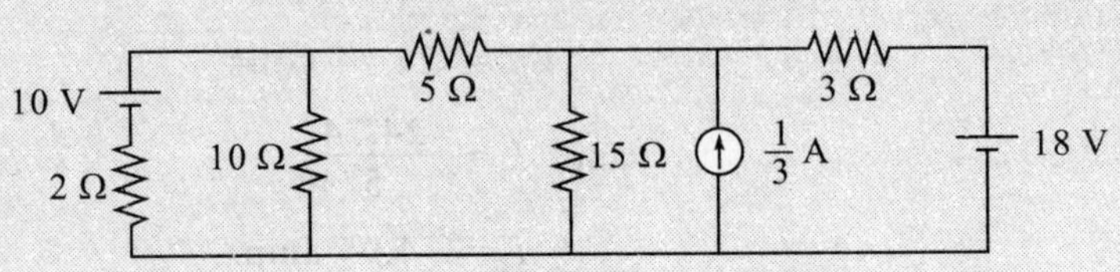

Fig. 1.43

Solution : Refer Fig. 1.43(a).

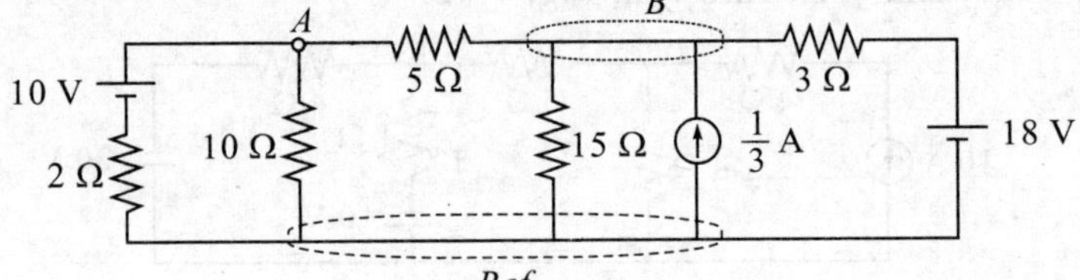

Fig. 1.43(a)

KCL at *A*

$$\frac{V_A - 10}{2} + \frac{V_A}{10} + \frac{V_A - V_B}{5} = 0$$

$$\text{or } 8V_A - 2V_B = 50 \quad \text{.... (i)}$$

KCL at *B*

$$\frac{V_B - V_A}{5} + \frac{V_B}{15} - \frac{1}{3} + \frac{V_B - 18}{3} = 0$$

$$-3V_A + 9V_B = 95 \quad \text{.... (ii)}$$

$$\therefore \begin{bmatrix} 8 & -2 \\ -3 & 9 \end{bmatrix} \begin{bmatrix} V_A \\ V_B \end{bmatrix} = \begin{bmatrix} 50 \\ 95 \end{bmatrix}$$

$$\therefore V_A = 9.69 \text{ volts and } V_B = 13.79 \text{ volts}$$

From Fig.1.43(a),

$$\therefore I_{2\,\Omega} = \frac{V_A - 10}{2} = \frac{9.69 - 10}{2} = \boxed{-0.155 \text{ A}}$$

$$I_{3\,\Omega} = \frac{V_B - 18}{3} = \frac{13.79 - 18}{3} = \boxed{-1.4 \text{ A}}$$

i.e. both the currents are towards their respective nodes *A* and *B*.

Ex. 1.31 : Find V_X using nodal analysis in Fig. 1.44.

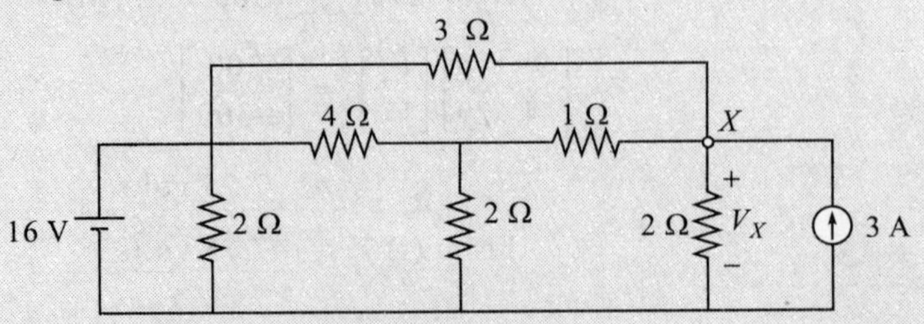

Fig. 1.44

Solution :

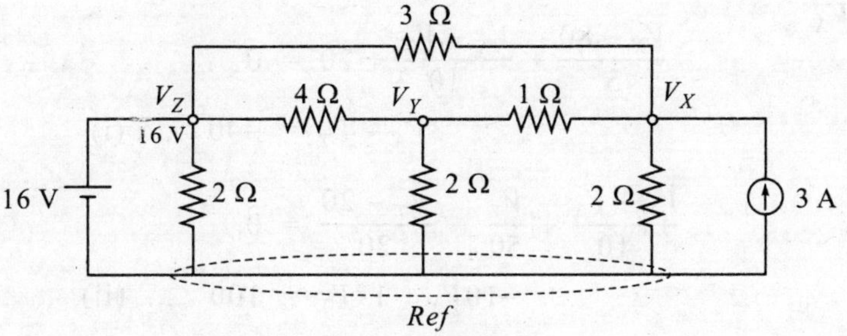

Fig. 1.44(a)

Note that the 16 V source is connected between terminal Z and reference and there is no resistance in series with 16 V source.

$$\therefore V_Z = 16 \text{ V}$$

There are only two unknowns i.e. V_X and V_Y

$\therefore$ **KCL at V_X**

$$\frac{V_X}{2} - 3 + \frac{V_X - V_Y}{1} + \frac{V_X - 16}{3} = 0$$

$$\text{or } 11V_X - 6V_Y = 50 \quad .... \text{(i)}$$

KCL at V_Y

$$\frac{V_Y - 16}{4} + \frac{V_Y}{2} + \frac{V_Y - V_X}{1} = 0$$

$$-4V_X + 7V_Y = 16 \quad .... \text{(ii)}$$

$$\therefore \begin{bmatrix} 11 & -6 \\ -4 & 7 \end{bmatrix} \begin{bmatrix} V_X \\ V_Y \end{bmatrix} = \begin{bmatrix} 50 \\ 16 \end{bmatrix}$$

$$\therefore V_X = \boxed{8.41 \text{ volts}}$$

Ex. 1.32 : Find current through 10 Ω resistance using nodal analysis in Fig. 1.45.

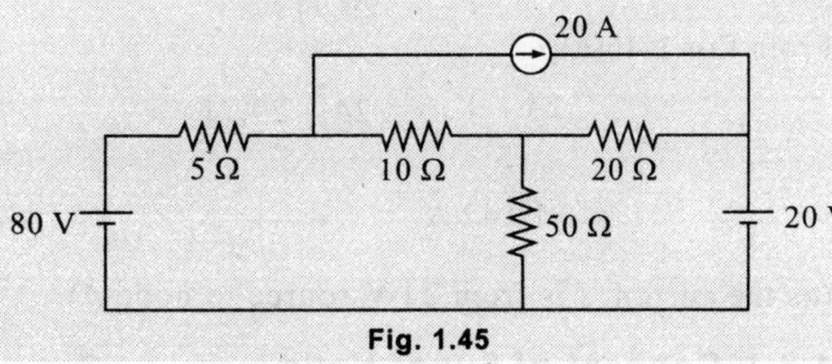

Fig. 1.45

Solution :

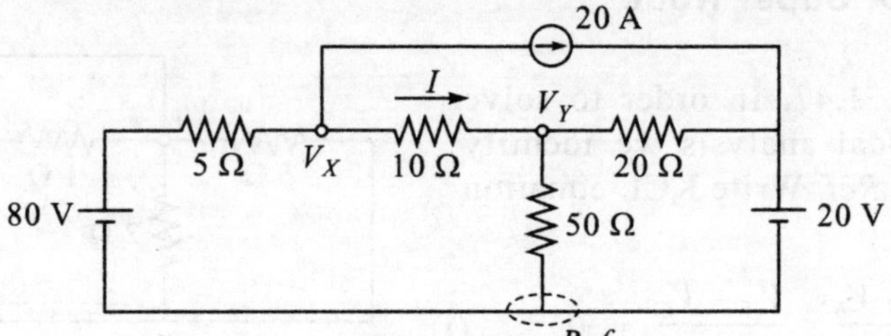

Fig. 1.45(a)

$\therefore$ **KCL at V_X**

$$\frac{V_X - 80}{5} + \frac{V_X - V_Y}{10} + 20 = 0$$

$$\therefore \quad 3V_X - V_Y = -40 \quad .... \text{(i)}$$

KCL at V_Y

$$\frac{V_Y - V_X}{10} + \frac{V_Y}{50} + \frac{V_Y - 20}{20} = 0$$

$$\therefore \quad -10V_X + 17V_Y = 100 \quad .... \text{(ii)}$$

$$\therefore \begin{bmatrix} 3 & -1 \\ -10 & 17 \end{bmatrix} \begin{bmatrix} V_X \\ V_Y \end{bmatrix} = \begin{bmatrix} -40 \\ 100 \end{bmatrix}$$

$$\therefore \quad V_X = \boxed{-14.15 \text{ volts}} \qquad V_Y = \boxed{-2.44 \text{ volts}}$$

From Fig.1.45(a),

$$I = \frac{V_X - V_Y}{10} = \frac{-14.15 - (-2.44)}{10} = \boxed{-1.17 \text{ A}}$$

i.e. current is opposite to the marked polarity.

Ex. 1.33 : Using nodal analysis find I in Fig. 1.46.

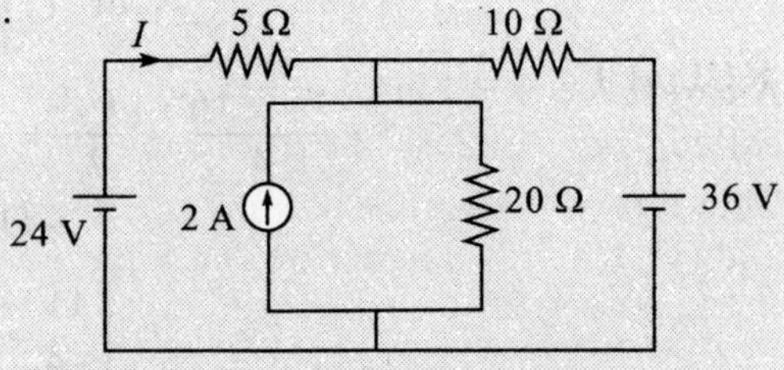

Fig. 1.46

Solution : Refer Fig. 1.43(a).

KCL at A

$$\frac{V_A - 24}{5} - 2 + \frac{V_A}{20} + \frac{V_A - 36}{10} = 0$$

Multiplying both sides by 20, we get

$$4V_A - 24 \times 4 - 2 \times 20 + V_A + 2V_A - 36 \times 2 = 0$$

$$\therefore \quad V_A = 29.71$$

From Fig.1.46(a),

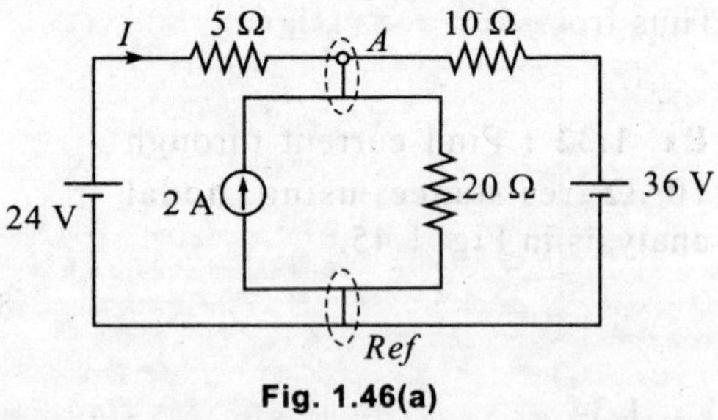

Fig. 1.46(a)

$$I = \frac{24 - V_A}{5} = \frac{24 - 29.71}{5}$$

$$I = \boxed{-1.142 \text{ A}}$$

(as the current I is from 24 V source to node A)

1.8.1 Concept of Super Node

Consider Fig. 1.47. In order to solve this circuit by nodal analysis we identify nodes A, B, C and Ref. Write KCL equation at node A

$$\frac{V_A}{5} + \frac{V_A}{2} + \frac{V_A - V_B}{1} + \frac{V_A - V_C}{4} = 0 \quad .... \text{(i)}$$

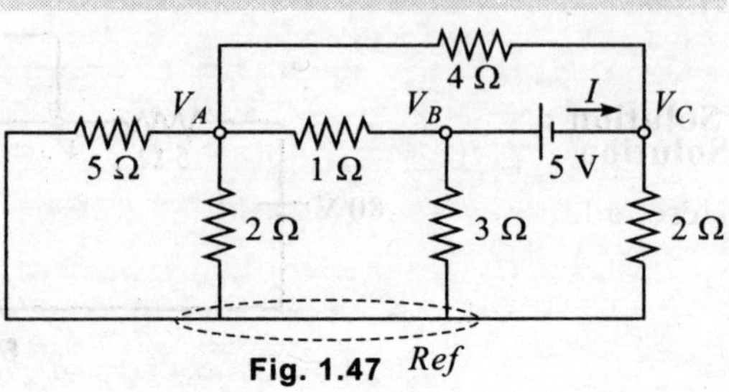

Fig. 1.47

Now, when we write KCL equation at B, the problem is branch BC. We know there is a voltage source of 5 V with terminal B at a higher potential than C. But the current through branch BC is not known. Similarly, at C we cannot write the KCL equation. So for the time being let us assume there is a current of I as marked in Fig. 1.47.

∴ KCL at B will give us

$$\frac{V_B - V_A}{1} + \frac{V_B}{3} + I = 0 \quad .... \text{(ii)}$$

and KCL at C will be

$$\frac{V_C}{2} + \frac{V_C - V_A}{4} - I = 0 \quad .... \text{(iii)}$$

Adding equations (ii) and (iii), we get

$$\frac{V_B - V_A}{1} + \frac{V_B}{3} + I + \frac{V_C}{2} + \frac{V_C - V_A}{4} - I = 0 \quad .... \text{(iv)}$$

From equation (iv) I gets cancelled off and new equation will be

$$\frac{V_B - V_A}{1} + \frac{V_B}{3} + \frac{V_C}{2} + \frac{V_C - V_A}{4} = 0 \quad .... \text{(v)}$$

A careful inspection of equation (v) reveals that if we consider node B and C as one node called "*super node*", the question of defining current in the branch BC does not arise.

This circuit has three unknowns, V_A, V_B and V_C where as we have got just equations (i) and (v). The third equation for super node will be

$$V_B - V_C = 5 \quad .... \text{(vi)}$$

(Node B is at a higher potential)

Thus from equations (i), (v) and (vi), we get

$$\begin{bmatrix} \frac{1}{5} + \frac{1}{2} + 1 + \frac{1}{4} & -1 & -\frac{1}{4} \\ -1 - \frac{1}{4} & 1 + \frac{1}{3} & \frac{1}{2} - \frac{1}{4} \\ 0 & 1 & -1 \end{bmatrix} \begin{bmatrix} V_A \\ V_B \\ V_C \end{bmatrix} = \begin{bmatrix} 0 \\ 0 \\ 5 \end{bmatrix} \quad \text{which can be simplified.}$$

Ex. 1.34 : Using Nodal analysis find current through 5 Ω resistance in Fig. 1.48.

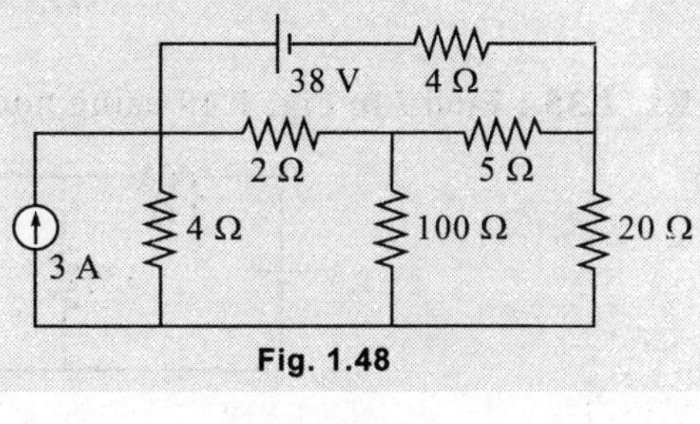

Fig. 1.48

Solution : Refer Fig. 1.48(a).

Here, additional node D is defied for super node.

KCL at super node A, D

$$-3 + \frac{V_A}{4} + \frac{V_A - V_B}{2} + \frac{V_D - V_C}{4} = 0$$

$$\therefore \; 3V_A - 2V_B + V_D - V_C = 12 \quad .... \text{(i)}$$

$$\text{and} \quad V_A - V_D = 38 \quad .... \text{(ii)}$$

$$\text{or} \quad V_D = V_A - 38 \quad .... \text{(iii)}$$

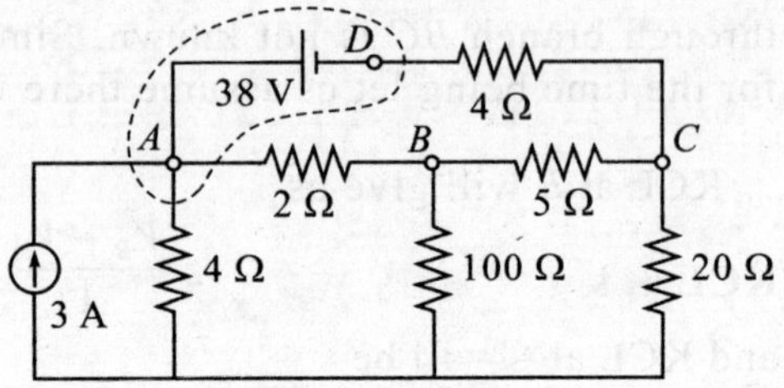

Fig. 1.48(a)

Substituting V_D from (iii) in (i), we get

$$4V_A - 2V_B - V_C = 50 \quad .... \text{(iv)}$$

KCL at B

$$\frac{V_B - V_A}{2} + \frac{V_B}{100} + \frac{V_B - V_C}{5} = 0$$

$$\text{or} \; -50V_A + 71V_B - 20V_C = 12 \quad .... \text{(v)}$$

KCL at C

$$\frac{V_C - V_B}{5} + \frac{V_C}{20} + \frac{V_C - V_D}{4} = 0$$

$$\text{or} \; -4V_B + 10V_C - 5V_D = 0 \quad .... \text{(vi)}$$

Substituting for V_D from (iii), we get

$$-4V_B + 10V_C - 5(V_A - 38) = 0$$

$$-5V_A - 4V_B + 10V_C = -190 \quad .... \text{(vii)}$$

$\therefore$ from equations (iv), (v) and (vii), we get

$$\begin{bmatrix} 4 & -2 & -1 \\ -50 & 71 & -20 \\ -5 & -4 & 10 \end{bmatrix} \begin{bmatrix} V_A \\ V_B \\ V_C \end{bmatrix} = \begin{bmatrix} 50 \\ 0 \\ -190 \end{bmatrix}$$

$$\therefore \; V_A = 13.61 \text{ V} \; ; \; V_B = 6.93 \text{ V} \; ; \; V_C = -9.42 \text{ V} \; ;$$

Current through 5 Ω will be from B to C as V_B is a higher potential as compared to V_C.

$$\therefore \; I = \frac{V_B - V_C}{5} = \frac{6.93 - (-9.42)}{5} = 3.27 \text{ A}$$

$$\therefore \; \boxed{I_{5\,\Omega} = 3.27 \text{ A from B to C}}$$

Ex. 1.35 : Find *I* in Fig. 1.49 using nodal analysis.

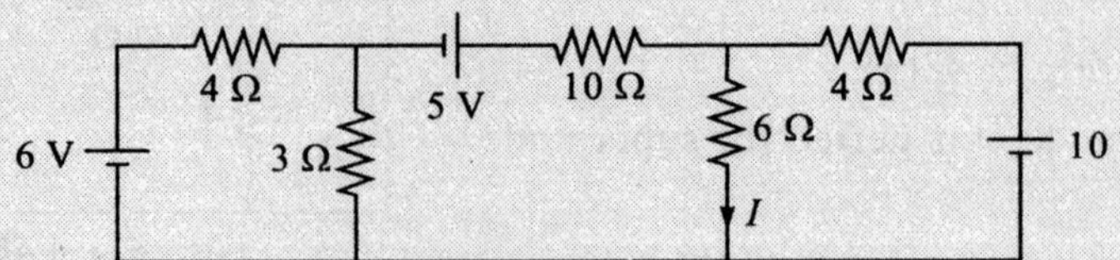

Fig. 1.49

Solution :

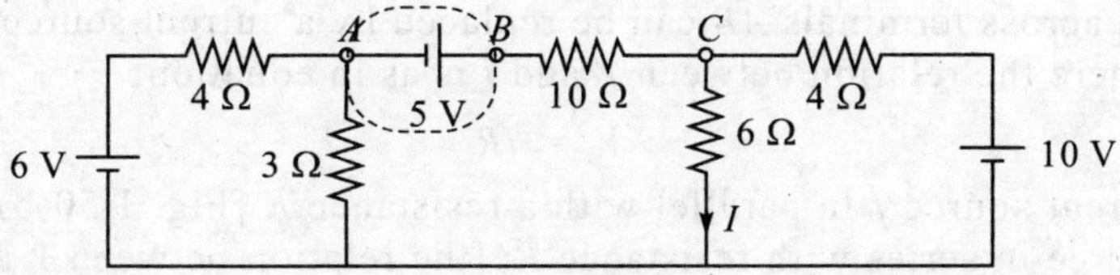

Fig. 1.49(a)

KCL at super node *A*, *B*

$$\frac{V_A - 6}{4} + \frac{V_A}{3} + \frac{V_B - V_C}{10} = 0 \quad \text{[Multiplying by 120]}$$

$$30V_A - 180 + 40V_A + 12V_B - 12V_C = 0$$

$$\therefore \quad 70V_A + 12V_B - 12V_C = 180 \quad .... \text{(i)}$$

$$\text{and } V_B - V_A = 5 \quad .... \text{(ii)}$$

KCL at node *C*

$$\frac{V_C - V_B}{10} + \frac{V_C}{6} + \frac{V_C - 10}{4} = 0 \quad \text{[Multiplying by 120]}$$

$$12V_C - 12V_B + 20V_C + 30V_C - 300 = 0$$

$$\therefore \quad -12V_B + 62V_C = 300 \quad .... \text{(iii)}$$

From equations (i), (ii) and (iii), we get

$$\begin{bmatrix} 70 & 12 & -12 \\ -1 & 1 & 0 \\ 0 & -12 & 62 \end{bmatrix} \begin{bmatrix} V_A \\ V_B \\ V_C \end{bmatrix} = \begin{bmatrix} 180 \\ 5 \\ 300 \end{bmatrix}$$

$$\therefore \quad V_C = 6.27 \text{ V}$$

$$\therefore \quad I = \frac{V_C}{6} = \boxed{1.045 \text{ A}}$$

1.9 Source Transformation

If a resistance R is connected in series with a voltage source V across terminals A and B (as shown in Fig. 1.50).

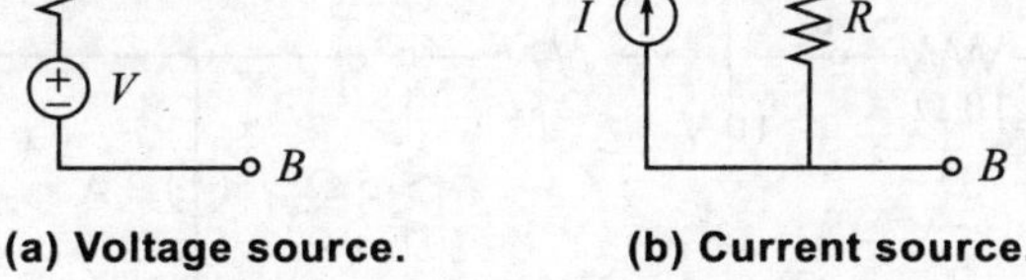

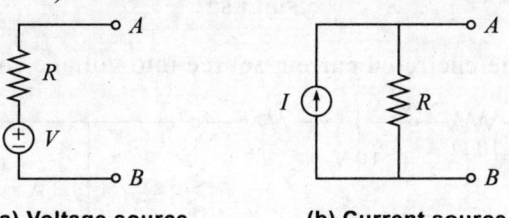

(a) Voltage source. **(b) Current source.**

Fig. 1.50 : Source transformation.

Then the circuit across terminals *AB* can be replaced by a current source *I* in parallel with resistance *R*, where the relation between *V* and *I* is as in equation,

$$V = IR \qquad \text{..... (1.28)}$$

Similarly, a current source *I* in parallel with a resistance *R* [Fig. 1.50(b)] can be replaced by a voltage source in series with resistance *R*, [the relation between *V* and *I* will be as in equation (1.28)] across the same pair of terminals *A* and *B*.

Note :

(1) If a voltage source V_1 is shown parallel to a resistance R_1 [Fig. 1.51(a)] then R_1 is redundant and R_1 can be replaced by open circuit.

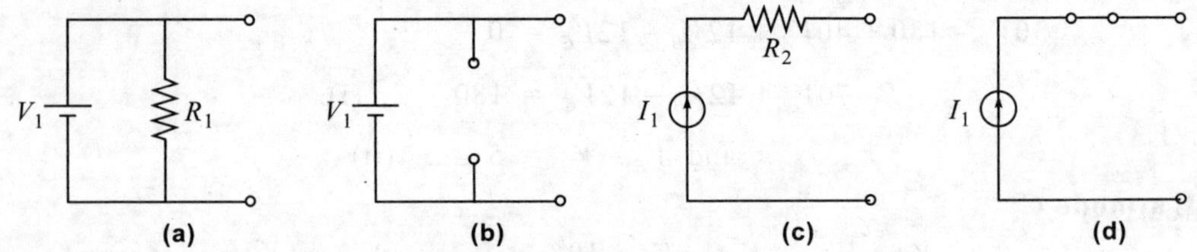

Fig. 1.51 : Redundant resistances.

Similarly, if R_2 is shown in series with a current source I_1, then R_2 is redundant and can be replaced by short circuit.

(2) In solving sums by source transformation always label the junctions and do not carry out transformation o the element where the desired current or voltage is to be calculated. All the steps except the last must be solved by source transformation or series-parallel combinations of resistances and sources.

(3) When we convert the voltage source to current source, the direction of current source is towards the positive terminal of voltage source and vice-versa.

Ex. 1.36 : Using source transformation in Fig. 1.52. find *I*.

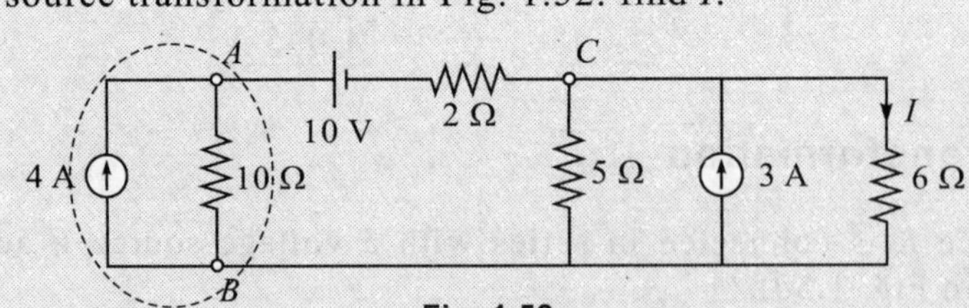

Fig. 1.52

Solution : Converting the encircled current source into voltage source.

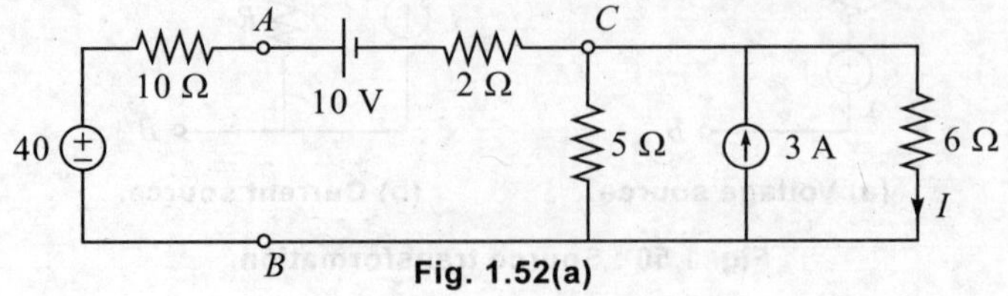

Fig. 1.52(a)

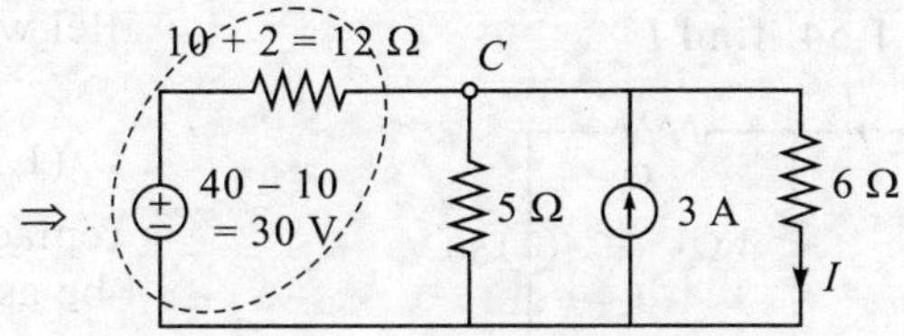

Fig. 1.52(b)

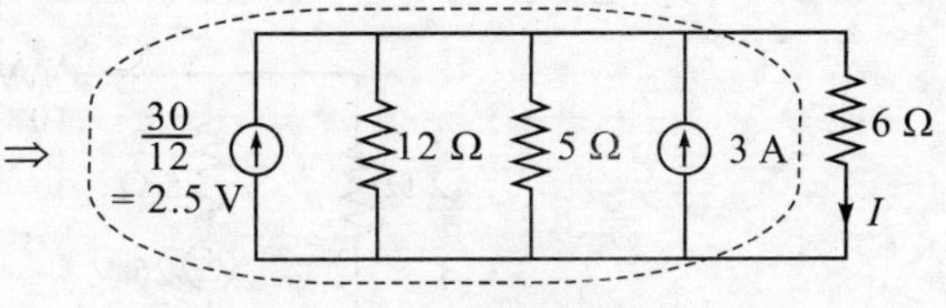

Fig. 1.52(c)

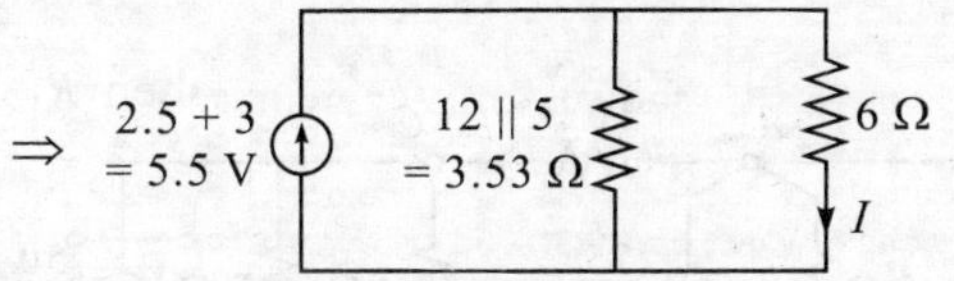

Fig. 1.52(c)

Using current division rule

$$\therefore \quad I = \frac{3.53}{6 + 3.53} \times 5.5 = \boxed{2.03 \text{ A}}$$

Ex. 1.37 : Using source transformation in Fig. 1.53 find power delivered by 50 V source.

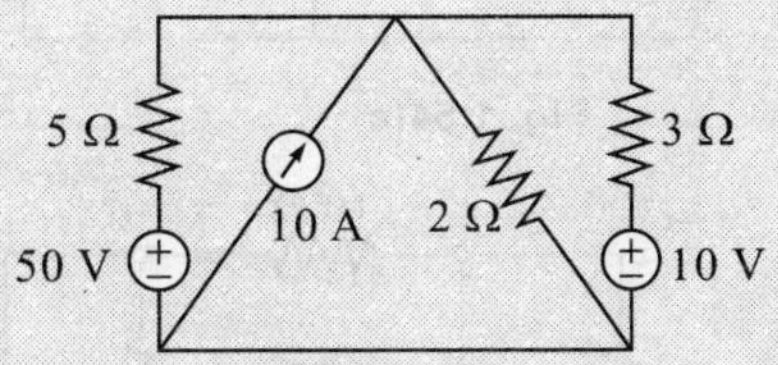

Fig. 1.53

Solution : Careful observation of the circuit indicates that all four branches are in parallel to each other across *A* and *B*.

Power delivered by 50 V source means product of 50 V and *I*, where *I* is the current through 50 V source. Refer Fig. 1.53(a).

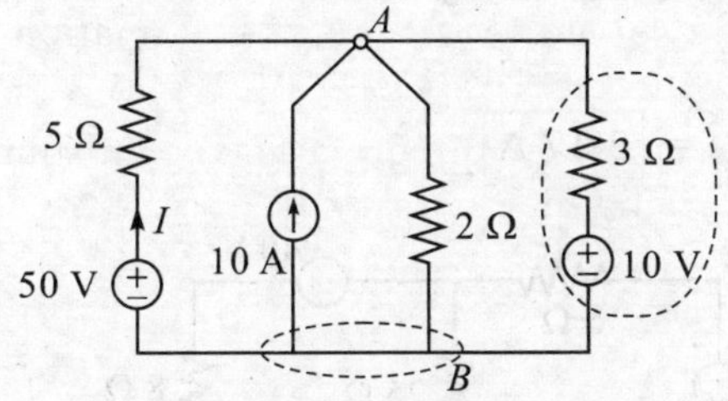

Fig. 1.53(a)

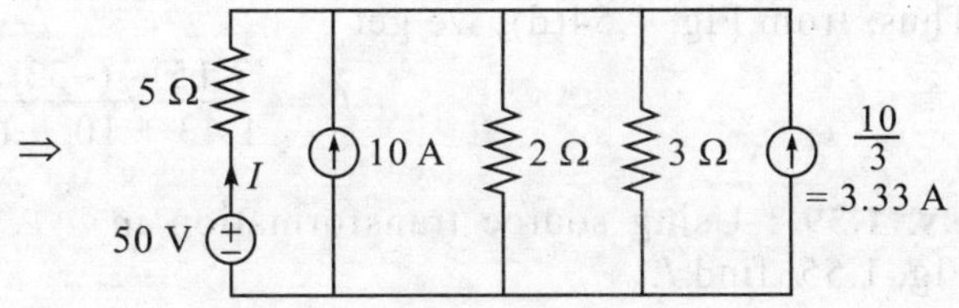

Fig. 1.53(b)

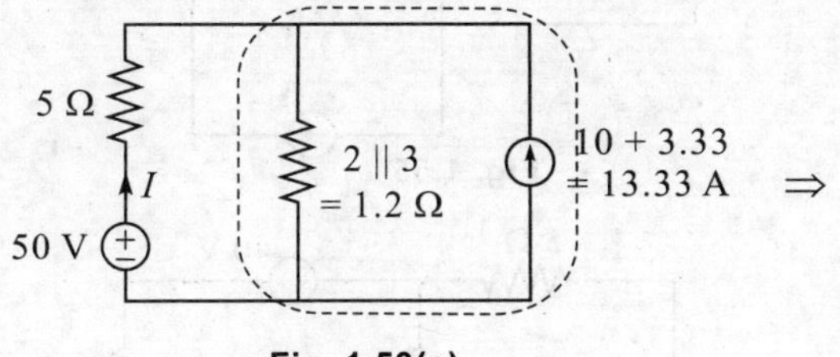

Fig. 1.53(c)

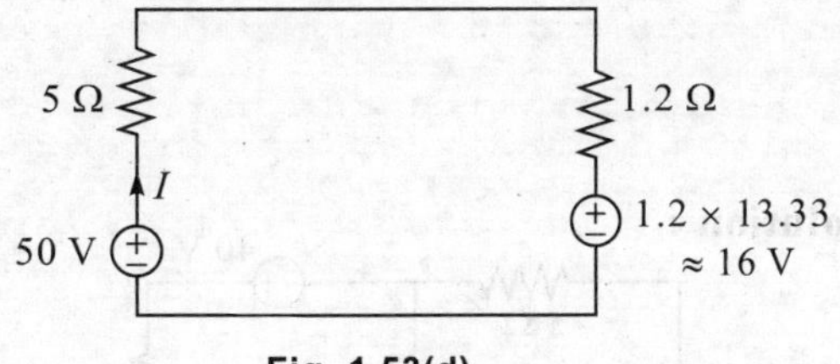

Fig. 1.53(d)

Thus, from Fig. 1.53(d), we get

$$\therefore \quad I = \frac{50 - 16}{5 + 1.2} = \boxed{5.48 \text{ A}}$$

$$\therefore \quad \text{Power delivered} = V \times I = 50 \times 5.48 = \boxed{274.19 \text{ watts}}$$

Ex. 1.38 : Using source transformation in Fig. 1.54. find I.

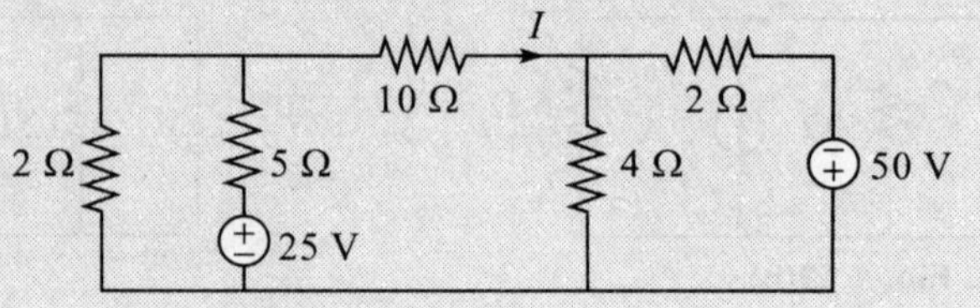

Fig. 1.54

Solution :

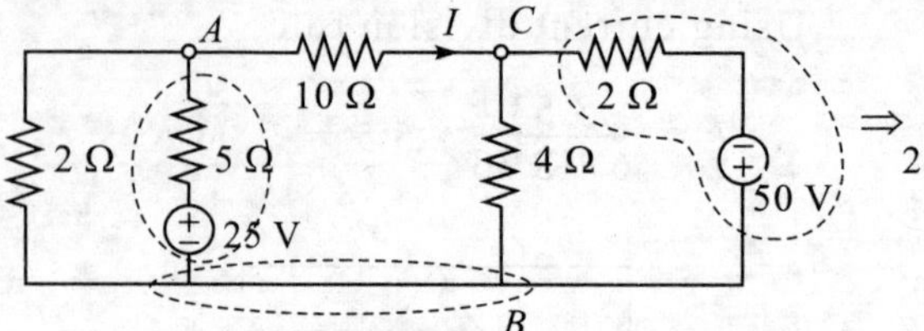

Fig. 1.54(a)

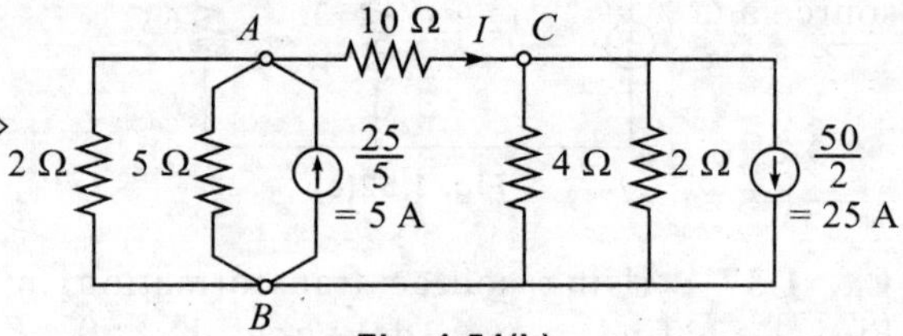

Fig. 1.54(b)

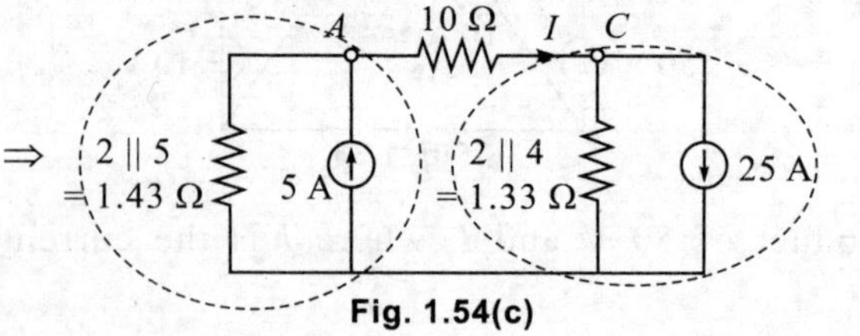

Fig. 1.54(c)

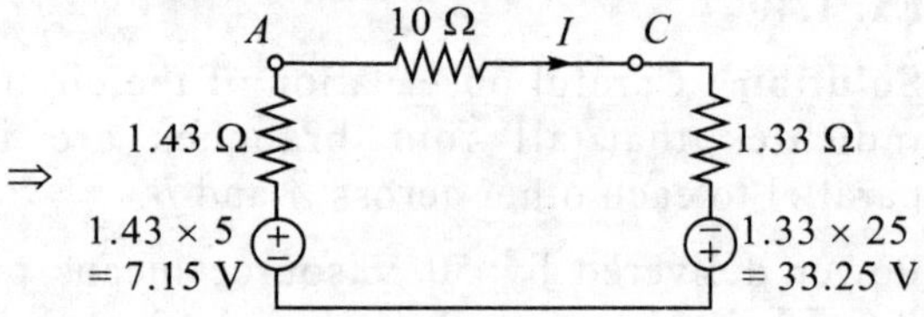

Fig. 1.54(d)

Thus, from Fig. 1.54(d), we get

$$\therefore \quad I = \frac{7.15 - (-33.25)}{1.43 + 10 + 1.33} = \boxed{3.17 \text{ A}}$$

Ex. 1.39 : Using source transformation in Fig. 1.55. find I.

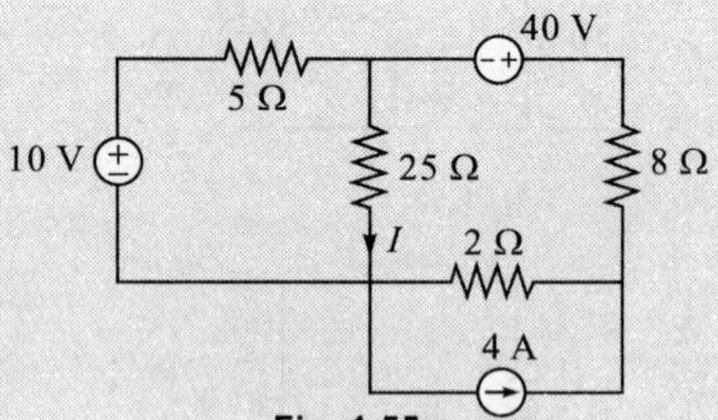

Fig. 1.55

Solution :

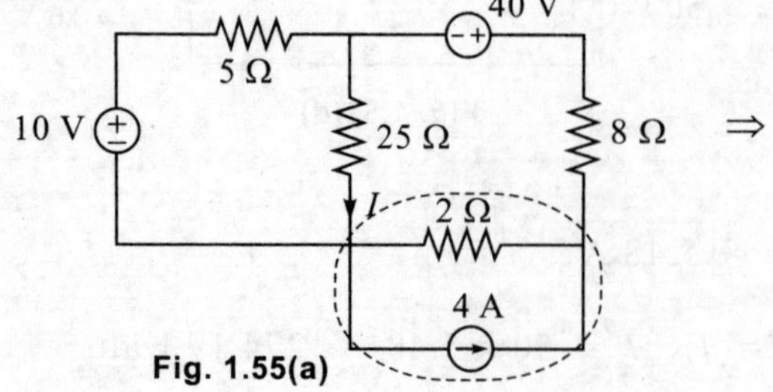

Fig. 1.55(a)

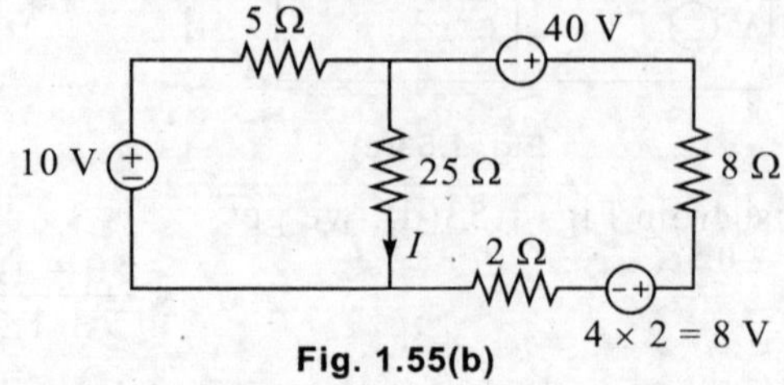

Fig. 1.55(b)

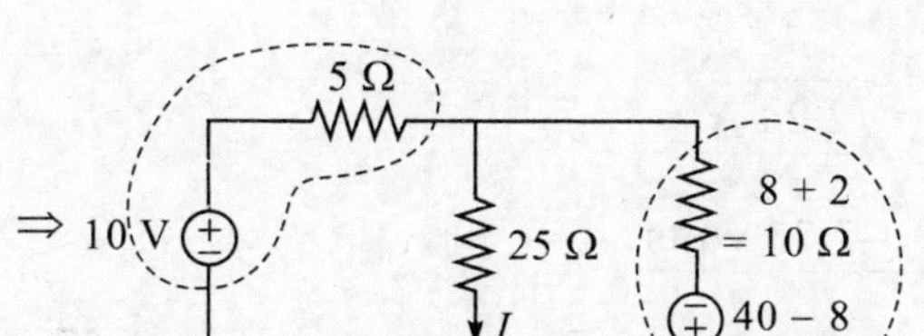

Fig. 1.55(c)

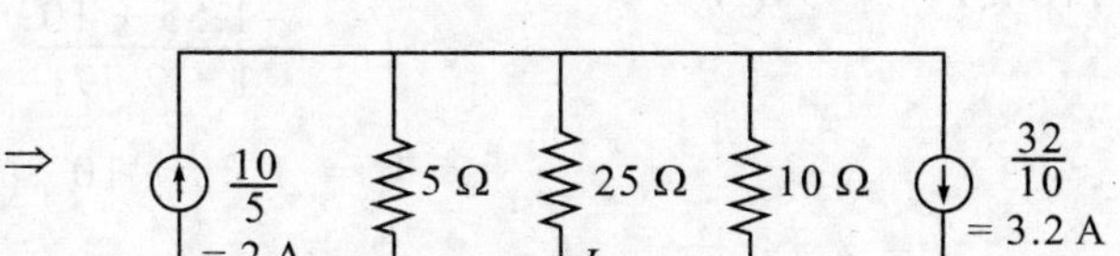

Fig. 1.55(d)

In Fig. 1.55(d) 2 A and 3.2 are in parallel but in opposite directions, taking sign of 2 A source and 5 Ω and 10 Ω are in parallel, we get Fig. 1.55(e).

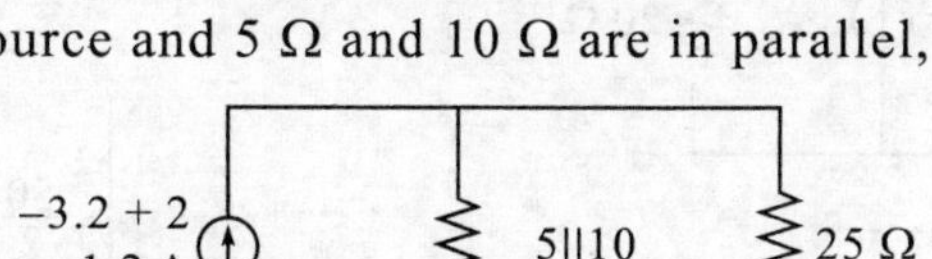

Fig. 1.55(e)

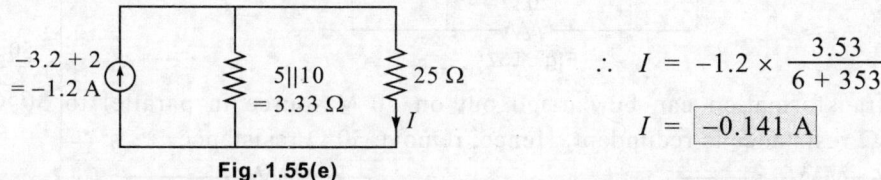

$$\therefore \quad I = -1.2 \times \frac{3.53}{6 + 353}$$

$$I = \boxed{-0.141 \text{ A}}$$

Ex. 1.40 : Using source transformation in Fig. 1.56 find V.

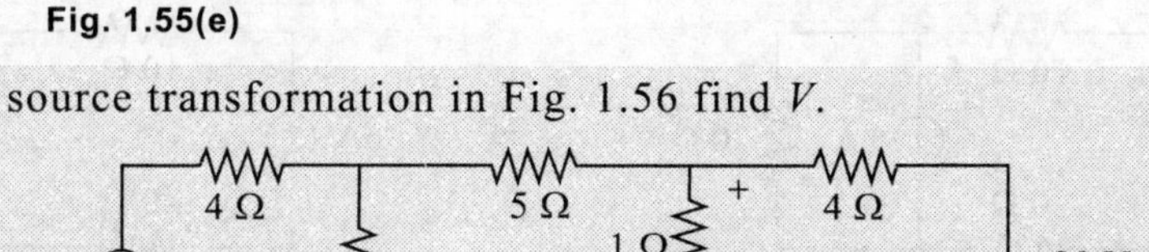

Fig. 1.56

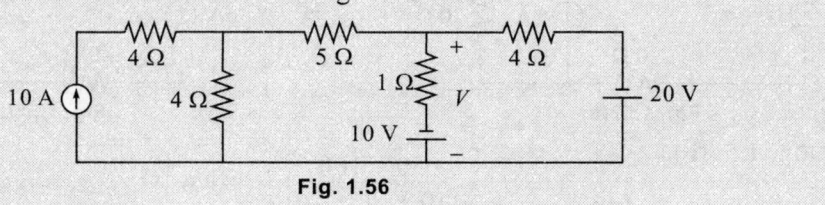

Solution : Here, 4 Ω resistance in series with current source is redundant. Thus removing that we get Fig. 1.56(a).

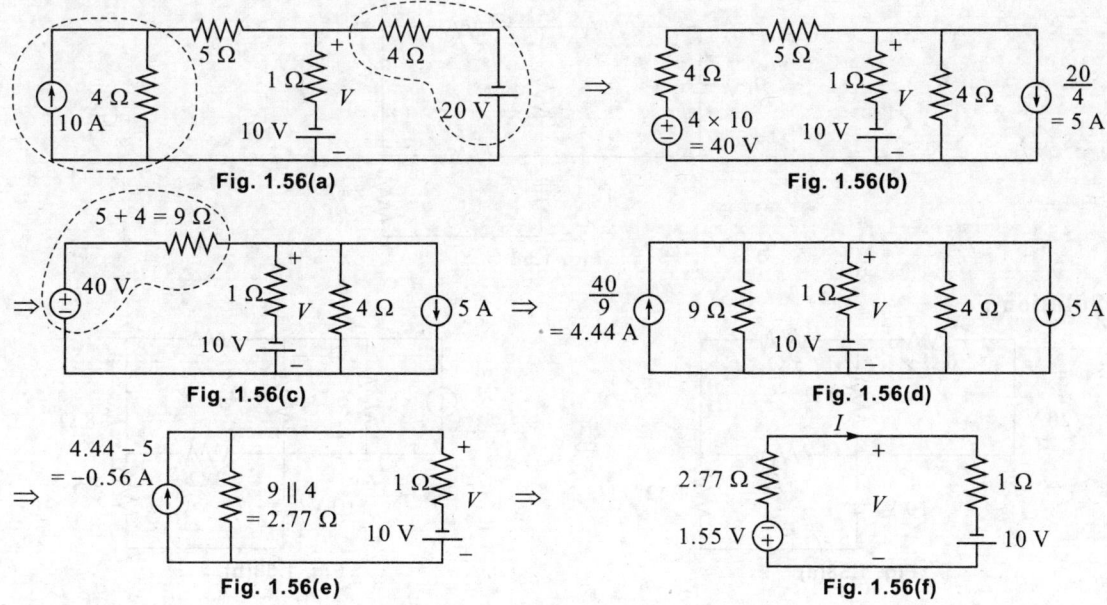

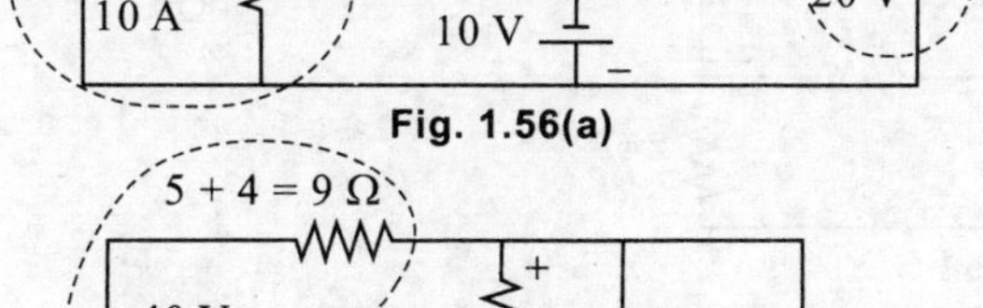

Fig. 1.56(a)

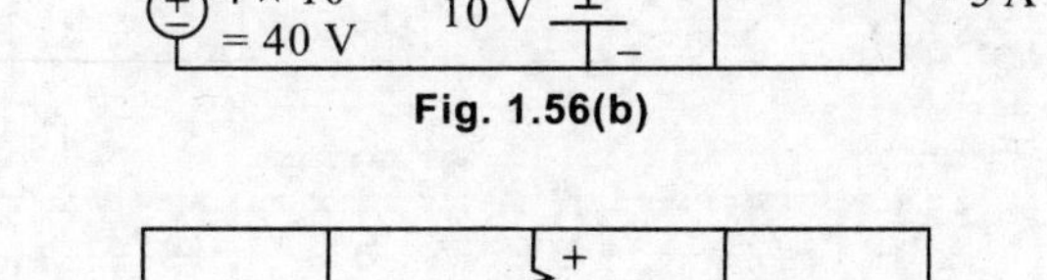

Fig. 1.56(b)

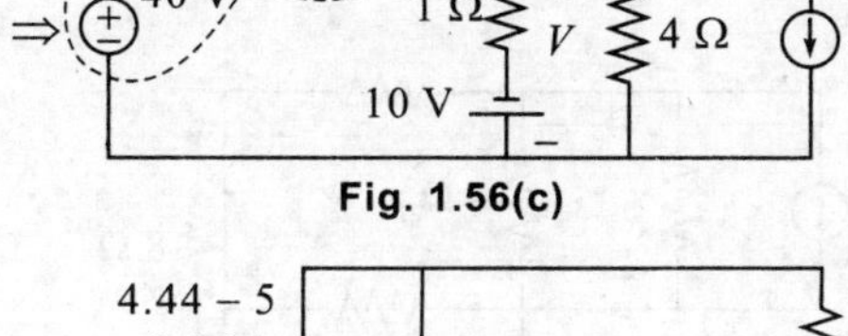

Fig. 1.56(c)

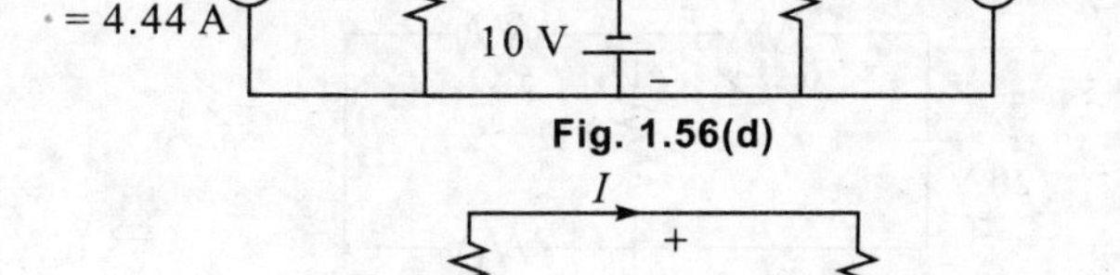

Fig. 1.56(d)

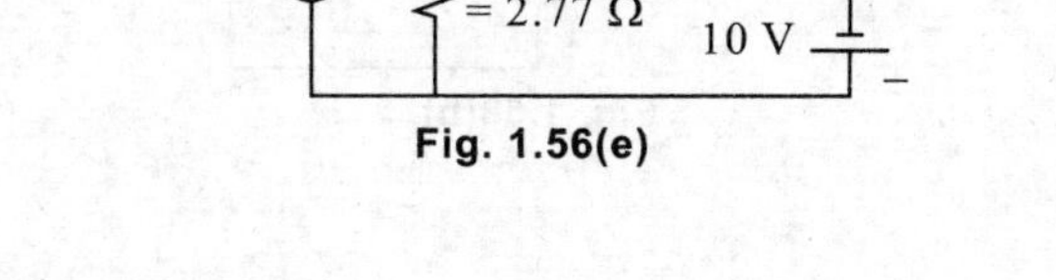

Fig. 1.56(e)

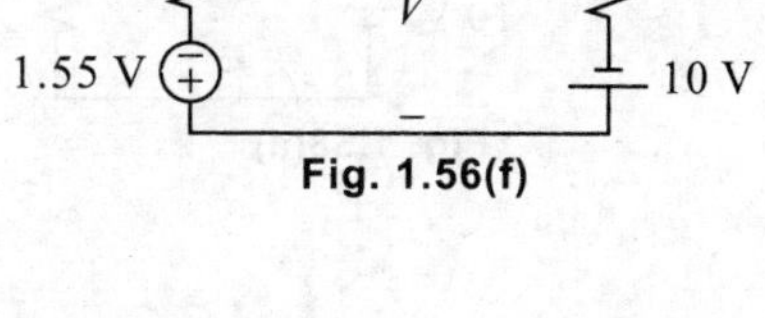

Fig. 1.56(f)

From Fig. 1.56(f)

$$I = \frac{-1.55 + 10}{1 + 2.77} = \boxed{2.24 \text{ A}}$$

$$\therefore \quad V = 1 \times I - 10 = \boxed{-7.75 \text{ volts}}$$

Ex. 1.41 : Using source transformation find current through 10 Ω resistance in Fig. 1.57.

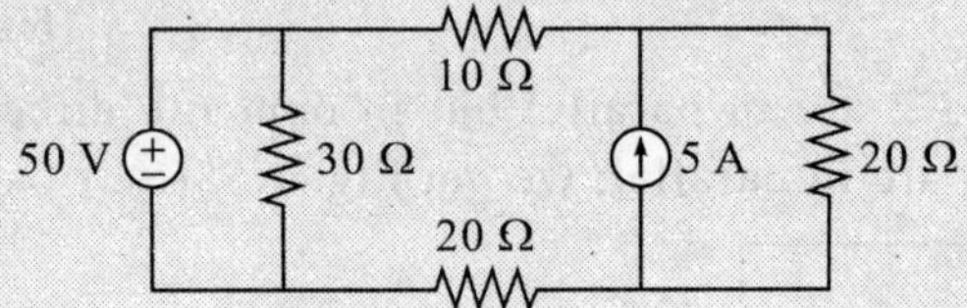

Fig. 1.57

Solution : No transformation can be carried out on 50 V source in parallel to 30 Ω resistance as 30 Ω resistance is redundant. Hence, remove 30 Ω resistance.

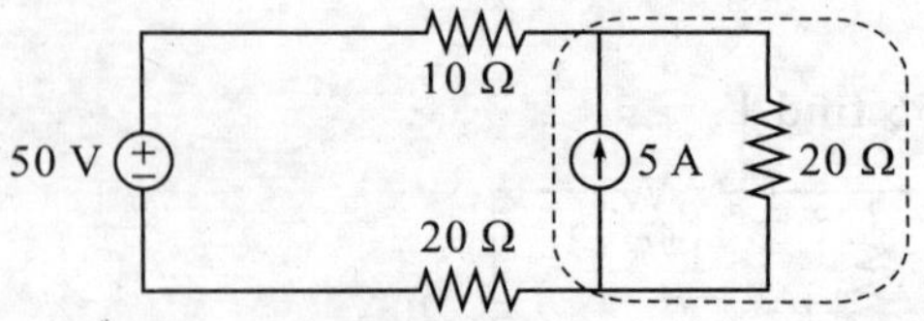

Fig. 1.57(a)

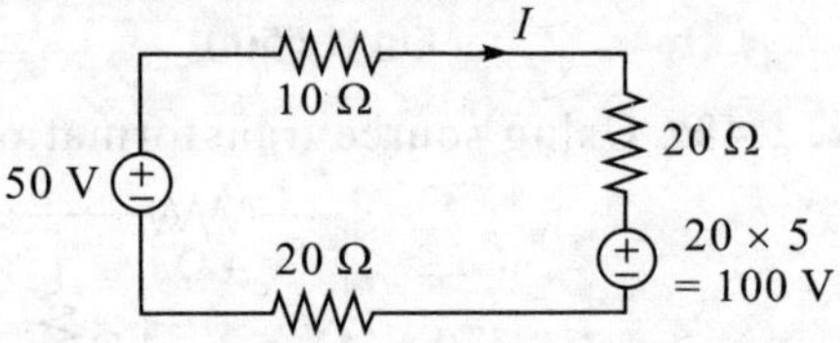

Fig. 1.57(b)

From Fig. 1.57(b)

$$I = \frac{50 - 100}{10 + 20 + 20} = \boxed{-1 \text{ A}}$$

i.e. current is opposite to the marked direction.

Ex. 1.42 : Using source transformation in Fig. 1.58 find $I_{2\,\Omega}$.

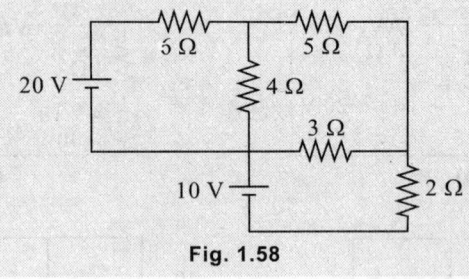

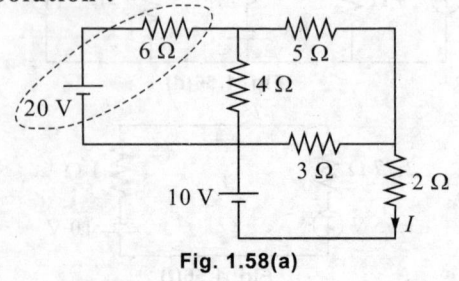

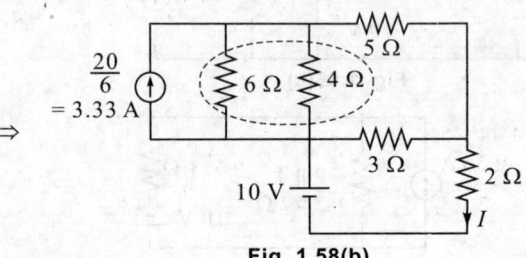

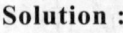

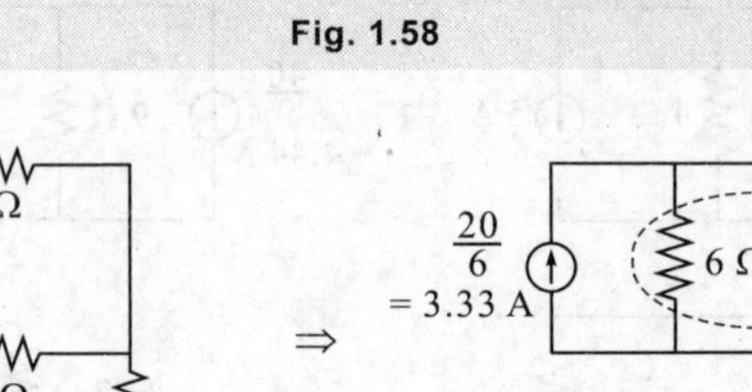

Fig. 1.58

Solution :

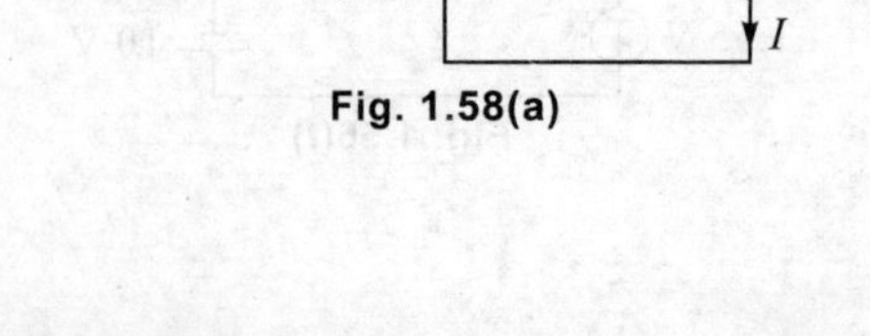

Fig. 1.58(a)

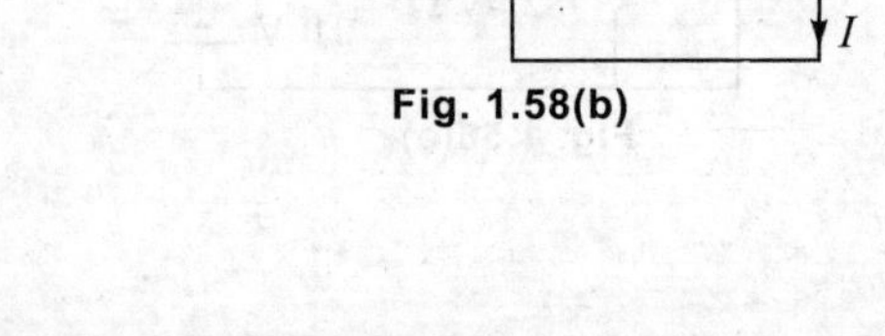

Fig. 1.58(b)

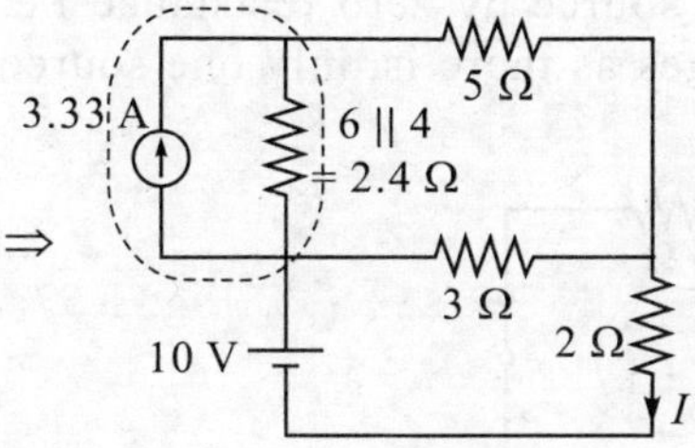

Fig. 1.58(c)

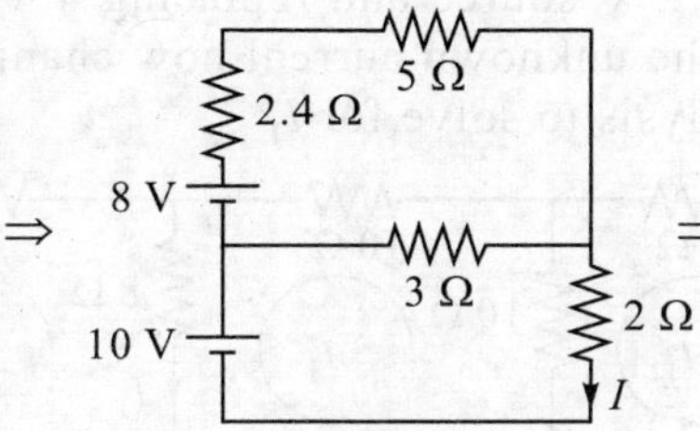

Fig. 1.58(d)

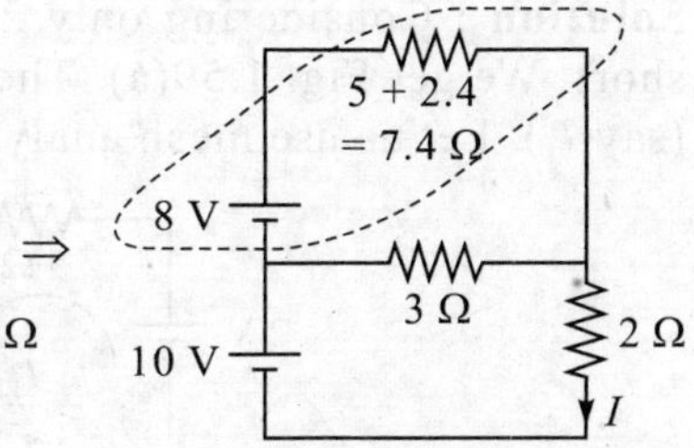

Fig. 1.58(e)

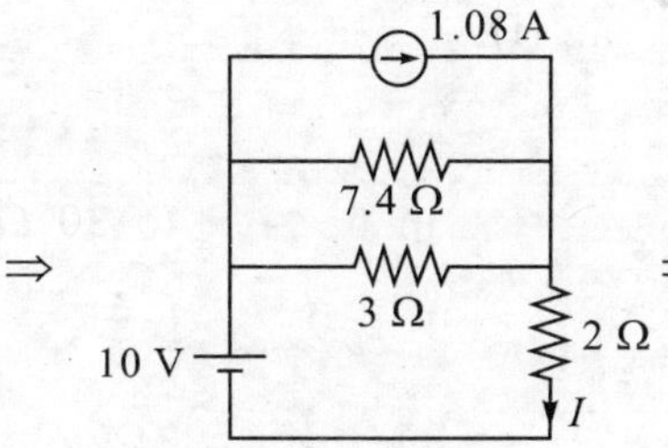

Fig. 1.58(f)

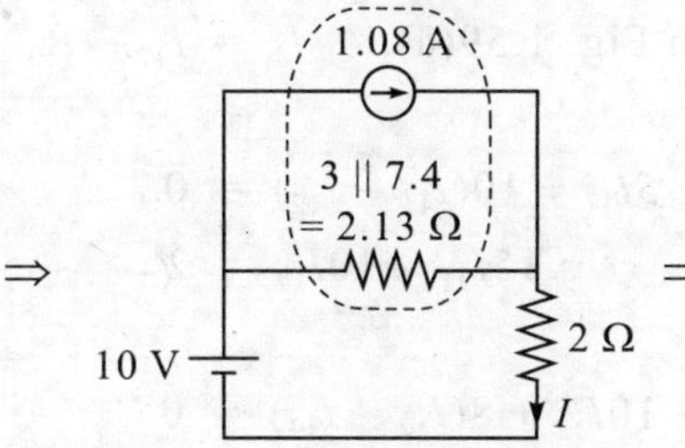

Fig. 1.58(g)

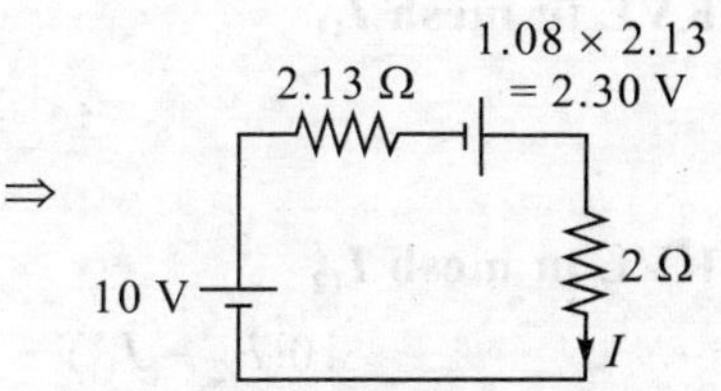

Fig. 1.58(h)

$$I = \frac{10 + 2.30}{2 + 2.13}$$

$$\therefore \; I = \boxed{2.98 \text{ A}}$$

1.10 Superposition Theorem

This theorem states that "*In a linear bilateral network containing more than one generator (or source of emf) the current which flows at any point is the algebraic sum of all currents which would flow at that point if each generator was considered separately and all other generators are replaced for the time being by their internal resistances.*"

This means that if any linear bilateral circuit has more than one emf source acting simultaneously, then each emf acts independent of other emfs i.e. as if other sources did not exist. The value of current at any point is the sum of all currents due to each emf sources and all other sources replaced by their internal resistance. Remember, the ideal internal resistance of a voltage source is zero [section 1.1(i)] and the ideal internal resistance of a current source is infinity (open circuit) [section 1.1(k)].

Ex. 1.43 : Using superposition theorem find *I* in Fig. 1.59.

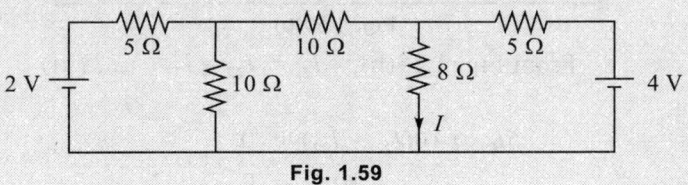

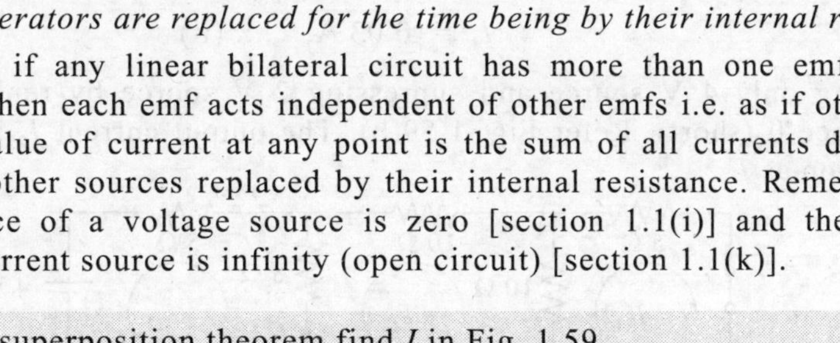

Fig. 1.59

Solution : Considering only 2 V source and replacing 4 V source by zero resistance i.e. short. We get Fig. 1.59(a). The unknown current now changes as there is only one source (say I_1). Let us use mesh analysis to solve for I_1

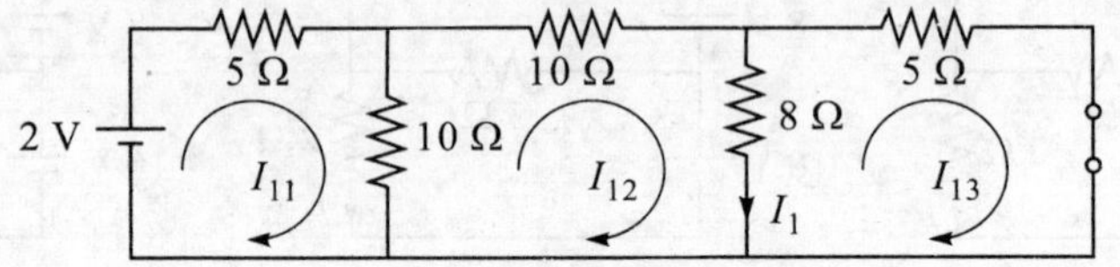

Fig. 1.59(a)

From Fig. 1.59(a), $I_1 = I_{12} - I_{13}$ .... (i)

KVL in mesh I_{11}

$$-2 + 5I_{11} + 10(I_{11} - I_{12}) = 0$$

$$\therefore 15I_{11} - 10I_{12} = 2$$

KVL in mesh I_{12}

$$10(I_{12} - I_{11}) + 10I_{12} + 8(I_{12} - I_{13}) = 0$$

$$-10\,I_{11} + 28I_{12} - 8I_{13} = 0$$

KVL in mesh I_{13}

$$8(I_{13} - I_{12}) + 5I_{13} = 0$$

$$\therefore -8I_{12} + 13I_{13} = 0$$

$$\therefore \begin{bmatrix} 15 & -10 & 0 \\ -10 & 28 & -8 \\ 0 & -8 & 13 \end{bmatrix} \begin{bmatrix} I_{11} \\ I_{12} \\ I_{13} \end{bmatrix} = \begin{bmatrix} 2 \\ 0 \\ 0 \end{bmatrix}$$

$$\therefore I_{12} = 0.08 \text{ and } I_{13} = 0.05$$

From equation (i) $I_1 = I_{12} - I_{13} = 0.08 - 0.05$

$$I_1 = \boxed{0.03\text{ A}} \quad \text{.... (ii)}$$

Now considering only 4 V source and supressing 2 V source by replacing it with its internal resistance 0 (short). Refer Fig. 1.59(b). The output current I_2 should also be in the same direction as I.

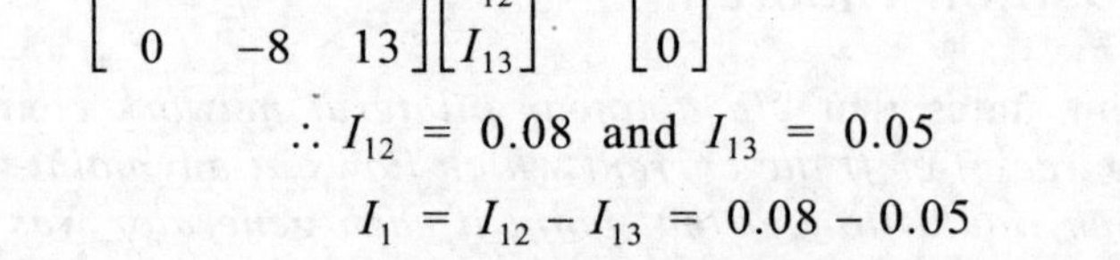

Fig. 1.59(b)

From Fig. 1.59(b), $I_2 = I_{22} - I_{23}$ .... (iii)

KVL in mesh I_{21}

$$5I_{21} + 10(I_{21} - I_{22}) = 0$$

$$\therefore 15I_{21} - 10I_{22} = 0$$

KVL in mesh I_{22}

$$10I_{22} + 8(I_{22} - I_{23}) + 10(I_{22} - I_{21}) = 0$$

$$\therefore 10I_{21} + 28I_{22} - 8I_{23} = 0$$

KVL in mesh I_{23}

$$5I_{23} + 4 + 8(I_{23} - I_{22}) = 0$$

$$-8I_{22} + 13I_{23} = -4$$

$$\therefore \begin{bmatrix} 15 & -10 & 0 \\ -10 & 28 & -8 \\ 0 & -8 & 13 \end{bmatrix} \begin{bmatrix} I_{21} \\ I_{22} \\ I_{23} \end{bmatrix} = \begin{bmatrix} 0 \\ 0 \\ -4 \end{bmatrix}$$

$$\therefore I_{22} = -0.15 \text{ and } I_{23} = -0.4$$

From equation (iii)

$$I_2 = I_{22} - I_{23} = -0.15 - (-0.4)$$

$$I_2 = \boxed{0.25 \text{ A}} \quad .... \text{(iv)}$$

$\therefore$ when both sources are connected together

$$I = I_1 + I_2 = 0.03 + 0.25$$

$$I = \boxed{0.28 \text{ A}}$$

Ex. 1.44 : Using superposition theorem find power dissipated in 10 Ω resistance in Fig. 1.60.

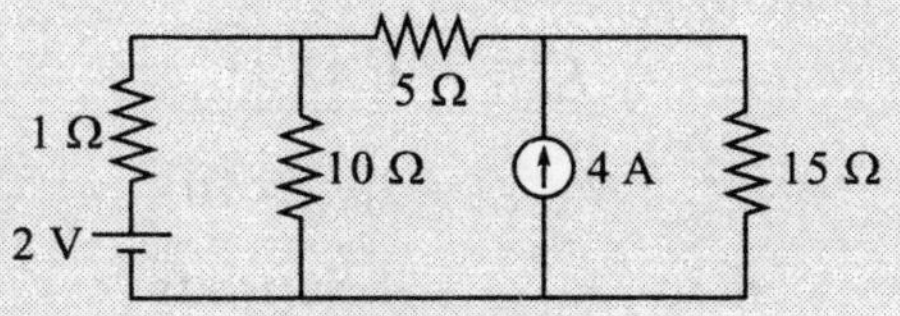

Fig. 1.60

Solution : In order to find power dissipated in 10 Ω resistance, we should know current in 10 Ω resistance.

Note : To suppress a current source it should be replaced by open circuit (infinite resistance) keep large distance between the open terminals as in Fig. 1.60(i).

Consider 2 V source

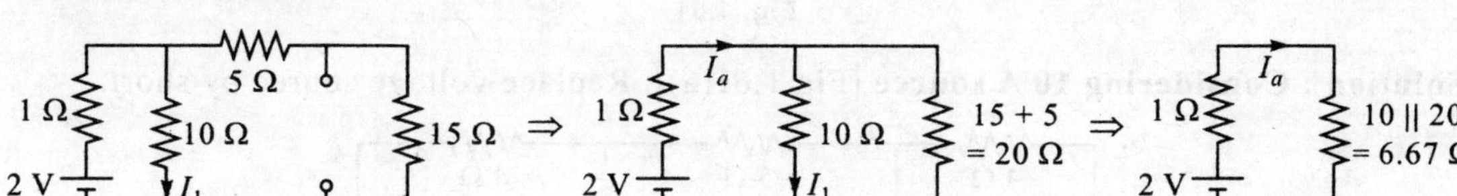

Fig. 1.60(a) **Fig. 1.60(b)** **Fig. 1.60(c)**

From Fig. 1.60(b)

$$I_1 = I_a \frac{20}{20 + 10} \quad .... \text{(i)}$$

$\therefore$ From Fig. 1.60(c) $\quad I_a = \dfrac{2}{1 + 6.67} = 0.26 \text{ A}$

From (i), we get $\quad I_1 = \boxed{0.17 \text{ A}}$ .... (ii)

Consider 4 A source

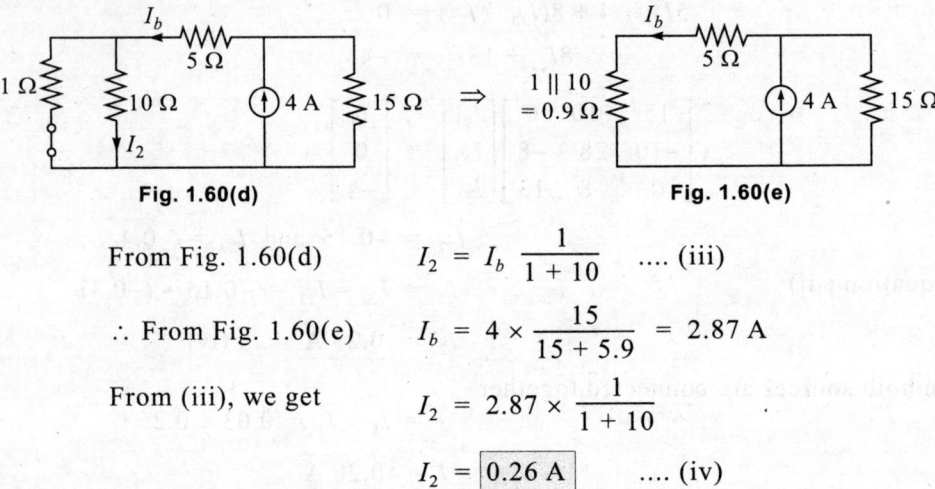

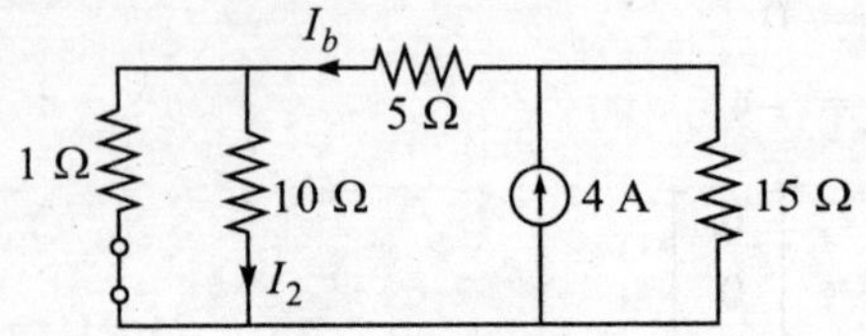

Fig. 1.60(d)

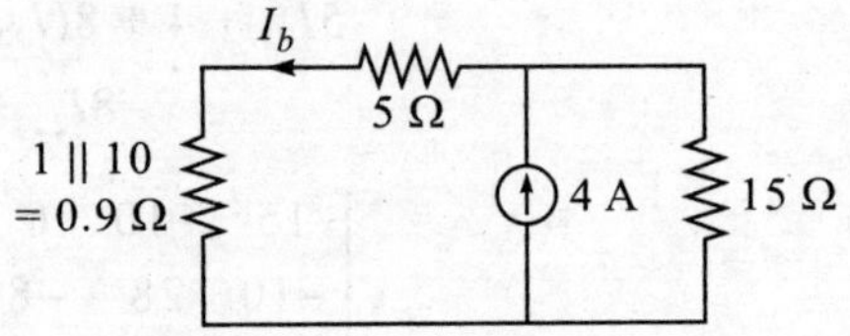

Fig. 1.60(e)

From Fig. 1.60(d) $\quad I_2 = I_b \dfrac{1}{1 + 10}$ .... (iii)

$\therefore$ From Fig. 1.60(e) $\quad I_b = 4 \times \dfrac{15}{15 + 5.9} = 2.87 \text{ A}$

From (iii), we get $\quad I_2 = 2.87 \times \dfrac{1}{1 + 10}$

$I_2 = \boxed{0.26 \text{ A}}$ .... (iv)

Thus considering both sources we get

$$I_{10\,\Omega} = I_1 + I_2 = 0.17 + 0.26$$

$$I_{10\,\Omega} = \boxed{0.43 \text{ A}}$$

$$\therefore \; P_{10\,\Omega} = I^2_{10\,\Omega} \times 10$$

$$P_{10\,\Omega} = \boxed{1.86 \text{ watts}}$$

Ex. 1.45 : Using super position theorem find V in Fig. 1.61.

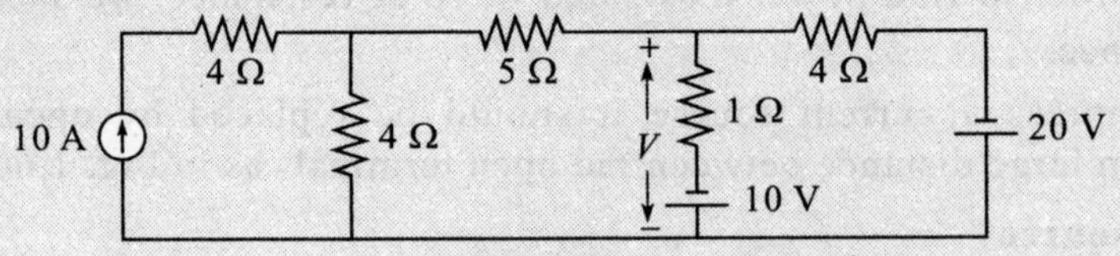

Fig. 1.61

Solution : Considering 10 A source [Fig 1.61(a)]. Replace voltage source by short.

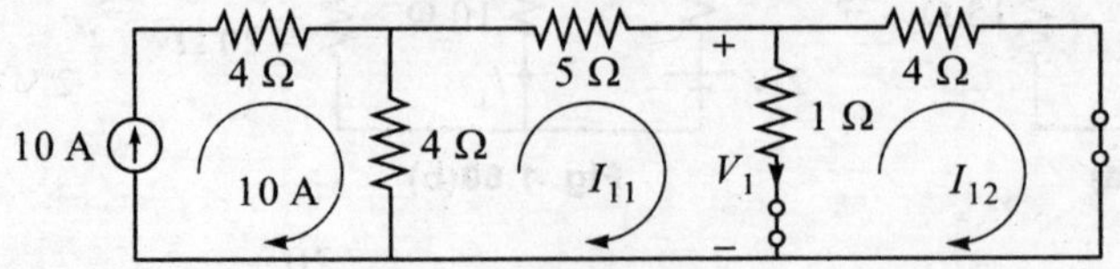

Fig. 1.61(a)

KVL in mesh I_{11}

$$4(I_{11} - 10) + 5I_{11} + 1(I_{11} - I_{12}) = 0$$

$$\therefore 10I_{11} - I_{12} = 40$$

KVL in mesh I_{12}

$$1(I_{12} - I_{11}) + 4I_{12} = 0$$

$$\therefore -I_{11} + 5I_{12} = 0$$

$$\therefore \begin{bmatrix} 10 & -1 \\ -1 & 5 \end{bmatrix} \begin{bmatrix} I_{11} \\ I_{12} \end{bmatrix} = \begin{bmatrix} 40 \\ 0 \end{bmatrix}$$

$$\therefore I_{11} = 4.08 \text{ and } I_{12} = 0.82$$

$$V_1 = 1(I_{11} - I_{12})$$

$$V_1 = \boxed{3.26 \text{ V}} \quad .... \text{(i)}$$

Considering 10 V source [Fig 1.61(b)]. Replace voltage source by short circuit and current source by open circuit.

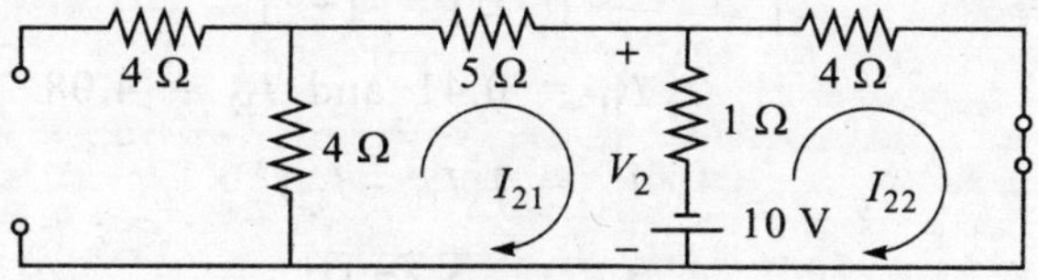

Fig. 1.61(b)

KVL in mesh I_{21}

$$4I_{21} + 5I_{21} + 1(I_{21} - I_{22}) - 10 = 0$$

$$\therefore 10I_{21} - I_{22} = 10$$

KVL in mesh I_{22}

$$4I_{22} + 10 + 1(I_{22} - I_{21}) = 0$$

$$\therefore -I_{21} + 5I_{22} = -10$$

$$\therefore \begin{bmatrix} 10 & -1 \\ -1 & 5 \end{bmatrix} \begin{bmatrix} I_{21} \\ I_{22} \end{bmatrix} = \begin{bmatrix} 10 \\ -10 \end{bmatrix}$$

$$\therefore I_{21} = 0.82 \text{ and } I_{22} = -1.84$$

$$V_2 = 1(I_{21} - I_{22}) - 10$$

$$V_2 = \boxed{-7.34 \text{ V}} \quad .... \text{(ii)}$$

Considering 20 V source [Fig 1.61(c)]. Replace current source by open circuit and voltage source by short circuit.

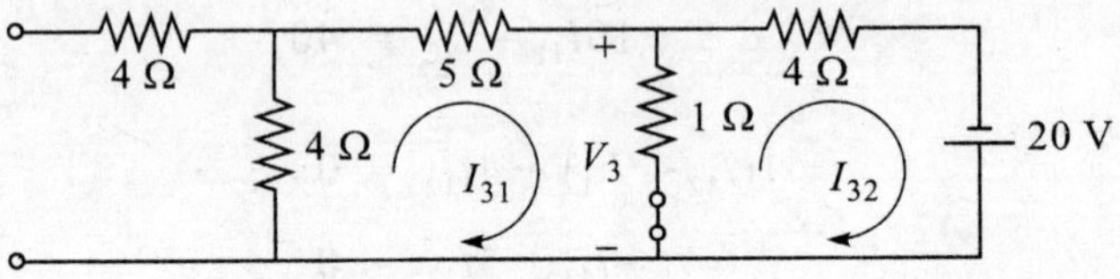

Fig. 1.61(c)

KVL in mesh I_{31}

$$4I_{31} + 5I_{31} + 1(I_{31} - I_{32}) = 0$$

$$\therefore\ 10I_{31} - I_{32} = 10$$

KVL in mesh I_{32}

$$1(I_{32} - I_{31}) + 4I_{32} - 20 = 0$$

$$\therefore\ -I_{31} + 5I_{32} = 20$$

$$\therefore\ \begin{bmatrix} 10 & -1 \\ -1 & 5 \end{bmatrix}\begin{bmatrix} I_{31} \\ I_{32} \end{bmatrix} = \begin{bmatrix} 0 \\ 20 \end{bmatrix}$$

$$\therefore\ I_{31} = 0.41 \text{ and } I_{32} = 4.08$$

$$V_3 = 1(I_{31} - I_{32})$$

$$V_3 = \boxed{-3.67 \text{ V}} \quad \text{.... (iii)}$$

Considering all sources together.

From (i), (ii) and (iii),

$$V = V_1 + V_2 + V_3 = 3.26 - 7.34 - 3.67$$

$$V = \boxed{-7.75 \text{ V}}$$

Ex. 1.46 : Find I_X using super position theorem in Fig. 1.62.

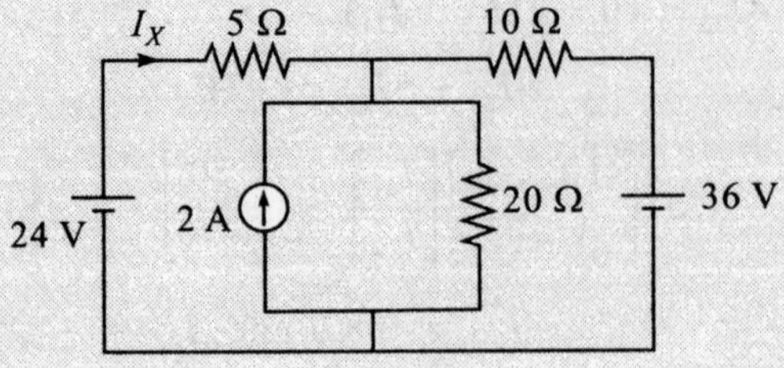

Fig. 1.62

Solution : Considering 24 V source. Replace current source by open circuit and voltage source by short circuit.

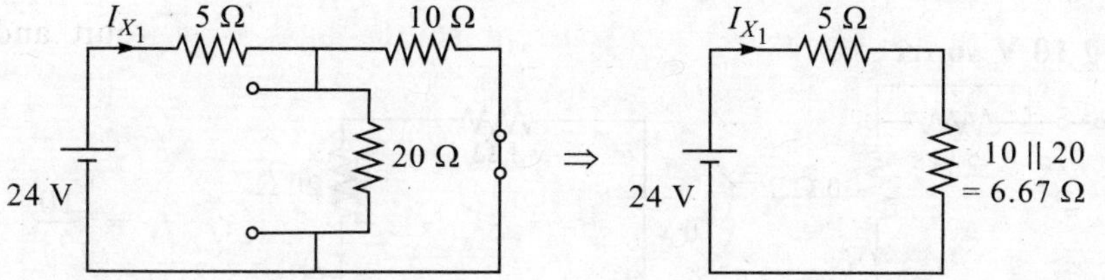

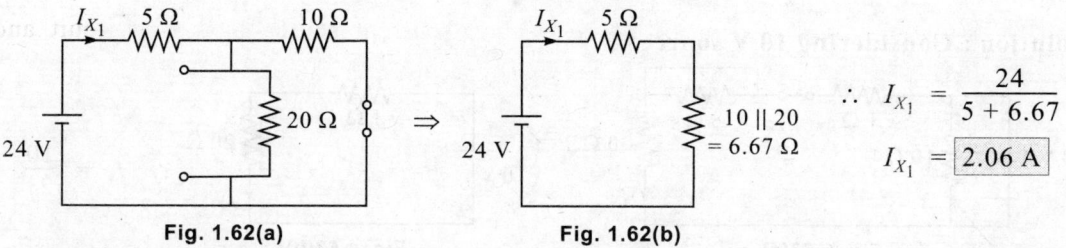

Fig. 1.62(a) Fig. 1.62(b)

$$\therefore I_{X_1} = \frac{24}{5 + 6.67}$$

$$I_{X_1} = \boxed{2.06 \text{ A}}$$

Considering 36 V source. Replace current source by open circuit and voltage source by short circuit.

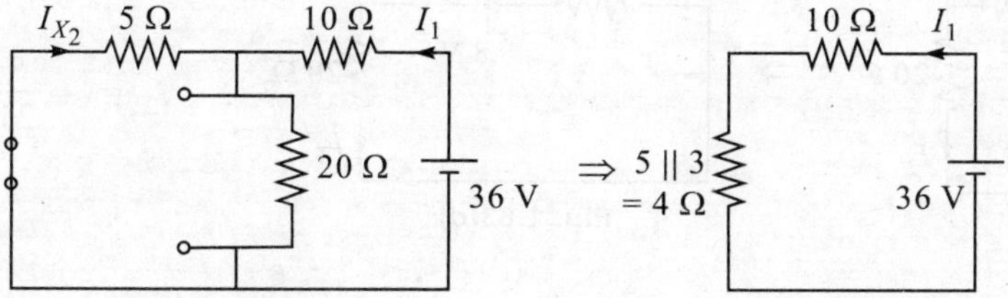

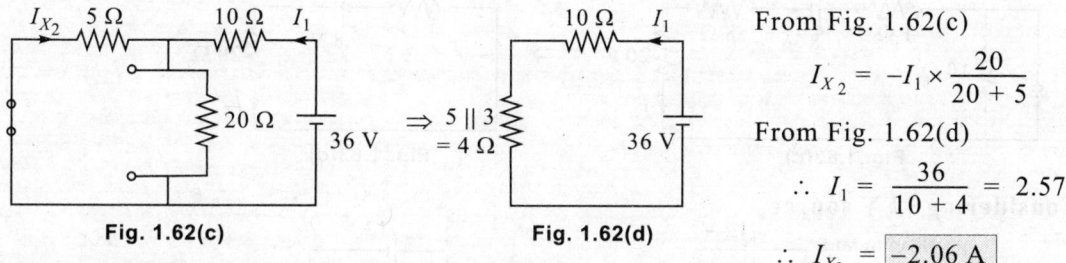

Fig. 1.62(c) Fig. 1.62(d)

From Fig. 1.62(c)

$$I_{X_2} = -I_1 \times \frac{20}{20 + 5}$$

From Fig. 1.62(d)

$$\therefore I_1 = \frac{36}{10 + 4} = 2.57$$

$$\therefore I_{X_2} = \boxed{-2.06 \text{ A}}$$

Considering 2 A source. Replace voltage sources by short circuit.

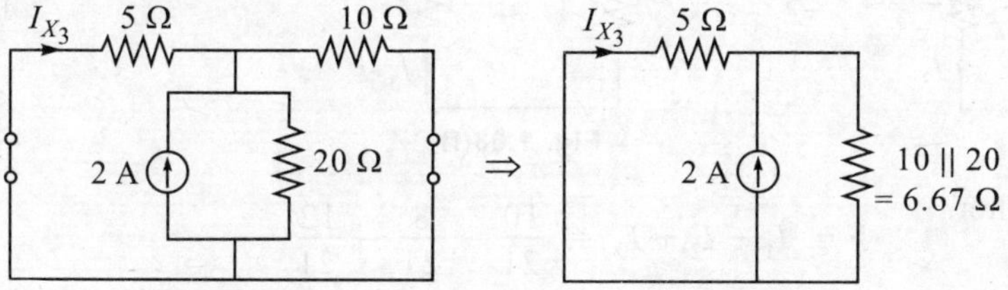

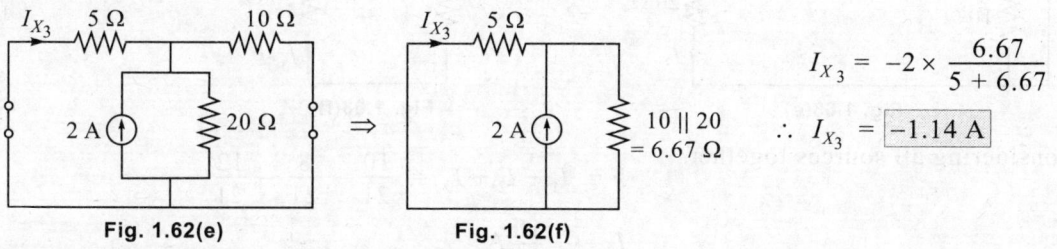

Fig. 1.62(e) Fig. 1.62(f)

$$I_{X_3} = -2 \times \frac{6.67}{5 + 6.67}$$

$$\therefore I_{X_3} = \boxed{-1.14 \text{ A}}$$

Considering all sources together,

$$\therefore I_X = I_{X_1} + I_{X_2} + I_{X_3} = 2.06 - 2.06 - 1.14$$

$$I_X = \boxed{-1.14 \text{ A}}$$

Ex. 1.47 : Using super position theorem, find I in Fig. 1.63.

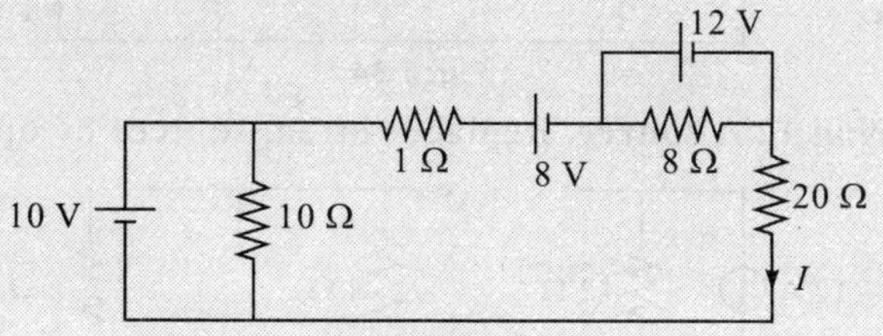

Fig. 1.63

Solution : Considering 10 V source

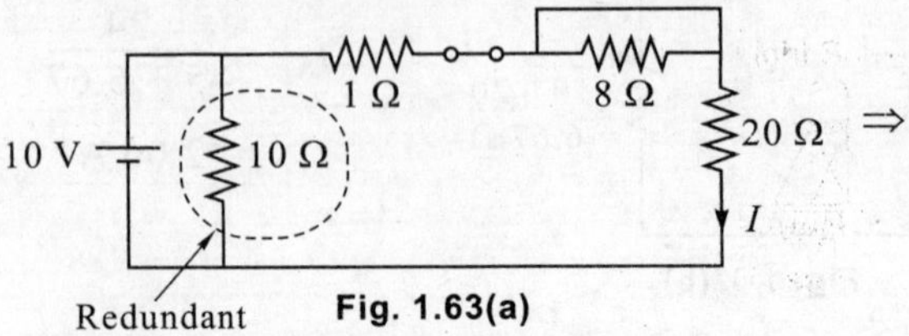

Fig. 1.63(a)

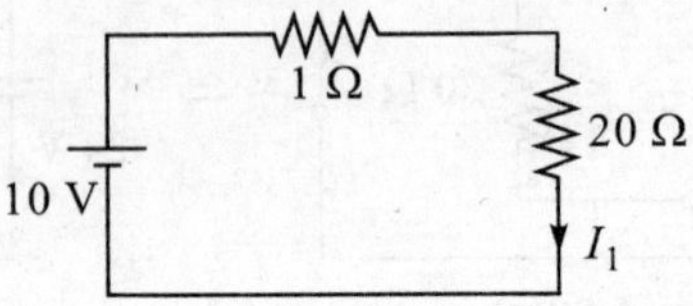

Fig. 1.63(b)

$$\therefore \quad I_1 = \boxed{\frac{10}{21}}$$

Considering 8 V source

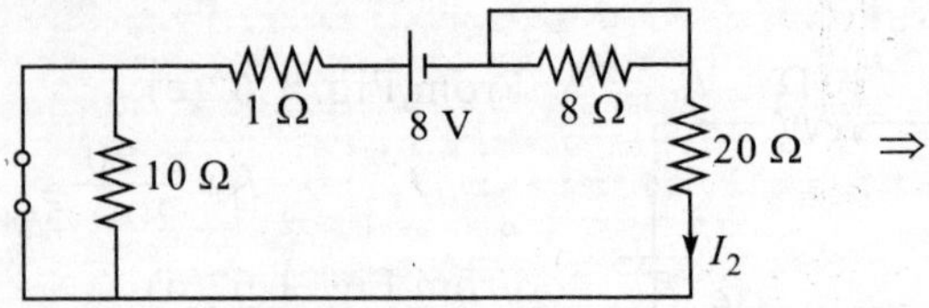

Fig. 1.63(c)

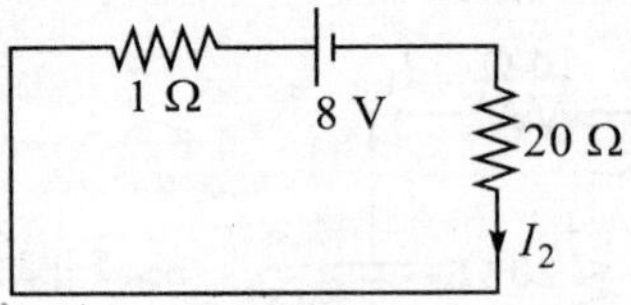

Fig. 1.63(d)

$$\therefore \quad I_2 = \boxed{-\frac{8}{21}}$$

Considering 12 V source

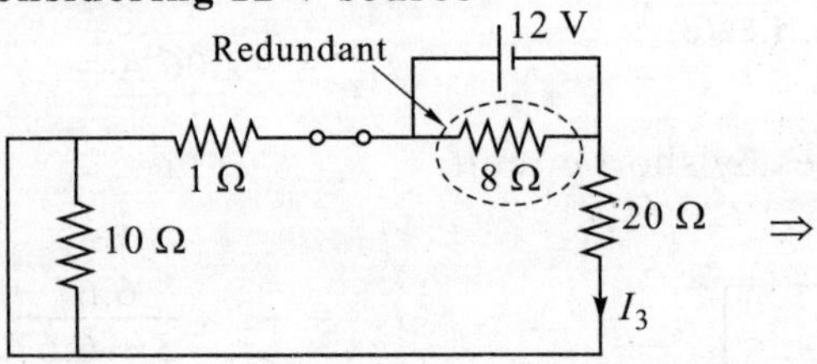

Fig. 1.63(e)

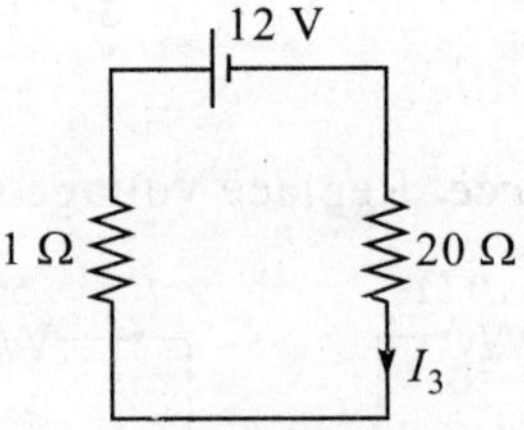

Fig. 1.63(f)

$$\therefore \quad I_3 = \boxed{-\frac{12}{21}}$$

Considering all sources together.

$$\therefore \quad I = I_1 + I_2 + I_3 = \frac{10}{21} - \frac{8}{21} - \frac{12}{21}$$

$$I = \boxed{-\frac{10}{21}\ \text{A}}$$

Ex. 1.48 : Using super position theorem find *I* in Fig. 1.64.

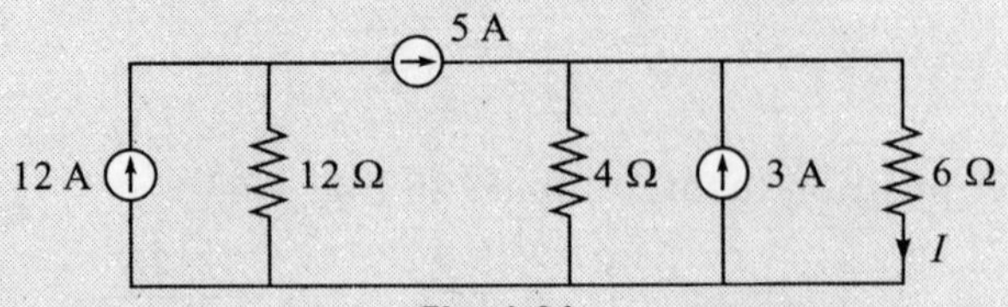

Fig. 1.64

Solution : Considering 12 A source. Replace current sources by open circuit.

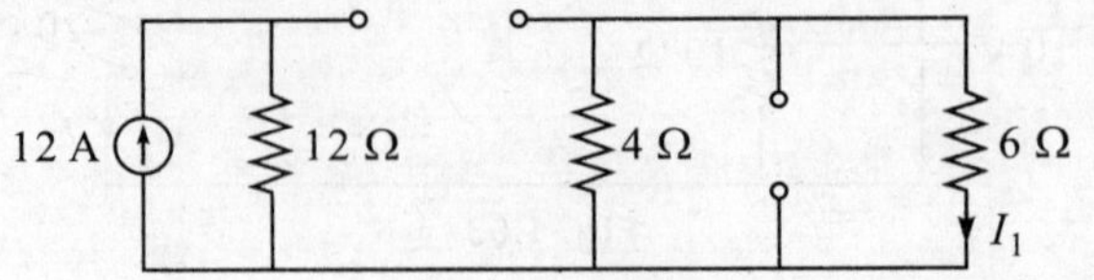

Fig. 1.64(a)

$$\therefore \quad I_1 = 0$$

Considering 5 A source

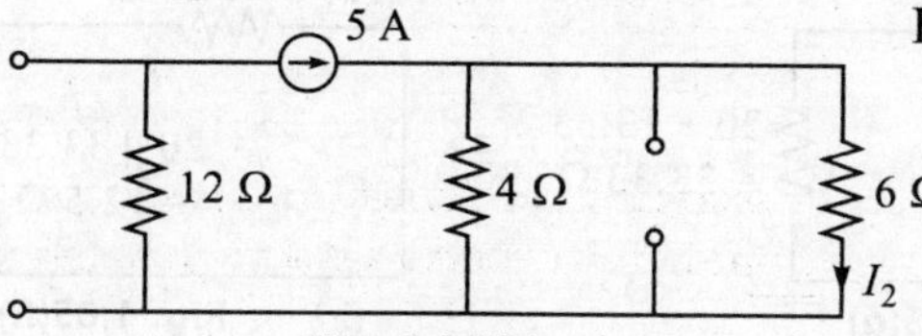

Fig. 1.64(b)

By current division rule,

$$\therefore\ I_2 = 5 \times \frac{4}{4+6}$$

$$I_2 = 2\text{ A}$$

Considering 3 A source

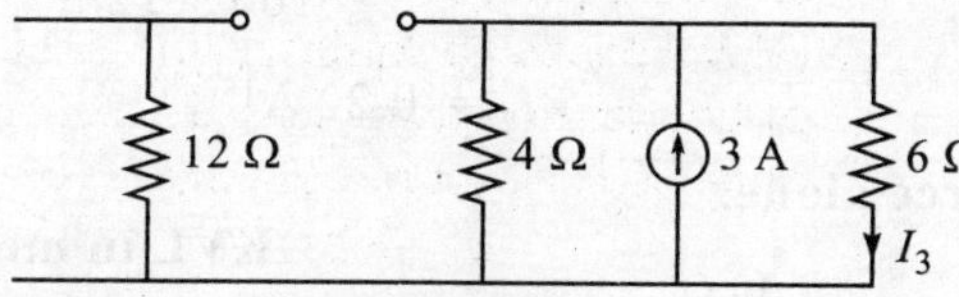

Fig. 1.64(d)

By current division rule,

$$\therefore\ I_3 = 3 \times \frac{4}{6+4}$$

$$I_3 = 1.2\text{ A}$$

Considering all sources together,

$$\therefore\ I = I_1 + I_2 + I_3 = 0 + 2 + 1.2$$

$$I = \boxed{3.2\text{ A}}$$

Ex. 1.49 : Find $I_{100\,\Omega}$ using super position theorem in Fig. 1.65.

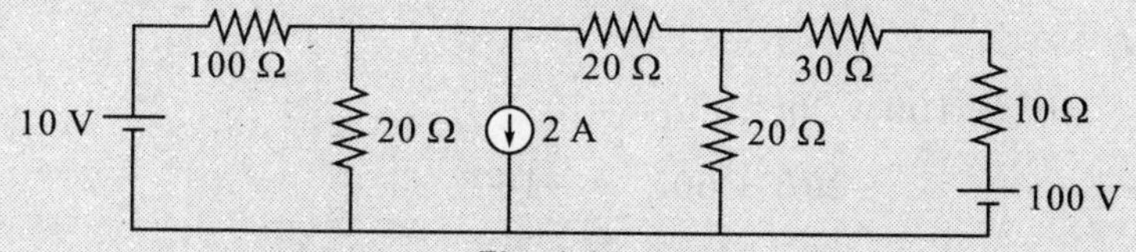

Fig. 1.65

Solution : Considering 10 V source and suppressing all other sources.

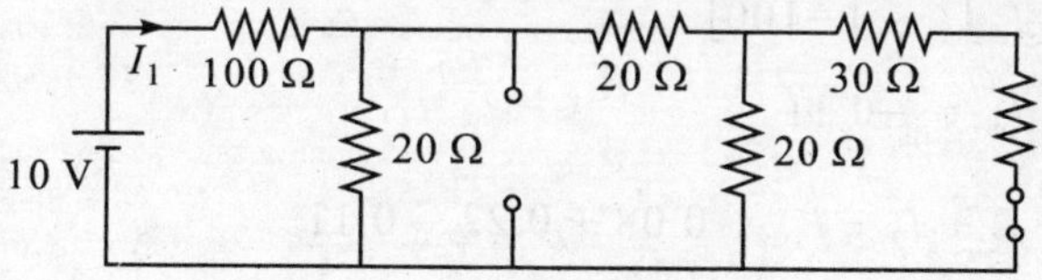

Fig. 1.65(a)

⇒

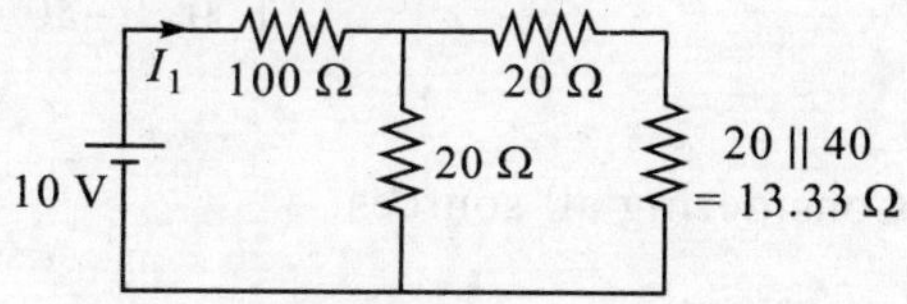

Fig. 1.65(b)

⇒

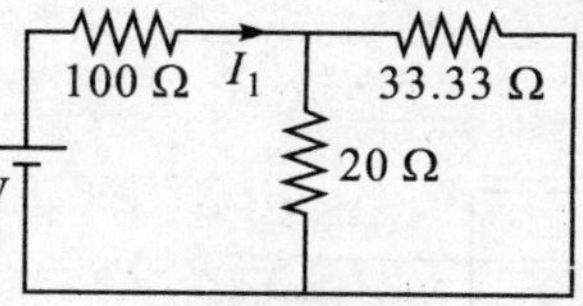

Fig. 1.65(c)

⇒

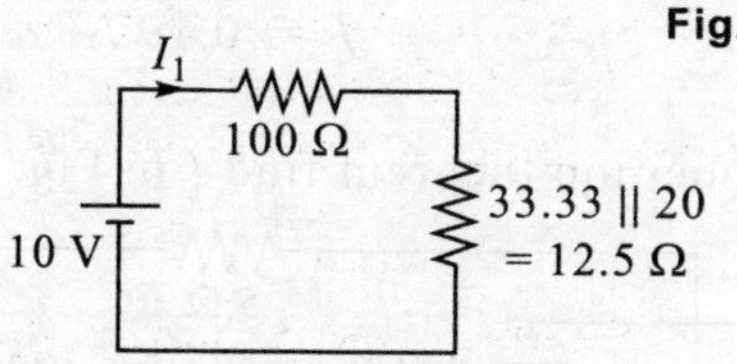

Fig. 1.65(d)

$$\therefore\ I_1 = \frac{10}{100 + 12.5}$$

$$I_1 = \boxed{0.08\text{ A}}$$

Considering 2A source and suppressing all other sources.

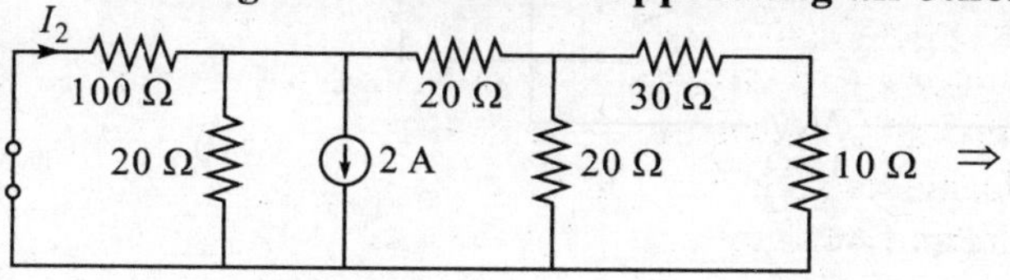

Fig. 1.65(e)

⇒

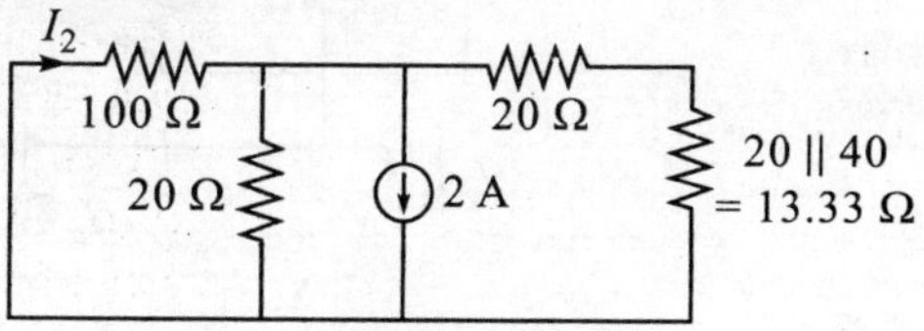

Fig. 1.65(f)

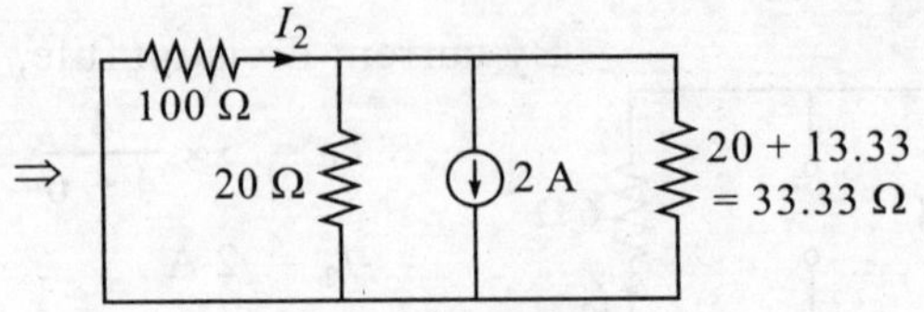

Fig. 1.65(g)

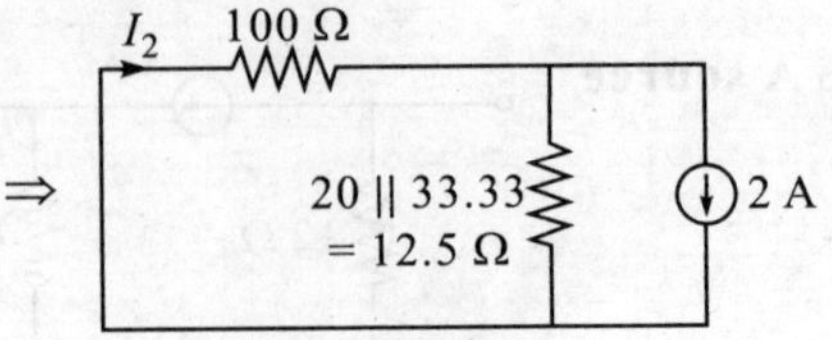

Fig. 1.65(h)

$$\therefore \; I_2 = 2 \times \frac{12.5}{100 + 12.5}$$

$$I_2 = \boxed{0.22 \text{ A}}$$

Considering 100 V source alone.

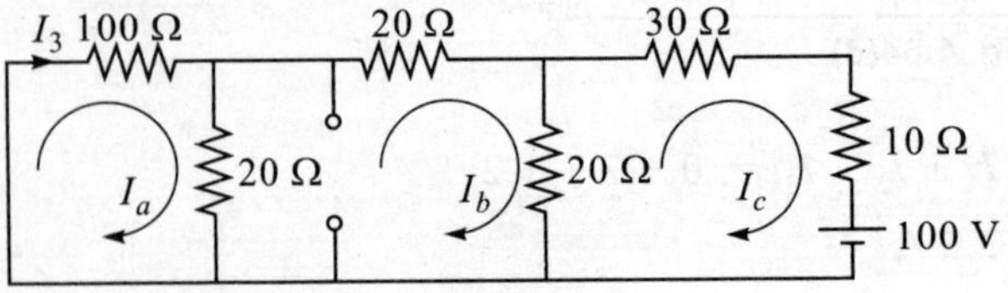

Fig. 1.65

KVL in mesh I_a

$$100I_a + 20(I_a - I_b) = 0$$

$$120I_a - 20I_b = 0$$

KVL in mesh I_b

$$20I_b + 20(I_b - I_c) + 20(I_b - I_a) = 0$$

$$-20I_a + 60I_b - 20I_c = 0$$

KVL in mesh I_c

$$40I_c + 100 + 20(I_c - I_b) = 0$$

$$-20I_b + 60I_c = -100$$

$$\therefore \begin{bmatrix} 120 & -20 & 0 \\ -20 & 60 & -20 \\ 0 & -20 & 60 \end{bmatrix} \begin{bmatrix} I_a \\ I_b \\ I_c \end{bmatrix} = \begin{bmatrix} 0 \\ 0 \\ -100 \end{bmatrix}$$

$$\therefore I_3 = I_a = -0.11$$

Considering all sources

$$\therefore \; I = I_1 + I_2 + I_3 = 0.08 + 0.22 - 0.11$$

$$I = \boxed{0.19 \text{ A}}$$

Ex. 1.50 : Using super position theorem find I in Fig. 1.66

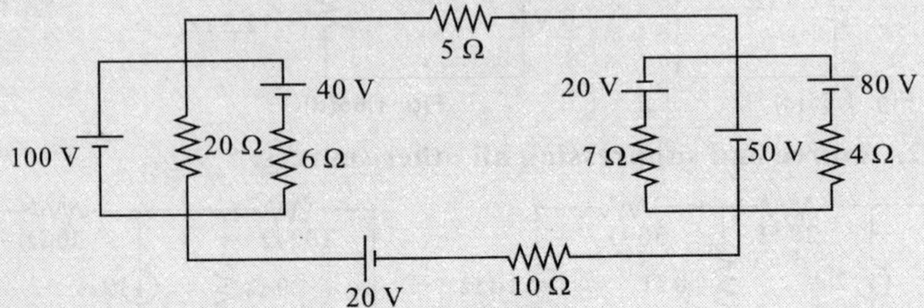

Fig. 1.66

Solution : Consider 100 V source alone.

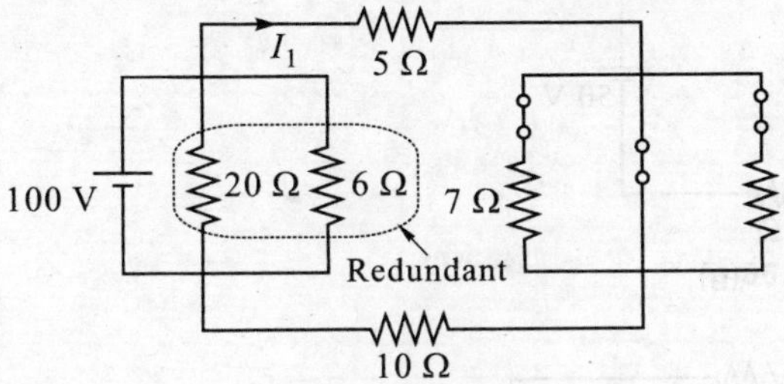

Fig. 1.66(a)

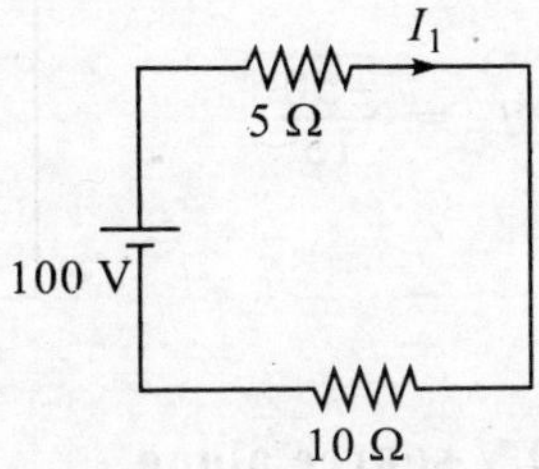

Fig. 1.66(b)

20 Ω and 6 Ω resistances are redundant as they are parallel to 10 V source.

7 Ω and 4 Ω are in parallel to 0 Ω therefore there equivalent resistance is zero.

$$\therefore I_1 = \frac{100}{15}$$

Consider 40 V source alone.

As 40 V source is shorted Fig. 1.66(c)

$$I_2 = 0$$

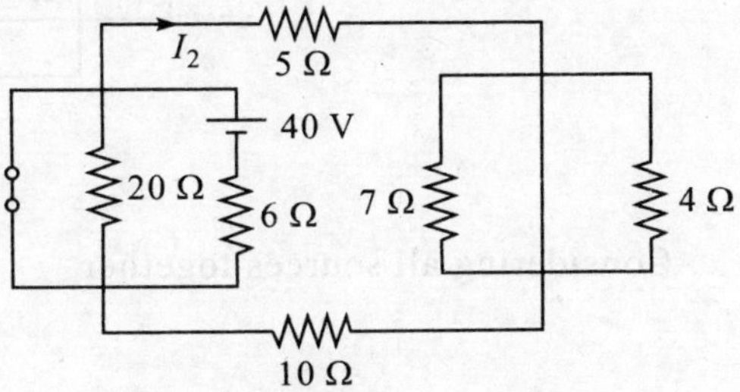

Fig. 1.66(c)

Consider 20 V source alone.

As 20 V source is shorted

Fig. 1.66(d)

$$I_3 = 0$$

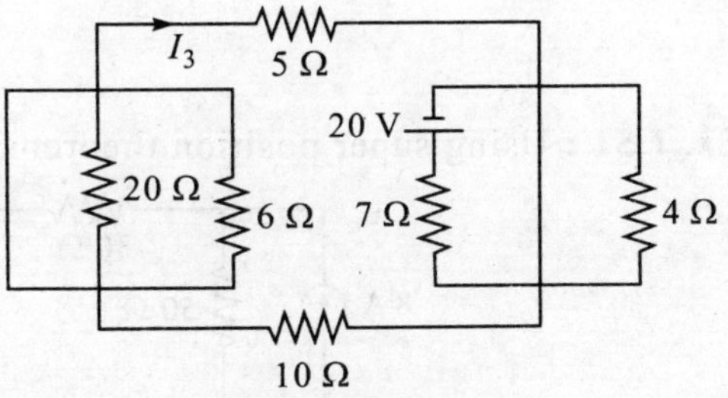

Fig. 1.66(d)

Consider 80 V source alone.

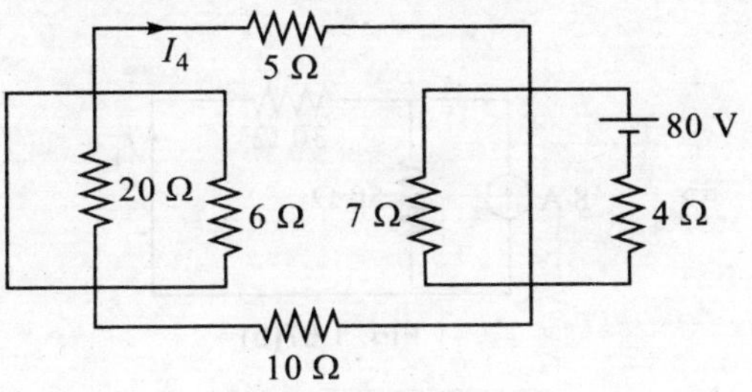

Fig. 1.66(e)

$$I_4 = 0$$

Consider 50 V source

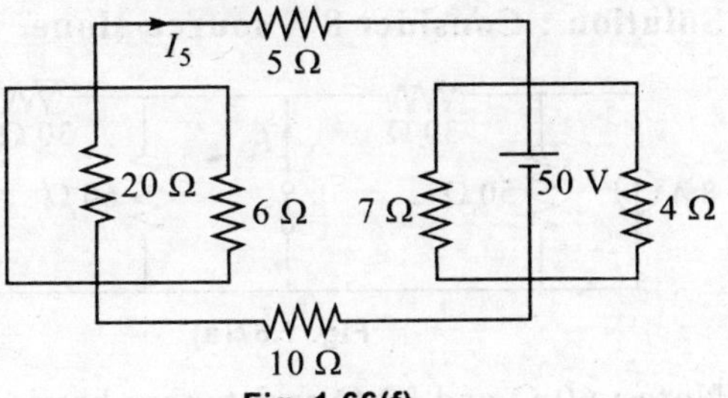

Fig. 1.66(f)

$$I_5 = \frac{-50}{15}$$

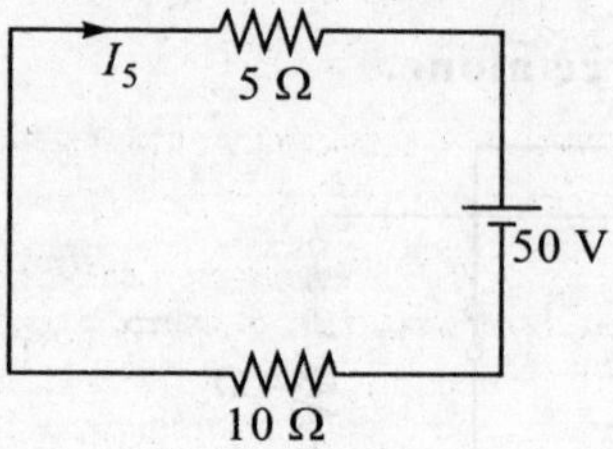

Fig. 1.66(g)

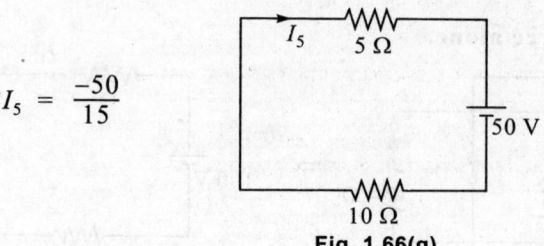

Consider 20 V source alone.

$$I_6 = \frac{20}{15}$$

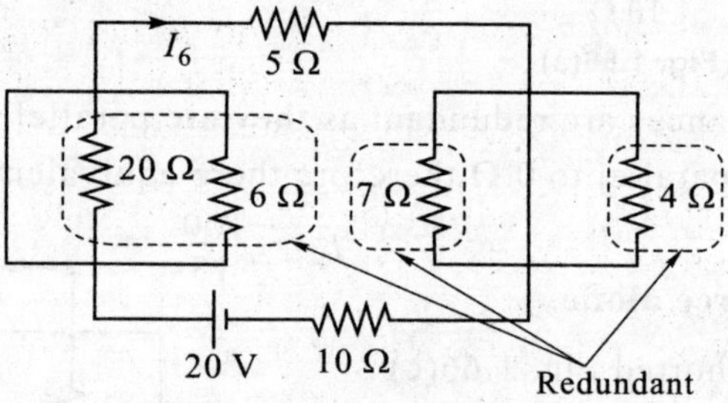

Fig. 1.66(h)

∴ Considering all sources together

$$I = I_1 + I_2 + I_3 + I_4 + I_5 + I_6$$

$$= \frac{100}{15} + 0 + 0 + 0 + \frac{-50}{15} + \frac{20}{15}$$

$$I = \frac{70}{15} = \boxed{4.67 \text{ A}}$$

Ex. 1.51 : Using super position theorem, find *I* in Fig. 1.67

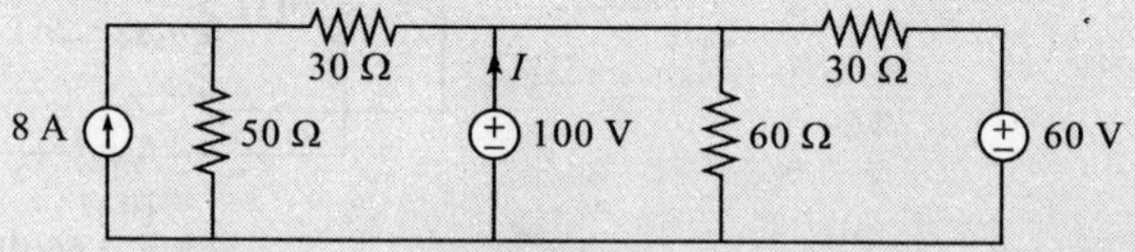

Fig. 1.67

Solution : Consider 8 A source alone.

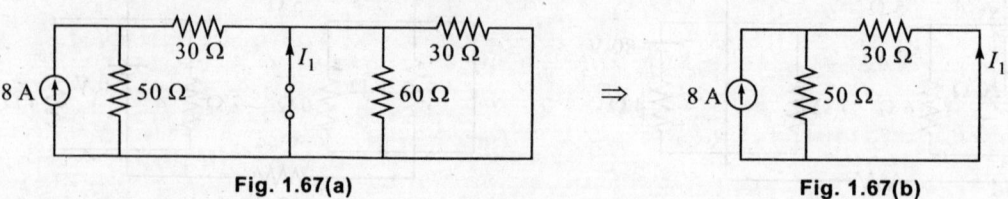

Fig. 1.67(a)

⇒

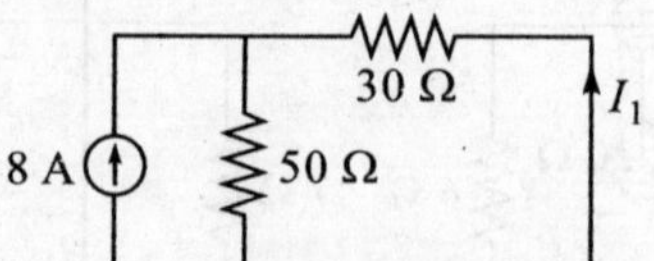

Fig. 1.67(b)

Note : 60 Ω and 30 Ω resistances have got shorted.

$$\therefore\ I_1 = -8 \times \frac{50}{50+30} = \boxed{-5 \text{ A}}$$

Consider 100 V source alone.

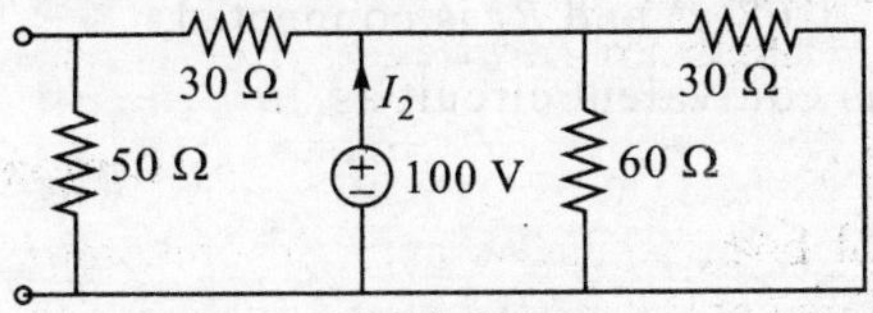

Fig. 1.67(c)

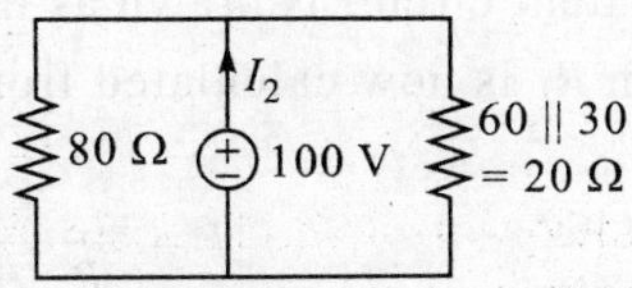

Fig. 1.67(d)

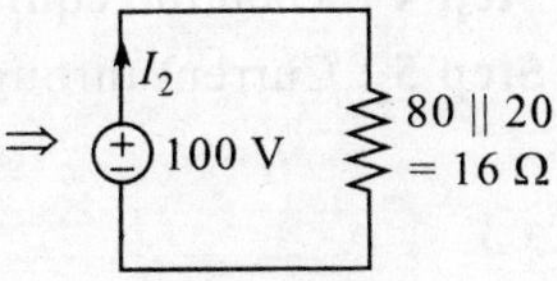

Fig. 1.67(e)

$$\therefore\ I_2 = \frac{100}{16} = \boxed{6.25\text{ A}}$$

Consider 60 V source alone.

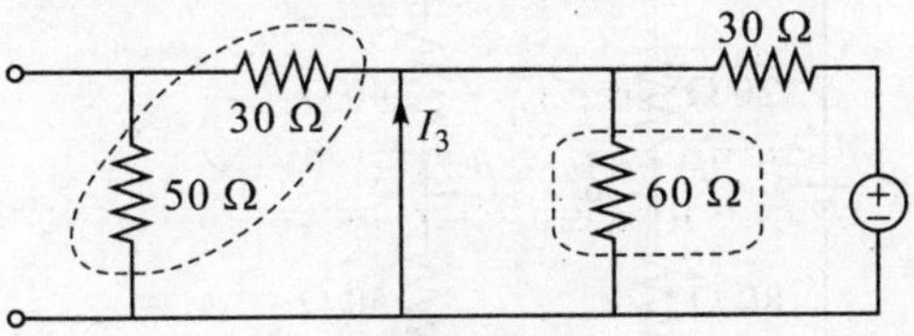

Fig. 1.67(f)

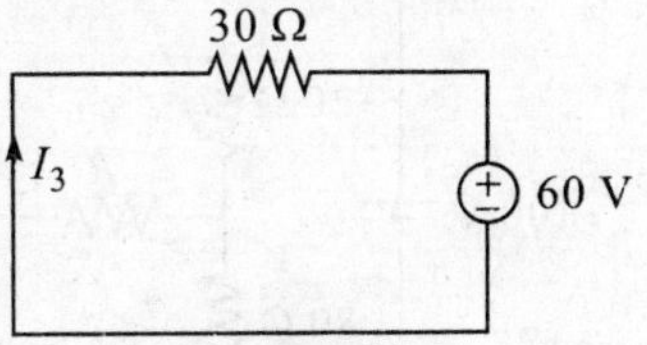

Fig. 1.67(g)

Here 30 Ω, 50 Ω, 60 Ω are shorted (Redundant)

$$\therefore\ I_3 = \frac{-60}{30} = \boxed{-2\text{ A}}$$

Consider all sources

$$I = I_1 + I_2 + I_3$$

$$= -5 + 6.25 - 2 = \boxed{-0.75\text{ A}}$$

1.11 Thevenin's Theorem

Thevenin's theorem states that "*Any linear bilateral circuit across any two terminals of a network can be replaced by a voltage sound (V_{th}) in series with a resistance (R_{eq}), where V_{th} is the open circuit voltage across those terminals after removing the element and R_{eq} is the equivalent resistance between those pair of terminals after supressing all the sources.*"

For example consider a simple circuit of Fig. 1.68(a).

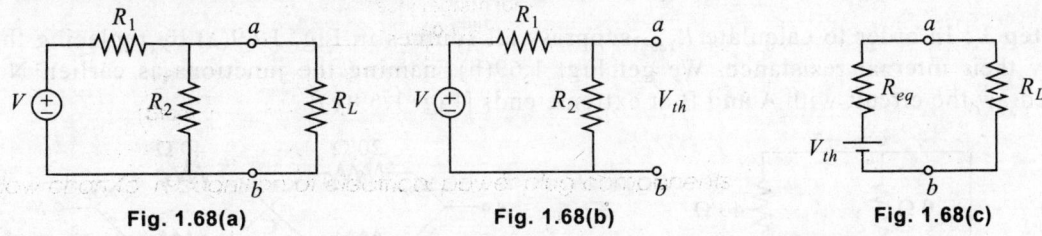

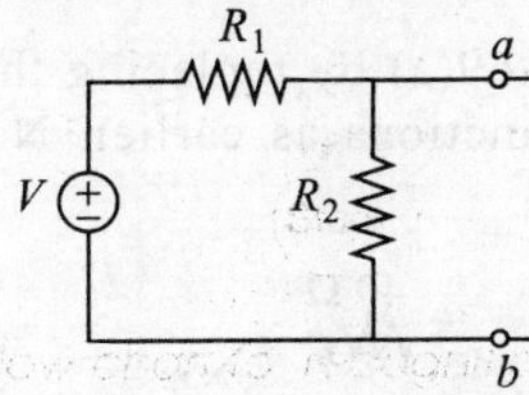

Fig. 1.68(a)

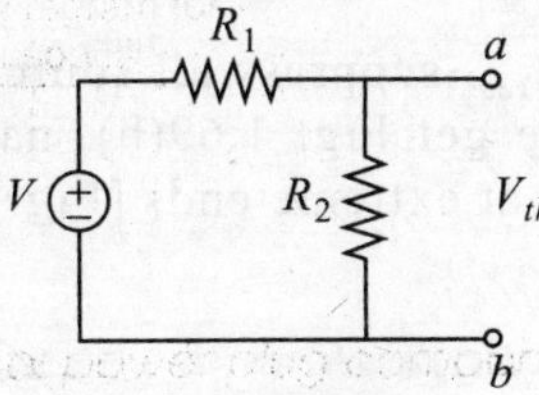

Fig. 1.68(b)

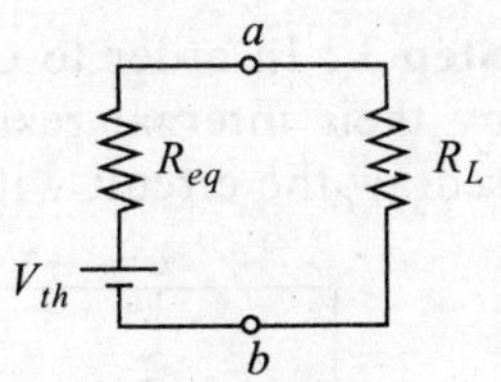

Fig. 1.68(c)

To find Thevenin's equivalent circuit we have to find V_{th} and R_{eq}. Thus

Step 1 : Remove R_L across which Thevenin's equivalent circuit is to be calculated.

Step 2 : Consider the circuit Fig. 1.68(b) and find V_{th} for this circuit which is V_{ab}.

Step 3 : Suppress all sources of step 2 and find R_{eq} between terminals *ab*.

Step 4 : Then the equivalent circuit is drawn as in Fig. 1.68(c) and R_L is connected.

Step 5 : Current through R_L is now calculated from this equivalent circuit as

$$I = \frac{V_{th}}{R_{eq} + R_L}$$

Ex. 1.52 : Find Thevenin's equivalent across R in Fig. 1.69.

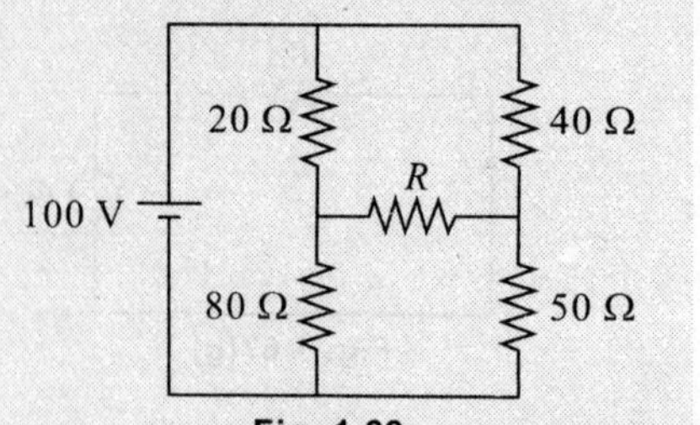

Fig. 1.69

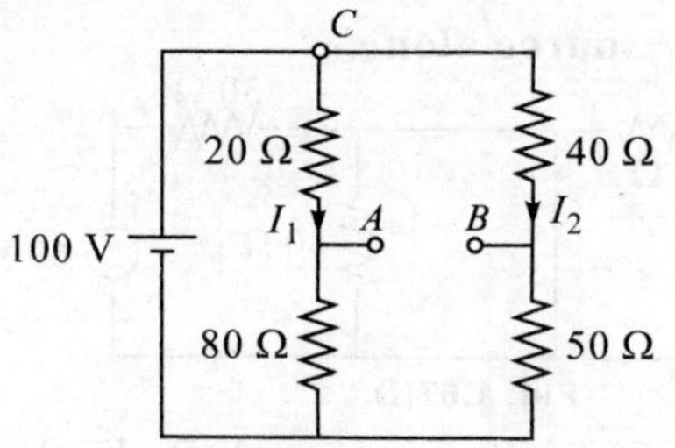

Fig. 1.69(a)

Solution : Step 1 : Remove R and name terminals A and B [Fig. 1.69(a)]

Step 2 : To define $V_{th} = V_{AB}$ we first assume currents in all branches (say I_1 and I_2) [Fig. 1.69(a)].

Then to define V_{AB}, start from A and end on B via C, we get

$$V_{th} = V_{AB} = -20\, I_1 + 40\, I_2 \qquad \text{.... (i)}$$

Now to find I_1 and I_2, we can use KVL in the inner and outer loop respectively.

$$I_1 = \frac{100}{20+80} = 1 \text{ A} \quad \text{and} \quad I_2 = \frac{100}{40+50} = 1.11 \text{ A}$$

From equation (i)

$$V_{th} = V_{AB} = -20 I_1 + 40 I_2$$

$$= -20 \times 1 + 40 \times 1.11$$

$$V_{AB} = \boxed{24.44 \text{ volts}} \qquad \text{.... (ii)}$$

Step 3 : In order to calculate R_{1eq}, suppress all sources in Fig. 1.69(a) by replacing them by their internal resistance. We get Fig. 1.69(b), naming the junctions as earlier. Now, redraw the circuit with A and B at extreme ends [Fig. 1.69(c)].

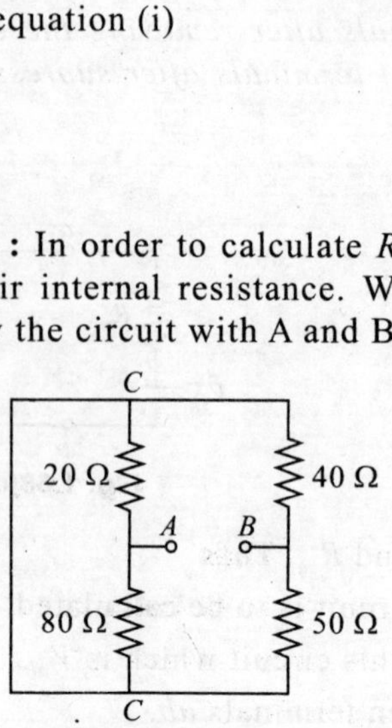

Fig. 1.69(b)

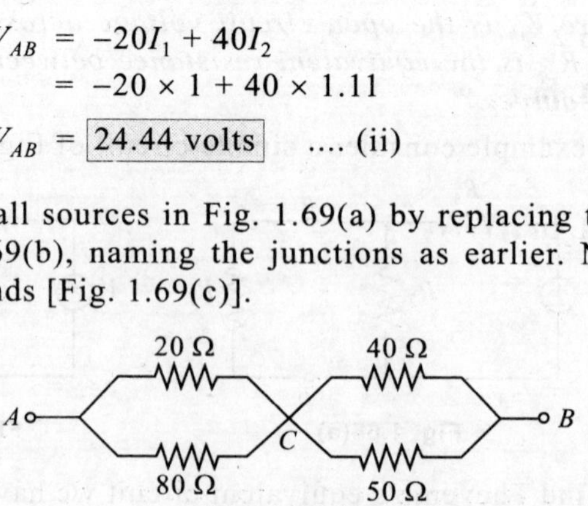

Fig. 1.69(c)

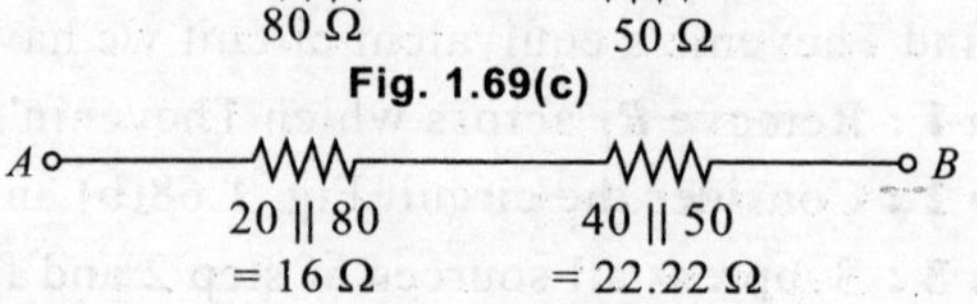

Fig. 1.69(d)

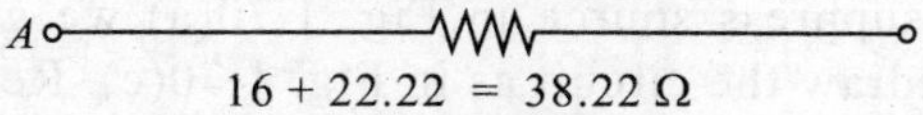

Fig. 1.69(e)

$$\therefore \ R_{eq} = \boxed{38.22 \ \Omega}$$

Step 4 : Draw Thevenin's equivalent circuit as in Fig. 1.69(f).

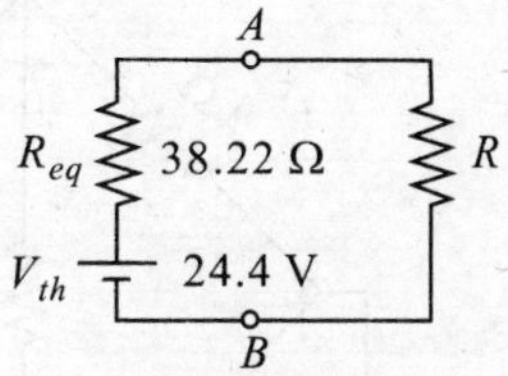

Fig. 1.68(f)

Ex. 1.53 : Using Thevenin's equivalent circuit find I in Fig. 1.70.

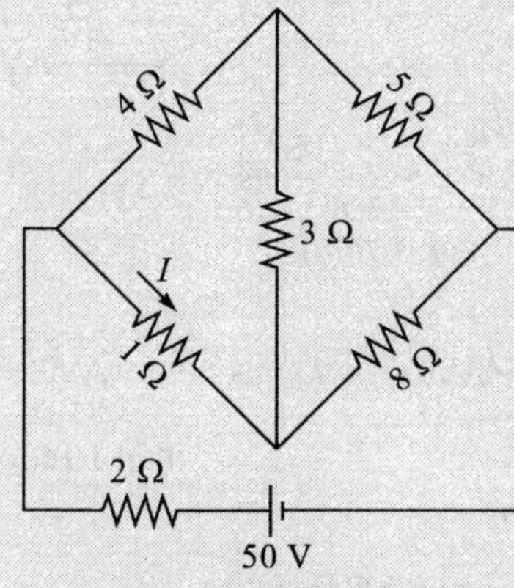

Fig. 1.70

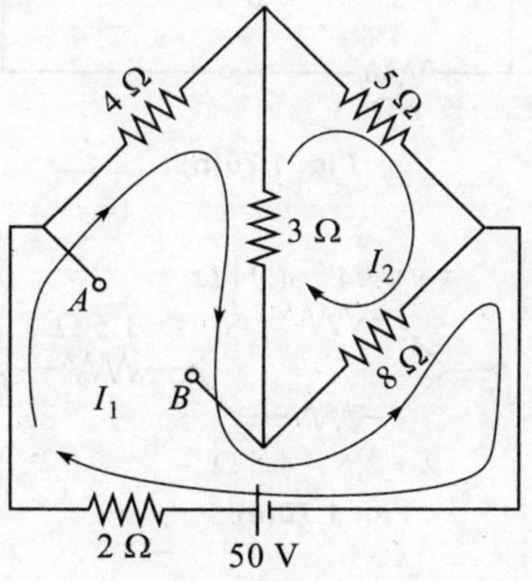

Fig. 1.70(a)

Solution : Step 1 : Remove resistance of 1 Ω and name terminals AB. [Fig. 1.70(a)]

Step 2 : Find $V_{th} = V_{AB}$. Let us use mesh analysis for this. Define two meshes I_1 and I_2.

KVL in mesh I_1

$$4I_1 + 3(I_1 - I_2) + 8(I_1 - I_2) - 50 + 2I_1 = 0$$

$$17I_1 - 11I_2 = 50 \quad \text{.... (i)}$$

KVL in mesh I_2

$$5I_2 + 8(I_2 - I_1) + 3(I_2 - I_1) = 0$$

$$-11I_1 + 16I_2 = 0 \quad \text{.... (ii)}$$

$$\therefore \begin{bmatrix} 17 & -11 \\ -11 & 16 \end{bmatrix} \begin{bmatrix} I_1 \\ I_2 \end{bmatrix} = \begin{bmatrix} 50 \\ 0 \end{bmatrix}$$

$$\therefore I_1 = 5.3 \text{ A and } I_2 = 3.64 \text{ A}$$

$$V_{th} = V_{AB} = 4I_1 + 3(I_1 - I_2)$$

$$= 4 \times 5.3 + 3(5.3 - 3.64)$$

$$\therefore V_{AB} = \boxed{26.18 \text{ V}}$$

Step 3 : To find R_{th}, suppress source in Fig. 1.70(a) we get Fig. 1.70(b). Name all the junctions carefully. Redraw the circuit as in Fig. 1.70(c). Reduce the circuit to find R_{eq}.

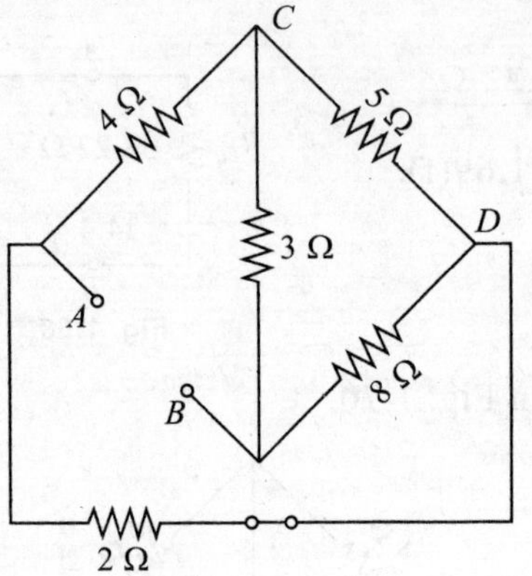

Fig. 1.70(b)

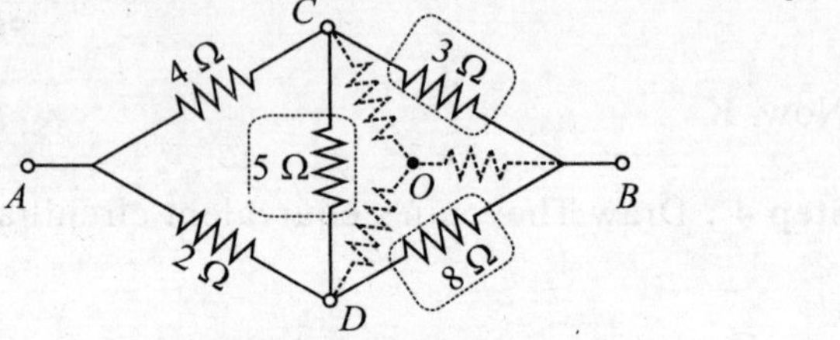

Fig. 1.70(c)

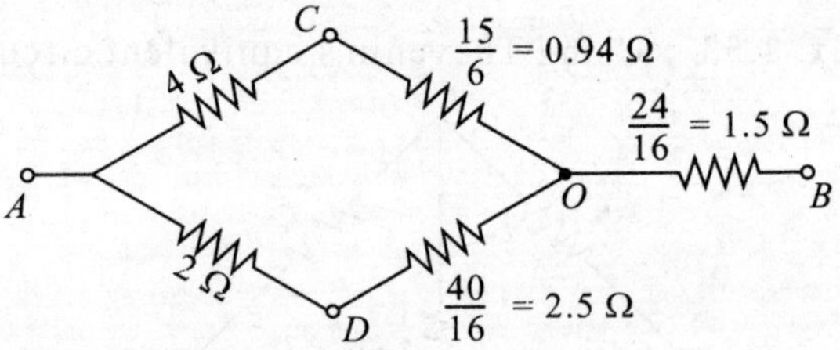

Fig. 1.70(d)

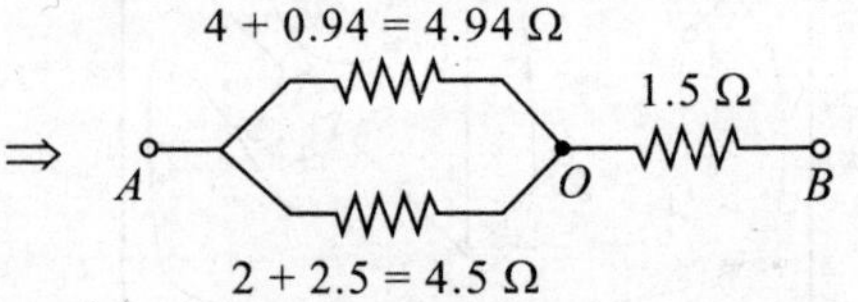

Fig. 1.70(e)

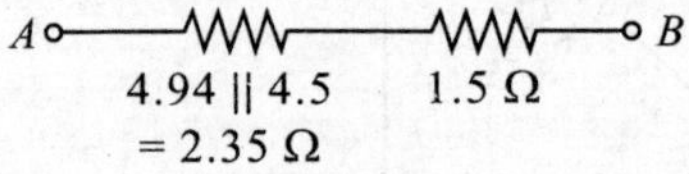

Fig. 1.70(f)

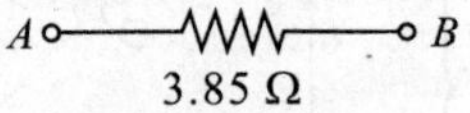

Fig. 1.70(g)

$$\therefore \; R_{eq} = R_{ab} = \boxed{3.85 \ \Omega}$$

Step 4 : Draw Thevenin's equivalent circuit across the 1 Ω resistance which was removed from terminals *AB*. Fig. 1.70(h).

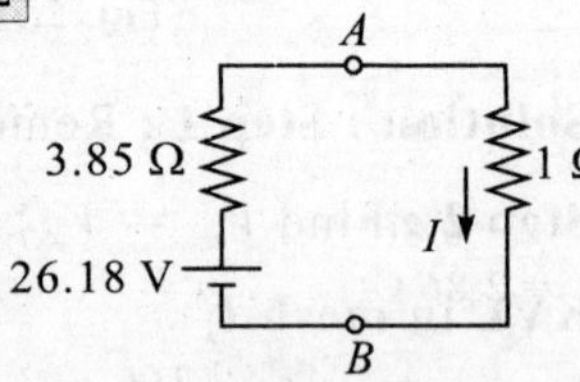

Fig. 1.70(h)

$$\therefore \; I = \frac{26.18}{3.85+1} = 5.4 \text{ A}$$

$$I = \boxed{5.4 \text{ A}}$$

Ex. 1.54 : Find *I* in Fig. 1.71 using Thenevin's theorem.

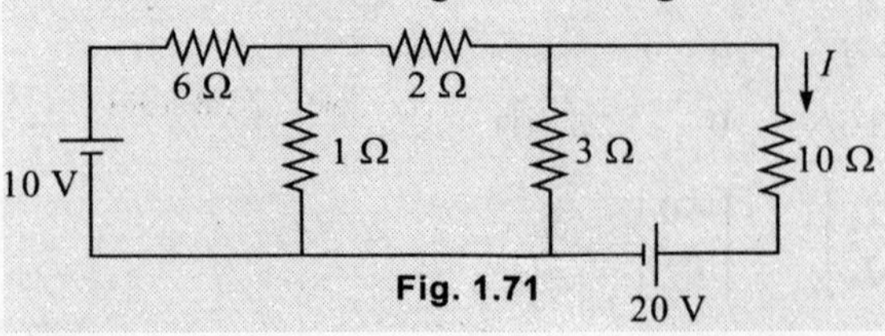

Fig. 1.71

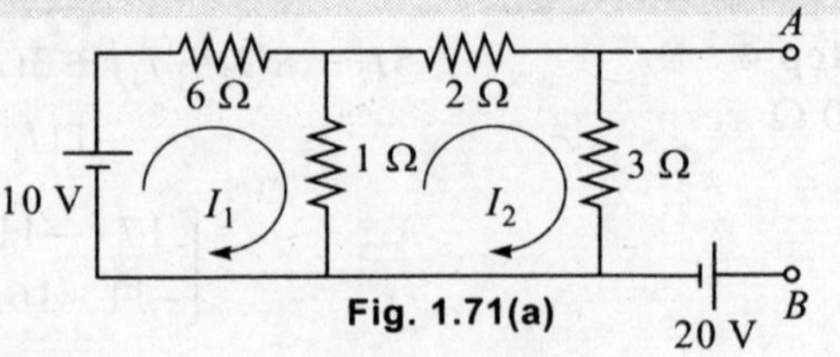

Fig. 1.71(a)

Solution : Step 1 : Remove 10 resistance and mark terminals *AB* [Fig. 1.71(a)]

Step 2 : Using mesh analysis find various currents in Fig. 1.71(a) define V_{AB} i.e. start from *A* and end on *B*.

$$V_{AB} = 3I_2 - 20 \quad \text{.... (i)}$$

Now, **KVL in mesh I_1**

$$-10 + 6I_1 + 1(I_1 - I_2) = 0$$

$$7I_1 - I_2 = 10 \quad \text{.... (ii)}$$

Now, **KVL in mesh I_2**

$$2I_2 + 3I_2 + 1(I_2 - I_1) = 0$$

$$-I_1 + 6I_2 = 0 \quad \text{.... (iii)}$$

$$\therefore \begin{bmatrix} 7 & -1 \\ -1 & 6 \end{bmatrix} \begin{bmatrix} I_1 \\ I_2 \end{bmatrix} = \begin{bmatrix} 10 \\ 0 \end{bmatrix}$$

$$\therefore I_2 = 0.24 \text{ A}$$

$\therefore$ from (i)

$$V_{AB} = 3I_2 - 20$$

$$= 3 \times 0.24 - 20$$

$$\therefore V_{AB} = \boxed{-19.28 \text{ V}}$$

Step 3 : To find R_{eq}, **suppress all sources by replacing them by their internal resistances.**

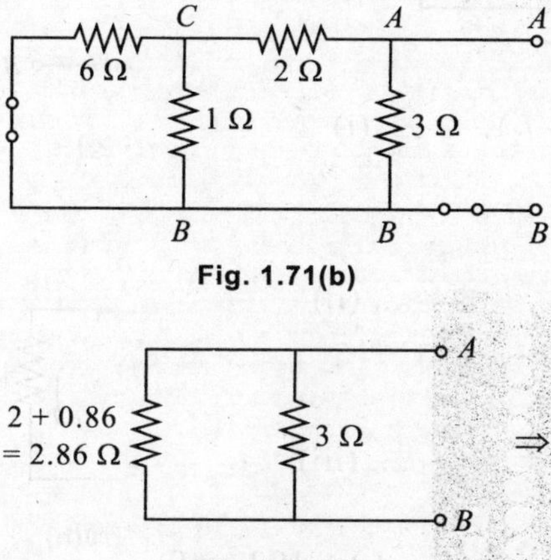

Fig. 1.71(b)

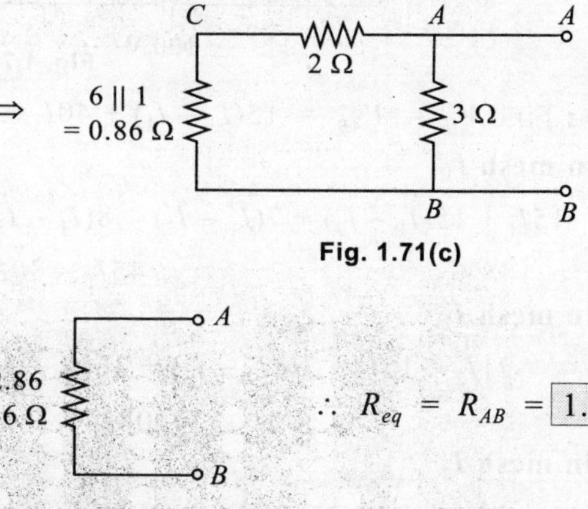

Fig. 1.71(c)

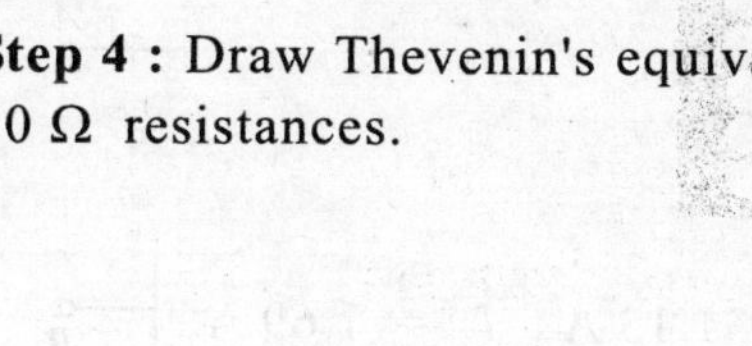

Fig. 1.71(d)

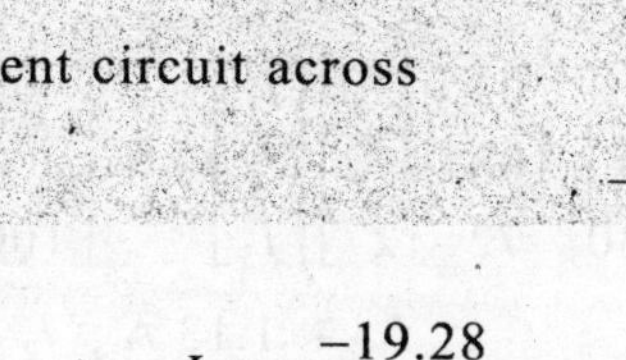

Fig. 1.71(e)

$$\therefore R_{eq} = R_{AB} = \boxed{1.46\ \Omega}$$

Step 4 : Draw Thevenin's equivalent circuit across 10 Ω resistances.

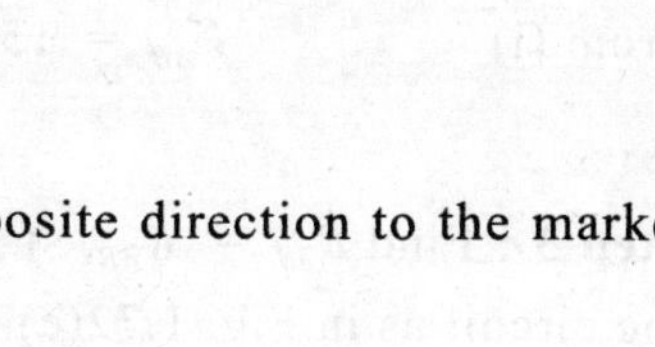

Fig. 1.71(f)

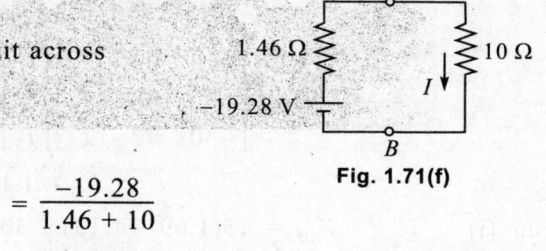

$$\therefore I = \frac{-19.28}{1.46 + 10}$$

$$I = \boxed{-1.68 \text{ A}}$$

i.e. current of 1.68 A flows through 10 Ω resistance in opposite direction to the marked value.

Ex. 1.55 : Using Thevenin's theorem find I in Fig. 1.72.

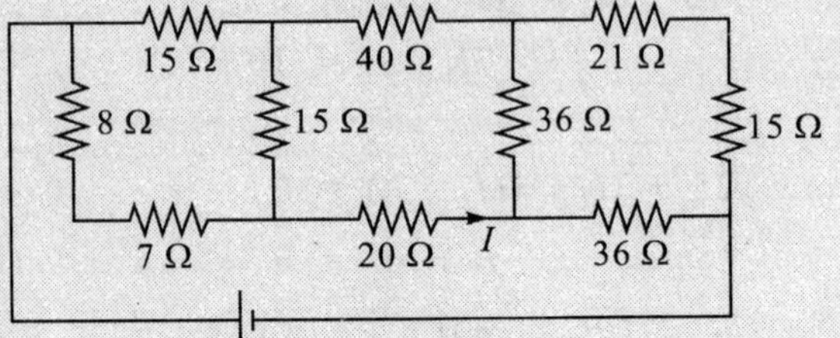

Fig. 1.72

Solution : Step 1 : Remove 20 Ω resistance [Fig 1.72(a)]

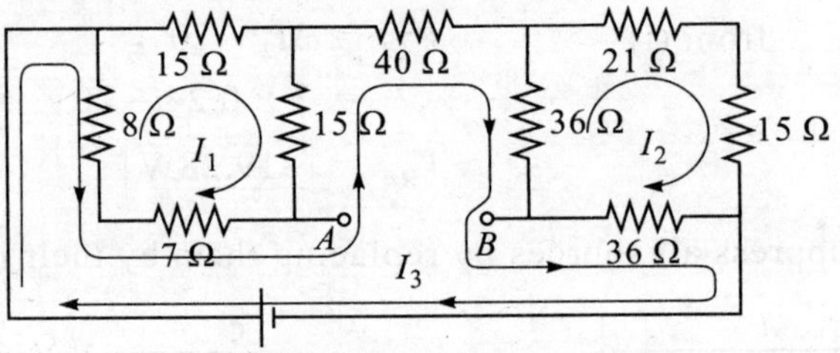

Fig. 1.72(a)

Step 2 : Find $V_{th} = V_{AB} = 15(I_3 - I_1) + 40I_3 + 36(I_3 - I_2)$ .... (i)

KVL in mesh I_1

$$15I_1 + 15(I_1 - I_3) + 7(I_1 - I_3) + 8(I_1 - I_3) = 0$$

$$45I_1 - 30I_3 = 0 \quad \text{.... (ii)}$$

KVL in mesh I_2

$$21I_2 + 15I_2 + 36(I_2 - I_3) + 36(I_2 - I_3) = 0$$

$$108I_2 - 72I_3 = 0 \quad \text{.... (iii)}$$

KVL in mesh I_3

$$8(I_3 - I_1) + 7(I_3 - I_1) + 15(I_3 - I_1) + 40I_3 + 36(I_3 - I_2) + 36(I_3 - I_2) - 100 = 0$$

$$\therefore \; -30I_1 - 72I_2 + 127I_3 = 100 \quad \text{.... (iv)}$$

$$\therefore \begin{bmatrix} 45 & 0 & -30 \\ 0 & 108 & -72 \\ -30 & -72 & 127 \end{bmatrix} \begin{bmatrix} I_1 \\ I_2 \\ I_3 \end{bmatrix} = \begin{bmatrix} 0 \\ 0 \\ 100 \end{bmatrix}$$

$$\therefore I_1 = 1.13 \text{ A} ; \; I_2 = 1.13 \text{ A} ; \; I_3 = 1.69 \text{ A}$$

From (i) $\quad V_{AB} = 15(1.69 - 1.13) + 40 \times 1.69 + 36\,(1.69 - 1.13)$

$$V_{AB} = \boxed{96.16 \text{ V}}$$

Step 3 : Find $R_{eq} = R_{AB}$, suppress all sources in Fig. 1.72(a) [Fig. 1.72(b)]. Now, redraw the circuit as in Fig. 1.72(c) with A and B on extreme ends.

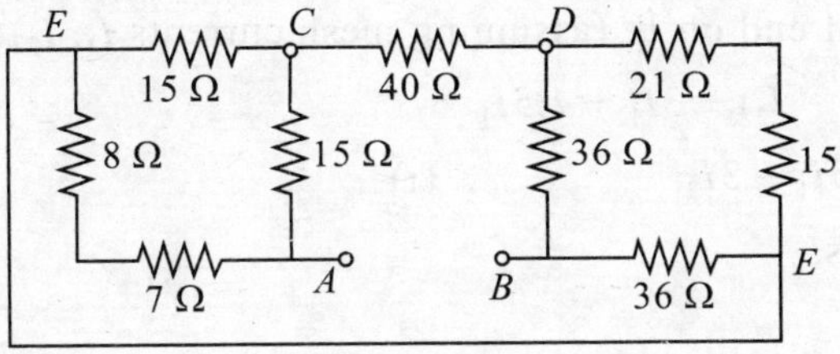

Fig. 1.72(b)

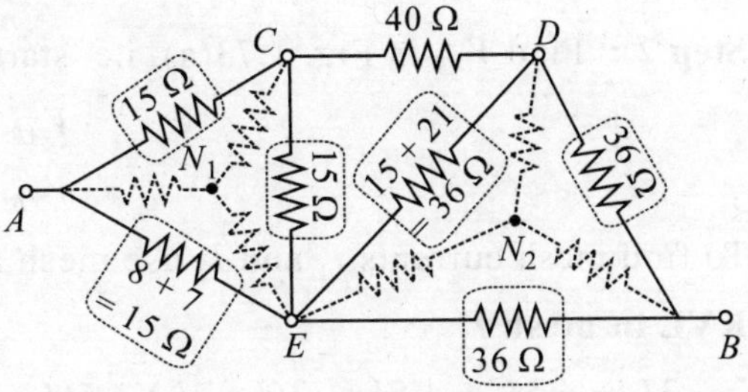

Fig. 1.72(c)

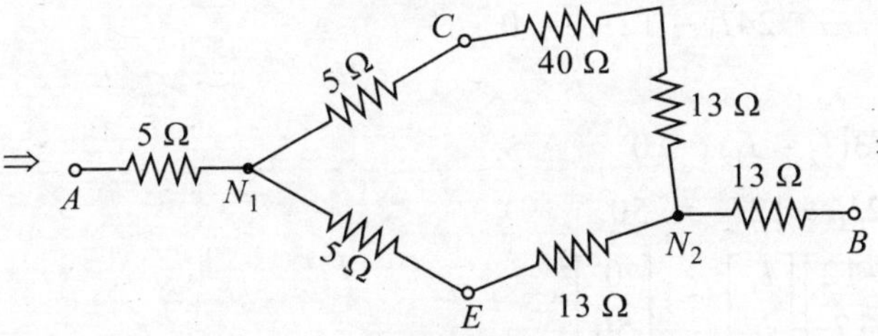

Fig. 1.72(d)

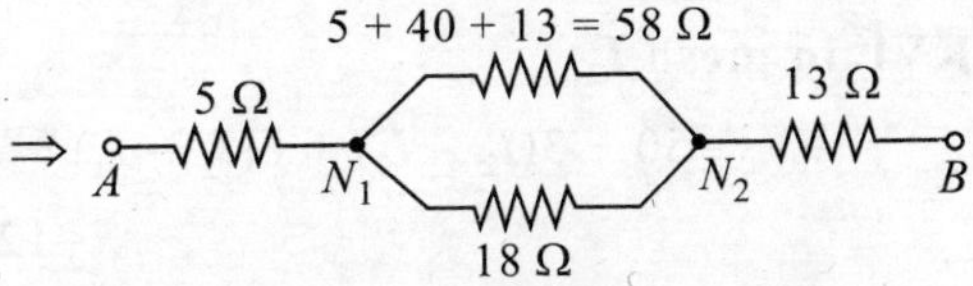

Fig. 1.72(e)

Fig. 1.72(f)

$$\therefore \; R_{AB} = \boxed{31.74\ \Omega}$$

Step 4 : Use Thevenin's equivalent circuit to find I

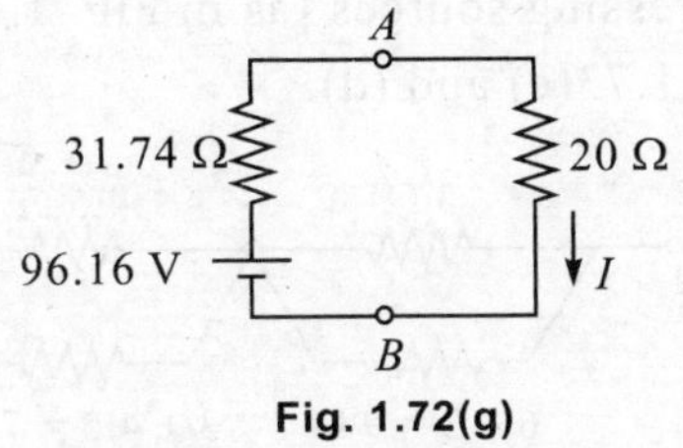

Fig. 1.72(g)

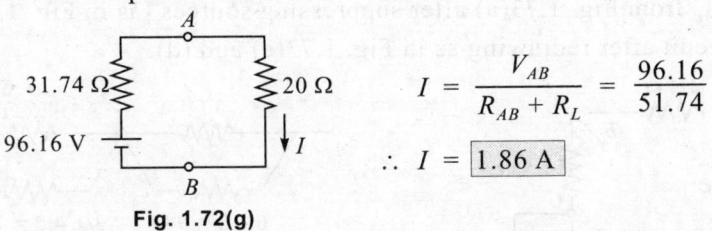

$$I = \frac{V_{AB}}{R_{AB} + R_L} = \frac{96.16}{51.74}$$

$$\therefore \; I = \boxed{1.86\ \text{A}}$$

Ex. 1.56 : Find I using Thevenin's Theorem in Fig. 1.73.

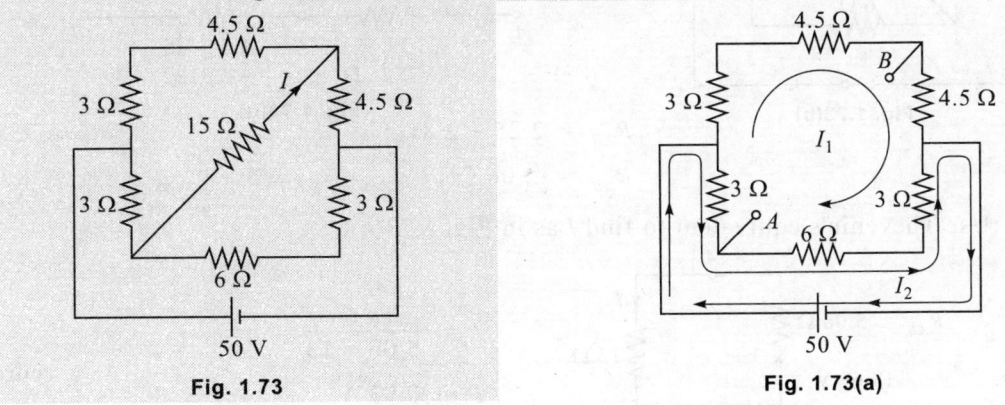

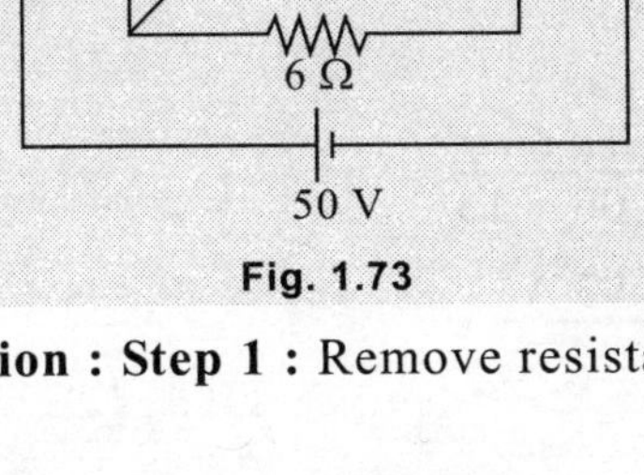

Fig. 1.73

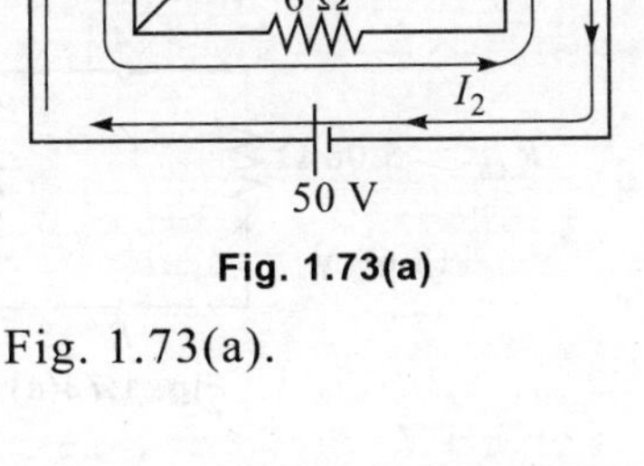

Fig. 1.73(a)

Solution : Step 1 : Remove resistance of 15 Ω, draw Fig. 1.73(a).

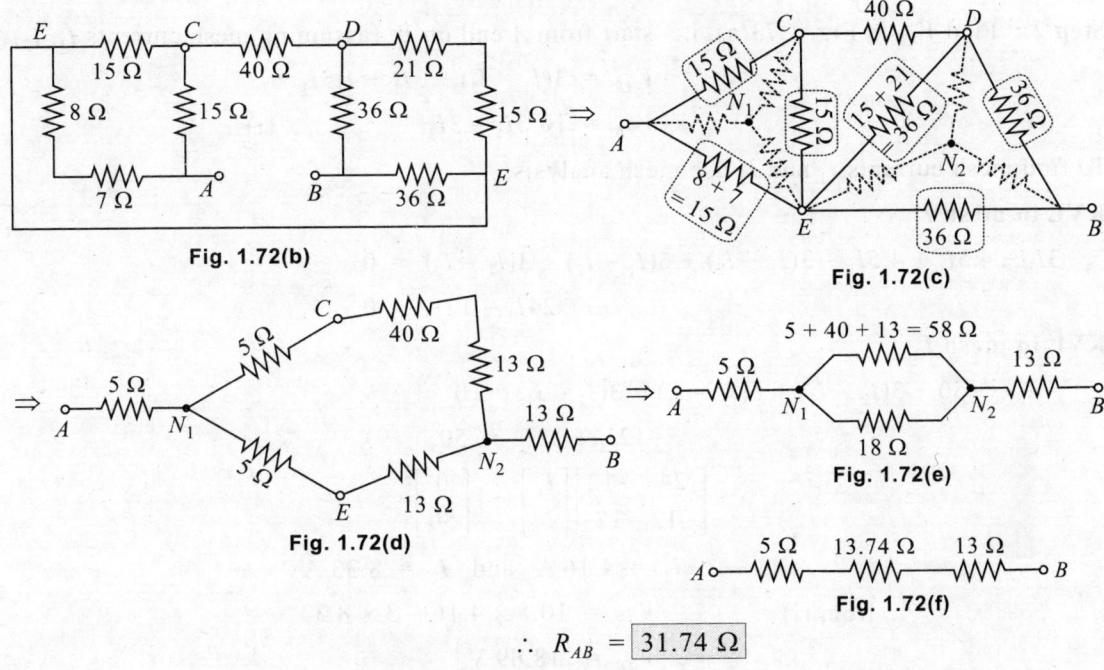

Step 2 : Find V_{AB} in Fig. 1.73(a), i.e. start from A end on B. (assuming mesh currents I_1, I_2)

$$V_{AB} = 3(I_1 - I_2) + 3I_1 + 4.5I_1$$

$$V_{AB} = 10.5I_1 - 3I_2 \quad \text{.... (i)}$$

To find mesh currents I_1 and I_2 use mesh analysis.

KVL in mesh I_1

$$3I_1 + 4.5I_1 + 4.5I_1 - 3(I_1 - I_2) + 6(I_1 - I_2) + 3(I_1 - I_2) = 0$$

$$24I_1 - 12I_2 = 0$$

KVL in mesh I_2

$$-50 + 3(I_2 - I_1) + 6(I_2 - I_1) + 3(I_2 - I_1) = 0$$

$$\therefore -12I_1 + 12I_2 = 50$$

$$\therefore \begin{bmatrix} 24 & -12 \\ -12 & 12 \end{bmatrix} \begin{bmatrix} I_1 \\ I_2 \end{bmatrix} = \begin{bmatrix} 0 \\ 50 \end{bmatrix}$$

$$\therefore I_1 = 4.16 \text{ A} \quad \text{and} \quad I_2 = 8.33 \text{ A}$$

$\therefore$ from (i)

$$V_{AB} = 10.5 \times 4.16 - 3 \times 8.33$$

$$\therefore V_{AB} = \boxed{18.69 \text{ V}}$$

Step 3 : Find R_{AB} from Fig. 1.73(a) after suppressing sources [as in Fig. 1.73(b)]. Reducing the circuit after redrawing as in Fig. 1.73(c) and (d).

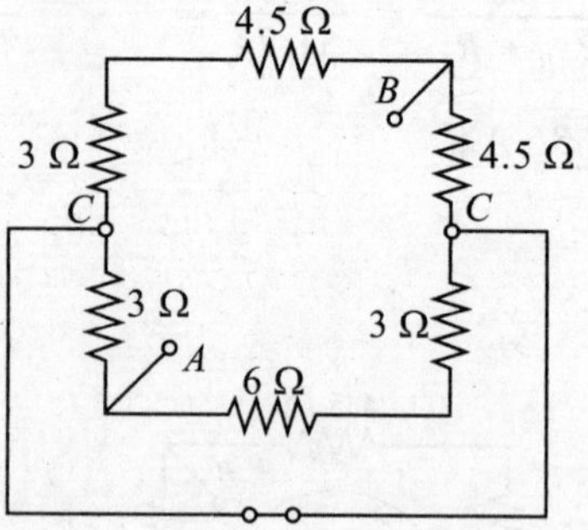

Fig. 1.73(b)

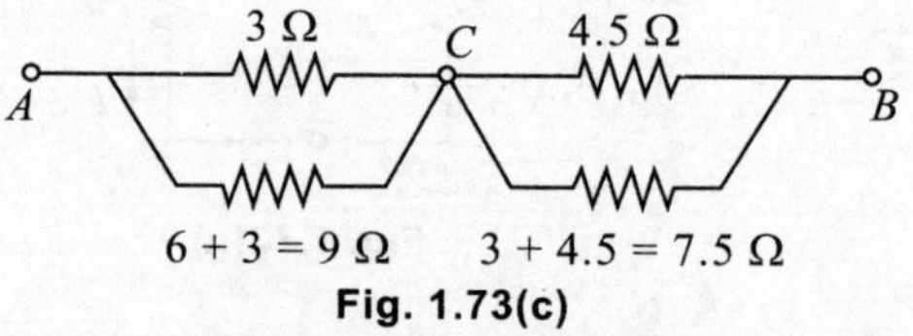

Fig. 1.73(c)

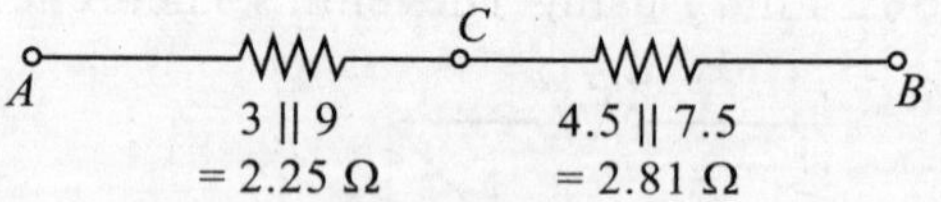

Fig. 1.73(d)

$$R_{AB} = 2.25 + 2.81$$

$$R_{AB} = \boxed{5.06 \ \Omega}$$

Step 4 : Use Thevenin's equivalent to find I as in Fig. 1.73(e).

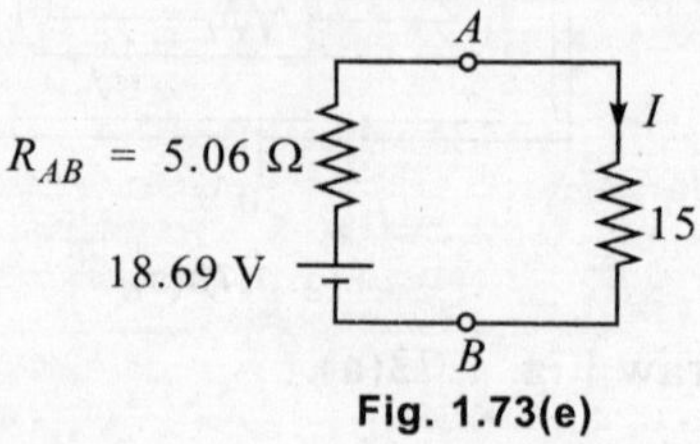

Fig. 1.73(e)

$$I = \frac{18.69}{5.06 + 15}$$

$$\therefore I = \boxed{0.93 \text{ A}}$$

Ex. 1.57 : Find I using Thevenin's theorem in Fig. 1.74.

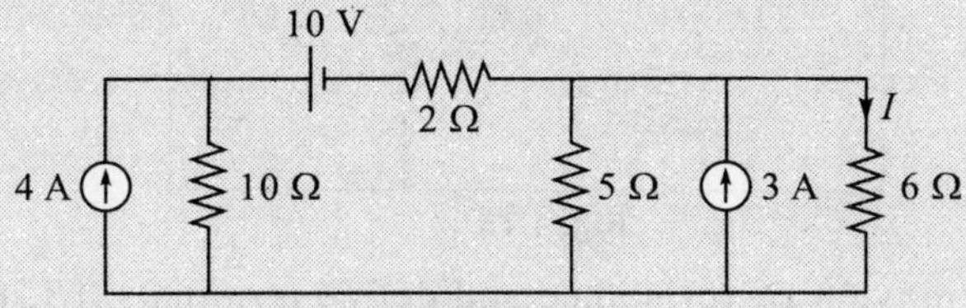

Fig. 1.74

Solution : Step 1 : Remove 6 Ω resistance and label terminals AB [Fig. 1.74(a)].

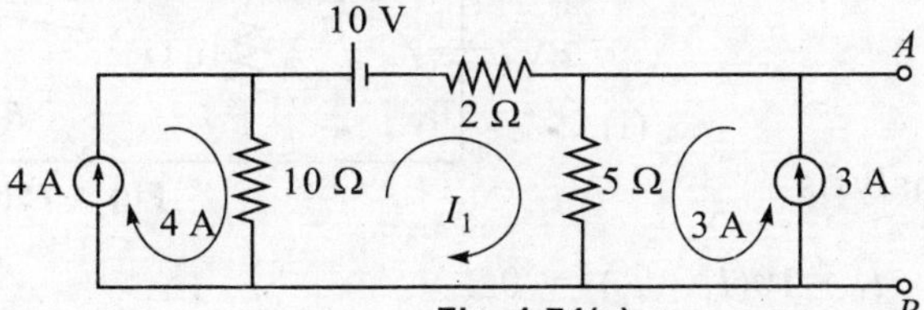

Fig. 1.74(a)

Step 2 : Find V_{AB} using mesh analysis V_{AB} here can be defined as

$$V_{AB} = 5(I_1 + 3)$$

KVL in mesh I_1

$$10 + 2I_1 + 5(I_1 + 3) + 10(I_1 - 4) = 0$$

$$\therefore 17I_1 = 15$$

$$I_1 = \frac{15}{17} = 0.88 \text{ A}$$

$$\therefore V_{AB} = 5(0.88 + 3) = 19.41 \text{ V}$$

Step 3 : Find $R_{eq} = R_{AB}$ by suppressing sources of Fig. 1.74(a).

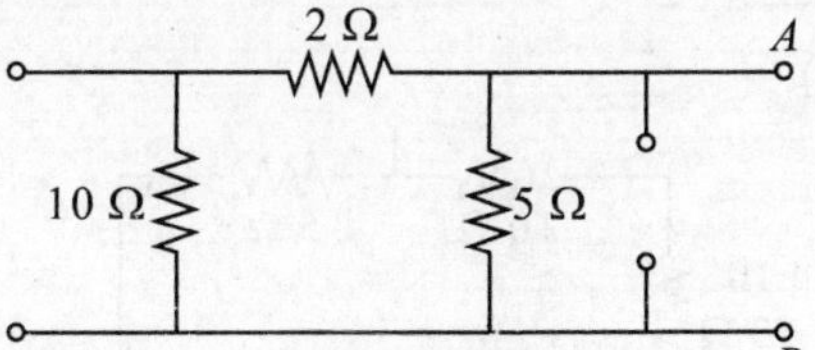

Fig. 1.74(b)

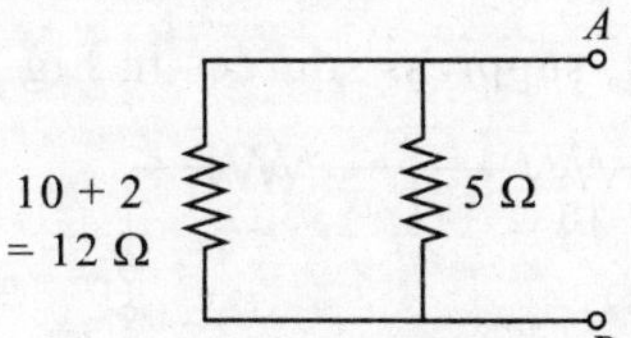

Fig. 1.74(c)

$$\therefore R_{AB} = \boxed{3.53\ \Omega}$$

Step 4 : Draw Thevenin's equivalent circuit as in Fig. 1.74(d).

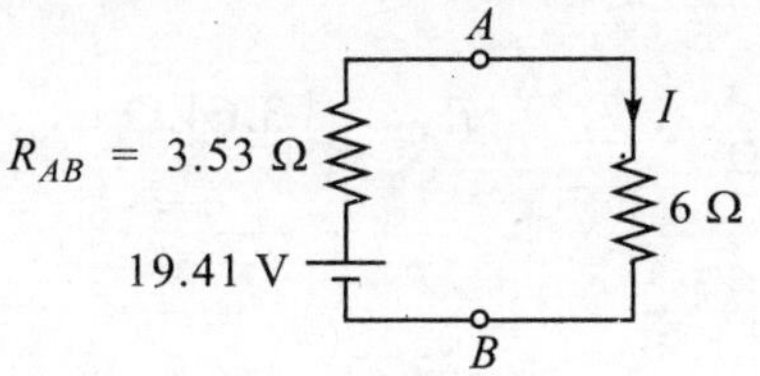

Fig. 1.74(d)

$$I = \frac{19.41}{3.53 + 6}$$

$$\therefore I = \boxed{2.04 \text{ A}}$$

Ex. 1.58 : Using Thevenin's Theorem, find I in Fig. 1.75.

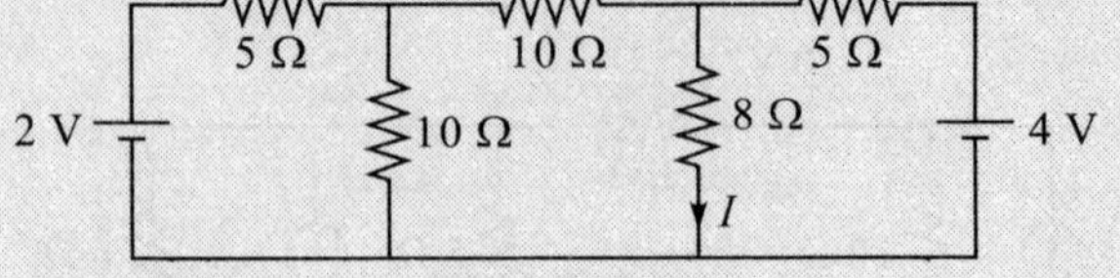

Fig. 1.75

Solution : Step 1 : Remove 8 Ω resistance and define terminals AB [Fig. 1.75(a)]

Step 2 : Find V_{AB} the open circuit voltage in Fig. 1.75(a)

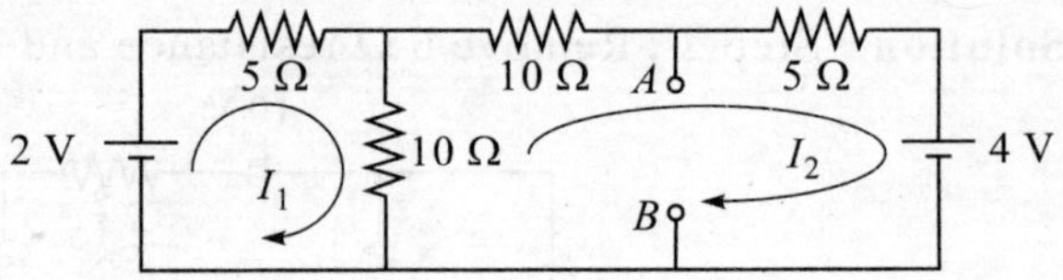

Fig. 1.75(a)

Assume currents I_1 and I_2.

$$\therefore \; V_{AB} = 5I_2 + 4 \qquad \text{.... (i)}$$

To find I_2, we use mesh analysis

KVL in mesh I_1

$$-2 + 5I_1 + 10(I_1 - I_2) = 0$$

$$15I_1 - 10I_2 = 2 \qquad \text{.... (ii)}$$

KVL in mesh I_2

$$10I_2 + 5I_2 + 4 + 10(I_2 - I_1) = 0$$

$$\therefore \; -10I_1 + 25I_2 = 4 \qquad \text{.... (iii)}$$

∴ from (ii) and (iii) we get

$$\therefore \; \begin{bmatrix} 15 & -10 \\ -10 & 25 \end{bmatrix} \begin{bmatrix} I_1 \\ I_2 \end{bmatrix} = \begin{bmatrix} 2 \\ -4 \end{bmatrix}$$

$$\therefore \; I_2 = -0.145 \text{ A}$$

∴ from (i)

$$V_{AB} = 5I_2 + 4 = 5 \times (-0.145) + 4$$

$$\therefore \; V_{AB} = \boxed{3.275 \text{ V}}$$

Step 3 : To find R_{AB}, suppress sources in Fig. 1.75(a).

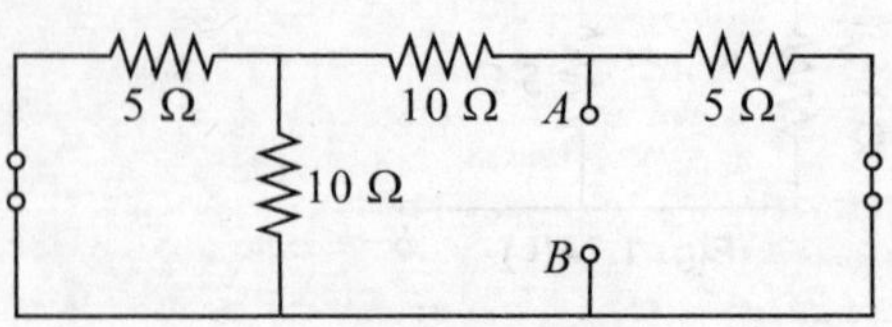

Fig. 1.75(b)

⇒

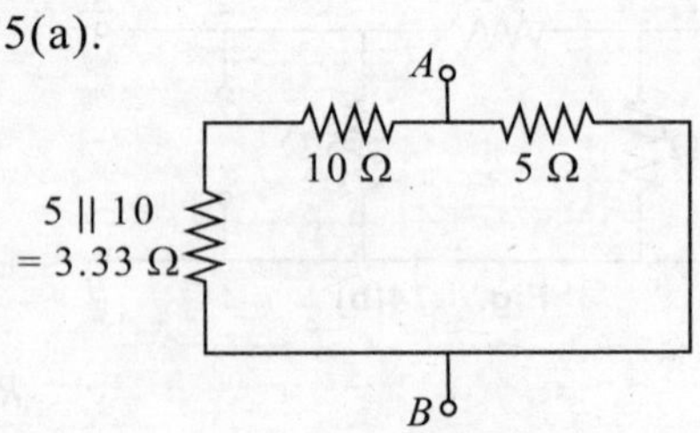

Fig. 1.75(c)

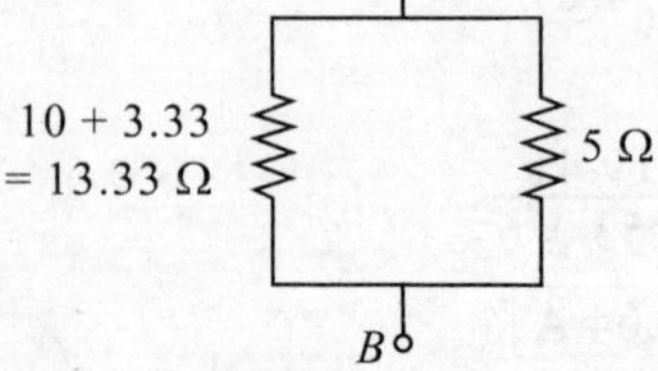

Fig. 1.75(d)

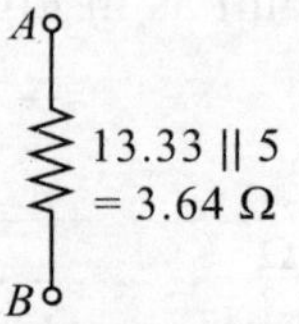

Fig. 1.75(e)

$$R_{AB} = \boxed{3.64 \; \Omega}$$

Step 4 : Draw Thevenin's equivalent circuit Fig. 1.75(f).

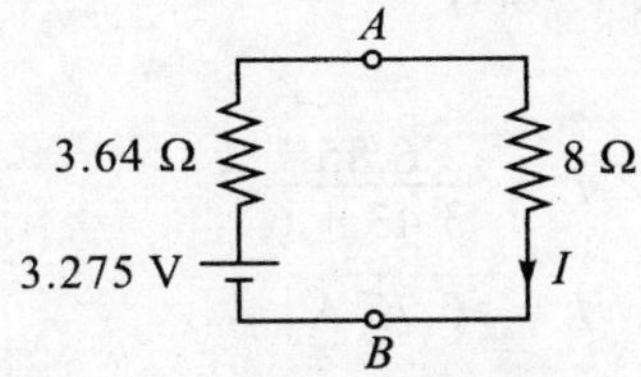

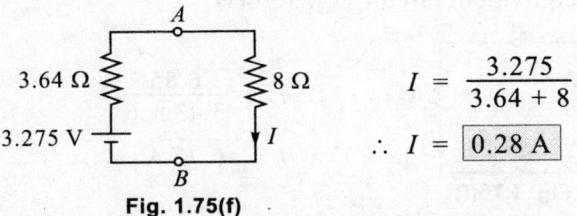

$$I = \frac{3.275}{3.64 + 8}$$

$$\therefore \; I = \boxed{0.28 \text{ A}}$$

Fig. 1.75(f)

Ex. 1.59 : Using Thevenin's equivalent circuit find I in Fig. 1.76.

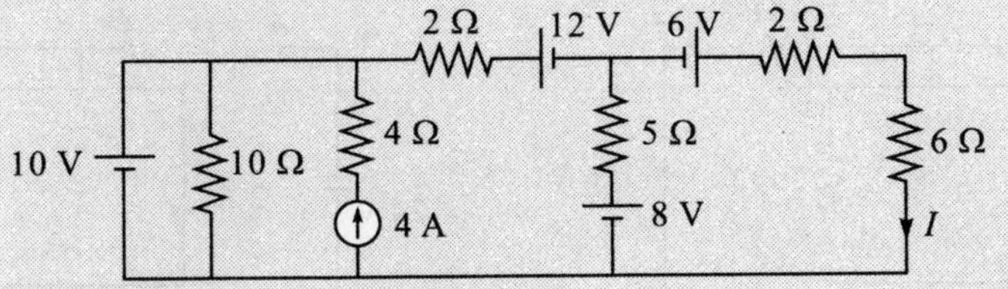

Fig. 1.76

Solution : Step 1 : Remove 6 Ω resistance [Fig. 1.76(a)]

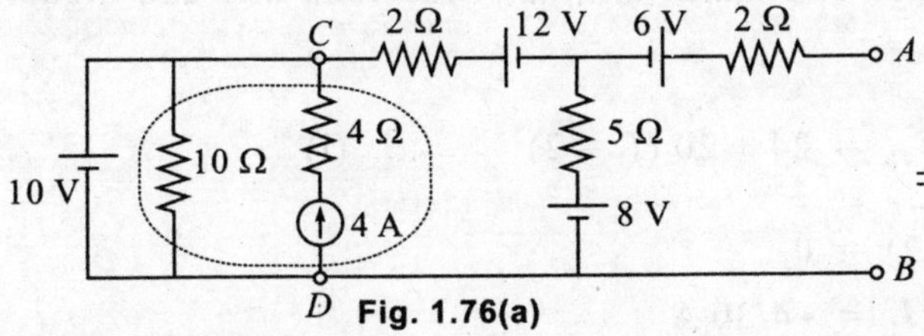

Fig. 1.76(a)

⇒

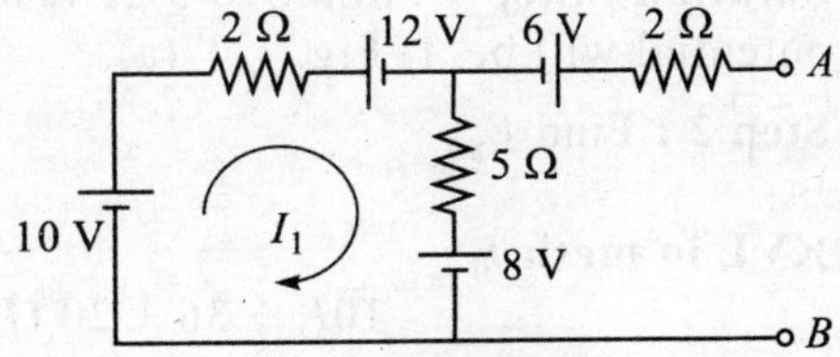

Fig. 1.76(b)

As encircled part of circuit is redundant, it can be eliminated because voltage across C and D remains 10 V only, as it is connected in parallel to 10 V source.

Step 2 : Find V_{AB}

$$V_{AB} = 6 + 5I_1 + 8 \quad \text{.... (i)}$$

KVL in mesh I_1

$$-10 + 2I_1 + 12 + 5I_1 + 8 = 0$$

$$I_1 = -1.43 \text{ A}$$

From (i) $\quad V_{AB} = \boxed{6.85 \text{ V}}$

Step 3 : Find R_{AB}, (suppress all sources) Fig. 1.76(c)

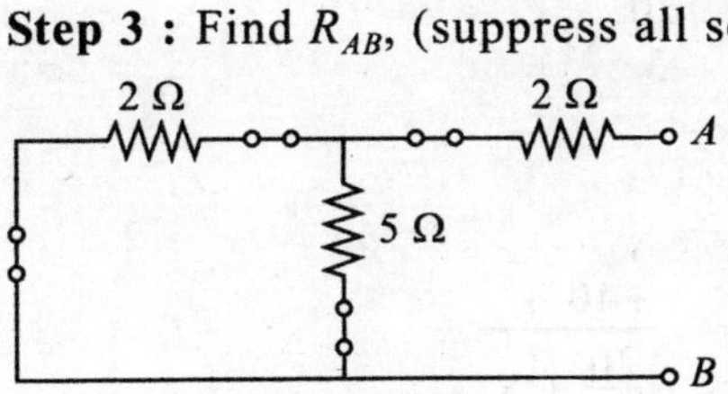

Fig. 1.76(c)

⇒

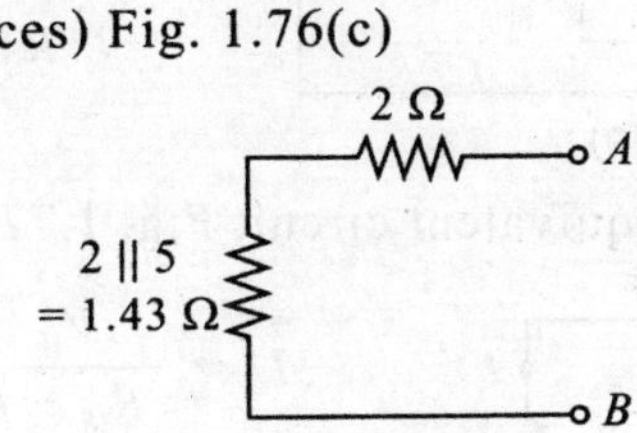

Fig. 1.76(d)

⇒

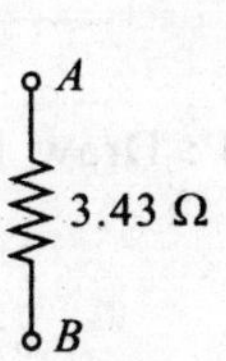

Fig. 1.76(e)

$$\therefore \; R_{AB} = \boxed{3.43 \; \Omega}$$

Step 4 : Draw Thevenin's equivalent circuit Fig. 1.76(f)

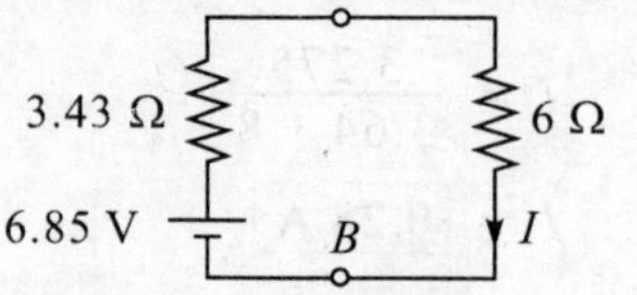

Fig. 1.76(f)

$$I = \frac{6.85}{3.43 + 6}$$

$$\therefore\ I = \boxed{0.73\ \text{A}}$$

Ex. 1.60 : Using Thevenin's theorem find I in Fig. 1.77.

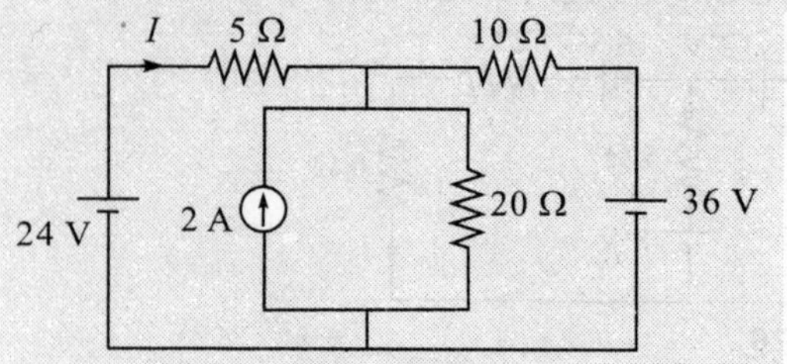

Fig. 1.77

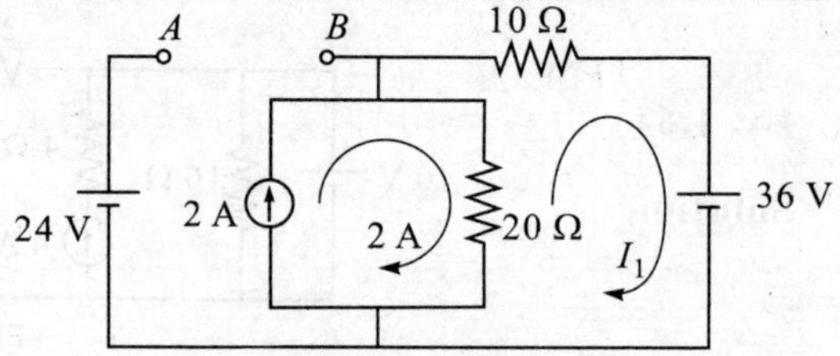

Fig. 1.77(a)

Solution : Step 1 : Remove 5 Ω resistance and mark terminals AB (look at I and higher potential will be A) Fig. 1.77(a).

Step 2 : Find V_{AB}

$$V_{AB} = 24 + 20\,(I_1 - 2) \qquad \text{.... (i)}$$

KVL in mesh I_1

$$10I_1 + 36 + 20\,(I_1 - 2) = 0$$

$$I_1 = -4/30\ \text{A}$$

$$\therefore \text{ from (i) } V_{AB} = 24 + 20I_1 - 40$$

$$V_{AB} = \boxed{-40/3\ \text{V}}$$

Step 3 : Find R_{AB} after suppressing sources Fig. 1.77(b).

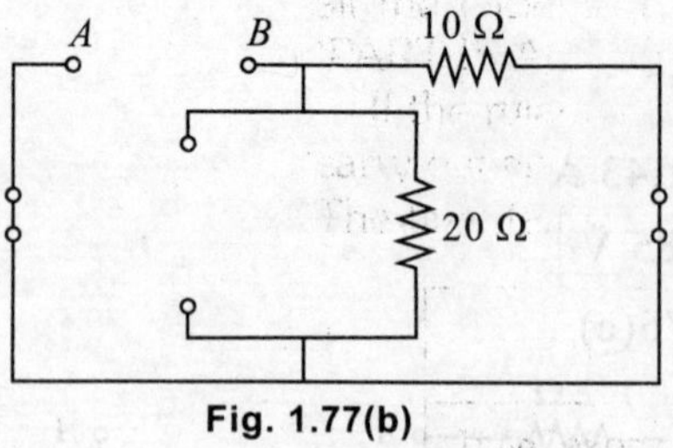

Fig. 1.77(b)

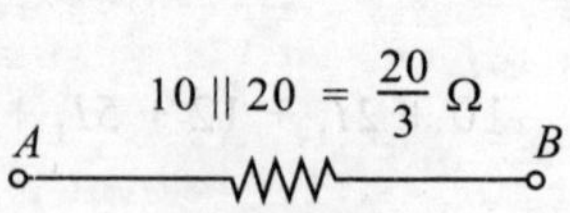

Fig. 1.77(c)

$$R_{AB} = \boxed{\frac{20}{3}\ \Omega}$$

Step 4 : Draw Thevenin's equivalent circuit Fig. 1.77(f).

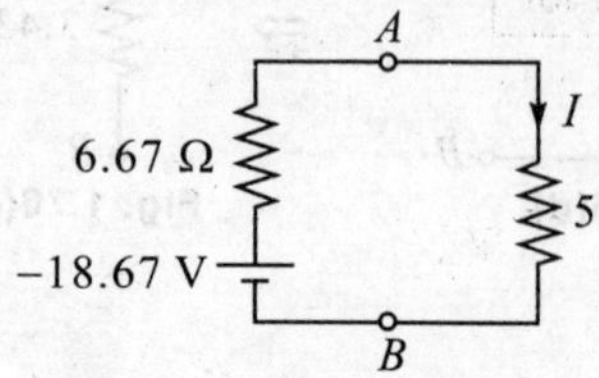

Fig. 1.77(d)

$$I = \frac{V_{th}}{R_{th} + R} = \frac{-40/3}{\frac{20}{3} + 5}$$

$$\therefore\ I = \boxed{-1.14\ \text{A}}$$

Negative sign of I indicates current is in opposite direction to the marked I.

Ex. 1.61 : Find V_{AB} in Fig. 1.78.

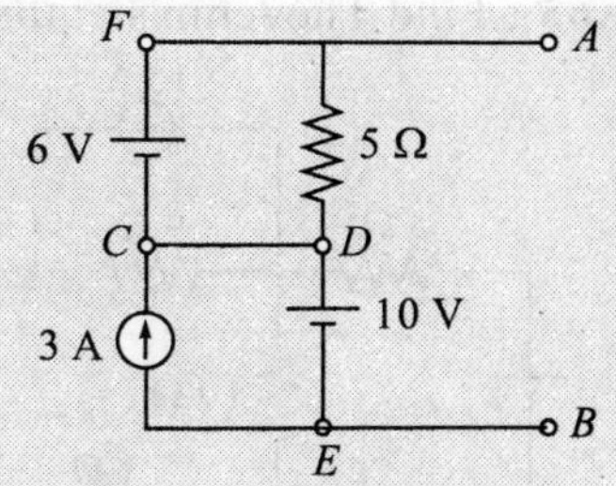

Fig. 1.78

Solution : To find V_{AB}, start from *A* and end on *B* without repeating any node through a path where voltage can be defined (i.e. do not include the current source in that path as voltage across the current source is not defined). So trace *A - F - C - D - E - B*.

$$\therefore \; V_{AB} = 6 + 10 = \boxed{16 \text{ V}}$$

Ex. 1.62 : Find V_{AB} in Fig. 1.79.

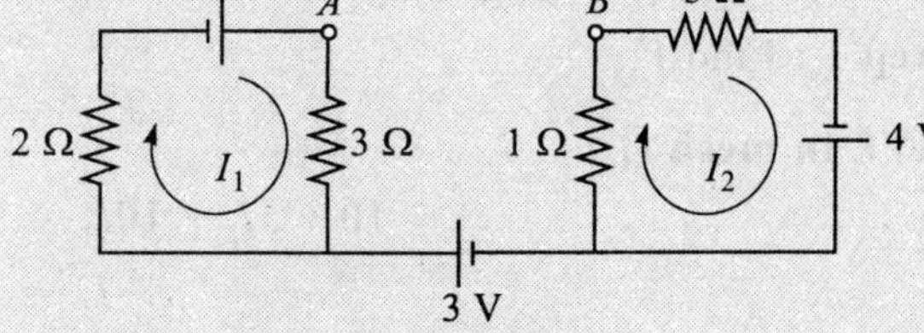

Fig. 1.79

Solution : KVL in mesh I_1

$$-5 + 3I_1 + 2I_1 = 0$$

$$\therefore \; I_1 = 1 \text{ A}$$

KVL in mesh I_2

$$3I_2 - 4 + 1I_2 = 0$$

$$\therefore \; I_2 = 1 \text{ A}$$

$$V_{AB} = 3I_1 + 3 + 1I_2$$

$$V_{AB} = \boxed{7 \text{ volts}}$$

Ex. 1.63 : Find V_{AB} in Fig. 1.80.

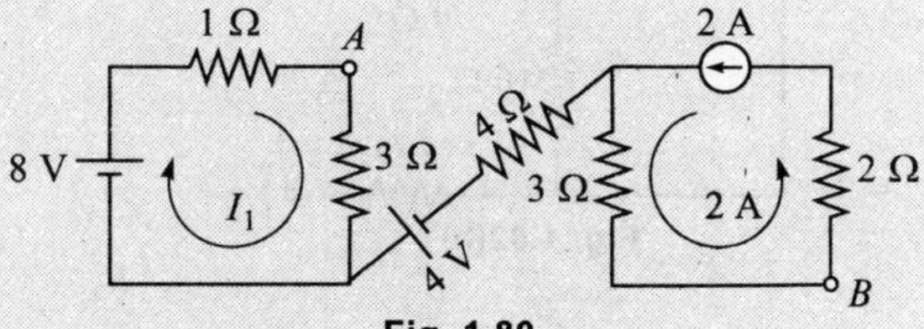

Fig. 1.80

Solution :

$$I_1 = \frac{8}{1+3} = 2 \text{ A}$$

$$V_{AB} = 3I_1 + 4 + 4 \times 0 + 3 \times 2$$

$$= 6 + 4 + 6$$

$$V_{AB} = \boxed{16 \text{ V}}$$

Ex. 1.64 : Find V_{AB} in Fig. 1.81.

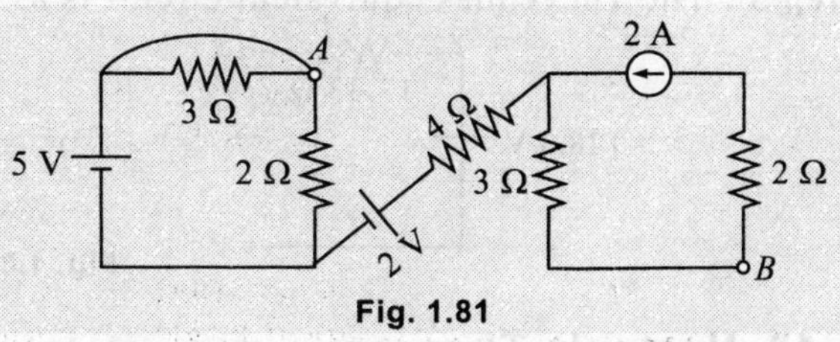

Fig. 1.81

Solution : Observe Fig. 1.81. 3 Ω resistance at *A* is shorted. Thus 3 Ω resistance is redundant. Fig. 1.81(a)

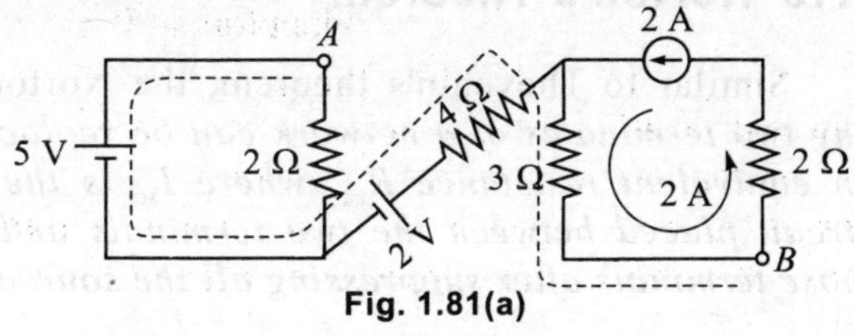

Fig. 1.81(a)

$$V_{AB} = 5 - 2 + 4 \times 0 + 3 \times 2$$

$$= 5 - 2 + 6$$

$$V_{AB} = \boxed{9 \text{ V}}$$

Ex. 1.65 : Find Thevenin's equivalent across xy in Fig. 1.82.

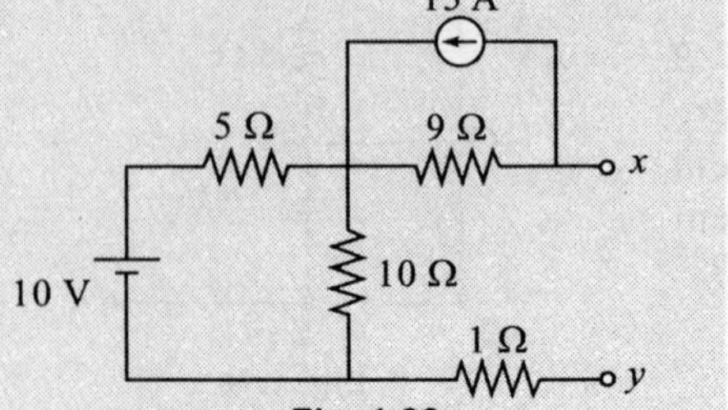

Fig. 1.82

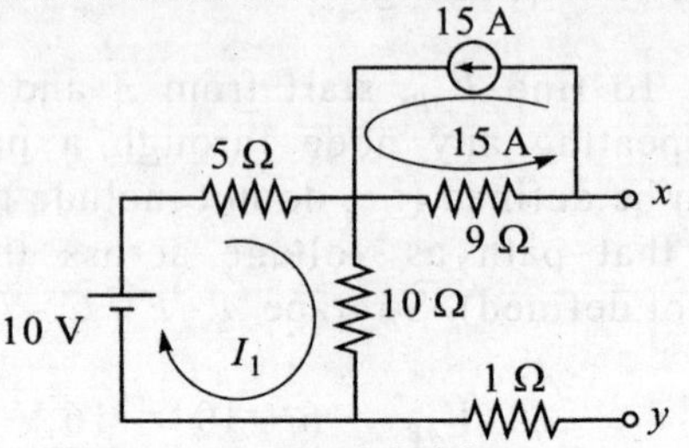

Fig. 1.82(a)

Solution : Observe Fig. 1.82(a).

Step 1 : Find V_{xy}

$$V_{xy} = -9 \times 15 + 10I_1 \quad \text{.... (i)}$$

KVL in mesh I_1

$$-10 + 5I_1 + 10I_1 = 0$$

$$\therefore \; I_1 = \frac{10}{15} = 0.67 \text{ A}$$

$\therefore$ From (i), we get $\quad V_{xy} = \boxed{-128.3 \text{ V}}$

Step 2 : Find R_{xy} after suppressing sources. Fig. 1.82(b)

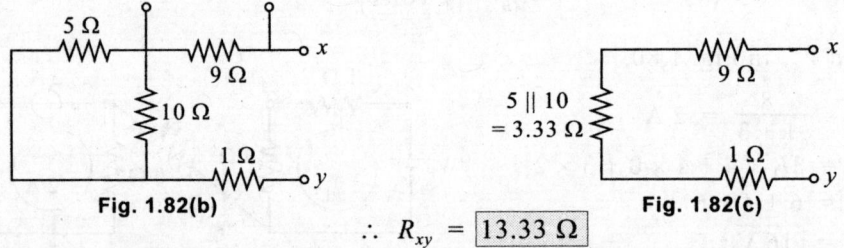

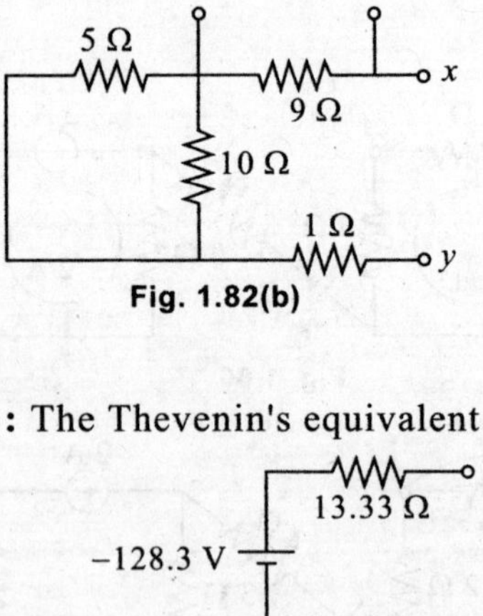

Fig. 1.82(b)

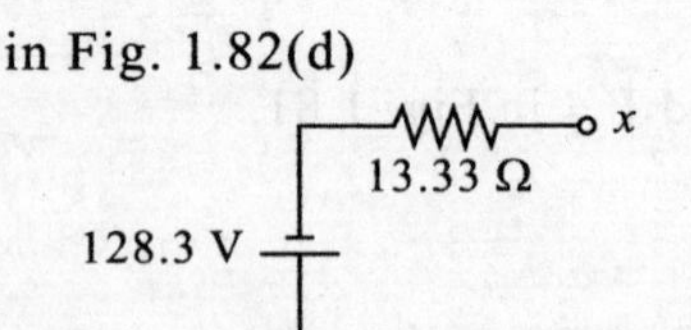

Fig. 1.82(c)

$$\therefore \; R_{xy} = \boxed{13.33 \; \Omega}$$

Step 3 : The Thevenin's equivalent circuit is as in Fig. 1.82(d)

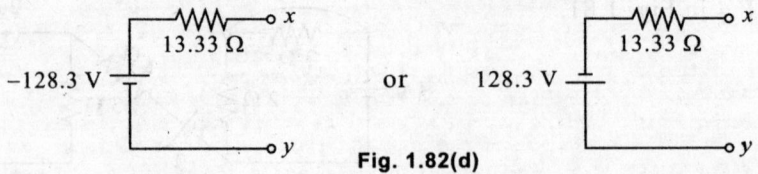

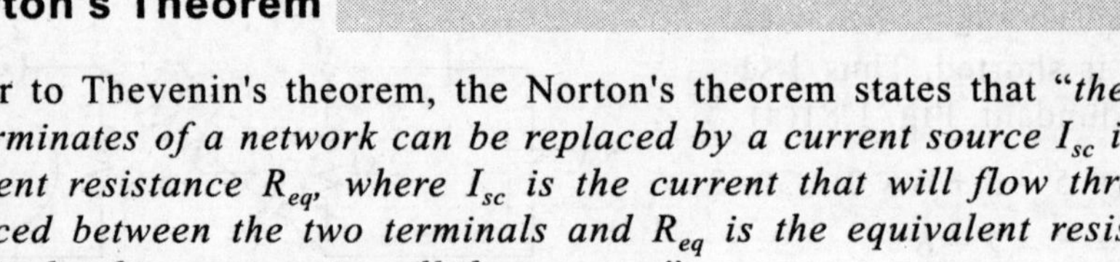

Fig. 1.82(d)

1.13 Norton's Theorem

Similar to Thevenin's theorem, the Norton's theorem states that "*the circuit across any two terminates of a network can be replaced by a current source I_{sc} in parallel with an equivalent resistance R_{eq}, where I_{sc} is the current that will flow through the short circuit placed between the two terminals and R_{eq} is the equivalent resistance between those terminals after suppressing all the sources.*"

In order to understand Norton's theorem follow the given steps :

Step 1 : Remove the resistance across which current is to calculated, name terminals say AB.

Step 2 : To find R_{eq}, suppress all sources, i.e. replace all the sources by their internal resistances and find R_{eq} between these terminals (AB).

Step 3 : Take the circuit of step 1. Connect terminals AB (i.e. short circuit terminals AB). Find current through this short circuit in the direction A to B. This current is I_{sc}.

Step 4 : Draw Norton's equivalent circuit as in Fig. 1.83. If the direction of current in step 3 is from A to B, I_{sc} in Fig. 1.83 will be towards A.

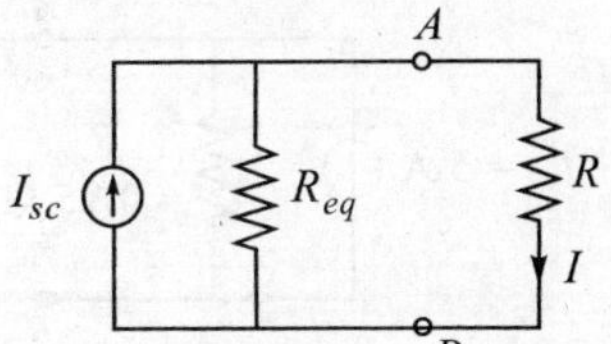

Fig. 1.83

If R is the load resistance then to find I current division rule can be applied as following:

$$I = I_{sc}\frac{R_{eq}}{R_{eq}+R}$$

Ex. 1.66 : Using Norton's equivalent circuit find I in Fig. 1.84.

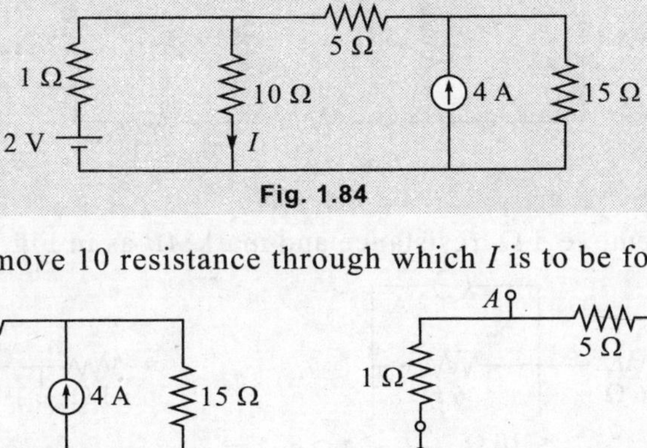

Fig. 1.84

Solution : Step 1 : Remove 10 resistance through which I is to be found [Fig. 1.84(a)].

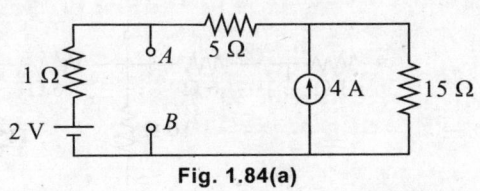

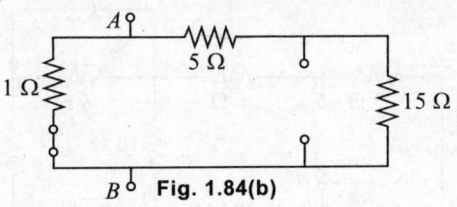

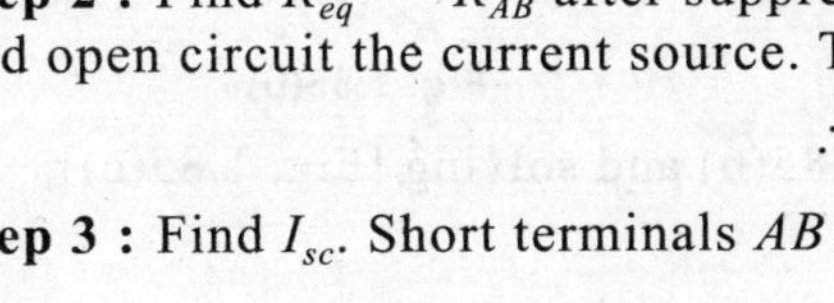

Fig. 1.84(a)

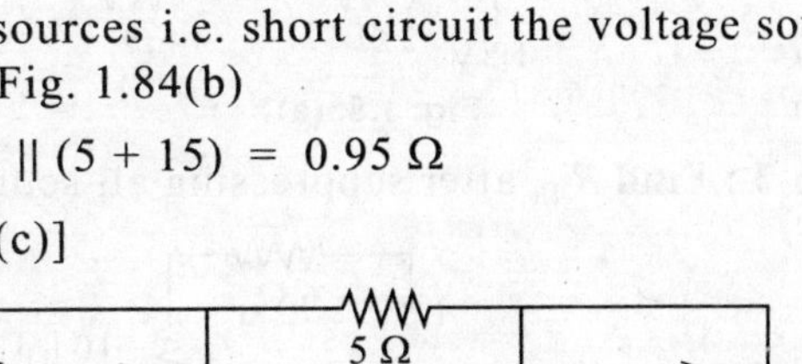

Fig. 1.84(b)

Step 2 : Find $R_{eq} = R_{AB}$ after suppressing the sources i.e. short circuit the voltage source and open circuit the current source. Thus from Fig. 1.84(b)

$$\therefore\ R_{AB} = 1 \parallel (5+15) = 0.95\ \Omega$$

Step 3 : Find I_{sc}. Short terminals AB [Fig. 1.84(c)]

$$I_{sc} = I_1 - I_2 \quad \text{.... (i)}$$

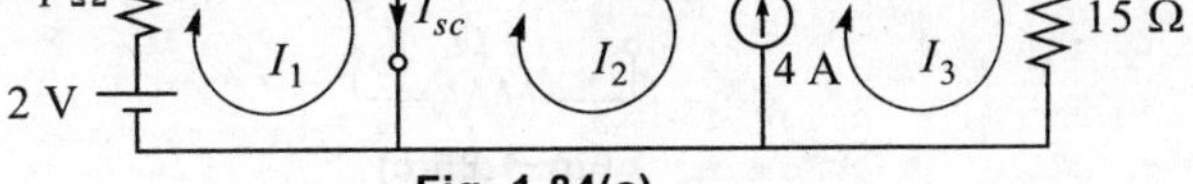

Fig. 1.84(c)

KVL in mesh I_1

$$-2 + 1I_1 = 0$$

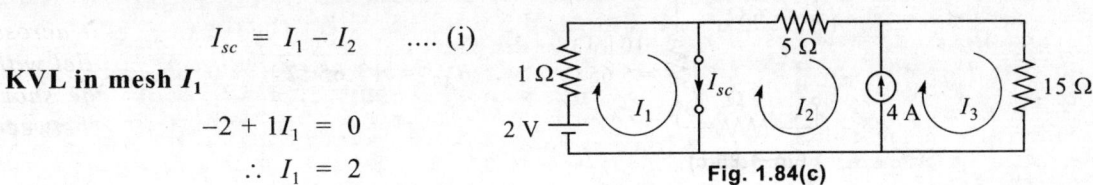

$$\therefore\ I_1 = 2$$

KVL in supermesh I_2-I_3 [current source between two meshes]

$$5I_2 + 15I_3 = 0 \quad .... \text{(ii)}$$

$$\text{and} \quad I_3 - I_2 = 4 \quad .... \text{(iii)}$$

$\therefore$ from (ii) and (iii) $\quad I_2 = -3 \text{ A}; I_3 = 1 \text{ A}$

$$I_{sc} = I_1 - I_2 = 2 - (-3) = 5 \text{ A}$$

Step 4 : Draw Norton's equivalent [Fig. 1.84(d)]

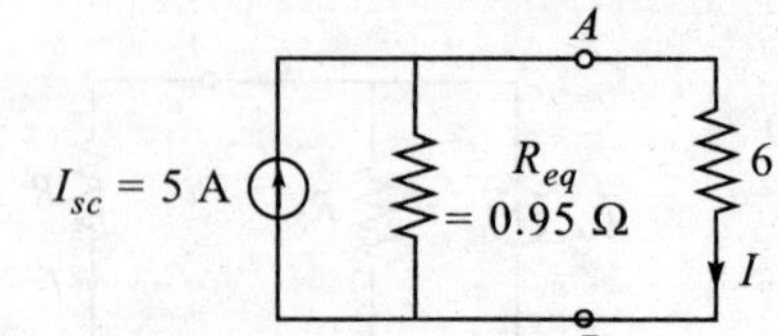

Fig. 1.84(d)

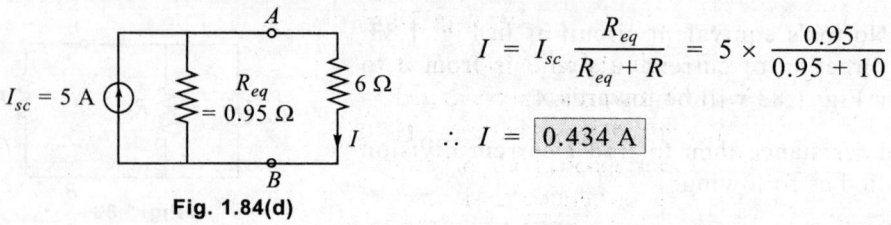

$$I = I_{sc} \frac{R_{eq}}{R_{eq} + R} = 5 \times \frac{0.95}{0.95 + 10}$$

$$\therefore I = \boxed{0.434 \text{ A}}$$

Ex. 1.67 : Using Norton's equivalent find I in Fig. 1.85.

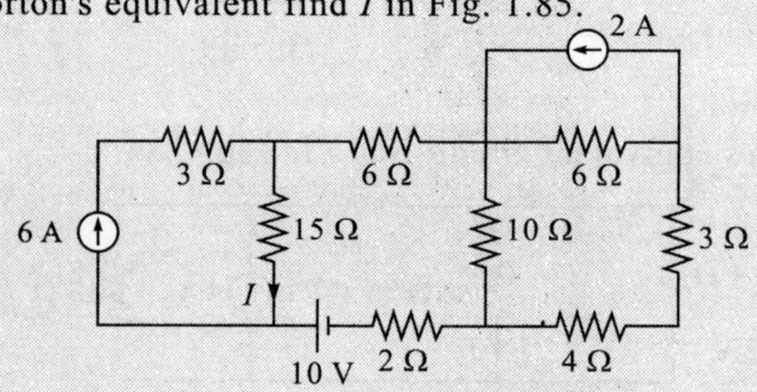

Fig. 1.85

Solution : Step 1 : Remove 5 Ω resistance and mark AB as in Fig. 1.85(a).

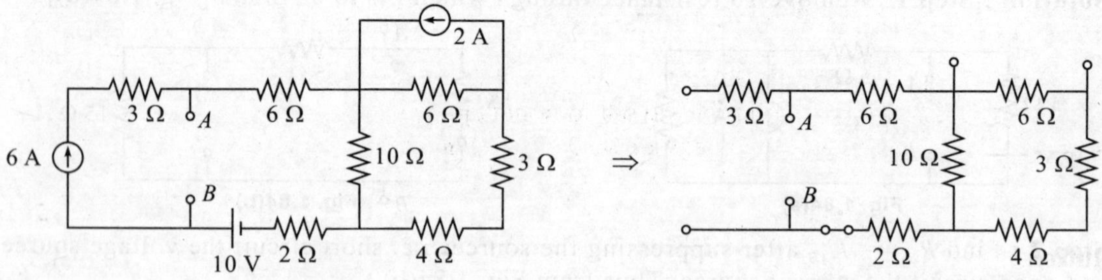

Fig. 1.85(a) **Fig. 1.85(b)**

Step 2 : Find R_{AB} after suppressing all sources Fig. 1.85(b) and solving [Fig. 1.85(c)]

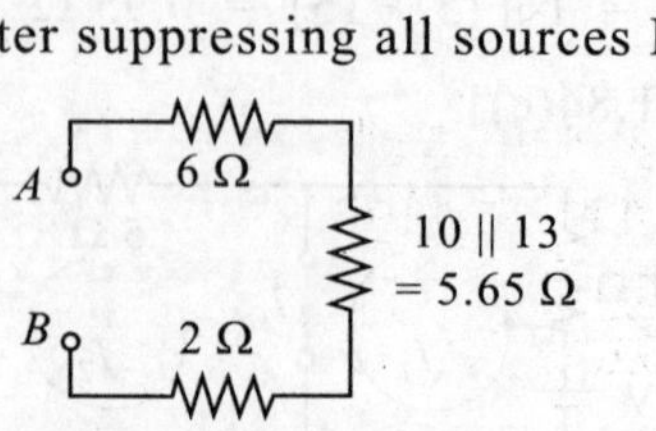

$$\therefore R_{AB} = \boxed{13.65\ \Omega}$$

Fig. 1.85(c)

Step 3 : To find I_{sc}, short terminals AB in Fig. 1.85(a) as in Fig. 1.85(d).

$$I_{sc} = 6 - I_1 \quad .... \text{(i)}$$

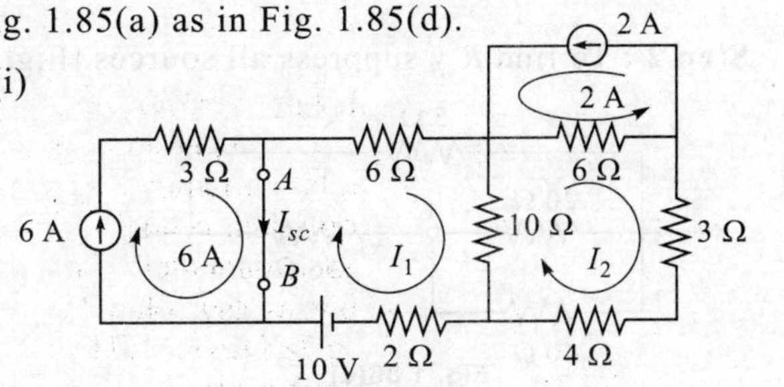

Fig. 1.85(d)

KVL in mesh I_1

$$6I_1 + 10(I_1 - I_2) + 2I_1 - 10 = 0$$

$$18I_1 - 10I_2 = 10 \quad .... \text{(ii)}$$

KVL in mesh I_2

$$10(I_2 - I_1) + 6(I_2 + 2) + 3I_2 + 4I_2 = 0$$

$$-10I_1 + 23I_2 = -12 \quad .... \text{(iii)}$$

Solving (ii) and (ii), we get

$$I_1 = 0.35 \text{ A} \; ; \; I_2 = -0.37 \text{ A}$$

$$\therefore \text{ from (i)} \quad I_{sc} = 6 - I_1$$

$$\therefore I_{sc} = \boxed{5.65 \text{ A}}$$

Step 4 : Draw Norton's equivalent as in Fig. 1.85(e).

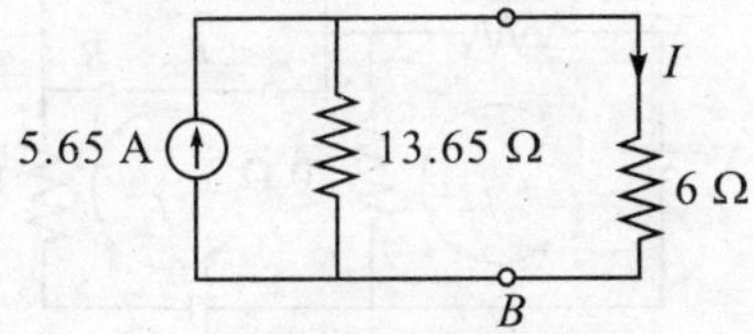

Fig. 1.85(e)

$$I = 5.65 \times \frac{13.65}{13.65 + 5}$$

$$\therefore I = \boxed{4.13 \text{ A}}$$

Ex. 1.68 : Find I in Fig. 1.86 using Norton's theorem.

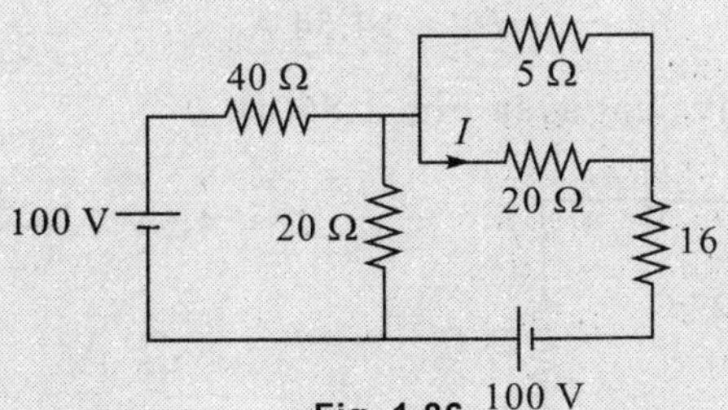

Fig. 1.86

Solution : Step 1 : Remove 20 Ω resistance and mark AB as in Fig. 1.86(a).

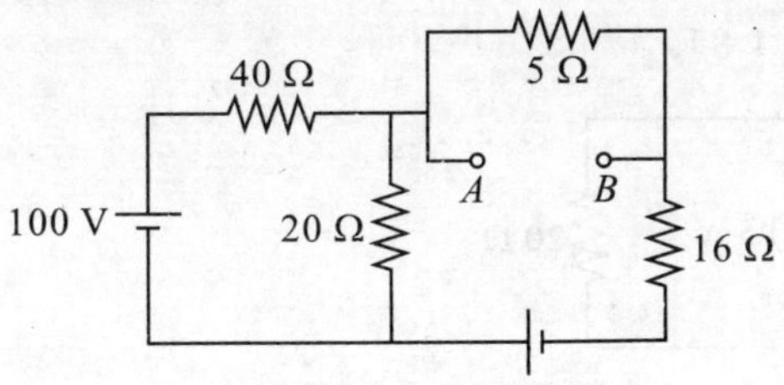

Fig. 1.86(a)

⇒

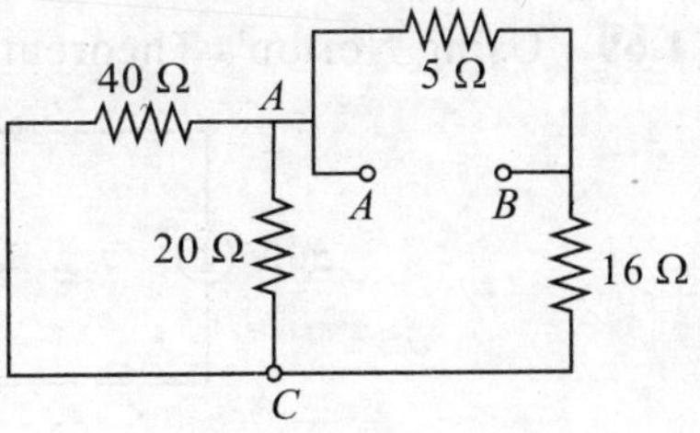

Fig. 1.86(b)

Step 2 : To find R_{AB} suppress all sources [Fig. 1.86(b)]

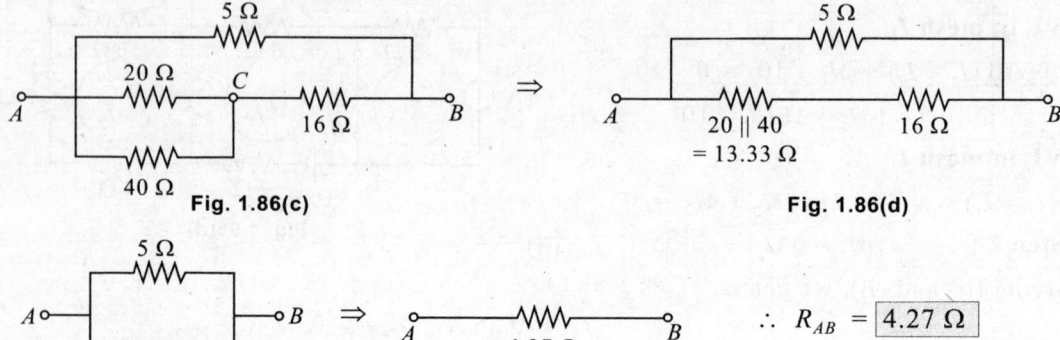

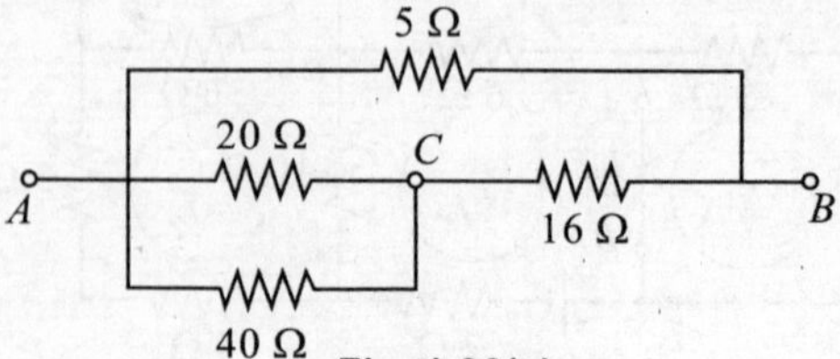

Fig. 1.86(c)

⇒

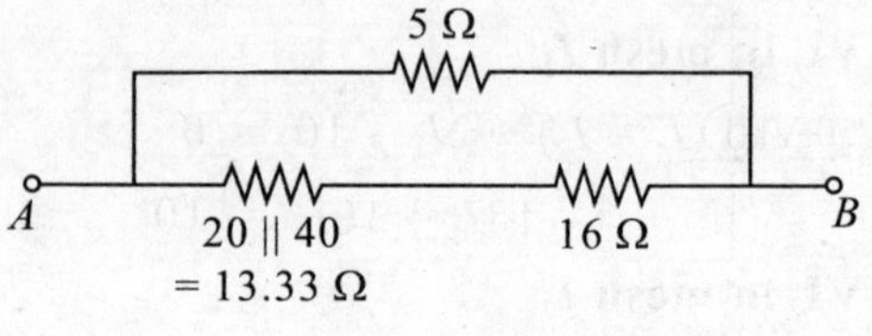

Fig. 1.86(d)

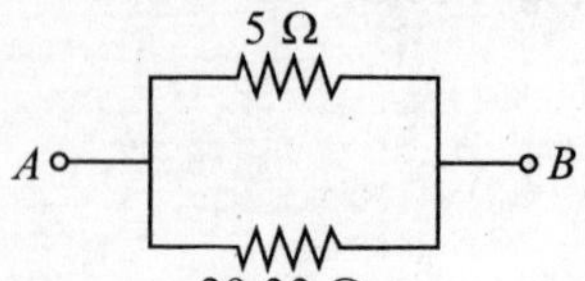

Fig. 1.86(e)

⇒

Fig. 1.86(f)

$\therefore \; R_{AB} = \boxed{4.27\ \Omega}$

Step 3 : To find I_{sc}. Short terminals *AB* Redundant

KVL in mesh I_1

$$-100 + 40I_1 + 20(I_1 - I_{sc}) = 0$$

$$60I_1 - 20I_{sc} = 100$$

KVL in mesh I_{sc}

$$16I_{sc} - 100 + 20(I_{sc} - I_1) = 0$$

$$\therefore \; -20I_1 + 36I_{sc} = 100$$

$$I_{sc} = \boxed{4.54\ \text{A}}$$

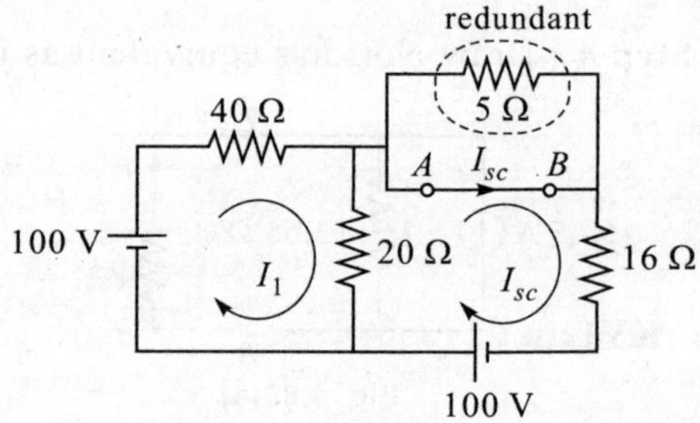

Fig. 1.86(g)

Step 4 : Draw Norton's equivalent as in Fig. 1.86(h).

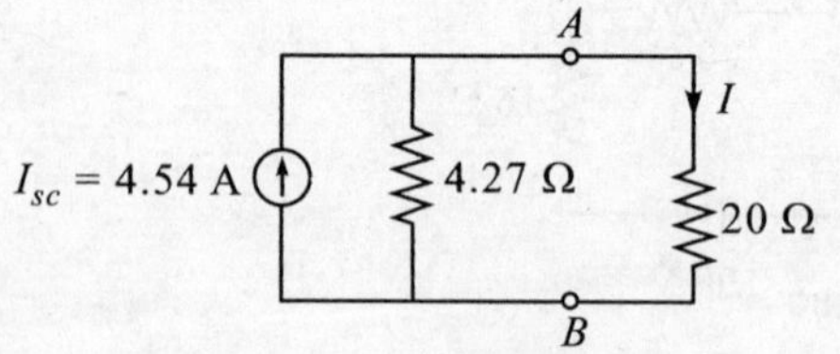

Fig. 1.86(h)

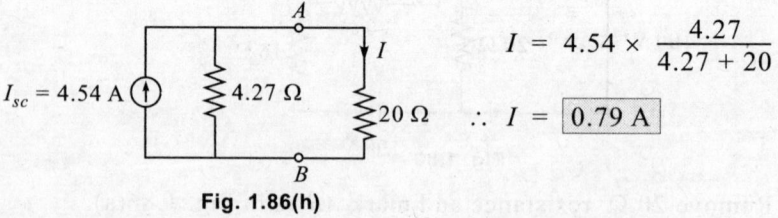

$$I = 4.54 \times \frac{4.27}{4.27 + 20}$$

$$\therefore \; I = \boxed{0.79\ \text{A}}$$

Ex. 1.69 : Using Norton's Theorem find $I_{10\,\Omega}$ in Fig. 1.87.

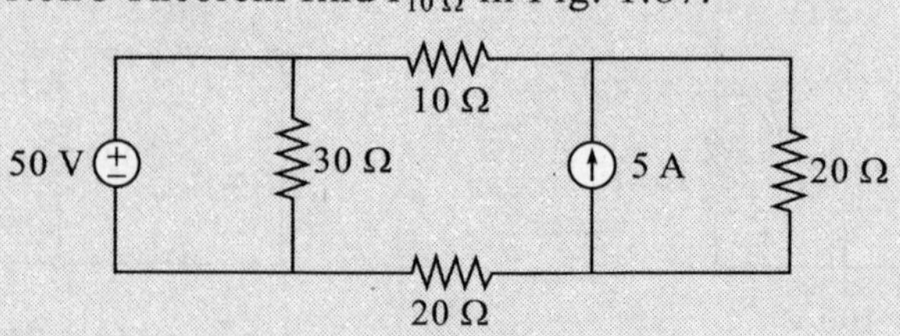

Fig. 1.87

Solution : Step 1 : Remove 10 Ω resistance and name terminals *AB* [Fig. 1.87(a)]

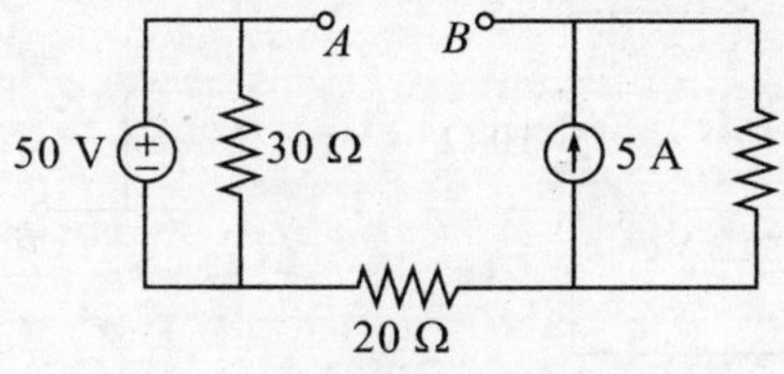

Fig. 1.87(a)

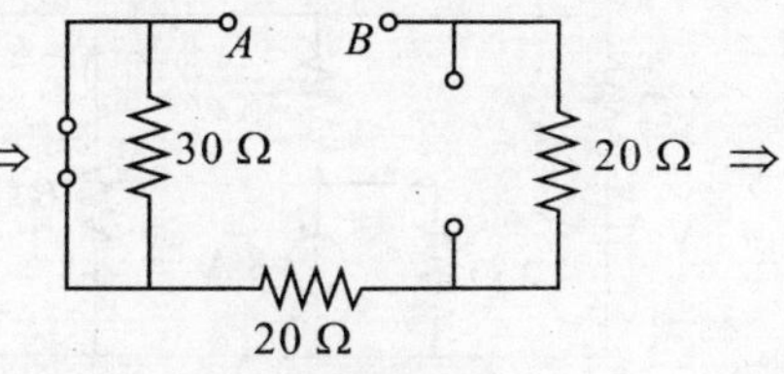

Fig. 1.87(b)

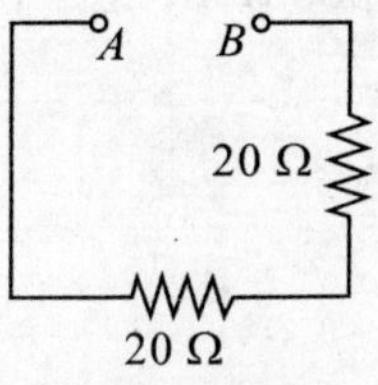

Fig. 1.87(c)

Step 2 : Find R_{AB} by suppressing all sources Fig. 1.87(b).

$$R_{AB} = \boxed{40\ \Omega}$$

Step 3 : Find I_{sc} from Fig. 1.87(a) by shorting *AB* as in Fig. 1.87(d)

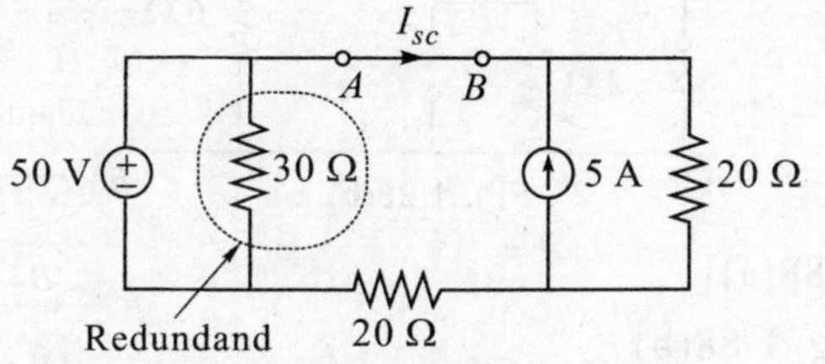

Fig. 1.87(d)

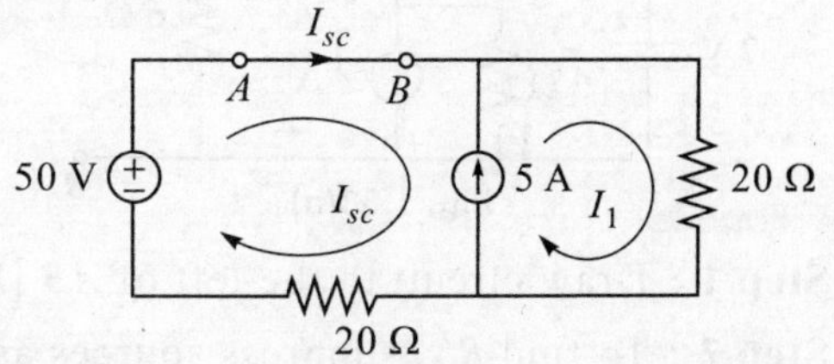

Fig. 1.87(e)

KVL in super mesh I_{sc}, I_1

$$-50 + 20I_1 + 20I_{sc} = 0$$

$$20I_1 + 20I_{sc} = 50 \quad .... \text{(i)}$$

and

$$I_1 - I_{sc} = 5 \quad .... \text{(ii)}$$

Solving (i) and (ii) we get

$$I_1 = 3.75\ \text{A}$$

$$I_{sc} = \boxed{-1.25\ \text{A}}$$

Step 4 : Draw Norton's equivalent circuit as in Fig. 1.87(f) as Fig. 1.87(g)

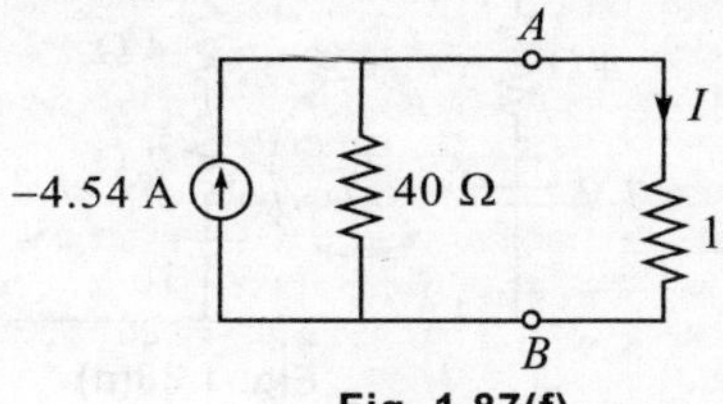

Fig. 1.87(f)

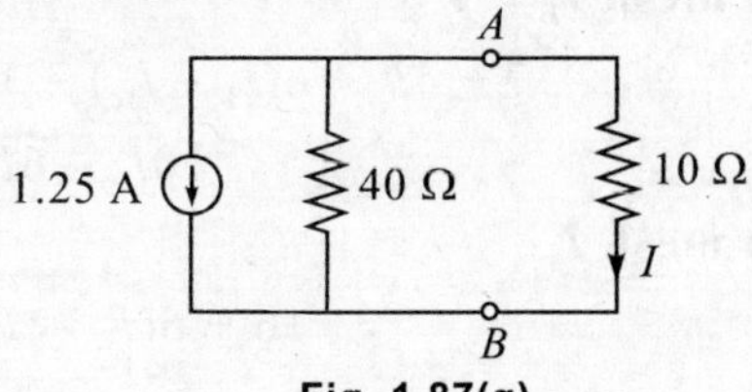

Fig. 1.87(g)

$$\therefore\ I = -1.25 \times \frac{40}{40 + 10}$$

$$I = \boxed{-1\ \text{A}}$$

Negative sign indicates current is from *B* to *A*.

Ex. 1.70 : Find Norton's equivalent to the left of AB in Fig. 1.88, then find I by super position.

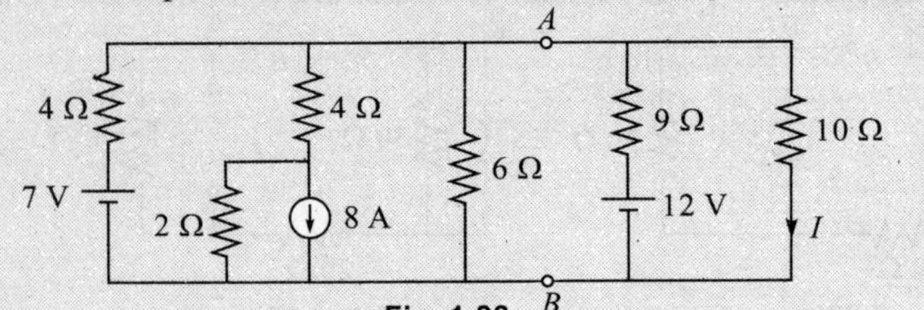

Fig. 1.88

Solution : Let us find Norton's equivalent of the circuit to the left of AB.

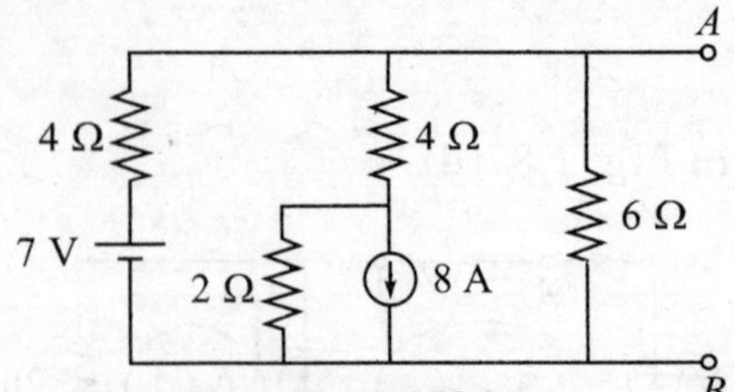

Fig. 1.88(a)

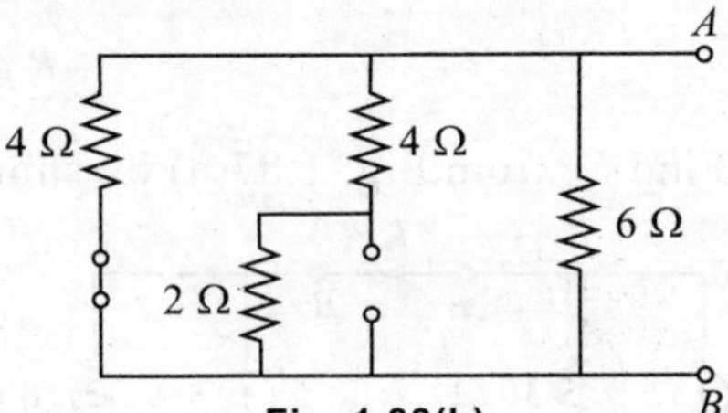

Fig. 1.88(b)

Step 1 : Draw circuit to the left of AB [Fig. 1.88(a)]

Step 2 : To find R_{eq}, suppress sources as in Fig. 1.88(b)

$$R_{AB} = 4 \parallel 6 \parallel 6$$

$$\therefore R_{AB} = \frac{12}{7} = 1.71\ \Omega$$

Step 3 : Find I_{sc} in Fig. 1.88(c). 6 Ω resistance is redundant as it is shorted.

Applying source transformation to 2 Ω in parallel with 8 A source we get Fig. 1.88(d)

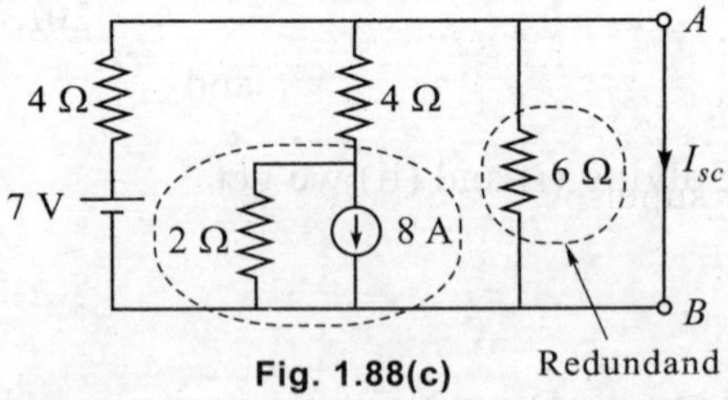

Fig. 1.88(c)

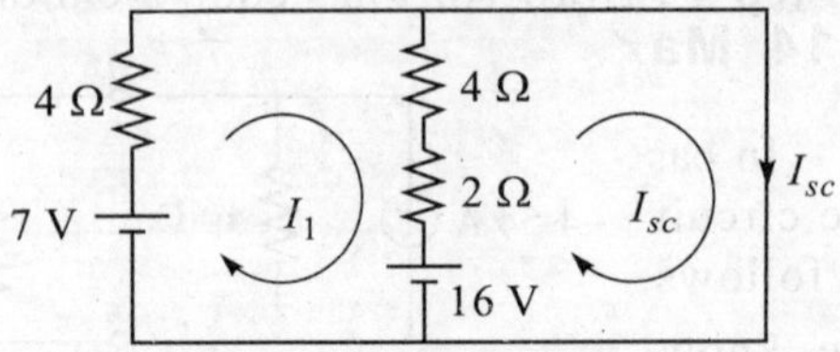

Fig. 1.88(d)

KVL in mesh I_1

$$7 + 4I_1 + 6(I_1 - I_{sc}) - 16 = 0$$

$$10I_1 - 6I_{sc} = 23$$

KVL in mesh I_{sc}

$$16 + 6(I_{sc} - I_1) = 0$$

$$-6I_1 + 6I_{sc} = -16$$

$$\therefore I_1 = 1.75\text{ A}; \quad I_{sc} = \boxed{-0.92\text{ A}}$$

Step 4 : Draw Norton's equivalent of the circuit to left of AB and the remaining circuit of Fig. 1.88, we get Fig. 1.88(e).

For using super position theorem consider 0.92 A source [Fig. 1.88(f)]

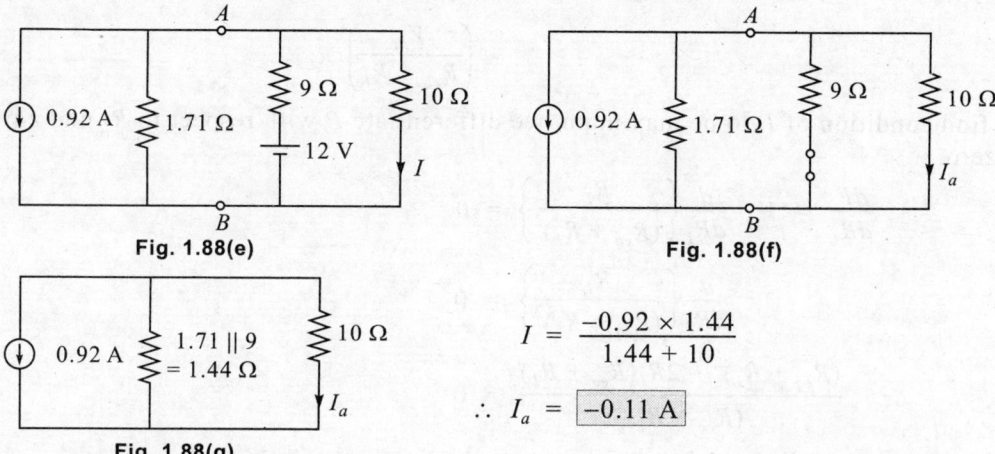

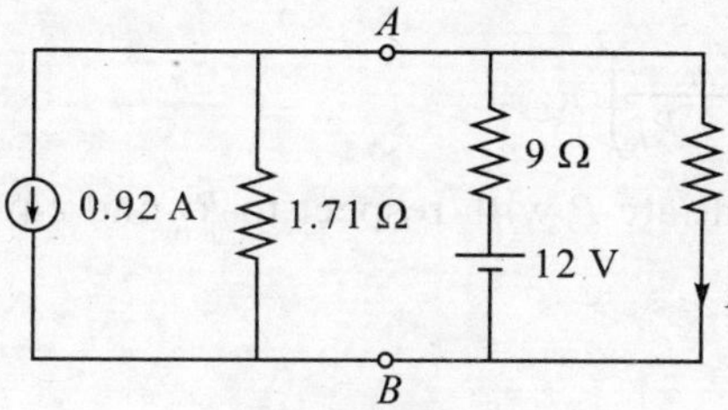

Fig. 1.88(e)

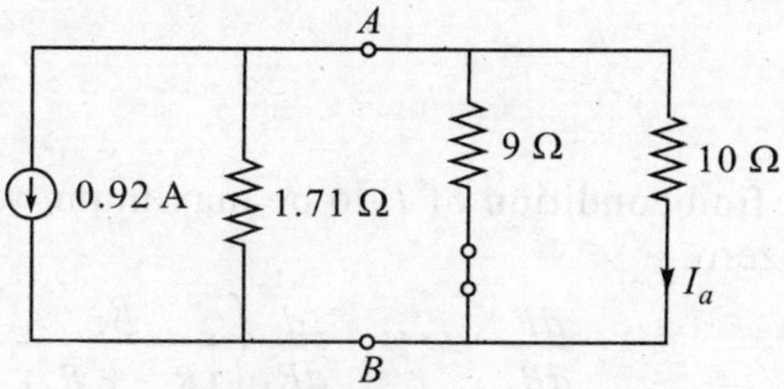

Fig. 1.88(f)

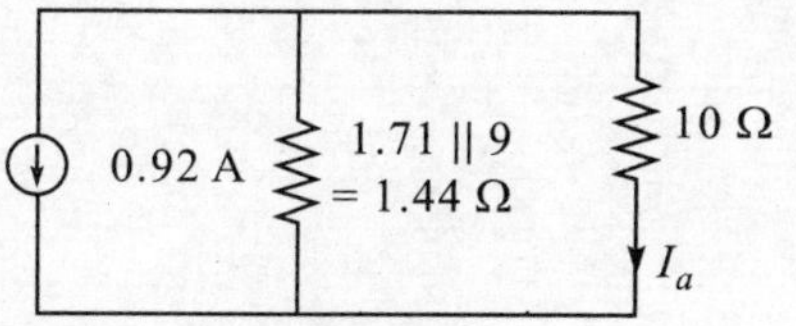

Fig. 1.88(g)

$$I = \frac{-0.92 \times 1.44}{1.44 + 10}$$

$$\therefore \; I_a = \boxed{-0.11 \text{ A}}$$

Consider 12 V source

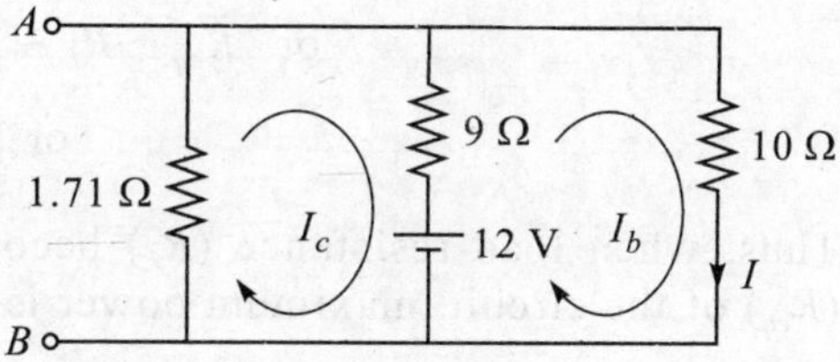

Fig. 1.88(h)

KVL in mesh I_c

$$1.71I_c + 9(I_c - I_b) + 12 = 0$$

$$10.71I_c - 9I_b = -12$$

KVL in mesh I_b

$$10I_b - 12 + 9(I_b - I_c) = 0$$

$$-9I_c + 19I_b = 12$$

$$\therefore \; I_b = 0.17 \text{ A and } I_c = -0.98\text{A}$$

By super position principle

$$I = I_a + I_b = -0.11 + 0.17$$

$$\therefore \; I = \boxed{0.06 \text{ A}}$$

1.14 Maximum Power Transfer Theorem

In case of circuits, very often, the aim is to transfer maximum power to some part of the circuit or to transfer maximum power to a component. This condition may be derived as follows:

We know that a circuit across any two terminals can be replaced by Thevenin's equivalent circuit as in Fig. 1.89. Now we want to derive a condition for resistance R_L such that maximum power is transferred to it.

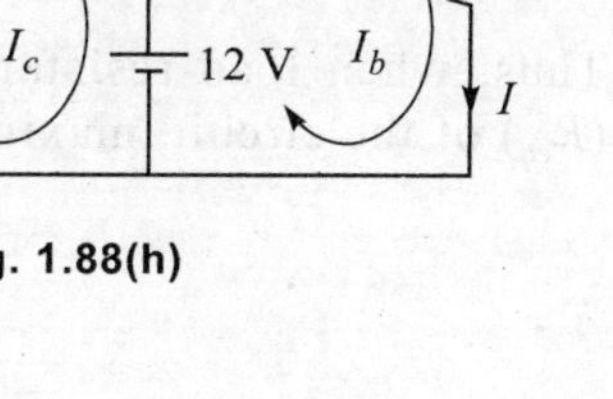

Fig. 1.89

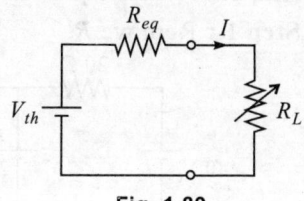

$$I = \frac{V_{th}}{R_{eq} + R_L} \qquad \text{..... (1.38)}$$

$$\text{Power consumed by } R_L = P = I^2 R_L$$

$$= \left(\frac{V_{th}}{R_{eq} + R_L}\right)^2 R_L$$

To find condition of P to be maximum, we differentiate P with respect to R_L and equate it to zero.

$$\frac{dP}{dR_L} = V_{th}^{\;2} \frac{d}{dR_L}\left\{\frac{R_L}{(R_{eq} + R_L)^2}\right\} = 0$$

$$\therefore \quad \frac{d}{dR_L}\left\{\frac{R_L}{(R_{eq} + R_L)^2}\right\} = 0$$

$$\text{or} \quad \frac{(R_{eq} + R_L)^2 - 2R_L(R_{eq} + R_L)}{(R_{eq} + R_L)^4} = 0$$

$$\text{or} \quad (R_{eq} + R_L)^2 - 2R_L(R_{eq} + R_L) = 0$$

$$\text{or} \quad R_{eq} + R_L - 2R_L = 0$$

$$\text{or} \quad \boxed{R_{eq} = R_L} \qquad \text{..... (1.39)}$$

Thus, when load resistance (R_L) becomes equal to the Thevenin's equivalent resistance (R_{eq}) of the circuit, maximum power is transferred to it. From equation (1.39).

$$\therefore \quad I = \frac{V_{th}}{2R_{eq}}$$

$$\therefore \quad P = I^2 R_L = \frac{V_{th}^{\;2}}{4R_{eq}^{\;2}} R_{eq}$$

$$\therefore \quad \boxed{P_{max} = \frac{V_{th}^{\;2}}{4R_{eq}}} \qquad \text{..... (1.40)}$$

Ex. 1.71 : Find R for maximum power transferred to it in Fig. 1.90. Also find the maximum power.

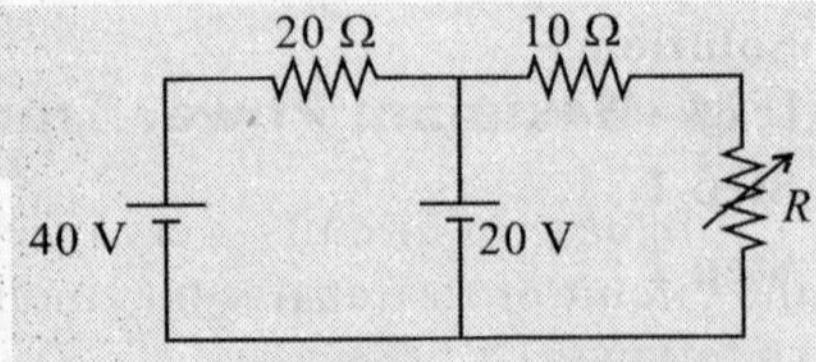

Fig. 1.90

Solution : To find condition for maximum power, first find Thevenin's equivalent across R.

Step 1 : Remove R.

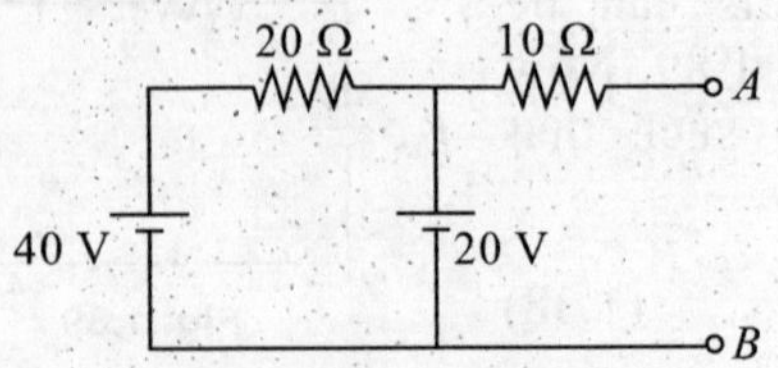

Fig. 1.90(a)

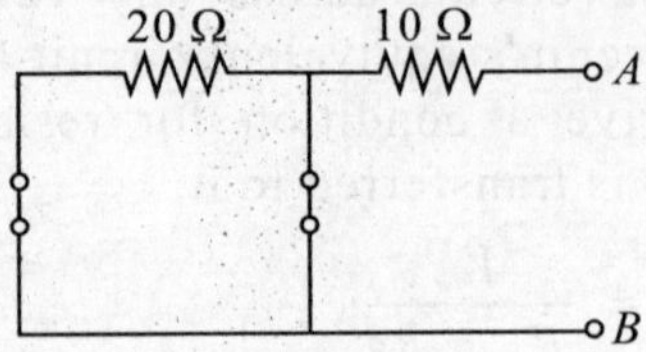

Fig. 1.90(b)

Step 2 : Find open circuit voltage in Fig. 1.90(a), $V_{th} = V_{AB}$.

$$\therefore \; V_{AB} = 20 \text{ V} \quad [\because \text{ no current in } 10\ \Omega]$$

Step 3 : Find equivalent resistance from Fig. 1.90(b).

$$\therefore \; R_{AB} = 10\ \Omega$$

Step 4 : Draw Thevenin's equivalent circuit across R. [Fig. 1.90(c)]

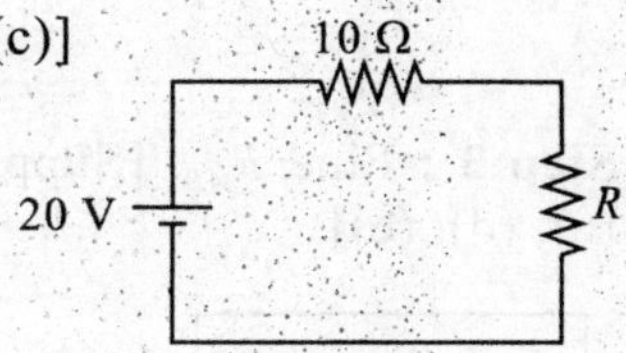

Fig. 1.90(c)

Condition for maximum power from equation (1.39).

$$R = \boxed{10\ \Omega}$$

Maximum power for this resistance R from equation (1.40) is

$$P_{max} = \frac{V_{th}^{\ 2}}{4R_{eq}} = \frac{20^2}{4 \times 10} = 10 \text{ watts}$$

$$P_{max} = \boxed{10 \text{ watts}}$$

Ex. 1.72 : Find R for maximum power transferred to it and also find the power transferred in Fig. 1.91.

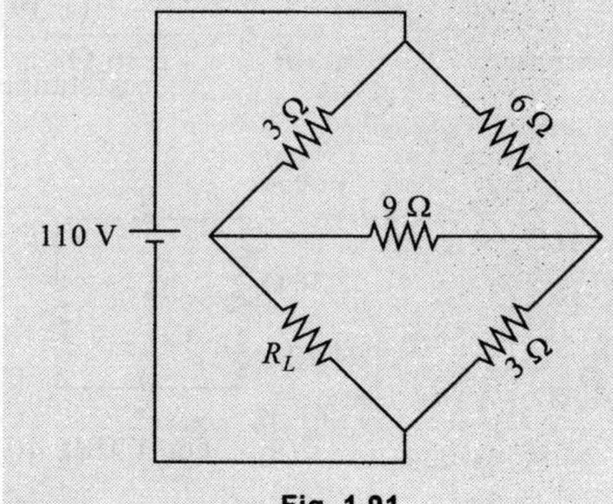

Fig. 1.91

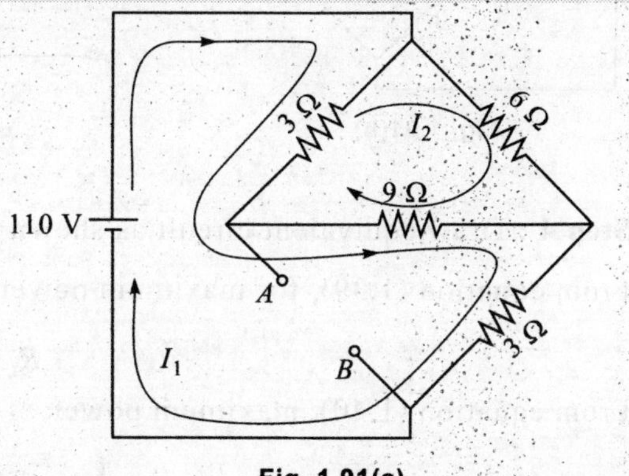

Fig. 1.91(a)

Solution : To find maximum power transferred first find Thevenin's equivalent circuit. [Fig. 1.91(a)]

Step 1 : Remove R_L from circuit Fig. 1.91(a).

Step 2 : Find V_{AB}

$$V_{AB} = 9(I_1 - I_2) + 3I_1 \quad \text{.... (i)}$$

KVL in mesh I_1

$$-110 + 3(I_1 - I_2) + 9(I_1 - I_2) + 3I_1 = 0$$

$$\therefore \; 15I_1 - 12I_2 = 110 \quad \text{.... (ii)}$$

KVL in mesh I_2

$$6I_2 + 9(I_2 - I_1) + 3(I_2 - I_1) = 0$$

$$\therefore \; -12I_1 + 18I_2 = 0 \quad \text{.... (iii)}$$

From (ii) and (ii), we get

$$I_1 = 15.71 \text{ A}; \qquad I_2 = 10.48 \text{ A}$$

$$\therefore \text{ from (i)} \quad V_{AB} = 12I_1 - 9I_2$$

$$V_{AB} = \boxed{94.2 \text{ V}}$$

Step 3 : Find R_{AB}. [Suppress all sources, name junction and simplify as in Fig. 1.91(b), (c), (d), (e)]

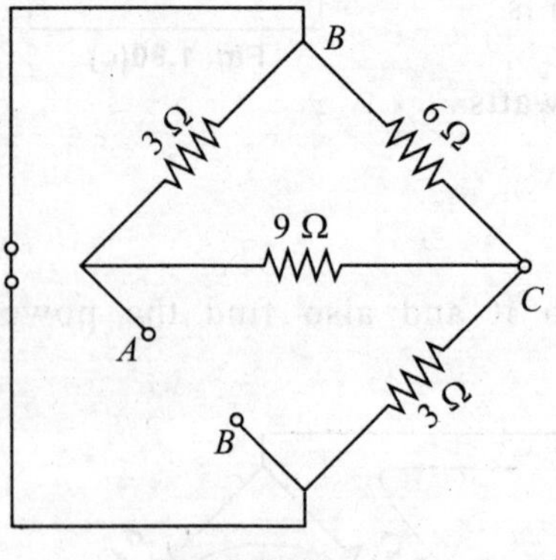

Fig. 1.91(b)

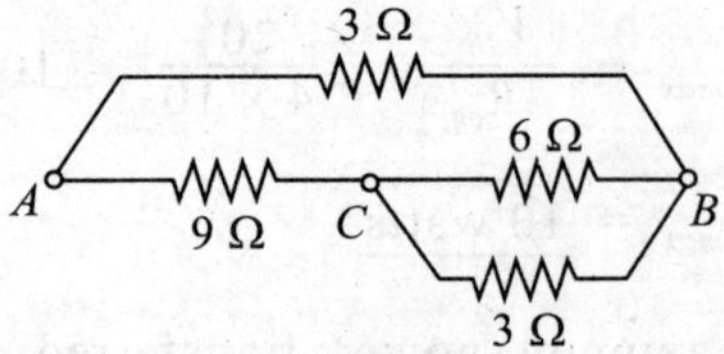

Fig. 1.91(c)

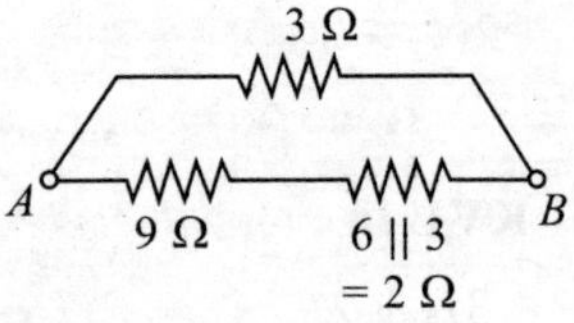

Fig. 1.91(d)

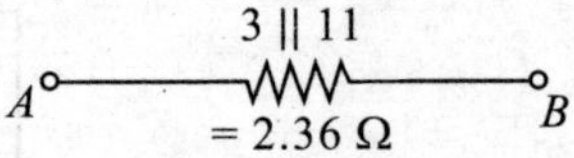

Fig. 1.91(e)

$$\therefore \; R_{AB} = \boxed{2.36 \; \Omega}$$

Step 4 : Draw equivalent circuit as shown in Fig. 1.91(f).

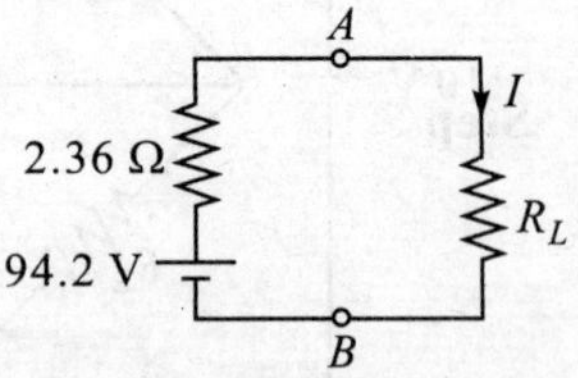

Fig. 1.91(f)

From equation (1.39), for maximum power

$$R_L = \boxed{2.36 \; \Omega}$$

From equation (1.40), maximum power

$$P_{max} = \frac{V_{th}^2}{4R_{eq}} = \frac{94.2^2}{4 \times 2.36} = 940 \text{ watts}$$

$$P_{max} = \boxed{940 \text{ watts}}$$

Ex. 1.73 : Find R for maximum power transferred to it and also find the power transferred in Fig. 1.92.

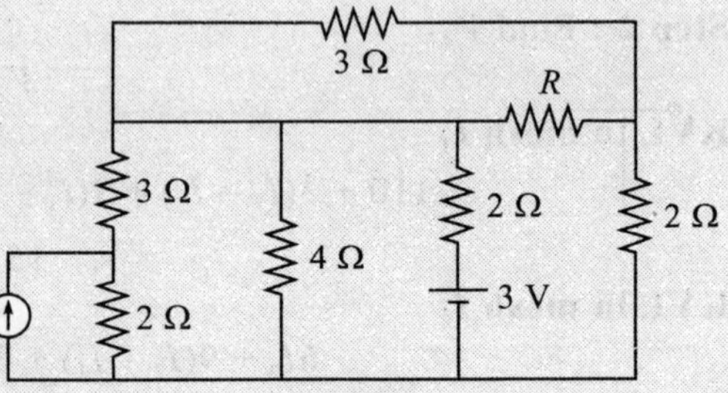

Fig. 1.92

Solution : Step 1 : Remove R

Step 2 : Find V_{AB} in Fig. 1.92(a) using mesh currents.

$$V_{AB} = 3I_3 \quad .... \quad (i)$$

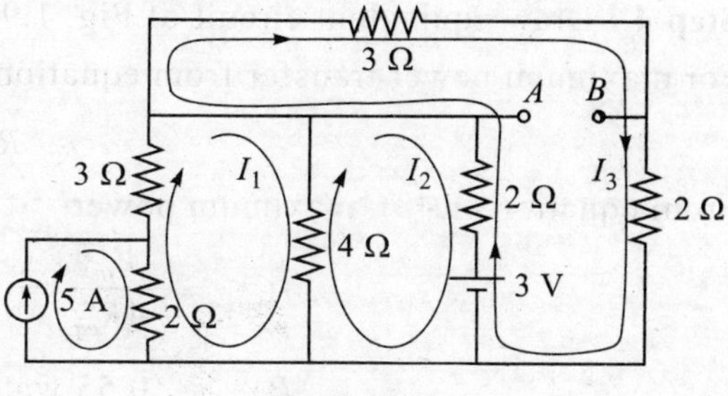

Fig. 1.92(a)

KVL in mesh I_1

$$2(I_1 - 5) + 3I_1 + 4(I_1 - I_2) = 0$$

$$9I_1 - 4I_2 = 10 \quad .... \quad (ii)$$

KVL in mesh I_2

$$2(I_2 - I_3) + 3 + 4(I_2 - I_1) = 0$$

$$-4I_1 + 6I_2 - 2I_3 = -3 \quad .... \quad (iii)$$

KVL in mesh I_3

$$3I_3 + 2I_3 - 3 + 2(I_3 - I_2) = 0$$

$$-2I_2 + 7I_3 = 3 \quad .... \quad (iv)$$

From (ii), (iii) and (iv), we get

$$I_1 = 1.39 \text{ A}; \; I_2 = 0.63 \text{ A}; \; I_3 = 0.61 \text{ A}$$

$\therefore$ from (i)

$$V_{AB} = 3I_3$$

$$V_{AB} = \boxed{1.83 \text{ V}}$$

Step 3 : To find R_{AB}, follow Fig. 1.92(b) to Fig. 1.92(f).

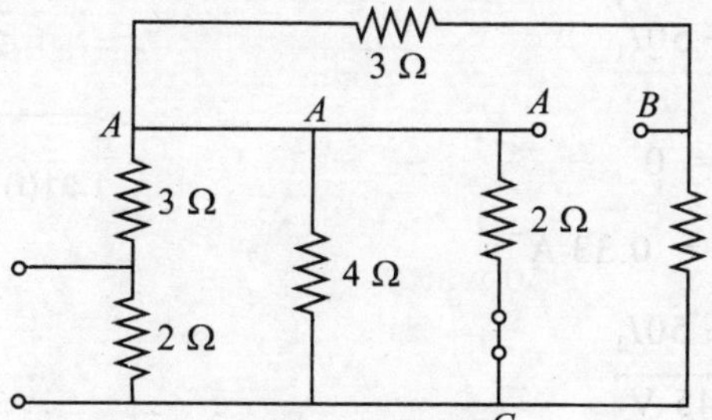

Fig. 1.92(b)

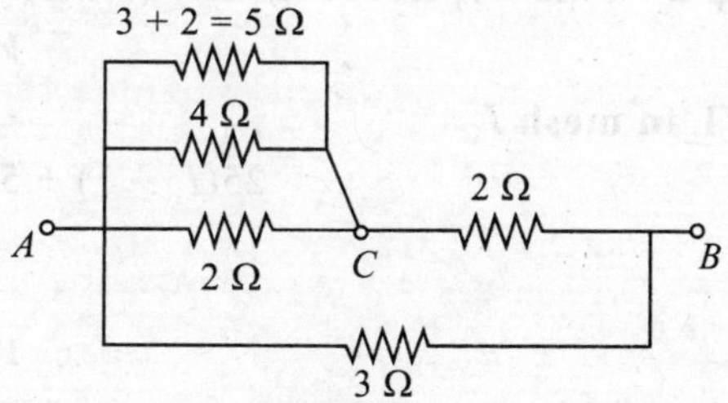

Fig. 1.92(c)

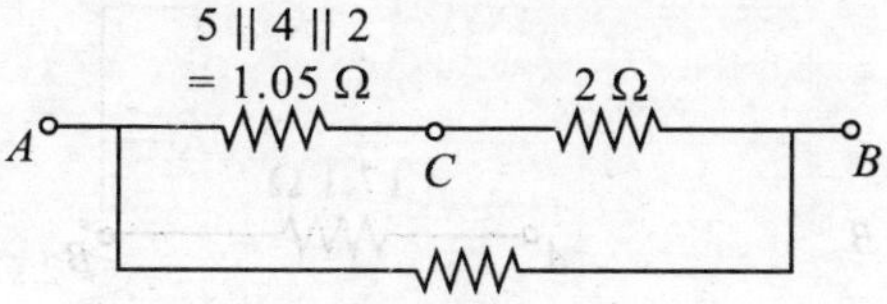

Fig. 1.92(d)

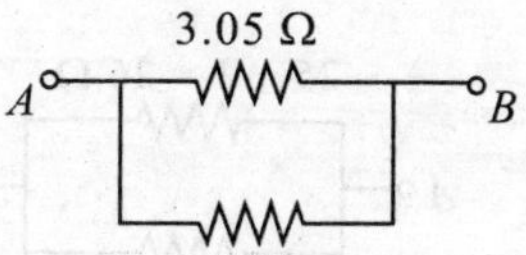

Fig. 1.92(e)

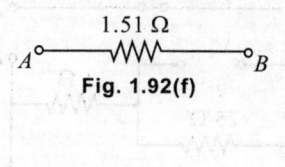

Fig. 1.92(f)

$$\therefore \; R_{AB} = \boxed{1.51 \, \Omega}$$

Step 4 : Draw equivalent circuit of Fig. 1.92 as in Fig. 1.92(g)

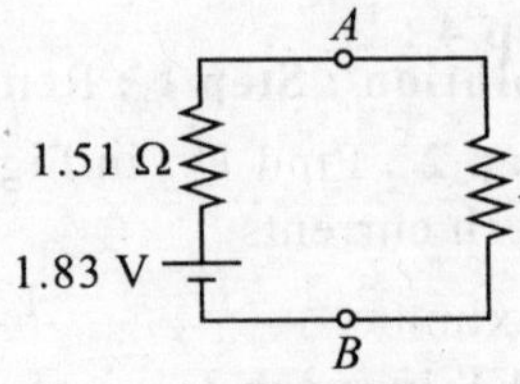

Fig. 1.92(g)

For maximum power transfer from equation (1.39)

$$\therefore \; R = \boxed{1.51 \; \Omega}$$

From equation (1.40), maximum power

$$P_{max} = \frac{V_{th}^2}{4R_{eq}} = \frac{1.83^2}{4 \times 2.36}$$

$$P_{max} = \boxed{0.55 \text{ watts}}$$

Ex. 1.74 : Find R for maximum power transferred to it in Fig. 1.93. Also find the maximum power transferred to it.

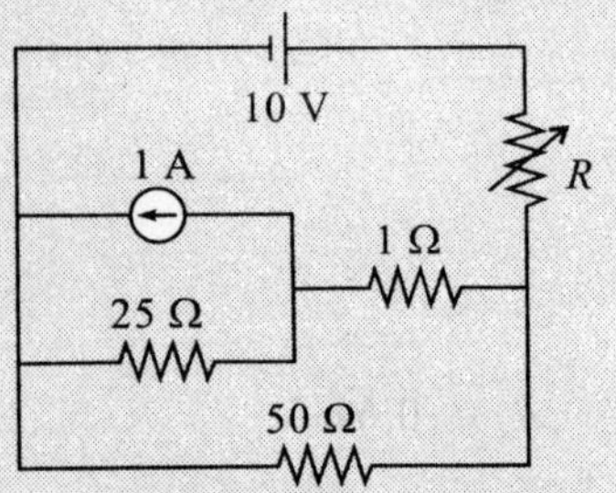

Fig. 1.93

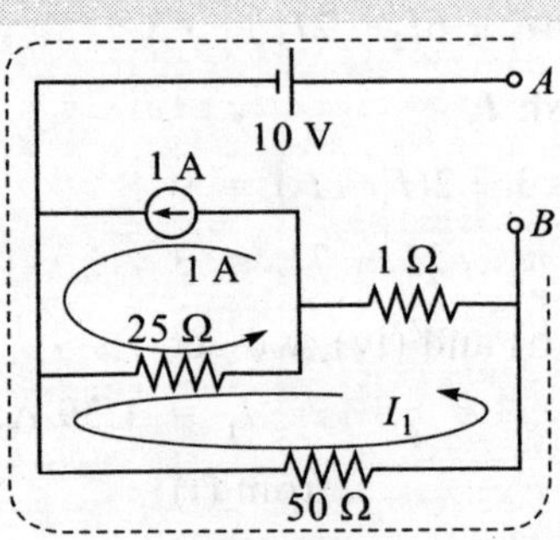

Fig. 1.93(a)

Solution : Step 1 : Remove R from the circuit

Step 2 : Find V_{AB} from Fig. 1.93(a), along the dotted path.

$$V_{AB} = 10 + 50I_1$$

KVL in mesh I_1

$$25(I_1 - 1) + 50I_1 + 1I_1 = 0$$

$$I_1 = \frac{25}{76} = 0.33 \text{ A}$$

$$\therefore \; V_{AB} = 10 + 50I_1$$

$$V_{AB} = \boxed{26.45 \text{ V}}$$

Step 3 : Supress all sources and find R_{AB} Fig. 1.93(b), (c)

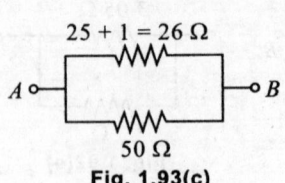

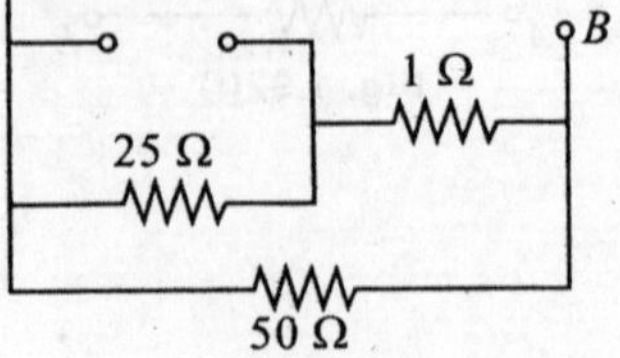

Fig. 1.93(b)

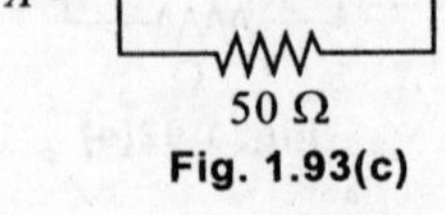

Fig. 1.93(c)

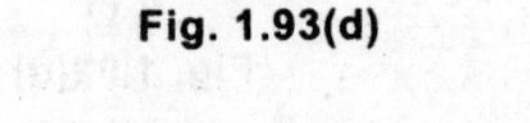

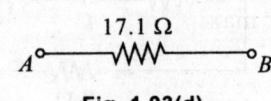

Fig. 1.93(d)

$$\therefore \; R_{AB} = \boxed{17.1 \; \Omega}$$

Step 4 : Draw equivalent circuit of Fig. 1.93 as in Fig. 1.93(e)

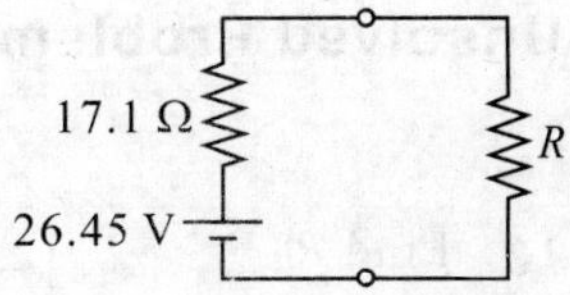

Fig. 1.93(e)

∴ For maximum power transfer

$$\therefore \; R = \boxed{17.1\ \Omega}$$

Maximum Power
$$P_{max} = \frac{V_{th}^2}{4R_{eq}} = \frac{26.45^2}{4 \times 17.1}$$

$$P_{max} = \boxed{10.23 \text{ watts}}$$

Ex. 1.75 : Find R for maximum power also find power in Fig. 1.94.

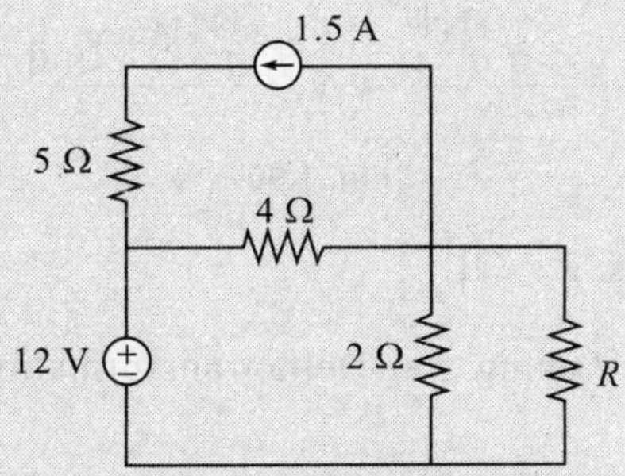

Fig. 1.94

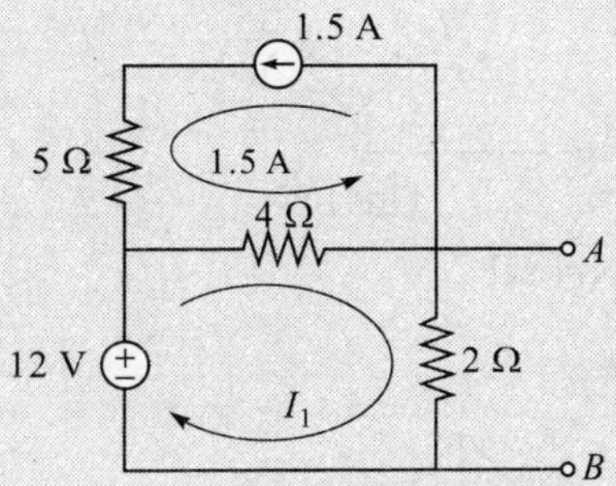

Fig. 1.94(a)

Solution : Step 1 : Remove R [Fig. 1.94(a)].

Step 2 : Define V_{AB}

$$V_{AB} = 2I_1$$

KVL in mesh I_1

$$4(I_1 + 1.5) + 2I_1 - 12 = 0$$

$$\therefore \; I_1 = 1 \text{ A}$$

$$V_{AB} = 2I_1$$

$$V_{AB} = \boxed{2 \text{ V}}$$

Step 3 : Find R_{AB} after suppressing sources [Fig. 1.94(b)].

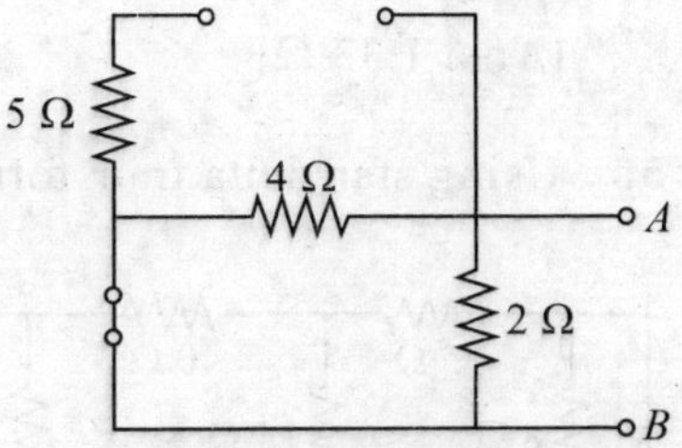

Fig. 1.94(b)

$$R_{AB} = 4 \parallel 2$$

$$\text{or } R_{AB} = \boxed{1.33\ \Omega}$$

Step 4 : Draw equivalent circuit as in Fig. 1.94(c).

For maximum power

$$R = \boxed{1.33\ \Omega}$$

$$\text{Maximum power} = P_{max} = \frac{2^2}{4 \times 1.33}$$

$$P_{max} = \boxed{0.75 \text{ watts}}$$

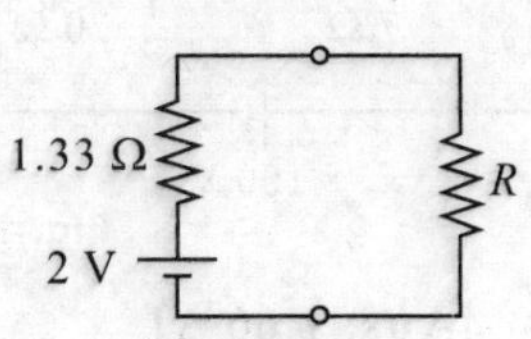

Fig. 1.94(c)

Unsolved Problems

1. Find R_{AB}.

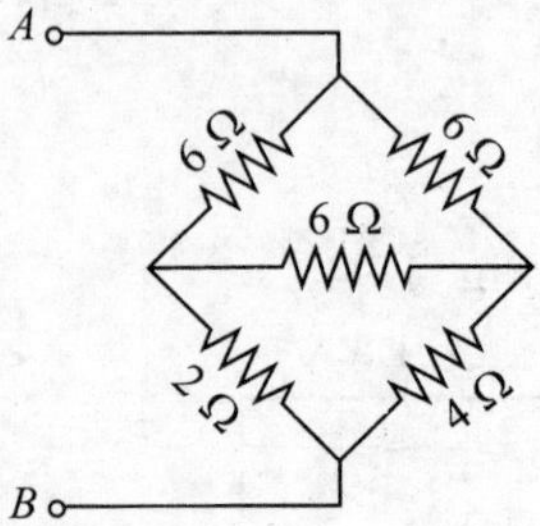

Fig. 1.95

[Ans. 4.4 Ω**]**

2. Find R_{AB}.

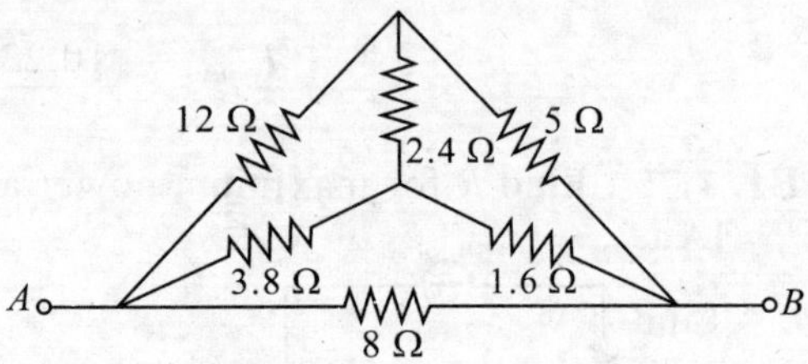

Fig. 1.96

[Ans. 2.7 Ω**]**

3. Find R_{AB}.

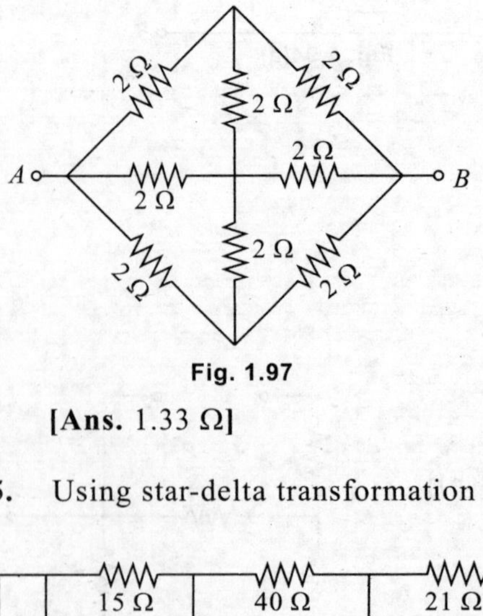

Fig. 1.97

[Ans. 1.33 Ω**]**

4. Find *I* using Star-Delta transformation.

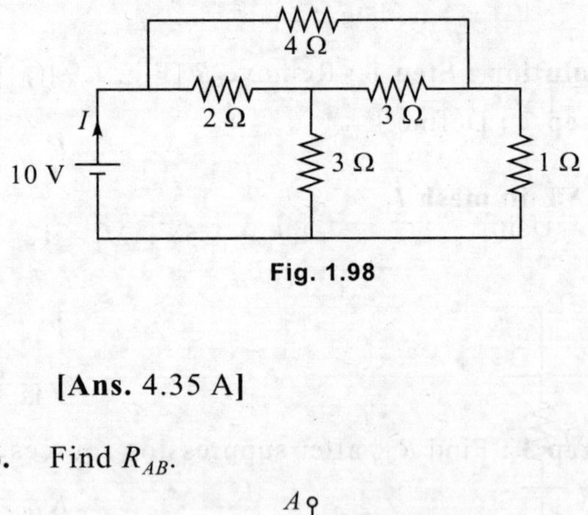

Fig. 1.98

[Ans. 4.35 A**]**

5. Using star-delta transformation find *I*.

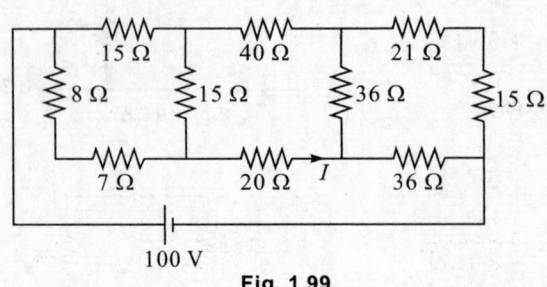

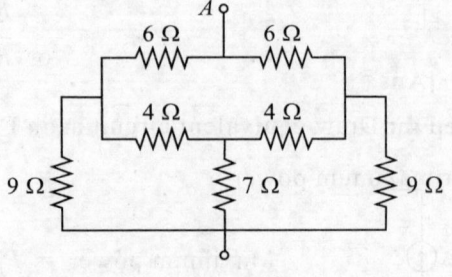

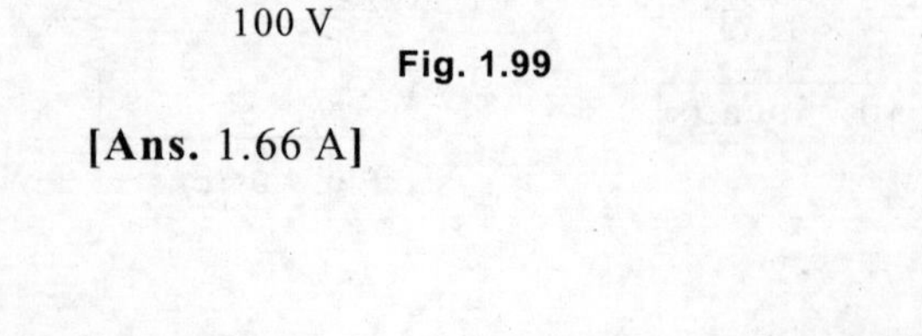

Fig. 1.99

[Ans. 1.66 A**]**

6. Find R_{AB}.

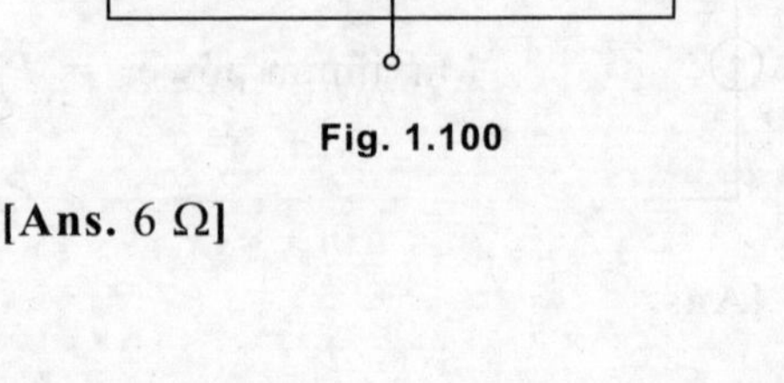

Fig. 1.100

[Ans. 6 Ω**]**

7. Find R_{AB}.

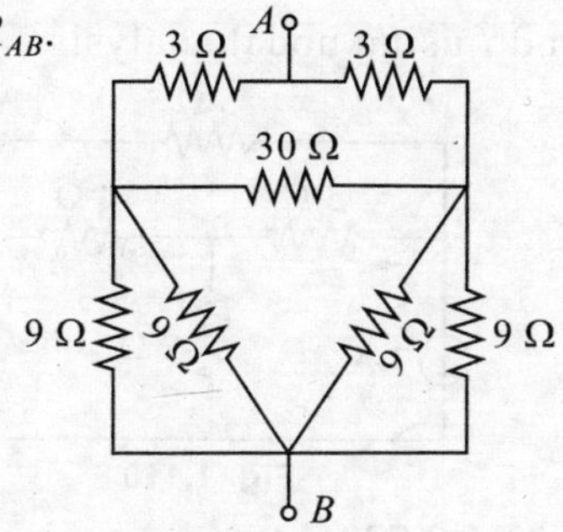

Fig. 1.101

[**Ans.** 3.75 Ω]

8. Find R_{xy}.

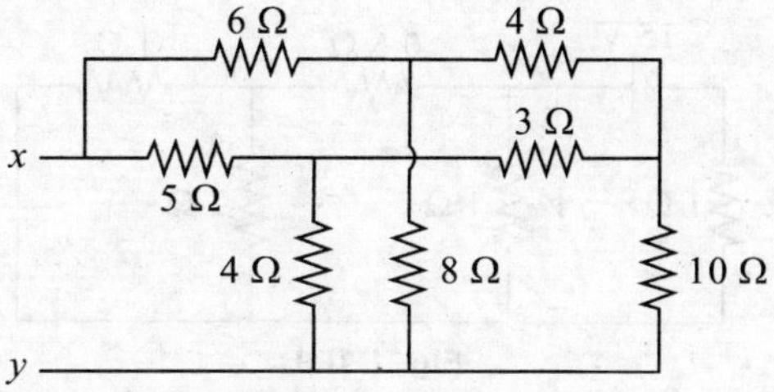

Fig. 1.102

[**Ans.** 4.93 Ω]

9. Find R_{xy}.

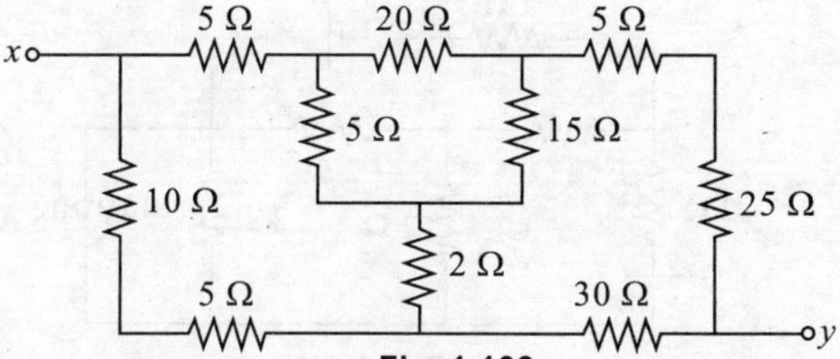

Fig. 1.103

[**Ans.** 21.81 Ω]

10. Using super position theorem find I.

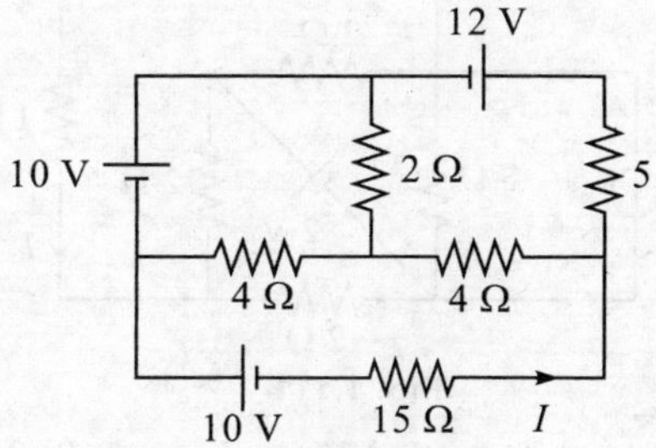

Fig. 1.104

[**Ans.** $I_{10\ V} = -0.477$ A, $I_{10\ V} = -0.569$ A, $I_{12\ V} = -0.352$ A, $I = -1.398$ A]

11. Using mesh analysis find I.

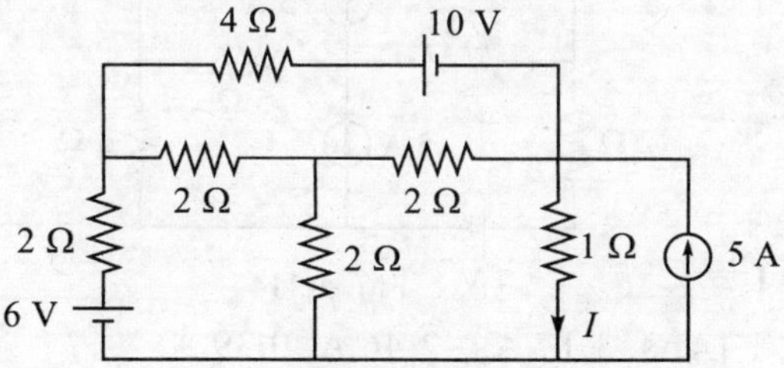

Fig. 1.105

[**Ans.** 5.40 A]

12. Using nodal analysis find I.

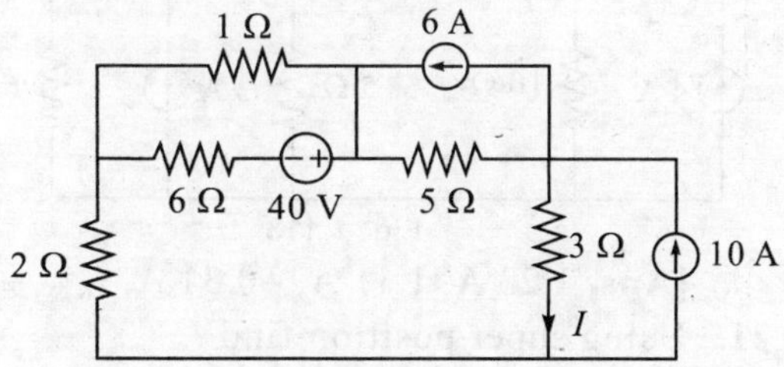

Fig. 1.106

[**Ans.** 4.94 A]

13. Find V using super position theorem.

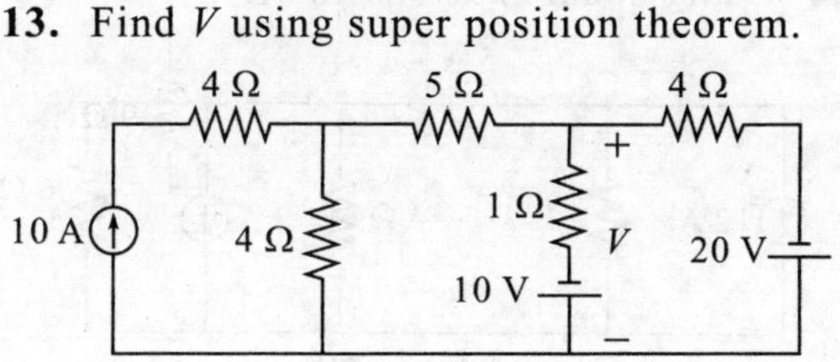

Fig. 1.107

[**Ans.** 3.26 V, –7.34 V, –3.67 V, –7.75 V]

14. Using nodal analysis find I.

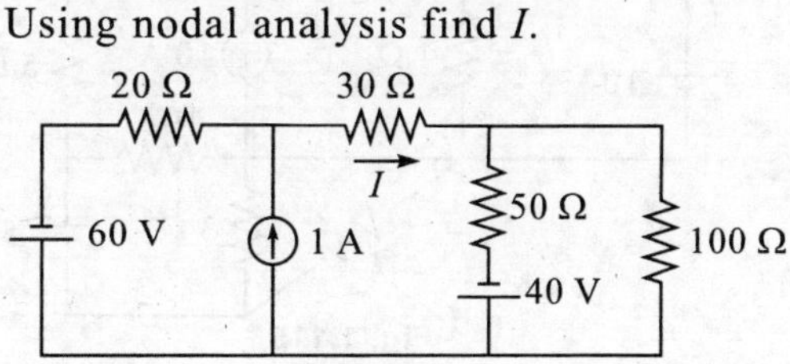

Fig. 1.108

[**Ans.** –0.15 A]

15. Find V using nodal analysis.

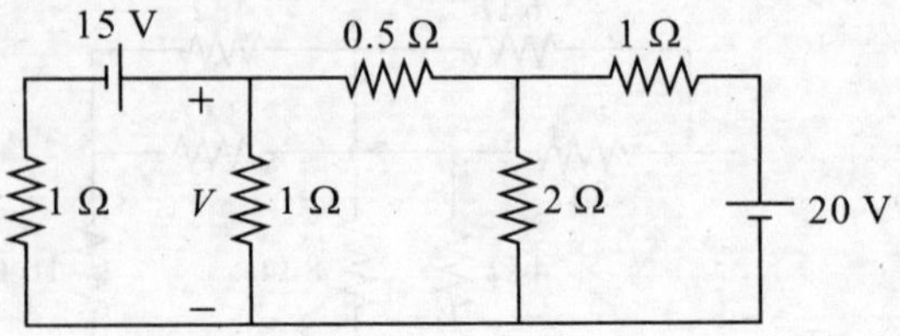

Fig. 1.109

[**Ans.** 9.25 V]

16. Find I using nodal analysis.

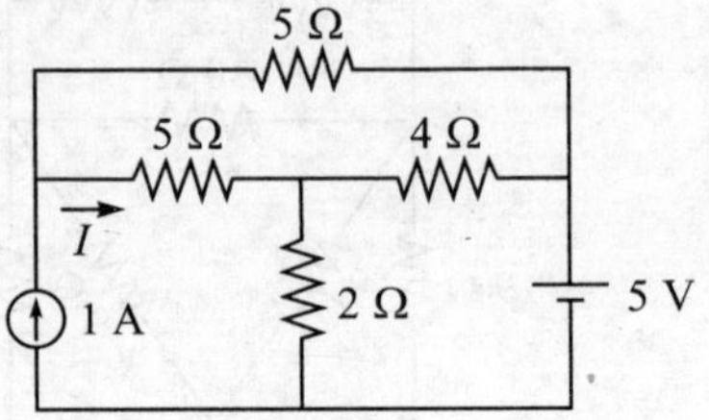

Fig. 1.110

[**Ans.** 0.734 A]

17. Find I using super position theorem.

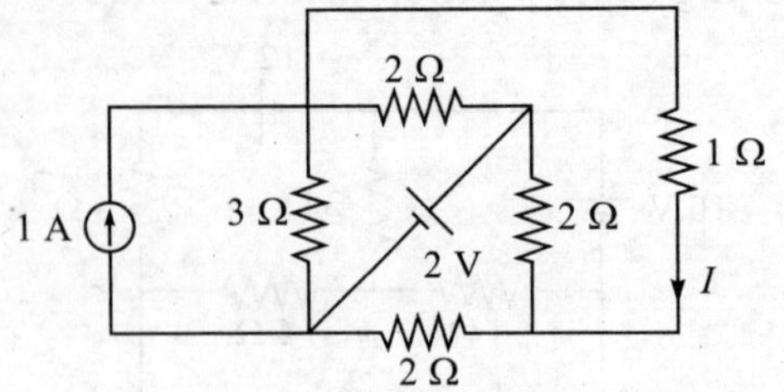

Fig. 1.111

[**Ans.** $I_{1\,A} = 0.375$ A, $I_{2\,V} = 0.0625$ A, $I = 0.437$ A]

18. Find $I_{4\,\Omega}$ super position theorem.

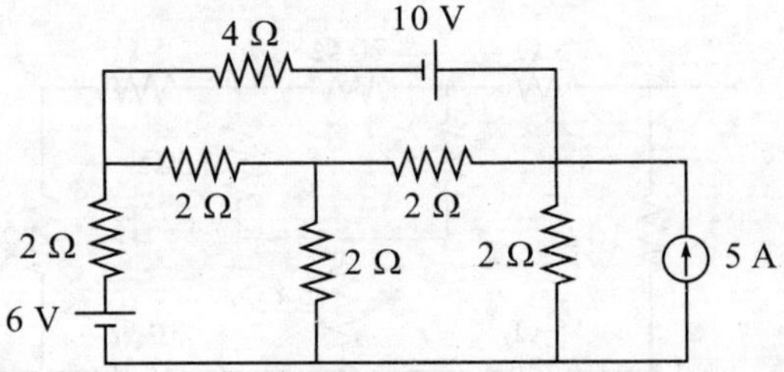

Fig. 1.112

[**Ans.** 0.5 A, 1.67 A, –0.83 A, $I = 1.34$ A]

19. Using super position theorem find $I_{6\,\Omega}$.

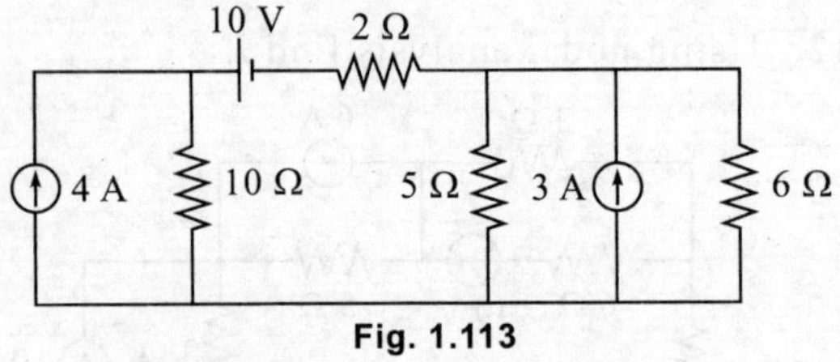

Fig. 1.113

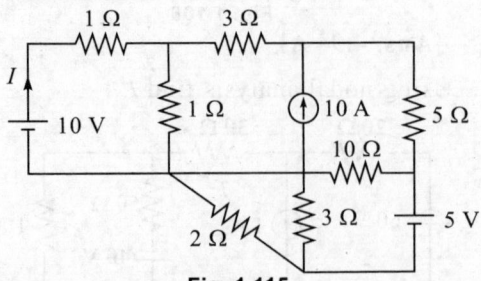

[**Ans.** 1.23 A, 1.11 A, –0.31 A, $I_{6\,\Omega} = 2.03$ A]

20. Using superposition theorem find $I_{3\,\Omega}$.

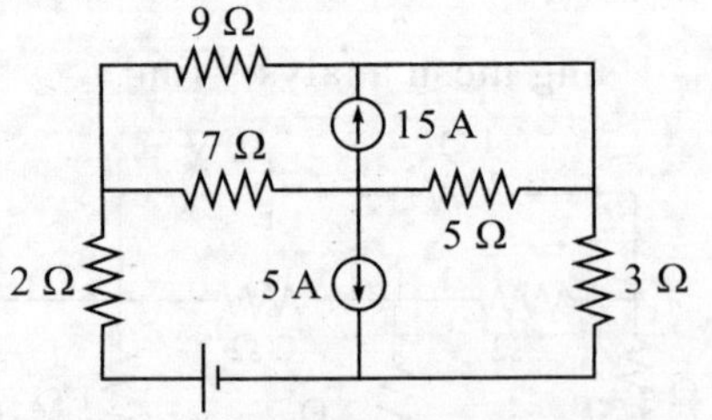

Fig. 1.114

[**Ans.** 3.17 A, –2.46 A, 0.39 A, $I_{3\,\Omega} = 1.1$ A]

21. Using super position find I.

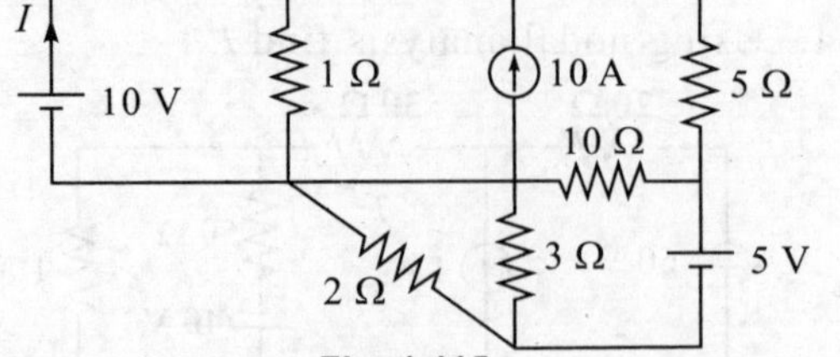

Fig. 1.115

[**Ans.** 5.26 A, –0.23 A, –3.17 A, $I = 1.86$ A]

22. Using nodal analysis find I.

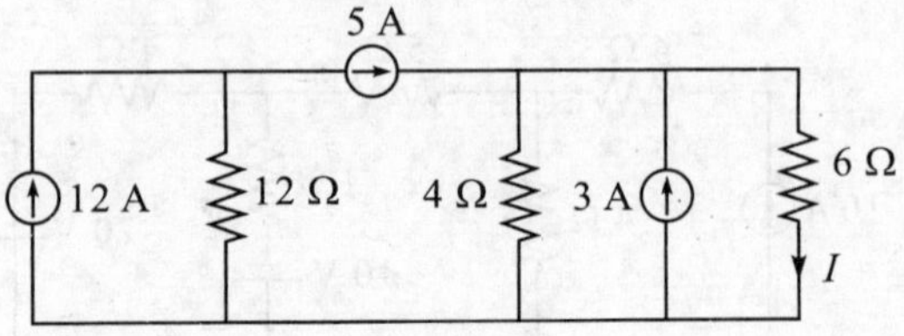

Fig. 1.116

[**Ans.** 3.26 A]

23. Using nodal analysis and super position theorem find I.

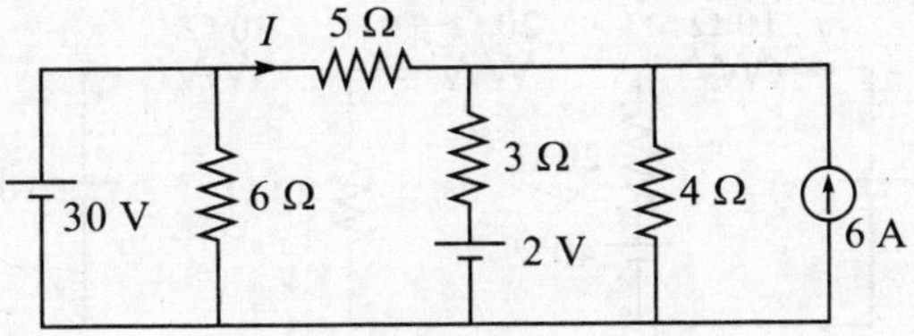

Fig. 1.117

[Ans. 2.76 A**]**

24. Convert the circuit to a single voltage source and resistance.

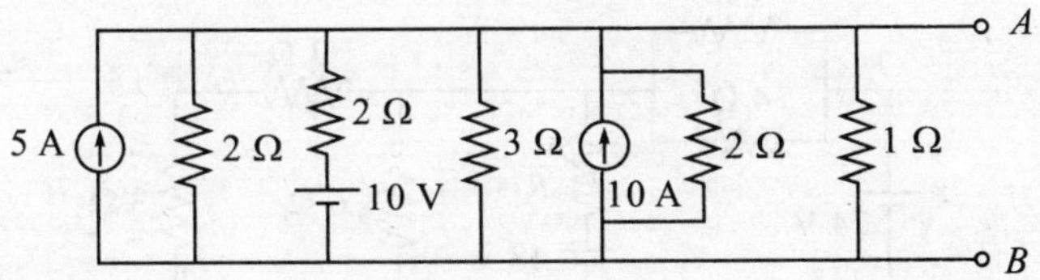

Fig. 1.118

[Ans. 0.35 Ω, 7.06 V**]**

25. Using source transformation and Thevenin's theorem find I.

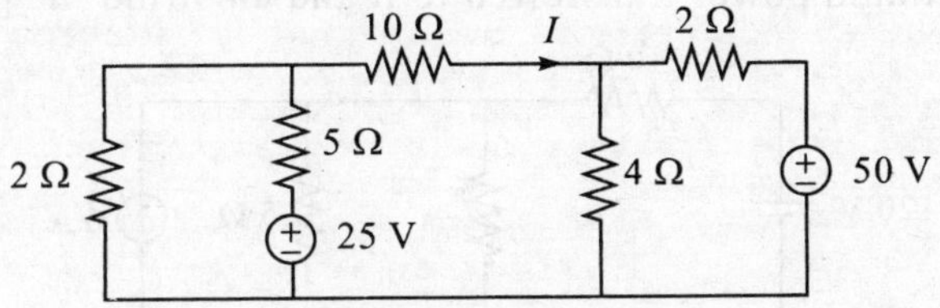

Fig. 1.119

[Ans. −2.05 A**]**

26. Using source transformation find I.

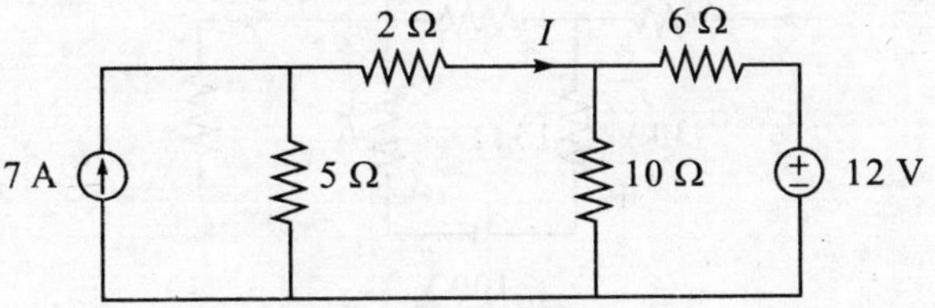

Fig. 1.120

[Ans. 2.56 A**]**

27. Using Norton's theorem find I.

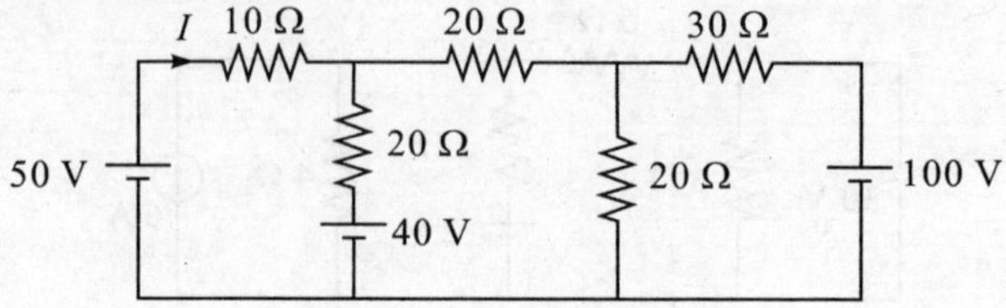

Fig. 1.121

[Ans. I_{sc} = 0.18 A, R_{eq} = 12.31 Ω, I = 0.45 A**]**

28. Find R for maximum power transferred to it and also find the power transferred.

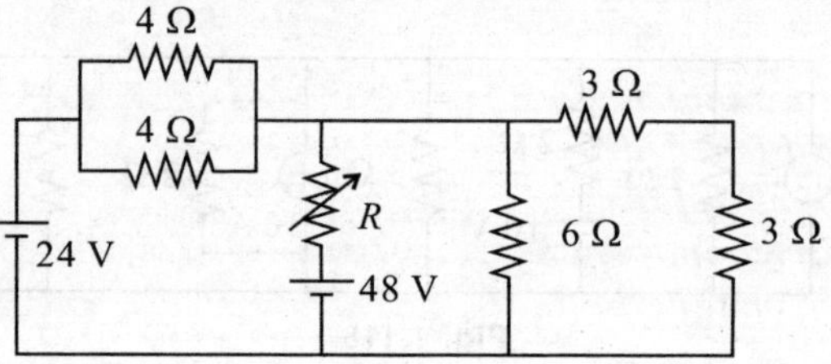

Fig. 1.122

[Ans. 1.2 Ω, 235.2 W**]**

29. Find R for maximum power transferred to it and also find the power transferred.

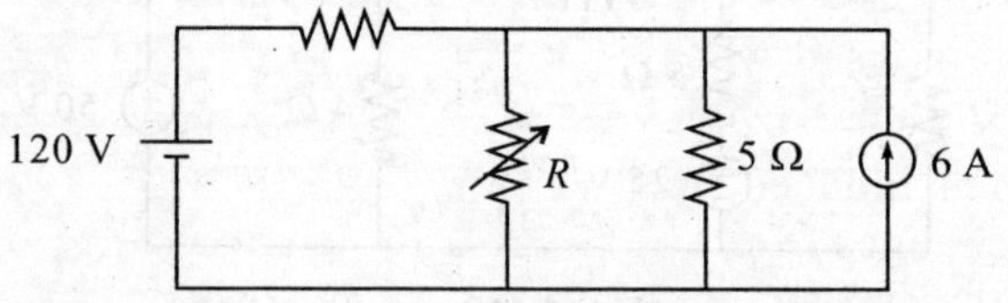

Fig. 1.123

[Ans. 3.33 Ω, 270.27 W**]**

30. Find R.

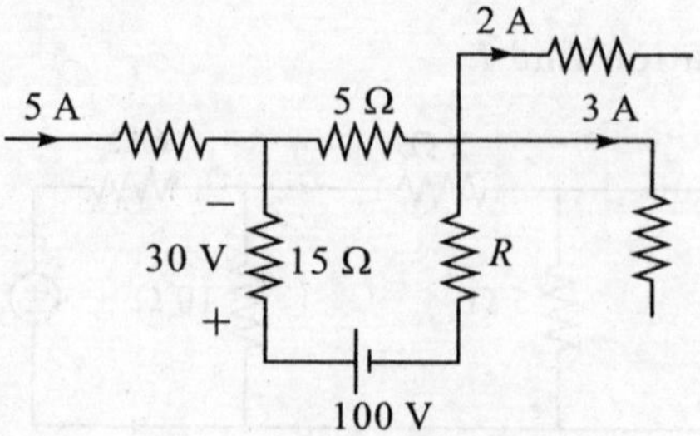

Fig. 1.124

[Ans. 17.5 Ω**]**

CHAPTER

2 ELECTROMAGNETIC INDUCTION

It is a well established fact that whenever an electric current flows through a conductor, a magnetic field is established around it. Conversely, when a magnetic field present around a conductor moves relative to conductor, it produces flow of electrons in the conductor. This phenomenon, where an emf and hence a current is induced in a conductor which is cut by magnetic flux, is known as ***electromagnetic induction***.

2.1 Direction of Induced emf and Current

The direction of induced current depends upon the direction of flux and direction of motion of conductor. It may be found by either *Flemings Right Hand Rule* or *Lenz's Law*. Fleming's right hand rule is used where induced emf is due to flux cutting or motion of conductor in magnetic field i.e. "*dynamically induced emf*".

Lenz's law's is used when induced emf is due to change in flux linkage or when flux which links with a coil changes. In this case there is no motion of the coil relative to the magnetic field and thus the emf so induced is "*statically induced emf*".

2.1.1 Dynamically Induced emf

Consider Fig. 2.1 three conductors *A*, *B* and *C* are shown in cross section in a magnetic field and the arrows on the conductors show their direction of movement. Conductor *A* is moving in the directions of the flux lines. As conductor *A* does not cut any lines of flux no emf induced in it.

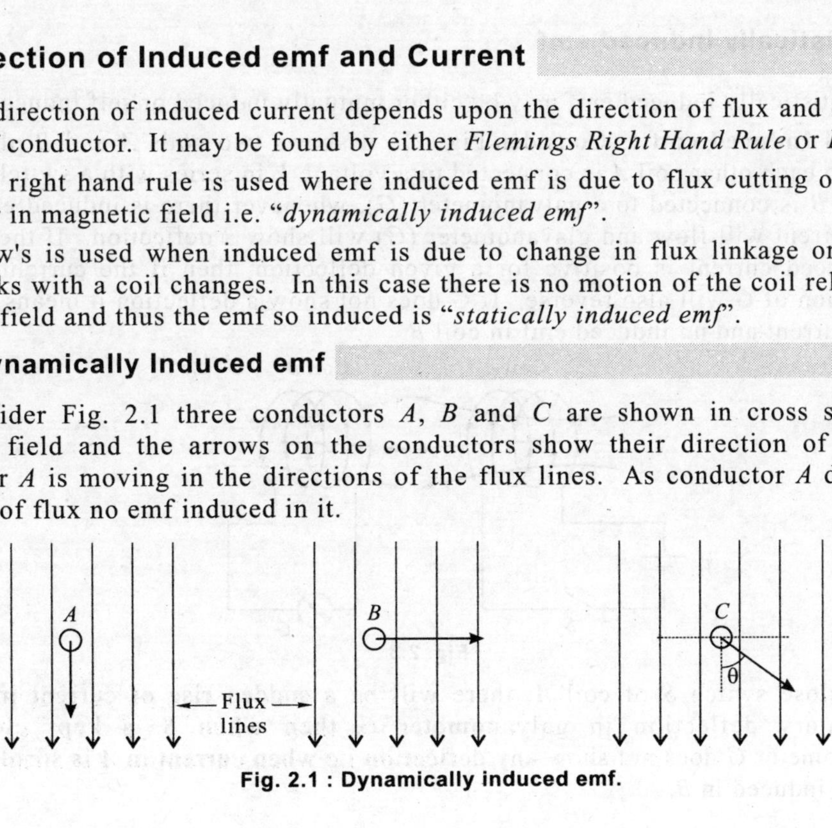

Fig. 2.1 : Dynamically induced emf.

Conductor B moves in a direction perpendicular to its length and perpendicular to the lines of flux, the induced emf in B is given by

$$e = Blv \qquad ..... (2.1)$$

where B is the flux density or field strength in webers per square meters,

l is length of conductor in meters and v is its velocity in meters per second.

The direction of this induced emf is given by Flemings' Right Hand Rules (Fig. 2.2).

Hold the thumb, fore finger and the central finger of your right hand in three mutually perpendicular directions. Then if the fore finger is pointed in the direction of field and the thumb in the direction of motion of the conductor then the central finger will point in the direction of induced emf.

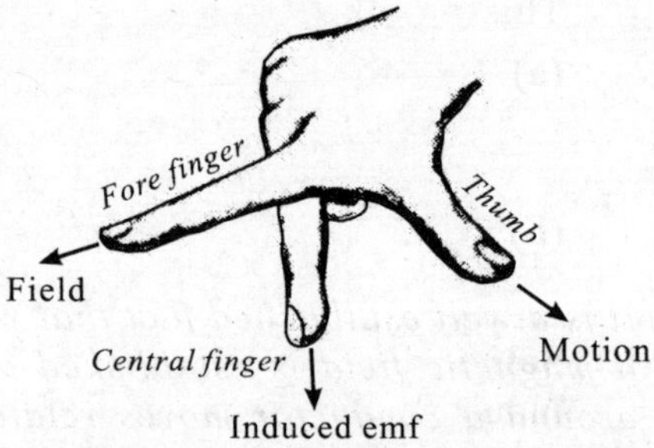

Fig. 2.2 : Fleming's right hand rule.

Conductor C in Fig. 2.1 is moving at an angle θ to the direction of the field. In this case the magnitude of the induced emf is given by

$$e = Blv \sin \theta \qquad ..... (2.2)$$

2.1.2 Statistically Induced emf

The statistically induced emf may be either mutually induced or self induced emf.

(1) Mutual Induced emf : Consider Fig. 2.3 it shows two coils A and B placed very close to each other coil A is connected to a voltage V in series with a switch S, where as coil B is connected to a galvanometer (G), whenever there is induced emf in coil B, a current will flow and glavanometer (G) will show a deflection. If the direction of induced current is positive for a given deflection, then if the current reverses, deflection of G will also reverse. If G does not show a deflection it means that there is no current and no induced emf in coil B

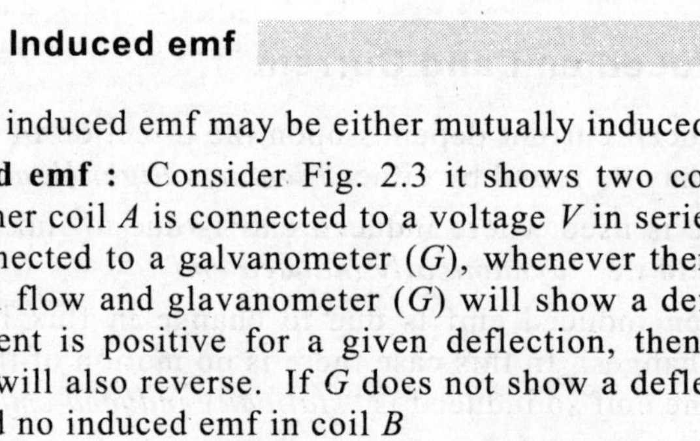

Fig. 2.3

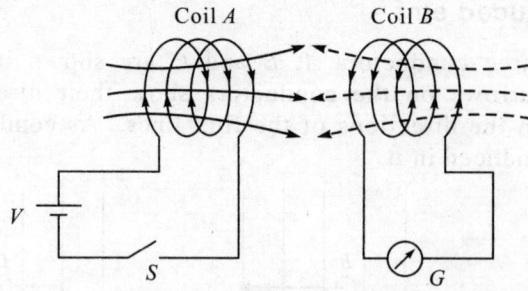

Now, close switch S of coil A. there will be a sudden rise of current in A and a momentary deflection in galvanometer G then when S is kept closed, the galvanometer G does not show any deflection i.e when current in A is steady, there is no emf induced in B.

If now, the switch S is opened suddenly, there is another momentary deflection in G in opposite direction, indicating reverse current, and G will again return to zero deflection position.

This experiment shows, that whenever, the current in coil A changes, there is an emf induced in B and no emf is induced in B if A has steady current. Also, the direction of induced emf by increasing current is opposite to the induced emf by decreasing current.

This can be explained by the following laws :

(a) **Faraday's Law of Electromagnetic Induction :** It states that whenever the number of lines of force linking with a circuit change, an emf is induced is the circuit proportional to the rate of change of flux.

(b) **Lenz's Law :** The direction of induced emf is such that the direction of current set up by it tends to oppose the change producing it.

(ii) **Self Induced emf :** We have learnt that whenever there is a change in flux emf is induced. In mutual induction flux linking in coil B changes due to change in flux produced by A. No matter how this flux is produced, an emf is induced if there is a change of flux linkage.

Thus, if a single coil carries a current it will produce flux, if the current changes the flux will also change. The change in flux will induce an emf in the coil, which in this case, will be called as self induced emf because it is set up by a change in its own current. If the current increases the self induced emf will oppose the current, where as if the current decreases it will act in the same direction as the current (Fig. 2.4).

Fig. 2.4

2.2 Magnetomotive Force (mmf)

For a current to flow in a circuit an *electromotive force (emf)* is a must. Similarly, to drive a flux through a magnetic circuit, a *magnetomotive force (mmf)* is a must.

When a current I flows through N turns, then magnetomotive force is produced and is given by

$$mmf = NI \text{ Amp-turns} \qquad \text{..... (2.3)}$$

2.3 Magnetic Field Strength

The magnetic field strength H is the magneto motive force per meter length of the magnetic circuit. If l is the length of magnetic flux path in meters, then

$$H = \frac{mmf}{l} = \frac{NI}{l} \text{ Amp-turns/m} \qquad \text{..... (2.4)}$$

2.4 Reluctance

Let us consider an iron ring of mean circumference l (Fig. 2.5), and area of cross section 'a' sq.m. with N turns of coil carrying I ampere current.

The total flux flowing in the dotted path of l is given by

$$\phi = \textit{Flux density} \times \textit{Area of cross section}$$

$$\text{or} \quad \phi = B \times a \qquad \text{..... (2.5)}$$

Also, $mmf = Hl$ from equation (2.4)

$$\therefore \quad \frac{\phi}{mmf} = \frac{Ba}{Hl} \qquad \text{..... (2.6)}$$

$$\text{But} \quad B = \mu_0 \mu_r H \qquad \text{..... (2.7)}$$

where, μ_0 and μ_r are constants and depend upon the magnetic material.

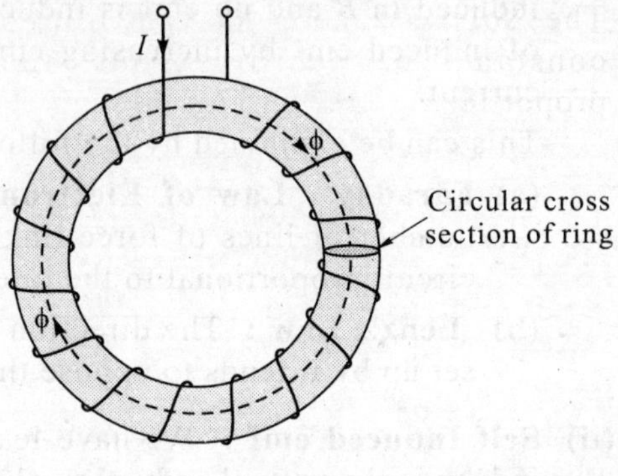

Fig. 2.5

For air and non-magnetic material $\mu_r = 1$.

From equations (2.6) and (2.7) we get

$$\frac{\phi}{mmf} = \mu_0 \mu_r \frac{a}{l}$$

$$\text{or} \quad \frac{mmf}{\phi} = \frac{l}{\mu_0 \mu_r a} \qquad \text{..... (2.8)}$$

This equation is similar to equation (2.9)

$$\frac{emf}{Current} = R = \rho \frac{l}{a} \qquad \text{..... (2.9)}$$

Thus from equation (2.8) and equation (2.9) an analogy between electric and magnetic circuits can be drawn i.e. *mmf* is analogous to *emf*,

flux to *current*

and $\frac{emf}{Current}$ is called *resistance*,

similarly, $\frac{mmf}{flux}$ can be called as *reluctance*.

It is a property of magnetic material which opposes the flow of the flux through it. It is denoted by S and given by equation (2.10) for magnetic materials.

$$\text{i.e. Reluctance} = S = \frac{l}{\mu_0 \mu_r a} \qquad \text{..... (2.10)}$$

2.5 Co-efficients of Self Inductance

Consider a solenoid of Fig. 2.6, with N turns, length l meters and area of cross section a m^2. Let, the current passing through the coil be I ampere. This current will produce a flux ϕ. If this current changes, the flux will change and hence emf will be induced in it.

This induced emf e as per Faraday's laws of electromagnetic induction, will be given by

$$e = -N\frac{d\phi}{dt} \qquad \text{..... (2.11)}$$

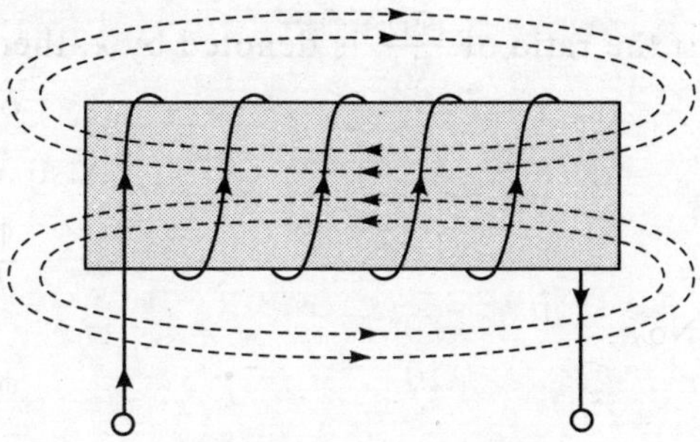

Fig. 2.6 : Self induced emf.

The solenoid here has an iron core with constant permeability. Thus, the flux is proportional to the current through the coil I

$$\therefore \phi \propto I$$

$$\text{or} \quad \frac{\phi}{I} = Constant$$

$$Flux = \frac{Flux}{Current} \times Current$$

$$\therefore \phi = \frac{\phi}{I} \times I$$

But $\frac{\phi}{I}$ = constant, if current is changing at a certain rate than flux will also change at the same rate.

$$\therefore \quad \frac{d\phi}{dt} = \frac{\phi}{I} \times \frac{dI}{dt} \qquad \text{..... (2.12)}$$

Thus, substituting $\frac{d\phi}{dt}$ from equation (2.12) in equation (2.11)

We, get

$$e = -N\frac{\phi}{I} \cdot \frac{dI}{dt} \qquad \text{..... (2.13)}$$

The term $\frac{N\phi}{I}$ is called *flux linkage per ampere* called *self inductance of the coil*, denoted by L.

Its practical unit is Henery.

$$\therefore L = \frac{N\phi}{I} \qquad \text{..... (2.14)}$$

$$\text{and } e = -L\frac{dI}{dt} \qquad \text{..... (2.15)}$$

The negative sign of equation (2.15) indicates that induced emf oppose the change in current i.e. if the current is increasing the induced emf will oppose this increase (Fig. 2.4) and if the current is a decreasing current than the induced emf will try to increase this current.

2.6 Co-efficient of Mutual Inductance

Consider two coils 1 and 2 be placed close to each other as in Fig. 2.7

Let N_1 = Number of turns in coil 1

ϕ_1 = Flux in coil 1 due to current I_1

N_2 = Number of turns in coil 2

ϕ_{12} = Flux in coil 2 due to flux ϕ_1

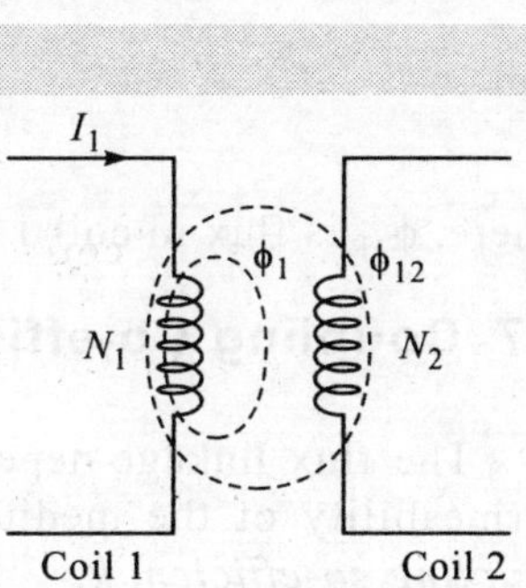

Fig. 2.7 : Mutually induced emf.

If the ratio of $\frac{\phi_{12}}{\phi_1}$ is denoted by k, then

$$\phi_{12} = k\phi_1 \quad \text{..... (2.16)}$$

$$\text{Also } \phi_1 \propto I_1$$

$$\text{or } \frac{\phi_1}{I_1} = \text{Constant} \quad \text{..... (2.17)}$$

Now,

$$\phi_{12} = \frac{\phi_{12}}{I_1} \times I_1$$

$$\phi_{12} = \frac{k\phi_1}{I_1} \times I_1 \quad \text{..... (2.18)}$$

i.e. when I_1 changes ϕ_{12} also changes with the same rate as $\frac{k\phi_1}{I_1}$ is a constant.

$$\therefore \frac{d\phi_{12}}{dt} = \frac{k\phi_1}{I_1}\frac{dI_1}{dt} \quad \text{..... (2.19)}$$

According to Faraday's laws of electromagnetic induction.

$$e_2 = N_2 \times \text{Rate of change of flux } \phi_{12}$$

$$= N_2 \frac{d\phi_{12}}{dt}$$

$$= N_2 \frac{k\phi_1}{I_1}\frac{dI_1}{dt}$$

$$\text{or } e_2 = M\frac{dI_1}{dt} \quad \text{..... (2.20)}$$

$$\text{where, } M = \frac{N_2 k\phi_1}{I_1} = \frac{N_2 \phi_{12}}{I_1} \quad \text{..... (2.21)}$$

$$= \frac{\text{Flux linkage of coil 2}}{\text{Current in coil 1}}$$

The constant M is called the *co-efficient of mutual induction* or *mutual inductance.* Mutual inductance is bilateral and analogous results are obtained if a time varying current I_2 is introduced in coil 2, thus

$$M = \frac{\text{Flux linkage of coil 1}}{\text{Current in coil 2}} \quad \text{..... (2.22)}$$

$$= \frac{N_1 k\phi_2}{I_2} = \frac{N_1 \phi_{21}}{I_2} \quad \text{..... (2.23)}$$

where, ϕ_{21} is flux in coil 1 due to flux ϕ_2 in coil 2.

2.7 Coupling Co-efficient

The flux linkage depends on spacing and orientation of the axes of the coils and on permeability of the medium. The fraction of total flux which links the coils in called *coupling co-efficient k*.

From equation (2.16),

$$k = \frac{\phi_{12}}{\phi_1} = \frac{\phi_{21}}{\phi_2} \qquad \text{..... (2.24)}$$

Since $\phi_{12} \leq \phi_1$ and $\phi_{21} \leq \phi_2$ the maximum value of k is unity. Now, multiply equations (2.21) and (2.23), we get

$$M^2 = \frac{N_2\,\phi_{12}}{I_1} \times \frac{N_1\,\phi_{21}}{I_2}$$

$$M^2 = \frac{N_2\,k\phi_1}{I_1} \times \frac{N_1\,k\phi_2}{I_2}$$

$$M^2 = k^2\left(\frac{N_1\,\phi_1}{I_1}\right)\left(\frac{N_2\,\phi_2}{I_2}\right) \qquad \text{..... (2.25)}$$

Substitute $L_1 = \dfrac{N_1\,\phi_1}{I_1}$ and $L_2 = \dfrac{N_2\,\phi_2}{I_2}$ in equation (2.25), we get

$$M^2 = k^2\,L_1 L_2$$

$$\therefore \quad M = k\sqrt{L_1 L_2} \qquad \text{..... (2.26)}$$

2.8 Rise of Current in Inductive Circuits

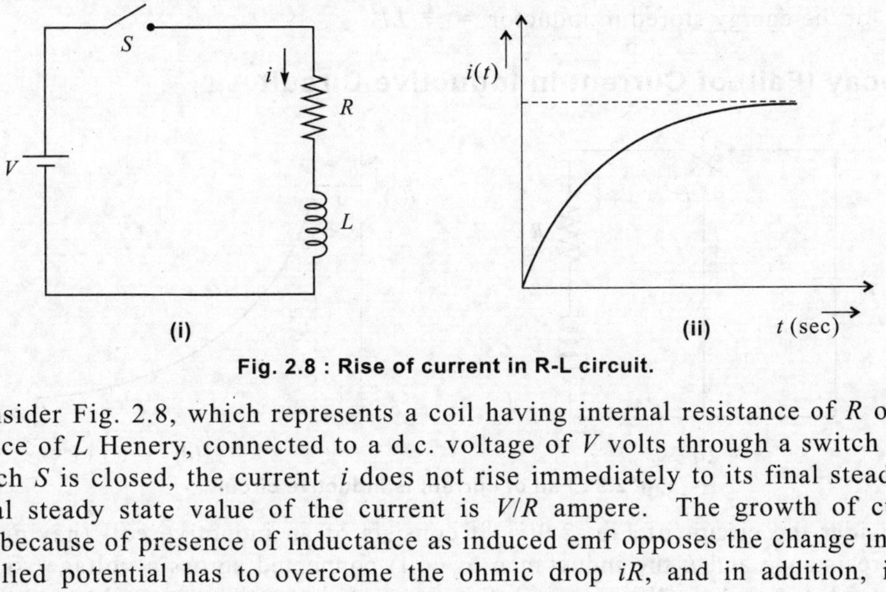

Fig. 2.8 : Rise of current in R-L circuit.

Consider Fig. 2.8, which represents a coil having internal resistance of R ohms and inductance of L Henery, connected to a d.c. voltage of V volts through a switch S. When the switch S is closed, the current i does not rise immediately to its final steady value. The final steady state value of the current is V/R ampere. The growth of current is delayed because of presence of inductance as induced emf opposes the change in current. The applied potential has to overcome the ohmic drop iR, and in addition, it has to overcome the back emf set-up by self inductance. This back emf will become zero only when the current becomes steady.

The self induced emf $= -L\,\dfrac{di}{dt}$ where i is the instantaneous value (small script letter) of current.

The applied potential difference (V) therefore has to possess a component equal and opposite to this as well as a component equal to the ohmic drop iR.

Hence, we have

$$V = iR + L\frac{di}{dt} \quad \text{..... (2.27)}$$

multiplying both sides of equation (2.27) by $i\,dt$ we get

$$Vi\,dt = i^2R\,dt + Li\,dt \quad \text{..... (2.28)}$$

$Vi\,dt$ represents the total energy supplied to the coil in time dt. $i^2R\,dt$ is converted into heat due to ohmic resistance of coil and $Li\,dt$ is the energy required to establish the magnetic field, whose presence is the cause of self induction. The solution of the differential equation (2.27) is

$$i(t) = \frac{V}{R}\left(1 - e^{\left(-\frac{R}{L}\right)t}\right) \quad \text{..... (2.29)}$$

$$i(t) = I\left(1 - e^{-\frac{Rt}{L}}\right) \quad \text{..... (2.30)}$$

where $I = \frac{V}{R}$ the steady value of current i. the plot of $i(t)$ is as shown in Fig. 2.8(ii).

From equation (2.28), the energy imparted to the magnetic field is $Li\,di$. Hence, when the current has attained a value I, the energy of the field will be

$$\int_0^I Li\,di = \frac{1}{2}LI^2$$

$$\text{or the energy stored in inductor} = \frac{1}{2}LI^2 \quad \text{..... (2.31)}$$

2.9 Decay (Fall) of Current in Inductive Circuit

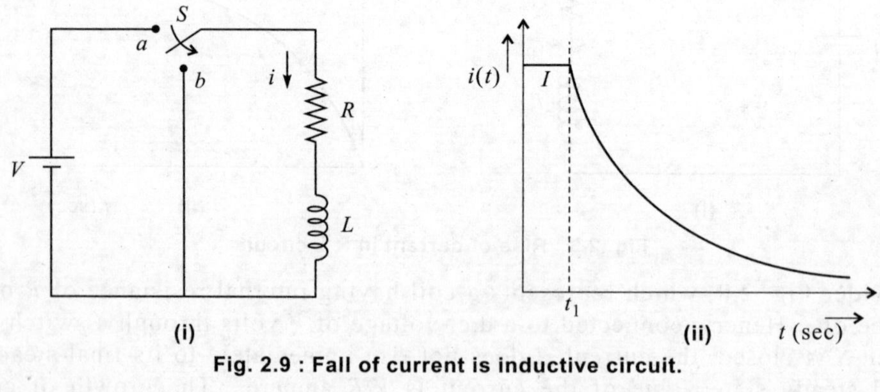

Fig. 2.9 : Fall of current is inductive circuit.

Consider the circuit of Fig. 2.9(i), it consists of an inductive coil (having R as its internal resistance and L the inductance of coil) connected across a voltage source of V volts through a switch S. When switch S is connected at a the source is connected to the coil. The current is now assumed to have reached a steady value ($I = V/R$). Now at instant t_1, the switch S is moved to position b, such that coil is shorted by the switch. The current I in the coil will not fall to zero immediately due to the presence of inductor. The applied voltage in this case is zero. Thus

$$0 = Ri + L\frac{di}{dt} \quad \text{..... (2.32)}$$

The solution of differential equation of equation (2.32) is as in equation (2.33).

$$i(t) = Ie^{-\left(\frac{R}{L}\right)t} \quad \text{..... (2.33)}$$

The plot of this decaying current of equation (2.33) is as shown in Fig. 2.9(ii). Figure shows that current decays and finally falls to zero.

Ex. 2.1 : A conductor 30.5 cm long rotates on the periphery of an armature of diameter 45 cm at 1000 rpm in a plane perpendicular to a magnetic field of strength 0.5 wb/m^2. Find the emf induced in it.

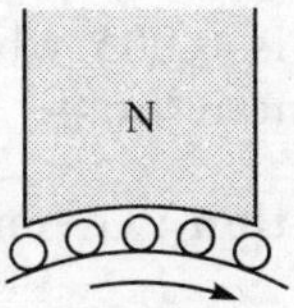

Solution : Given : Diameter $= 0.45$ m, $L = 0.305$ m,

rpm = 1000 revolutions per min.

$$\therefore \text{Revolution per sec} = \frac{1000}{60}$$

$$B = \text{Flux density} = 0.5 \text{ wb/m}^2$$

∴ from equation (2.1)

$$e = Blv$$

$$\text{Velocity } v = \pi D \times (\text{rev/sec}) = \pi \times 0.45 \times \frac{1000}{60}$$

$$= 23.56 \text{ m/s}$$

$$\therefore e = 0.5 \times 0.305 \times 23.56$$

$$= 3.59 \text{ volts}$$

Ex. 2.2 : A coil of resistance 10 Ω and inductance of 14 has a current which increases uniformly at the rate of 10000 A/sec. Find the value of applied voltage when

(a) The current is 10 A **(b)** The current is 50 A.

Solution : Given : $R = 10\ \Omega$, $L = 1$ H, $\frac{di}{dt} = 10{,}000$ A/s

Refer equation (2.27)

$$V = Ri + L\frac{di}{dt}$$

(a) When $i = 10$ A

$$V = 10 \times 10 + 1 \times 10000 = 10100 \text{ volts}$$

(b) When $i = 50$ A

$$V = 10 \times 50 + 1 \times 10000 = 10500 \text{ volts}$$

Ex. 2.3 : A certain choke coil has 1500 turns when 4 A are passed through it, the total magnetic flux in the coil. to 0.06 wb. The resistance of the coil is 20 Ω. Find an expression for the current in the coil immediately after it is switch on to a d.c. supply yielding 100 V. Assume that self inductance of the coil is constant.

Solution : Given : $N = 1500$, $I = 4$ A, $\phi = 0.06$ wb, $R = 20\ \Omega$, $V = 100$ V

$$L = \frac{N\phi}{I} \quad \text{... [from equation (2.14)]}$$

$$L = \frac{1500 \times 0.06}{4} = 22.5 \text{ H}$$

From equation (2.29)

$$i = \frac{V}{R}\left(1 - e^{-\frac{R}{L}t}\right)$$

$$= \frac{100}{20}\left(1 - e^{-\frac{20}{22.5}t}\right)$$

$$\therefore\ i = 5\left(1 - e^{-0.89\,t}\right)$$

Ex. 2.4 : The field winding of a d.c. machine is wound with 950 turns and has a resistance of 55 Ω. When the exciting voltage of 230 V, the magnetic flux linkage of the coil is 0.005 wb. Calculate the self-inductance of the coil and the energy stored in the magnetic field.

Solution : Given : $N = 550$ turns, $V = 230$ V, $R = 55\ \Omega$, $\phi = 0.005$ wb

From equation (2.14)

$$L = \frac{N\phi}{I} = \frac{550 \times 0.005}{4.18} = 0.657 \text{ H}$$

The energy stored is given by equation (2.31)

$$\text{Energy stored } W_i = \frac{1}{2}\,Li^2 = \frac{1}{2} \times 0.657 \times 4.18^2$$

$$= 5.74 \text{ Joules}$$

CHAPTER

3 A.C. FUNDAMENTALS

Alternating current transmission systems have great advantage over the direct current ones owing to great simplicity of increasing or decreasing the voltage by means of transformers both in transmission and distribution systems.

3.1 Introduction

The d.c. machines, having been developed, also presented many difficulties connected with obtaining larger unit powers and high voltages across the terminals. The first direct-current power transmission tests carried out by M. Deprez in 1883-86 proved the great importance but also showed the difficulties inherent in high voltage d.c. system. To obtain a high d.c. voltage at generating station several d.c. high voltage generators were connected in series. In the following period, practice showed the great advantage of alternating current transmission lines, which became almost universal. However, at present owing to modern highly developed ac to dc and dc to ac converters, direct current high voltage transmissions have again appeared.

Alternating current transmission systems have great advantage over the direct current ones owing to great simplicity of increasing or decreasing the voltage by means of transformers both in transmission and distribution systems.

Incidentally, sine curve occurs very commonly in nature (e.g. Pendulum, vibrating strings etc.). Apparently sine wave is natures standard. One may wonder why we should select only sinusoidal alternating current system.

There may be the following reasons for doing so :

(1) Applying sinusoidal voltage to properly designed coils results in production of rotating magnetic field which is utilized in motors useful in commercial and industrial applications.

(2) A.c. produces least disturbance.

(3) Use of sinusoidal a.c. underlines the use of transformers which enables bulk power transmission at high voltages over long distances.

(4) When current in elements like resistance inductance or capacitance is sinusoidal the voltage across these elements are also sinusoidal. This is not true with other wave forms.

(5) A sinusoidal wave remains sinusoidal (at same frequency) even after many integrations or differentiations i.e. mathematical computations over sinusoidal a.c. wave form results in a.c. sinusoids at same frequency but different amplitudes and phase angles.

Keeping in view the above importance of sinusoidal a.c., this chapter deals with generation of sinusoidal alternating currents and voltages. The general terms associated with the above wave forms are also discussed. Further, non sinusoidal output functions are also considered so as to provide a generalized approach to alternating quantities. This chapter also discusses about the vector representation of sinusoidal alternating quantities. It also throws light on vector algebra which will be helpful in solving a.c circuits and analysis.

In the first chapter, we have dealt with direct current (d.c.), which flows continuously in one direction. A constant d.c. source means the current flows in one direction with a constant magnitude with respect to time.

An **alternating quantity** is one which acts in alternate positive and negative direction, whose magnitude undergoes a definite series of changes in definite intervals of time, and the sequence of changes while negative is identical with the sequence while positive. The graphs of some such quantities are shown in Fig. 3.1.

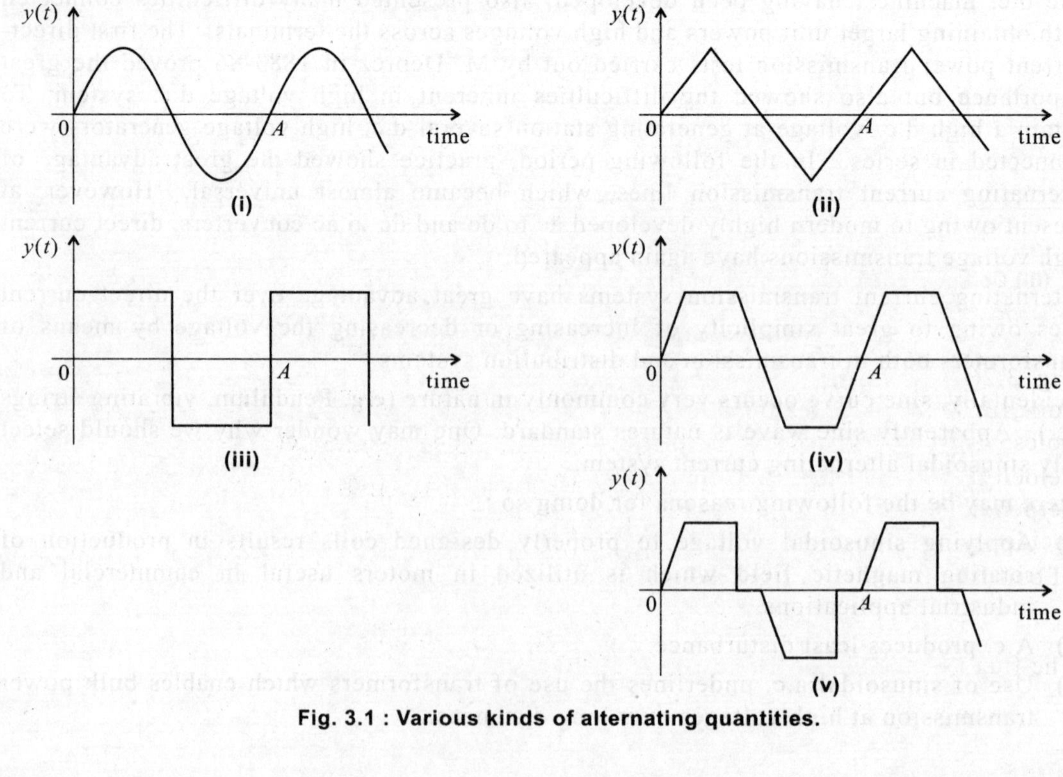

Fig. 3.1 : Various kinds of alternating quantities.

Fig. 3.1(i) shows a sinusoidal alternating quality which will be discussed in details and is the standard a.c. waveform. Some light is thrown on non-sinusoidal waveforms also in this chapter.

3.2 Generation of Alternating Voltages and Currents

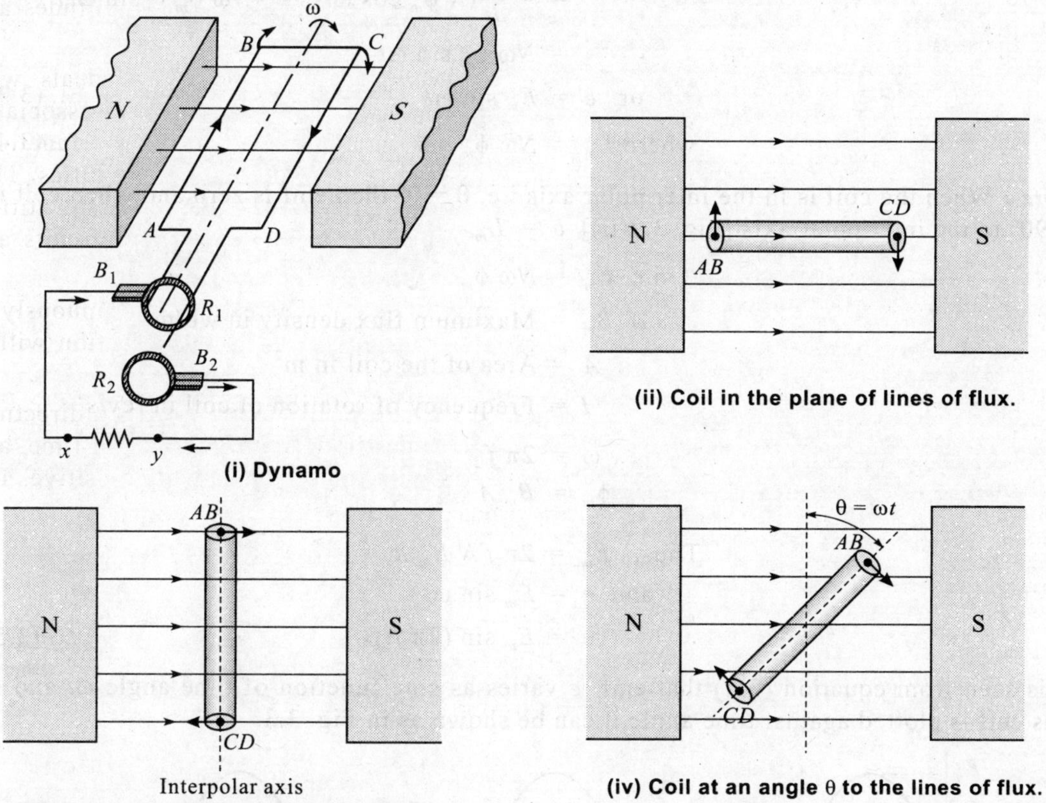

(i) Dynamo

(ii) Coil in the plane of lines of flux.

(iii) Coil perpendicular to lines of flux.

(iv) Coil at an angle θ to the lines of flux.

Fig. 3.2 : Generation of sinusoidal a.c. voltage.

Fig. 3.2(i) shows an a.c. dynamo (a.c. generator). It consists of a pair of magnets N-S. A coil *ABCD* with conductor's *AB* and *CD* placed within the magnetic field between the poles. This coil is rotated in the direction as shown along the axis with an angular velocity ω radian/sec. Let time t be measured from the inter polar axis (i.e. axis perpendicular to line of flux) Fig. 3.2(iv). Fig. 3.2(iii) shows the position of coil co-incidences with inter polar axis. Maximum flux passes through the coil i.e. flux linkage of coil is maximum. In t sec the coil rotates through angle θ.

$$\theta = \omega t \qquad ..... (3.1)$$

The flux linkage (ψ) of the coil with N turns will be

$$\psi = N \phi_m \cos \omega t \qquad ..... (3.2)$$

According to Faradays laws of induction the emf induced (e) in the coil is given by rate of change of flux linkage of coil.

$$e = -\frac{d\psi}{dt}$$

$$= -\frac{d}{dt}(N\,\phi_m \cos \omega t) = -N\omega\,\phi_m(-\sin \omega t)$$

$$= N\omega\,\phi_m \sin \omega t$$

$$\text{or}\quad e = E_m \sin \omega t \qquad \text{..... (3.3)}$$

$$\text{where } E_m = N\omega\,\phi_m \qquad \text{..... (3.4)}$$

Note : When the coil is in the inter polar axis i.e. $\theta = 0°$ then emf is zero and when coil is at 90° to the inter polar axis [Fig. 3.2(ii)] $e = E_m$

$$\text{i.e. } E_m = N\omega\,\phi_m$$

If B_m = Maximum flux density in wb/m^2

A = Area of the coil in m^2

f = Frequency of rotation of coil in rev/s

$$\therefore\ \omega = 2\pi f$$

$$\therefore\ \phi_m = B_m A$$

$$\text{Thus,}\quad E_m = 2\pi f N B_m A$$

$$\text{and}\quad e = E_m \sin \omega t$$

$$e = E_m \sin(2\pi ft) \qquad \text{..... (3.5)}$$

It is seen from equation (3.5) that emf e varies as sine function of time angle ωt and if this emf is plotted against time angle it can be shown as in Fig. 3.3.

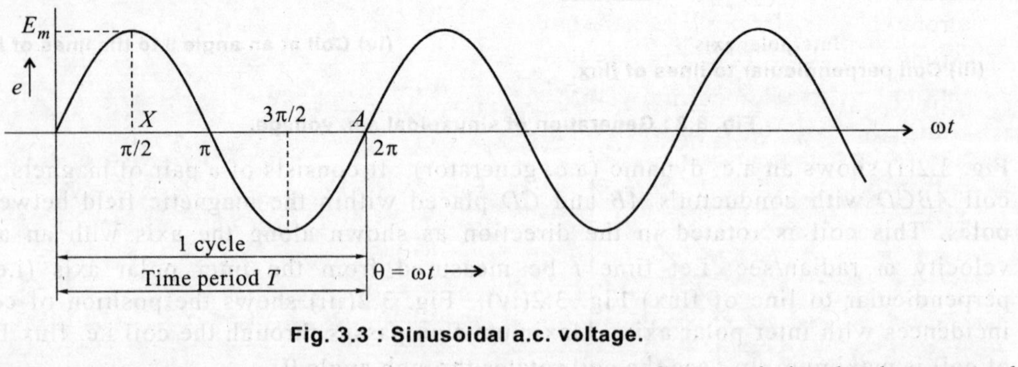

Fig. 3.3 : Sinusoidal a.c. voltage.

Similarly, the equation of alternating current can be given for a resistive load connected across this coil.

$$i = I_m \sin \omega t$$

The small case letters indicate the instantaneous value of the signal. E_m indicates the maximum value.

3.3 Terminologies of Sinusoidal Functions

As the sinusoidal quantity varies continuously with time, let us define certain terminologies associated with the a.c. quantities of Fig. 3.3.

(a) Cycle : One complete set of positive and negative values of the function which goes on repeating itself is called a *cycle*. [Refer Fig. 3.1, *OA* represents 1 cycle in each waveform].

(b) Time Period (*T*) : The time taken by an alternating quantity to complete one cycle is called its *time period T*, e.g. if supply frequency is 50 Hz the time period

$$T = \frac{1}{50} \text{ secs.}$$

(c) Frequency (*f*) : It is the number of cycles of the supply that occurs per second. It is denoted by *f*. Its unit is hertz (Hz). *Frequency* is reciprocal of time period,

$$\text{i.e. } f = \frac{1}{T} \qquad ..... (3.6)$$

(d) Amplitude (maximum or peak value) : The maximum positive or negative value of the alternating quantity is known as the its *amplitude*. Here, the amplitude is E_m.

(e) Angular Frequency (ω) : As seen in Fig 3.3 the values of sine function repeats itself after 2π radian. Angular frequency ω is the number of radian covered in one second. Its unit is radian per sec. The supply frequency has *f* cycles per second and one cycle covers 2π radian. Thus,

$$\omega = 2\pi f \qquad ..... (3.7)$$

$$\omega = \frac{2\pi}{T} \qquad \left(\because f = \frac{1}{T}\right)$$

(f) Phase : Phase of an alternating quantity means the fraction of the time period (*T*) elapsed by the quantity since it has last passed through the zero position of reference. Refer Fig. 3.3, the phase of voltage at point *X* is *T*/4 sec when *T* is the time period. If *T* = 2π radian then phase of voltage at *X* is π/2 radians.

In electrical engineering we are, however, more concerned about the relative phases or phase difference between alternating quantities rather that their absolute phases.

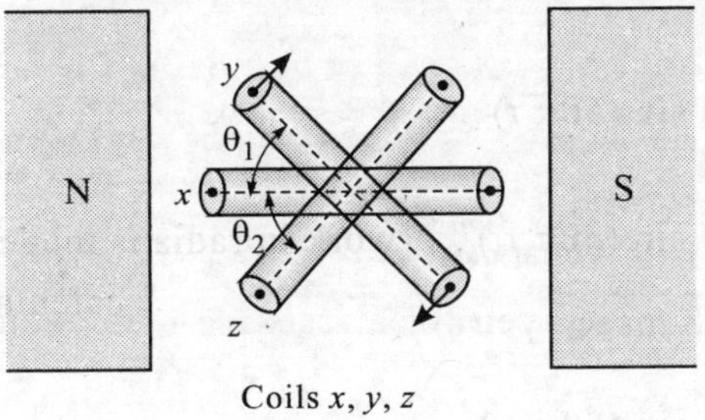

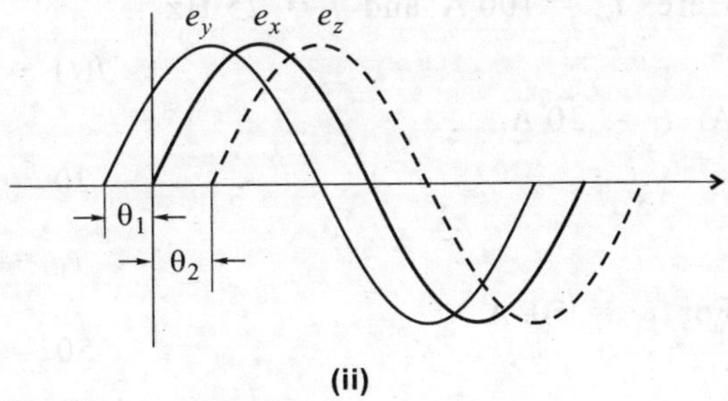

Fig. 3.4 : Three coils with a phase difference.

Consider Fig. 3.4, it shows three coils x, y and z fixed with respect to each other such that angle between x and y is θ_1 and that between x and z is θ_2. These coils are now rotated about their axis at a speed of ω rad/s in between the poles. If the emf in coil x is as shown in Fig. 3.4(ii), then as coil y is ahead of coil x its zero crossing will be θ_1 radians ahead of e_x. Similarly the emf of coil z which is behind x by θ_2 radian will have its zero crossing θ_2 radian after the zero crossing of emf in x.

(g) Phase Difference : As seen in Fig. 3.4 the three coils x, y and z are displaced by angles θ_1 and θ_2 and are rotating in the *same uniform field* with the *same angular frequency*. All the three induced emf are same but have an *important difference*. All the three emf do not reach their zero values or maximum values together. It is seen that *phase difference* between coils x and y is θ_1 and emf e_y leads e_x by θ_1. Similarly e_z lags behind e_x by angle θ_2.

A leading alternating quantity is one which reaches its zero or maximum value earlier as compared to the other quantity.

Similarly, a lagging alternating quantity is one whose zero or maximum value is reached later as compared to the other quantity. Thus, e_y leads e_x by angle θ_1 and e_z lags behind e_x by angle θ_2.

The three equations for e_x, e_y and e_z are given by

$$e_x = E_m \sin \omega t \quad \text{..... (3.8)}$$

$$e_y = E_m \sin (\omega t + \theta_1) \quad \text{..... (3.9)}$$

$$e_z = E_m \sin (\omega t - \theta_2) \quad \text{..... (3.10)}$$

Positive sign in angle θ_1 denotes *lead* in phase whereas negative sign with θ_2 denotes a phase *lag*.

Ex. 3.1 : A sinusoidal alternative current of frequency 25 Hz has the maximum value of 100 A. How long will it take to attain values of 20 A, 50 A and 100 A from the instant it crosses 0 A in the positive direction. What is the time period of this wave.

Solution : Let the expression for current be

$$i(t) = I_m \sin 2\pi f t$$

Here, $I_m = 100$ A and $f = 25$ Hz

$$\therefore \quad i(t) = 100 \sin (50\pi t)$$

At $i_1 = 20$ A

$$20 = 100 \sin (50\pi t_1) \text{ ... [work in radians mode of calculator]}$$

$$\therefore t_1 = \boxed{1.28 \text{ msec}}$$

For $i_2 = 50$ A

$$50 = 100 \sin (50\pi t_2)$$

$$\therefore t_2 = \boxed{3.33 \text{ msec}}$$

For $i_3 = 100$ A

$$100 = 100 \sin (50\pi\, t_3)$$
$$\therefore\ t_3 = 0.01 \text{ sec}$$
$$T = \text{Time period} = \frac{1}{f} = \frac{1}{25}$$
$$\therefore\ T = \boxed{0.04 \text{ sec}}$$

Ex. 3.2 : A 50 Hz sinusoidal voltage wave shape has maximum value of 350 V. Calculate its instantaneous value 0.005 seconds after the wave passes through zero in the positive direction and 0.009 seconds after the wave passes through 0 V in negative direction.

Solution : Let $v(t) = V_m \sin 2\pi f t$.

Here, $V_m = 350$ and $f = 50$ Hz ... (given)

$$\therefore\ v(t) = 350 \sin (100\pi\, t)$$

At $t_1 = 0.005$ sec

$$v_1 = 350 \sin (100\pi \times 0.005) = \boxed{350 \text{ V}}$$

At $t_2 = 0.009$ sec

$$\therefore\ t_3 = 0.01 + 0.009 = 0.019$$
$$v_2 = 350 \sin (100\pi\, t_3) = 350 \sin (100\pi \times 0.019) = \boxed{-108.15 \text{ V}}$$

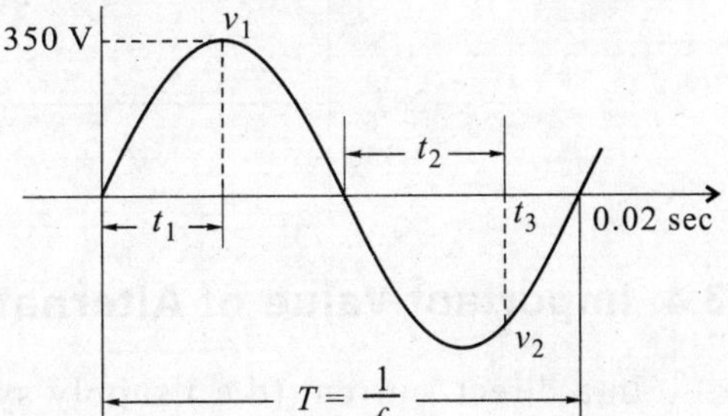

Fig. 3.5

Ex. 3.3 : Draw the following waveforms over one cycle.

$$v_1 = 330 \cos (\omega t - \pi/6)$$
$$v_2 = 330 \sin \omega t$$
$$v_3 = 330 \cos (\omega t - 2\pi/3)$$
$$v_4 = 100 \cos 2\omega t.$$

Solution : Let us calculate all voltage at different instants

ωt (rad)	0	$\pi/6$	$\pi/3$	$\pi/2$	$2\pi/3$	$5\pi/6$	π
$v_1 = 330 \cos (\omega t - \pi/6)$	285.7	330	285.7	165	0	−165	−285.7
$v_2 = 330 \sin \omega t$	0	165	285.7	330	285.7	165	0
$v_3 = 330 \cos (\omega t - 2\pi/3)$	165	285.7	330	285.7	165	0	−165
$v_4 = 100 \cos 2\omega t$	100	50	−50	−100	−50	50	100

Now plot these as in Fig. 3.6.

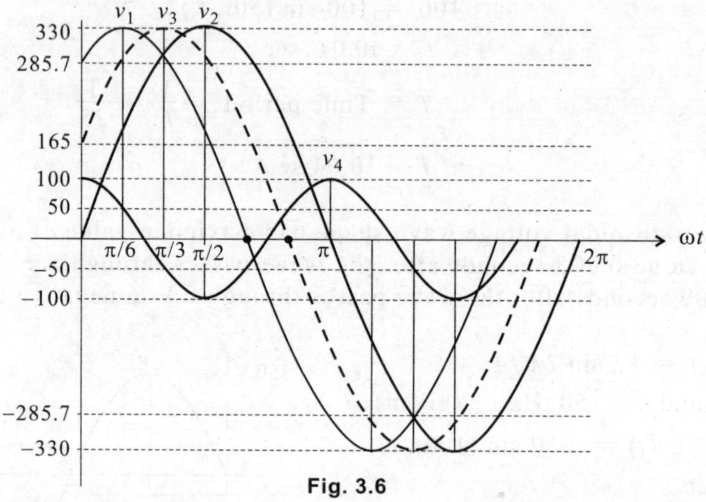

Fig. 3.6

3.4 Important Value of Alternating Voltage and Currents

In a direct current (d.c.) supply system the applied voltage and current under steady state are constant with respect to time, so in order to express these quantities we use those values directly. However, as seen earlier, the alternating voltages and currents continuously show a change in their magnitudes with respect to time. In order to indicate their values these different parameters are used.

(1) Peak value or amplitude

(2) Average value

(3) Effective or rms value.

3.4.1 Average Value

Average value, by definition, *is the algebraic sum of all the values, divided by the total number of values*. This is exactly how we find average marks. A waveform is a continuous variations of values of a certain parameter Y (here current or voltage) with respect to time (or angle θ) over a given cycle.

Thus, the average value of waveform can also be found by first identifying the cycle. Then finding the area under the curve by integrating the given function for a complete cycle and dividing it by its time period T.

Thus average value of a function $y(t)$, where y here is either current or voltage, with a time period of T given by

$$Y_{av} = \frac{1}{T}\int_0^T \textit{Area under full cycle}$$

$$Y_{av} = \frac{1}{T}\int_0^T y(t)\,dt \quad \text{..... (3.11)}$$

Consider an alternating waveform of voltage as in Fig. 3.3. It has same areas of positive and negative half cycles. Hence, **the average value of full cycle alternating quantity will be zero**. This average value does not convey any useful information about the waveforms. Therefore, for alternating waveforms we define half cycle average. Thus, the **half cycle average** of sinusoidal waveform is defined as

$$Y_{av} \text{ (half cycle)} = \frac{1}{T/2} \int_0^{T/2} y(t)\, dt \qquad \text{..... (3.12)}$$

3.4.2 Effective or RMS Value

The rms value or effective value of an alternating current is given by *that steady (d.c.) current which when flowing through a given circuit for a given time produces the same heat or same work done as produced by an alternating current when flowing through the same circuit for the same time.*

It is also called *the effective value of an alternating current.* For finding the effective value of a sinusoidal quantity we will first find the effective value for any general waveform so as to obtain general formula for effective value. Later, solved examples will show the method to find average value, effective values of various kinds of waveform, sinusoidal as well as non-sinusoidal.

Let us consider Fig. 3.7.

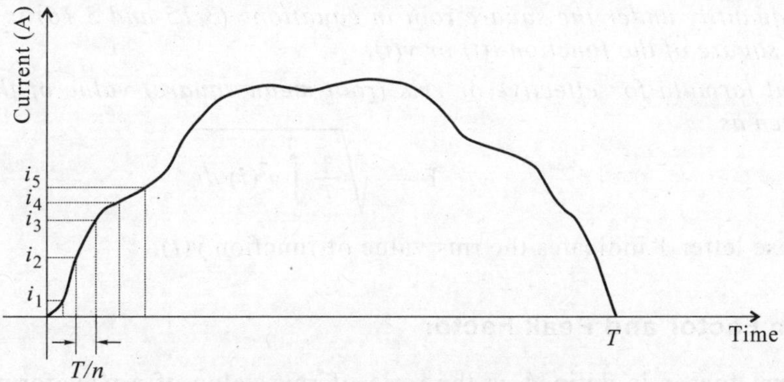

Fig. 3.7 : Effective value of current waveform.

It shown a current waveform randomly generated over a time period T. To find the heat produced by this waveform, divide this interval T in very small n intervals such that each interval has duration of (T/n) seconds. If this current is passed through a resistance R. Then work done in each interval can be given by

$$\text{Work done in first interval} = i_1^2 R \frac{T}{n}$$

$$\text{Work done in second interval} = i_2^2 R \frac{T}{n}$$

$$\vdots \qquad \vdots$$

$$\text{Work done in second interval} = i_n^2 R \frac{T}{n}$$

where i_1 is the average current in first interval, i_2 in the second interval and so on ...

$$\therefore \text{ Total work done in } T \text{ sec} = i_1^2 R \frac{T}{n} + i_2^2 R \frac{T}{n} + \ldots\ldots + i_n^2 R \frac{T}{n} \qquad \ldots\ldots (3.13)$$

Now, suppose a direct current of I (amp) produce the same work done while following through same resistance R for same interval T.

$$\text{The work done by } I \text{ amp d.c.} = I^2RT \qquad \ldots\ldots (3.14)$$

By definition, equating work done from equation (3.13) and (3.14) we get

$$I^2RT = i_1^2 R \frac{T}{n} + i_2^2 R \frac{T}{n} + \ldots\ldots + i_n^2 R \frac{T}{n}$$

$$I^2 = \frac{i_1^2 + i_2^2 + \ldots\ldots + i_n^2}{n}$$

$$\text{or } I = \sqrt{\frac{i_1^2 + i_2^2 + \ldots\ldots + i_n^2}{n}} \qquad \ldots\ldots (3.15)$$

Or effective value (I) is the root of mean of squares of instantaneous currents.
Similarly, the rms value of voltage will be given by the expression

$$V = \sqrt{\frac{v_1^2 + v_2^2 + \ldots\ldots + v_n^2}{n}} \qquad \ldots\ldots (3.16)$$

Note : *The quantity under the square root in equations (3.15 and 3.16) is the average or mean of the square of the function i(t) or v(t).*

Thus general formula for effective or rms (root mean square) value of the function y(t) can be written as

$$Y = \sqrt{\frac{1}{T}\int_0^T y^2(t)\, dt} \qquad \ldots\ldots (3.17)$$

The uppercase letter Y indicates the rms value of function $y(t)$.

3.4.3 Form Factor and Peak Factor

The **form factor** is defined as the ratio of rms value of a waveform to its average value i.e.

$$\text{Form factor } K_f = \frac{Y_{rms}}{Y_{av}} = \frac{\textit{rms value}}{\textit{Average value}} \qquad \ldots\ldots (3.18)$$

The form factor has its use in generation, instrument correction factors. It helps in finding hysteresis loss for different waveforms. An alternating current with higher form factor will amount to higher hysteresis loss. Its least value is 1 and highest maybe as high as 5. For sinusoidal ac its value is 1.11.

The **peak factor** or **crest factor** is defined as *the ratio of amplitude or peak value to rms value.*

$$K_p = \frac{Y_{max}}{Y_{rms}} = \frac{\textit{Maximum value}}{\textit{rms value}} \qquad \ldots\ldots (3.19)$$

The peak factor indicates the maximum voltage being applied to various parts of a circuit. It helps in deciding the ratings of components to the used in circuits. It also helps in deciding the dielectric insulation, since the dielectric stress produced depends upon the maximum value of voltage and not its rms value.

Ex. 3.4 : Find the half cycle average and rms value of a sinusoidal alternating voltage. Also find the form factor and peak factor.

Solution : The expression for sinusoidal voltage (refer Fig. 3.8) is

$$v = V_m \sin \omega t$$

$$T = 2\pi \text{ (period of cycle)}$$

$$\therefore V_{av}\text{(half cycle)} = \frac{1}{T/2}\int_0^{T/2} V_m \sin\theta \, d\theta$$

$$= \frac{1}{\pi}\int_0^{\pi} V_m \sin\theta \, d\theta$$

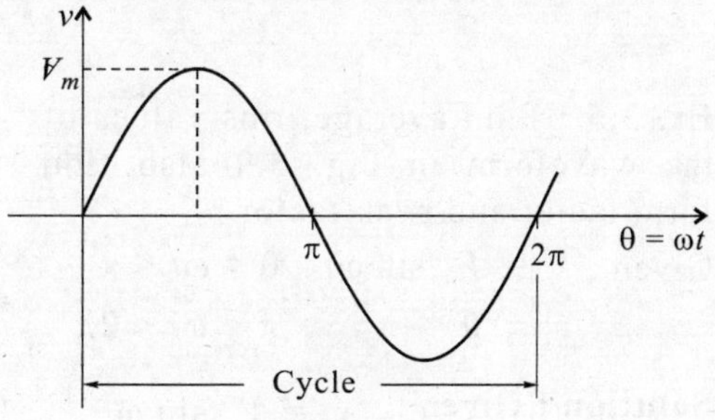

Fig. 3.8

$$\therefore V_{av} = \frac{1}{\pi}\left[V_m(-\cos\theta)_0^{\pi}\right] = \frac{V_m}{\pi}[1+1]$$

$$\boxed{V_{av} = \frac{2V_m}{\pi}} \qquad \text{..... (3.20)}$$

$$V_{rms} = V = \sqrt{\frac{1}{2\pi}\int_0^{2\pi} V_m^2 \sin^2\theta \, d\theta}$$

$$= \sqrt{\frac{V_m^2}{2\pi}\int_0^{2\pi}\frac{1-\cos 2\theta}{2}\, d\theta}$$

$$= \sqrt{\frac{V_m^2}{4\pi}\left[\theta - \frac{1}{2}\sin 2\theta\right]_0^{2\pi}}$$

$$= \sqrt{\frac{V_m^2}{4\pi}\left[2\pi - 0 - \frac{1}{2}(\sin 4\pi - \sin 0)\right]}$$

$$= \sqrt{\frac{V_m^2}{4\pi}[2\pi]}$$

$$\boxed{V_{rms} = \frac{V_m}{\sqrt{2}}} \qquad \text{..... (3.21)}$$

$$\text{Form factor } K_f = \frac{V_{rms}}{V_{av}} = \frac{\frac{V_m}{\sqrt{2}}}{\frac{2V_m}{\pi}} = \frac{\pi}{2\sqrt{2}}$$

$$\boxed{K_f = 1.11} \qquad \text{..... (3.22)}$$

$$\text{Peak factor } K_p = \frac{V_{max}}{V_{rms}} = \frac{V_m}{\frac{V_m}{\sqrt{2}}} = \sqrt{2}$$

$$\boxed{K_p = 1.414} \qquad \text{..... (3.23)}$$

Ex. 3.5 : Find average, rms values of the waveform in Fig. 3.9 also find form factor and peak factor.

Given : $v = V_m \sin \omega t \quad 0 < \omega t < \pi$

$= 0 \quad \pi < \omega t < 2\pi$

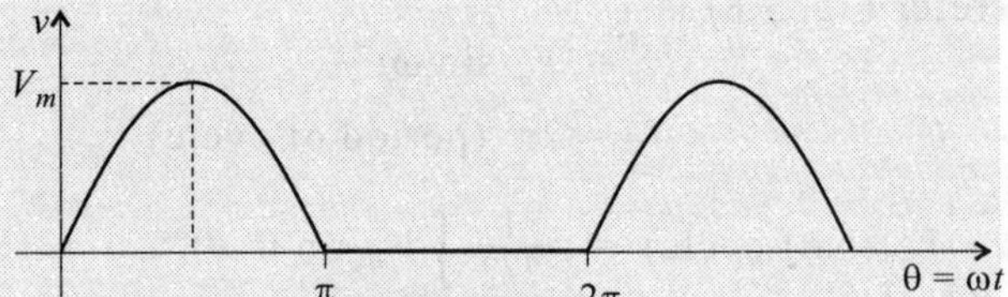

Fig. 3.9

Solution : Given : $v = V_m \sin \omega t \quad 0 < \omega t < \pi$

$= 0 \quad \pi < \omega t < 2\pi$

The interval here is $T = 2\pi$, as the waveform is not alternating we will find full cycle average.

$$V_{av} = \frac{1}{2\pi}\int_0^{2\pi} v(\theta)\, d\theta$$

$$= \frac{1}{2\pi}\left[\int_0^{\pi} V_m \sin\theta\, d\theta + \int_{\pi}^{2\pi} 0\, d\theta\right]$$

$$= \frac{1}{2\pi}\int_0^{\pi} V_m \sin\theta\, d\theta$$

$$= \frac{V_m}{2\pi}\left[-\cos\theta\right]_0^{\pi} = \frac{V_m}{2\pi}[2] = \boxed{\frac{V_m}{\pi}}$$

$$V_{rms} = V = \sqrt{\frac{1}{2\pi}\left[\int_0^{\pi} V_m^2 \sin^2\theta\, d\theta + \int_{\pi}^{2\pi} 0\, d\theta\right]}$$

$$= \sqrt{\frac{V_m^2}{2\pi}\int_0^{\pi}\frac{1-\cos 2\theta}{2}\, d\theta}$$

$$= \sqrt{\frac{V_m^2}{4\pi}\left[\theta - \frac{1}{2}\sin 2\theta\right]_0^{\pi}}$$

$$= \sqrt{\frac{V_m^2}{4\pi}\left[\pi - \frac{1}{2}(\sin 2\pi - \sin 0)\right]}$$

$$= \sqrt{\frac{V_m^2}{4\pi}[\pi]}$$

$$\boxed{V_{rms} = \frac{V_m}{2}}$$

$$\text{Form factor } K_f = \frac{V_{rms}}{V_{av}} = \frac{\frac{V_m}{2}}{\frac{V_m}{\pi}} = \frac{\pi}{2} = \boxed{1.57}$$

$$\text{Peak factor } K_p = \frac{V_{max}}{V_{rms}} = \frac{V_m}{\frac{V_m}{2}} = \boxed{2}$$

Ex. 3.6 : Find the form factor of the waveform in Fig. 3.10 the output of the full wave rectifier.

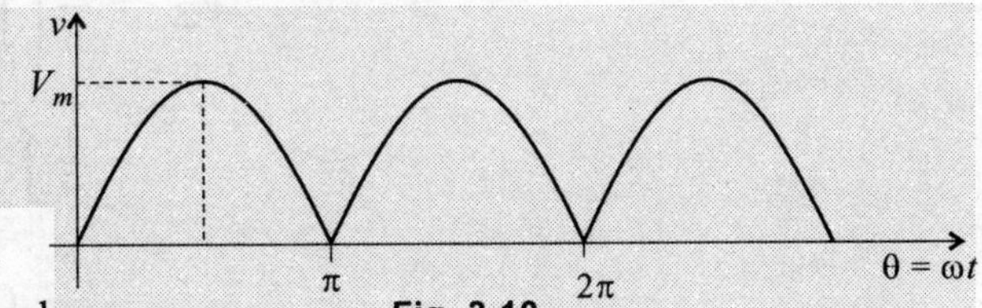

Fig. 3.10

Solution : The interval for this function is $T = \pi$ and $v = V_m \sin \omega t$ in this interval

$$\therefore \; V_{av} = \frac{1}{\pi}\int_0^{\pi} V_m \sin\theta \, d\theta$$

$$= \frac{V_m}{\pi}[-\cos\theta]_0^{\pi}$$

$$= \boxed{\frac{2V_m}{\pi}}$$

$$V_{rms} = \sqrt{\frac{1}{\pi}\int_0^{\pi} V_m^2 \sin^2\theta \, d\theta}$$

$$= \sqrt{\frac{V_m^2}{\pi}\int_0^{\pi}\frac{1-\cos 2\theta}{2}\, d\theta}$$

$$= \sqrt{\frac{V_m^2}{2\pi}\left[\theta - \frac{1}{2}\sin 2\theta\right]_0^{\pi}}$$

$$= \boxed{\frac{V_m}{\sqrt{2}}}$$

$$\text{Form factor } K_f = \frac{V_{rms}}{V_{av}} = \frac{\frac{V_m}{\sqrt{2}}}{\frac{2V_m}{\pi}} = \frac{\pi}{2\sqrt{2}}$$

$$= \boxed{1.11}$$

Ex. 3.7 : Find the average and rms value of the waveform in Fig. 3.11 for $\alpha = \pi/4$.

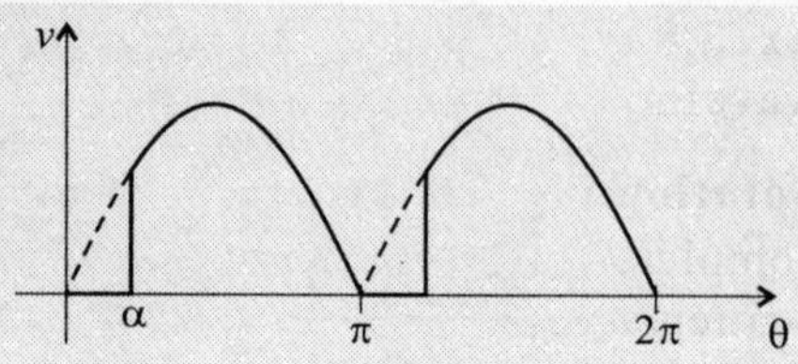

Fig. 3.11

Solution : The function here can be defined as

$$v = 0 \qquad 0 < \theta < \alpha$$

$$v = V_m \sin\theta \qquad \alpha < \theta < \pi$$

The interval here is $T = \pi$.

$$V_{av} = \frac{1}{\pi}\left[\int_0^{\alpha} 0\, d\theta + \int_{\alpha}^{\pi} V_m \sin\theta\, d\theta\right]$$

$$= \frac{1}{\pi}\int_{\alpha}^{\pi} V_m \sin\theta\, d\theta = \frac{V_m}{\pi}\left[-\cos\theta\right]_{\alpha}^{\pi}$$

$$= \frac{V_m}{\pi}(1 + \cos\alpha)$$

For $\alpha = \frac{\pi}{4}$

$$V_{av} = \frac{V_m}{\pi}\left(1 + \cos\frac{\pi}{4}\right) = 0.54\, V_m$$

$$V_{rms} = \sqrt{\frac{1}{\pi}\left[\int_0^{\alpha} 0\, d\theta + \int_{\alpha}^{\pi} V_m^2 \sin^2\theta\, d\theta\right]}$$

$$= \sqrt{\frac{V_m^2}{2\pi}\int_{\alpha}^{\pi}(1 - \cos 2\theta)\, d\theta}$$

$$= \sqrt{\frac{V_m^2}{2\pi}\left[\theta - \frac{1}{2}\sin 2\theta\right]_{\alpha}^{\pi}}$$

$$= \sqrt{\frac{V_m^2}{4\pi}\left[\pi - \alpha - \frac{1}{2}(\sin 2\pi - \sin 2\alpha)\right]}$$

For $\alpha = \frac{\pi}{4}$ [*when solving this expression on calculator work in radians mode*]

$$\therefore\ V_{rms} = \sqrt{\frac{V_m^2}{4\pi}\left[\pi - \frac{\pi}{4} - \frac{1}{2}\left(\sin 2\pi - \sin\frac{2\pi}{4}\right)\right]}$$

$$\boxed{V_{rms} = 0.674\, V_m}$$

Ex. 3.8 : Find the form factor for waveform in Fig. 3.12.

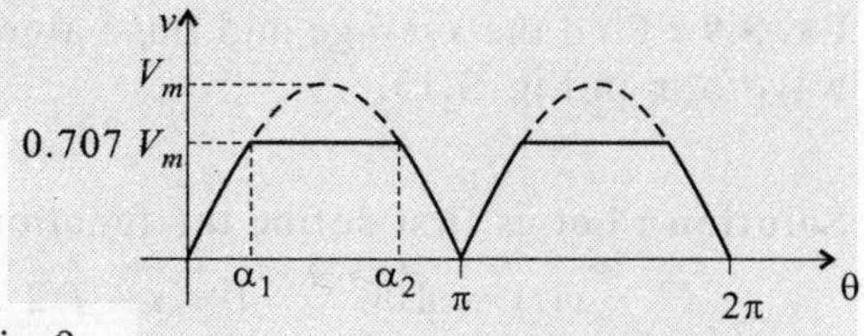

Fig. 3.12

Solution : The general expression for complete waveform between 0 to π can be written as

$$v = V_m \sin\theta$$

$$\text{At } \alpha_1 \text{ and } \alpha_2,\quad v = 0.707\ V_m$$

$$\therefore\quad 0.707\ V_m = V_m \sin\theta$$

$$\therefore\quad \theta = 45^\circ \text{ and } 135^\circ$$

$$\therefore\quad \alpha_1 = 45^\circ = \frac{\pi}{4} \text{ rad}$$

$$\text{and } \alpha_2 = 135^\circ = \frac{3\pi}{4} \text{ rad}$$

Thus defining the function

$$v = V_m \sin\theta \qquad 0 < \theta < \frac{\pi}{4}$$

$$= 0.707\ V_m \qquad \frac{\pi}{4} < \theta < \frac{3\pi}{4}$$

$$= V_m \sin\theta \qquad \frac{3\pi}{4} < \theta < \pi$$

Thus interval here is $T = \pi$

$$\therefore\quad V_{av} = \frac{1}{\pi}\left[\int_0^{\pi/4} V_m \sin\theta\, d\theta + \int_{\pi/4}^{3\pi/4} 0.707\ V_m\, d\theta + \int_{3\pi/4}^{\pi} V_m \sin\theta\, d\theta\right]$$

$$= \frac{V_m}{\pi}\left\{\left[-\cos\theta\right]_0^{\pi/4} + 0.707\left[\theta\right]_{\pi/4}^{3\pi/4} + \left[-\cos\theta\right]_{3\pi/4}^{\pi}\right\}$$

$$= \frac{V_m}{\pi}\left\{1 - \cos\frac{\pi}{4} + 0.707\left(\frac{3\pi}{4} - \frac{\pi}{4}\right) + 1 - \cos\frac{3\pi}{4}\right\}$$

[use radians mode of calculator]

$$\boxed{V_{av} = 0.54\ V_m}$$

$$V_{rms} = \sqrt{\frac{1}{\pi}\left[\int_0^{\pi/4} V_m^2 \sin^2\theta\, d\theta + \int_{\pi/4}^{3\pi/4} (0.707\ V_m)^2\, d\theta + \int_{3\pi/4}^{\pi} V_m^2 \sin^2\theta\, d\theta\right]}$$

$$= \sqrt{\frac{V_m^2}{\pi}\left[\int_0^{\pi/4} \frac{1-\cos 2\theta}{2} d\theta + 0.707^2 \int_{\pi/4}^{3\pi/4} d\theta + \int_{3\pi/4}^{\pi} \frac{1-\cos 2\theta}{2}\, d\theta\right]}$$

$$= \sqrt{\frac{V_m^2}{\pi}\left\{\frac{1}{2}\left[\theta - \frac{1}{2}\sin 2\theta\right]_0^{\pi/4} + 0.707^2\left(\frac{3\pi}{4} - \frac{\pi}{4}\right) + \frac{1}{2}\left[\theta - \frac{1}{2}\sin 2\theta\right]_{3\pi/4}^{\pi}\right\}}$$

$$\boxed{V_{rms} = 0.584\ V_m}$$

Ex. 3.9 : Find the average and rms value of waveform in Fig. 3.13.

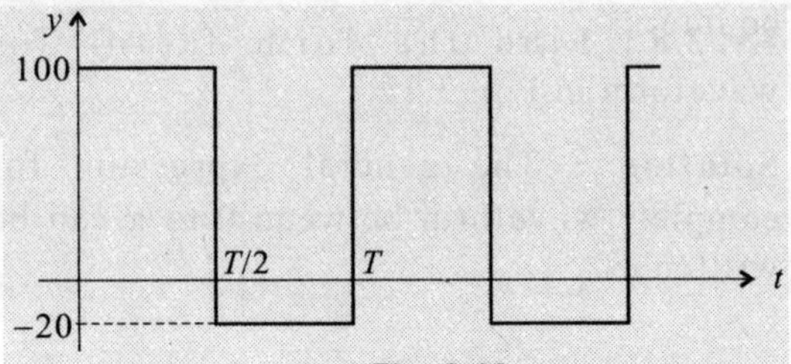

Fig. 3.13

Solution : Let us first define the function $y(t)$

$$y(t) = 100 \qquad 0 < t < T/2$$
$$= -20 \qquad T/2 < t < T$$

The time interval is T.

Here
$$y^2(t) = 10^4 \qquad 0 < t < T/2$$
$$= 400 \qquad T/2 < t < T$$

$$\therefore \quad Y_{av} = \frac{1}{T}\left[\int_0^{T/2} 100\, dt + \int_{T/2}^{T} -20\, dt\right]$$

$$= \frac{1}{T}\left[100\, t\Big|_0^{T/2} - 20\, t\Big|_{T/2}^{T}\right] = \frac{1}{T}\left[100\left(\frac{T}{2} - 0\right) - 20\left(T - \frac{T}{2}\right)\right]$$

$$= \frac{1}{T}\left[100\left(\frac{T}{2}\right) - 20\left(\frac{T}{2}\right)\right] = \boxed{40}$$

$$Y_{rms} = \sqrt{\frac{1}{T}\left[\int_0^{T/2} 10^4\, dt + \int_{T/2}^{T} 400\, dt\right]}$$

$$= \sqrt{\frac{1}{T}\left[10^4\, t\Big|_0^{T/2} + 400\, t\Big|_{T/2}^{T}\right]}$$

$$= \sqrt{\frac{1}{T}\left[10^4\left(\frac{T}{2} - 0\right) + 400\left(T - \frac{T}{2}\right)\right]}$$

$$= \sqrt{\frac{1}{T}\left[10^4\left(\frac{T}{2}\right) + 400\left(\frac{T}{2}\right)\right]} = \sqrt{5200}$$

$$\boxed{Y_{rms} = 72.11}$$

Ex. 3.10 : Find average and rms value of waveform in Fig. 3.14

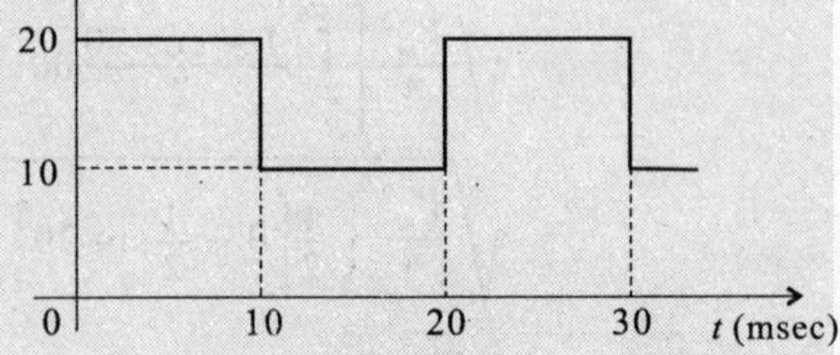

Fig. 3.14

Solution : Let us first define the function $v(t)$

$$v(t) = 20 \qquad 0 < t < 10 \text{ ms}$$
$$= 10 \qquad 10 < t < 20 \text{ ms}$$
$$v^2(t) = 400 \qquad 0 < t < 10 \text{ ms}$$
$$= 100 \qquad 10 < t < 20 \text{ ms}$$

The internal $T = 20$ ms

$$\therefore \; V_{av} = \frac{1}{T}\int_0^T v(t)\,dt$$

$$= \frac{1}{20}\left[\int_0^{10} 20\,dt + \int_{10}^{20} 10\,dt\right] = \frac{1}{20}\left[20\,t\Big|_0^{10} + 10\,t\Big|_{10}^{20}\right]$$

$$= \frac{1}{20}[20 \times 10 + 10 \times 10] = \boxed{15 \text{ volts}}$$

$$V_{rms} = \sqrt{\frac{1}{T}\int_0^t v^2(t)\,dt}$$

$$= \sqrt{\frac{1}{20}\left[\int_0^{10} 400\,dt + \int_{10}^{20} 100\,dt\right]} = \sqrt{\frac{1}{20}\left[400\,t\Big|_0^{10} + 100\,t\Big|_{10}^{20}\right]}$$

$$= \sqrt{\frac{1}{20}[400 \times 10 + 100 \times 10]} = \boxed{15.81 \text{ volts}}$$

Ex. 3.11 : Find the average and rms value of waveform in the Fig. 3.15.

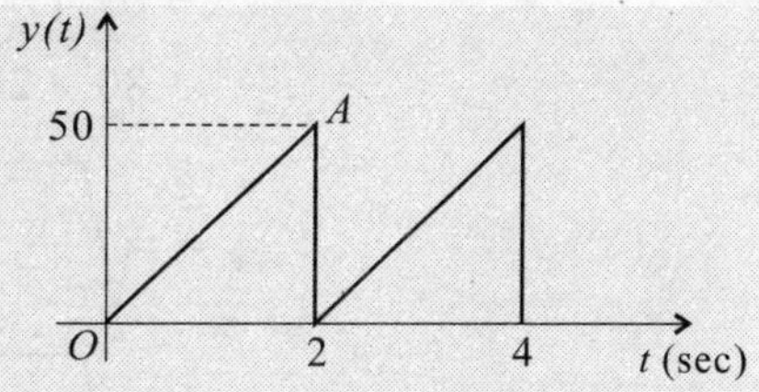

Fig. 3.15

Solution : This wave form consists of straight line with a slope. The general expression of line OA in Fig. 3.13 can be

$$y = mx + c$$

where $c = 0$ and $m = \frac{50-0}{2-0} = 25$

Here $x = t$, interval $T = 2$ sec

$$y(t) = 25\,t \qquad 0 < t < 2$$

$$\text{and} \; y^2(t) = 625\,t^2 \qquad 0 < t < 2$$

$$\therefore \; Y_{av} = \frac{1}{2}\int_0^2 25\,t\,dt$$

$$= \frac{1}{2}\left[20\,\frac{t^2}{2}\right]_0^2 = \frac{25}{4} \times 4 = \boxed{25}$$

$$Y_{rms} = \sqrt{\frac{1}{T}\int_0^T y^2(t)\,dt} = \sqrt{\frac{1}{2}\int_0^2 625\,t^2\,dt}$$

$$= \sqrt{\frac{1}{2} \times 625 \times \frac{t^3}{3}\Big|_0^2} = \sqrt{\frac{1}{2} \times 625 \times \frac{8}{3}}$$

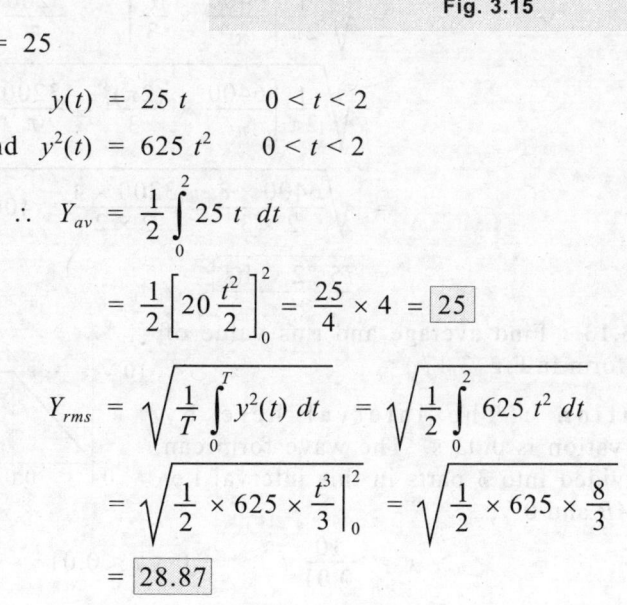

$$= \boxed{28.87}$$

Ex. 3.12 : Find average and rms value of waveform in Fig. 3.16.

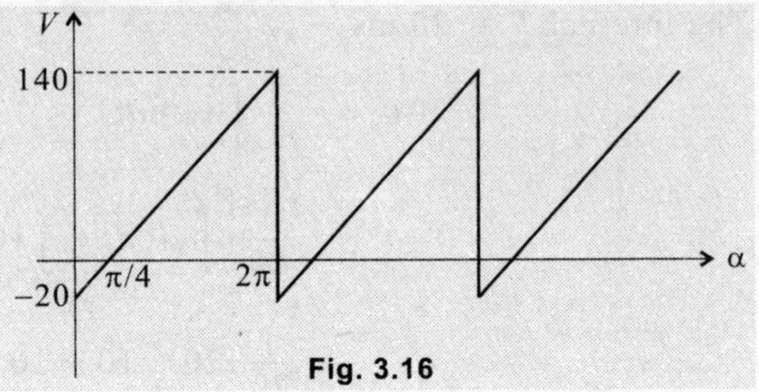

Fig. 3.16

Solution : Here, the interval $T = 2\pi$

Expression for voltage waveform is

$$v = m\alpha + c$$

where $c = -20$

$$\text{and } m \text{ (slope)} = \frac{140-(-20)}{2\pi} = \frac{160}{2\pi}$$

$$\therefore\ v = \frac{160}{2\pi}\alpha - 20 = \frac{80}{\pi}\alpha - 20$$

$$\text{and } v^2 = \frac{6400}{\pi^2}\alpha^2 - \frac{3200}{\pi}\alpha + 400$$

$$\therefore\ V_{av} = \frac{1}{2\pi}\int_0^{2\pi}\left(\frac{80}{\pi}\alpha - 20\right)d\alpha = \frac{1}{2\pi}\left\{\frac{80}{\pi}\left(\frac{\alpha^2}{\pi}\right)_0^{2\pi} - 20(\alpha)_0^{2\pi}\right\}$$

$$= \frac{1}{2\pi}\left\{\frac{80}{\pi}\times\frac{4\pi^2}{2} - 20\times 2\pi\right\}$$

$$= 80 - 20 = \boxed{60 \text{ volts}}$$

$$V_{rms} = \sqrt{\frac{1}{2\pi}\int_0^{2\pi}\left[\frac{6400}{\pi^2}\alpha^2 - \frac{3200}{\pi}\alpha + 400\right]d\alpha}$$

$$= \sqrt{\frac{1}{2\pi}\left[\frac{6400}{\pi^2}\times\left.\frac{\alpha^3}{3}\right|_0^{2\pi} - \frac{3200}{\pi}\times\left.\frac{\alpha^2}{2}\right|_0^{2\pi} + 400\,\alpha\Big|_0^{2\pi}\right]}$$

$$= \sqrt{\frac{1}{2\pi}\left[\frac{6400}{\pi^2}\times\frac{(2\pi)^3}{3} - \frac{3200}{\pi}\times\frac{(2\pi)^2}{2} + 400\times 2\pi\right]}$$

$$= \sqrt{\frac{6400\times 8}{2\times 3} - \frac{3200\times 4}{2\times 2} + 400}$$

$$= \boxed{75.72 \text{ volts}}$$

Ex. 3.13 : Find average and rms value of waveform in Fig. 3.17.

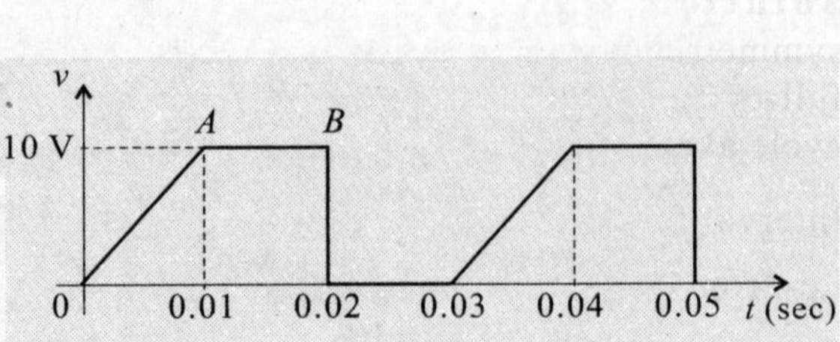

Fig. 3.17

Solution : The interval here by observation is 0.03 s. The wave form can be divided into 3 parts in this interval i.e. *OA*, *AB* and 0 V.

$$\therefore\ v = \frac{10}{0.01}t \qquad 0 < t < 0.01$$

$$\text{or } v = 1000\,t \qquad 0 < t < 0.01$$
$$= 10 \qquad 0.01 < t < 0.02$$
$$= 0 \qquad 0.02 < t < 0.03$$
$$\text{and } v^2 = 10^6\,t^2 \qquad 0 < t < 0.01$$
$$= 100 \qquad 0.01 < t < 0.02$$
$$= 0 \qquad 0.02 < t < 0.03$$

$$\therefore \quad V_{av} = \frac{1}{0.03}\left[\int_0^{0.01} 1000\,t\,dt + \int_{0.01}^{0.02} 10\,dt + \int_{0.02}^{0.03} 0\,dt\right]$$
$$= \frac{1}{0.03}\left[1000\,\frac{t^2}{2}\bigg|_0^{0.01} + 10\,t\bigg|_{0.01}^{0.02}\right]$$
$$= \frac{1}{0.03}\left[1000 \times \frac{0.01^2}{2} + 10 \times 0.01\right]$$
$$= \boxed{5 \text{ volts}}$$

$$V_{rms} = \sqrt{\frac{1}{0.03}\left[\int_0^{0.01} 10^6\,t^2\,dt + \int_{0.01}^{0.02} 100\,dt + \int_{0.02}^{0.03} 0\,dt\right]}$$
$$= \sqrt{\frac{1}{0.03}\left[10^6\,\frac{t^3}{3}\bigg|_0^{0.01} + 100\,t\bigg|_{0.01}^{0.02}\right]}$$
$$= \sqrt{\frac{1}{0.03}\left[10^6 \times \frac{0.01^3}{3} + 100 \times 0.01\right]}$$
$$= \boxed{6.67 \text{ volts}}$$

Ex. 3.14 : Find the average and rms value of the waveform in Fig. 3.18.

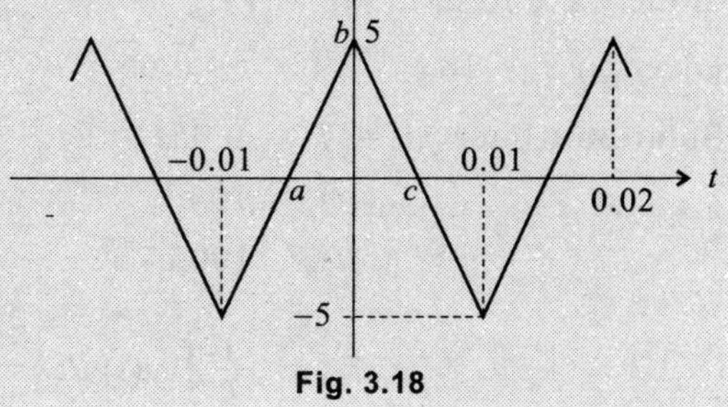

Fig. 3.18

Solution : As this wave form is symmetrical about time axis (x-axis), the full-cycle average will be zero. Hence half-cycle average will be calculated.

Interval for half-cycle $= T = 0.01$ s

i.e. from a (-0.005) to c (0.005).

$$\text{Equation for } ab \Rightarrow \ y = \frac{5}{0.05}\,t + 5$$
$$y = 1000\,t + 5 \qquad -0.005 < t < 0$$

Equation for $bc \Rightarrow y = -1000\,t + 5 \quad 0 < t < 0.005$

$$\text{Half-cycle average } Y_{av} = \frac{1}{0.01}\left[\int_{-0.005}^{0}(1000\,t+5)\,dt + \int_{0}^{0.005}(-1000\,t+5)\,dt\right]$$

$$= \frac{1}{0.01}\left[1000\left.\frac{t^2}{2}\right|_{-0.005}^{0} + 5\,t\Big|_{-0.005}^{0} - 1000\left.\frac{t^2}{2}\right|_{0}^{0.005} + 5\,t\Big|_{0}^{0.005}\right]$$

$$= \frac{1}{0.01}\left[-500 \times 0.005^2 + 5(0.005) - 500(0.005)^2 + 5(0.005)\right]$$

$$= \boxed{2.5}$$

$$Y_{rms} = \sqrt{\frac{1}{0.01}\left[\int_{-0.005}^{0}(1000\,t+5)^2\,dt + \int_{0}^{0.005}(-1000\,t+5)^2\,dt\right]}$$

$$= \sqrt{\frac{1}{0.01}\left[\int_{-0.005}^{0}(10^6\,t^2 + 10^4\,t + 25)\,dt + \int_{0}^{0.005}(10^6\,t^2 - 10^4\,t + 25)\,dt\right]}$$

$$= \sqrt{\frac{1}{0.01}\left[10^6\left.\frac{t^3}{3}\right|_{-0.005}^{0} + 10^4\left.\frac{t^2}{2}\right|_{-0.005}^{0} + 25\,t\Big|_{-0.005}^{0} + 10^6\left.\frac{t^3}{3}\right|_{0}^{0.005} - 10^4\left.\frac{t^2}{2}\right|_{0}^{0.005} + 25\,t\Big|_{0}^{0.005}\right]}$$

$$= \sqrt{\frac{1}{0.01}\left[\frac{1}{24} - \frac{1}{8} + \frac{1}{8} + \frac{1}{24} - \frac{1}{8} + \frac{1}{8}\right]}$$

$$= \boxed{2.88}$$

Ex. 3.15 : Find the average and rms value of the wave form in Fig. 3.19.

Given : $y(t) = 10\,e^{-200t}$, $0 < t < 0.05$

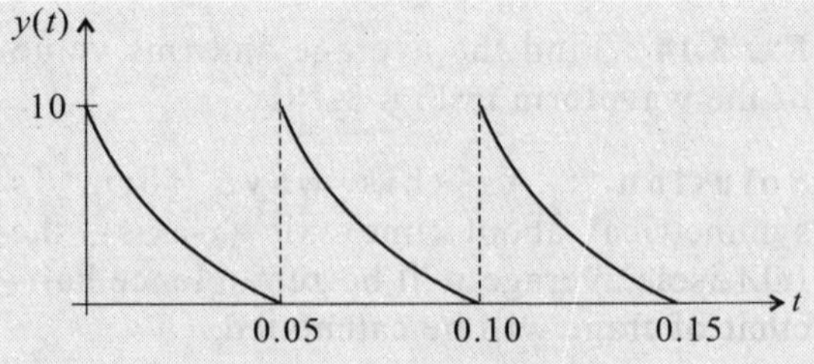

Fig. 3.19

Solution : Interval $= T = 0.05$

$$y(t) = 10\,e^{-200t}$$

$$y^2(t) = 100\,e^{-400t}$$

$$\therefore Y_{av} = \frac{1}{T}\int_0^T y(t)\,dt = \frac{1}{0.05}\int_0^{0.05} 10\,e^{-200t}\,dt$$

$$= \frac{10}{0.05}\left[\frac{e^{-200t}}{-200}\right]_0^{0.05} = -1\,[e^{-200 \times 0.05} - e^0] = \boxed{1}$$

$$Y_{rms} = \sqrt{\frac{1}{T}\int_0^T y^2(t)\,dt} = \sqrt{\frac{1}{0.05}\int_0^{0.05} 100\,e^{-400t}\,dt}$$

$$= \sqrt{\frac{100}{0.05}\left[\frac{e^{-400t}}{-400}\right]_0^{0.05}} = \sqrt{-5\,[e^{-20} - e^0]}$$

$$= \boxed{2.24}$$

3.5 Vector Representation of Sinusoidal A.C.

We have so far seen the various kinds of unidirectional and alternating waveforms. In any case, unless otherwise stated, the computations of a.c. circuits are based on the assumptions of sinusoidal voltages and currents, given by the equations

$$v(t) = V_m \sin \omega t$$

$$\text{or in general } v(t) = V_m \sin (\omega t + \phi)$$

These voltages (or currents) are continuously changing and it is cumbersome to handle varying parameters according to the instantaneous values. The conventional method is to represent these quantities by vector notations. If we consider any vector of length OA as in Fig. 3.20. Then the perpendicular from A on x-axis is given by $OA \sin \theta$, which is similar to the expression of the sinusoidal waveform.

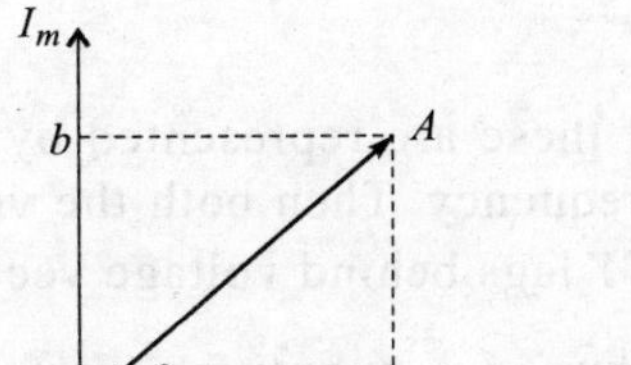

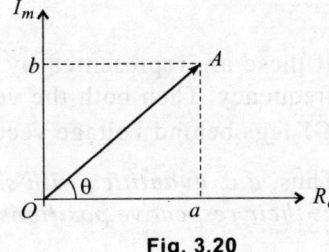

Fig. 3.20

Let us consider a sinusoidal waveform as in Fig. 3.21.

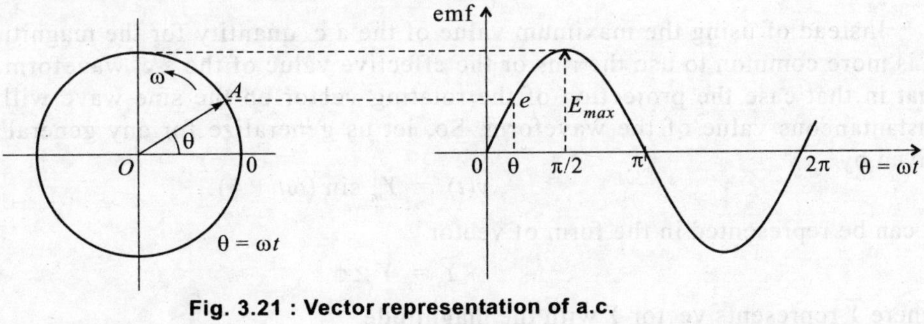

Fig. 3.21 : Vector representation of a.c.

OA is a vector which is rotating in anticlockwise direction with the "*same frequency*" as that of the sinusoidal quantity. The length of OA is equal to the maximum value of sine wave. At any instant $\theta = \omega t$, magnitudes of emf is e given by

$$e = E_{max} \sin \theta$$

$$e = E_{max} \sin \omega t$$

Thus, the vector OA can be used to represent the a.c. sine wave. These vectors then may be used, instead of the instantaneous values, to achieve the designed results.

Now, let us consider two a.c. quantities $v(t)$ and $i(t)$ of the same frequency but having a phase different of θ between them as in the Fig. 3.22. From e.g. 3.8 and 3.10.

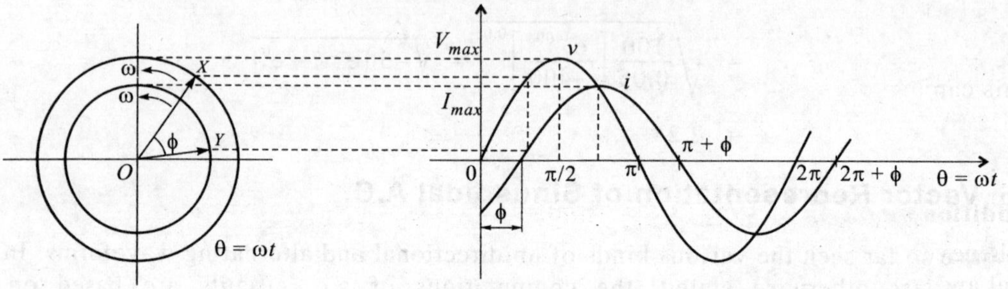

Fig. 3.22

We can write

$$v(t) = V_m \sin \omega t$$

$$\text{and} \quad i(t) = I_m \sin (\omega t - \phi)$$

If these are represented by vectors OX and OY respectively, both rotating with the same frequency. Then both the vectors are fixed with respect to each other and current vectors OY lags behind voltage vectors OX by the same angle ϕ.

Thus, *a.c. quantities with same frequency only can be drawn on common vector diagram as their respective positions will remain the same always.*

3.6 Vector Representation Using RMS Values

Instead of using the maximum value of the a.c. quantity for the magnitude of vector, it is more common to use the rms or the effective value of the a.c. waveform. Please note that in that case the projection of the rotating vector on the sine wave will not give the instantaneous value of the waveform. So, let us generalize for any general a.c. quantity given by

$$y(t) = Y_m \sin (\omega t + \phi)$$

It can be represented in the form of vector

$$\overline{Y} = Y \angle \phi$$

where $\overline{Y}$ represents vector Y with the magnitude

$$Y = \frac{Y_m}{\sqrt{2}} \qquad \text{[refer equation (3.21)]}$$

3.7 Mathematical Operation of Vectors

As a.c. quantities can now be represented by vector, we should first revise the mathematical operations like addition, subtraction, multiplication and division of vectors. Any vector Y can be represented in either rectangular or polar form.

$\overline{Y} = Y\angle\phi$ the polar form

$\overline{Y} = a + jb$ the rectangular form (Cartesian form)

where $a = Y\cos\phi$ and $b = Y\sin\phi$

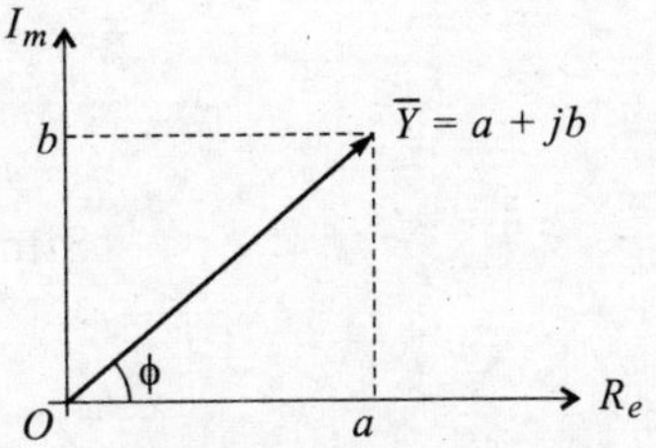

Fig. 3.23 : Representation of vector in complex plane.

This can be understood from Fig. 3.23.

$$Y = \sqrt{a^2 + b^2} \text{ and } \phi = \tan^{-1}\frac{b}{a}$$

Addition and Subtraction

Whenever we add or subtract two complex numbers (vectors or phasor) remember that real and imaginary parts should be kept separate.

Let $\overline{z}_1 = 3 + 4j$ and $\overline{z}_2 = -2 - 6j$

$$\text{Then } \overline{z}_1 + \overline{z}_2 = 3 + 4j + (-2 - 6j) = 1 - 2j$$

$$= \sqrt{1^2 + 2^2} \angle \tan^{-1}\frac{-2}{1} = 2.2\angle -63.43^\circ$$

$$\overline{z}_1 - \overline{z}_2 = (3 + 4j) - (-2 - 6j) = 3 + 4j + 2 + 6j$$

$$= 5 + 10j$$

$$= \sqrt{5^2 + 10^2} \angle \tan^{-1}\frac{10}{5} = \boxed{11.18\angle 63.43^\circ}$$

Multiplication and Division

For multiplication of complex numbers remember that $j^2 = -1$.

$$\overline{z}_1 \cdot \overline{z}_2 = (3 + 4j)(-2 - 6j) = -6 - 8j - 18j - 24j^2$$

$$= -6 - 26j + 24$$

$$= 18 - 26j$$

$$= \boxed{31.62\angle -55.3^\circ}$$

For division use complex conjugate of denominator as shown below

$$\overline{z}_1 \div \overline{z}_2 = \frac{3 + 4j}{-2 - 6j} \times \frac{-2 + 6j}{-2 + 6j}$$

$$= \frac{-6 - 8j + 18j - 24}{(-2)^2 - (6j)^2} = \frac{-30 + 10j}{40}$$

$$= -0.75 + 0.25j$$

$$= \boxed{0.79\angle 161.56^\circ}$$

***Note :** Modern day calculators allow all the operations directly on the calculator in the complex mode. They can convert complex numbers from polar to rectangular form and vice versa at the click of button. Only thing don't forget to use brackets for a complex number. These calculators also allow calculations in the mixed form i.e. let $\overline{z}_3 = 10\angle 45^\circ$ and $\overline{z}_4 = 4 + 5j$ then addition, subtraction, multiplication and division can be done directly.*

$$\overline{z}_3 + \overline{z}_4 = (10 \angle 45^\circ) + (4 + 5j) = 11.07 + 12.07j$$
$$= 16.38 \angle 47.47^\circ$$

Similarly $$\overline{z}_3 \div \overline{z}_4 = \frac{10 \angle 45^\circ}{4 + 5j} = 1.55 - 0.17j$$
$$= \boxed{1.56 \angle -6.34^\circ}$$

Addition and Subtraction of Vectors Graphically

If A and B are two vectors as shown in Fig 3.24(i) then to add $\overline{A}$ and $\overline{B}$ draw a parallelogram and the diagonal $\overline{C}$ is the resultant of $\overline{A}$ and $\overline{B}$.

If $|\overline{A}| = A$, $|\overline{B}| = B$ and $|\overline{C}| = C$

then $C = A^2 + B^2 + 2AB \cos \phi$

Similarly, the subtraction of $\overline{A}$ and $\overline{B}$ is done by first drawing $-\overline{B}$ (equal and opposite of $\overline{B}$). Then drawing the parallelogram between $\overline{A}$ and $-\overline{B}$. The resultant is $\overline{D}$ as in Fig. 3.24(ii).

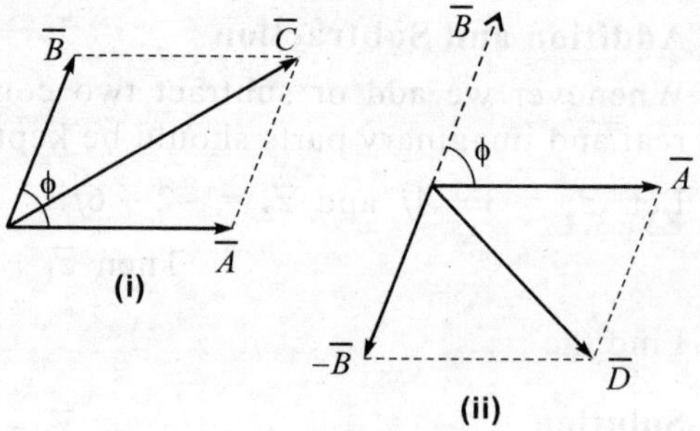

Fig. 3.24

If there are three or more vectors then, one way of finding the additions of all these vectors $\overline{z}_1$, $\overline{z}_2$, $\overline{z}_3$ and $\overline{z}_4$ graphically is draw one vector $\overline{z}_1$. On the head of $\overline{z}_1$ draw $\overline{z}_2$ (Fig. 3.25), similarly on the head of $\overline{z}_2$ draw $\overline{z}_3$ and so on. The resultant of all the vectors is $\overline{z}$ which is drawn from tail of $\overline{z}_1$ to head of $\overline{z}_4$.

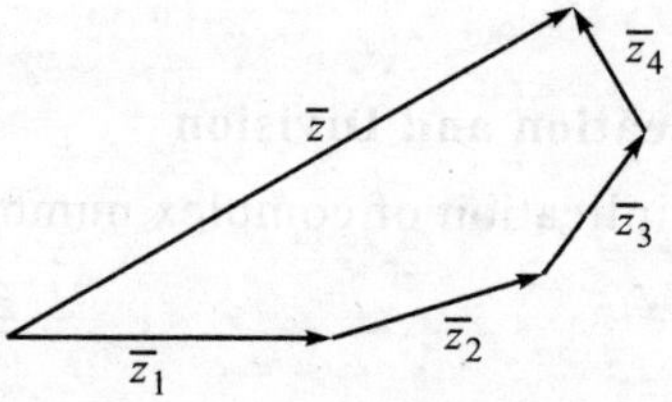

Fig. 3.25

Ex. 3.16 : Two sinusoidal currents are given as follows.

$$i_1 = 14.14 \sin \omega t$$
$$i_2 = 21.21 \sin (\omega t + 30^\circ)$$

Find the resultant of the two currents.

Solution : Let us find the vector representation of i_1 and i_2 as $\overline{I}_1$ and $\overline{I}_2$ respectively. [refer section 3.5, 3.6]

For any general waveform $$i = I_m \sin (\omega t + \phi)$$

$$\overline{I} = \frac{I_m}{\sqrt{2}} \angle \phi$$

$$\therefore \quad \overline{I}_1 = \frac{14.14}{\sqrt{2}} \angle 0^\circ = 10 \angle 0^\circ$$

and $$\overline{I}_2 = \frac{21.21}{\sqrt{2}} \angle 30^\circ = 15 \angle 30^\circ$$

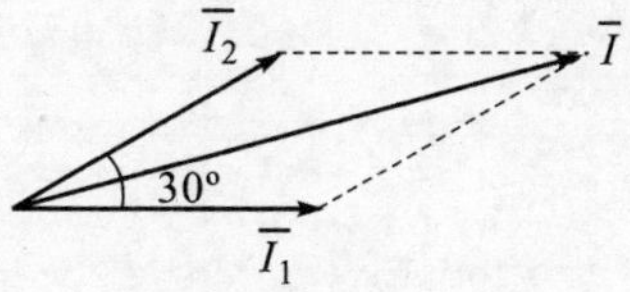

Fig. 3.26

$$\overline{I} = \overline{I_1} + \overline{I_2}$$
$$= (10 \angle 0^\circ) + (15 \angle 30^\circ) = 10 + 13 + 7.5j$$
$$= 23 + 7.5j$$
$$= \boxed{24.18 \angle 18.06^\circ}$$

∴ the resultant current can also be written as

$$i = \sqrt{2} \times 24.18 \sin(\omega t + 18.06^\circ)$$
$$= \boxed{34.19 \sin(\omega t + 18.06^\circ)}$$

Ex. 3.17 : Given : $i_1 = 5 \sin \omega t$; $i_2 = 10 \sin(\omega t - 30^\circ)$;

$i_3 = 5 \cos(\omega t - 30^\circ)$; $i_4 = -10 \sin(\omega t + 45^\circ)$

Find the resultant of all the currents.

Solution : To represent all the currents in the vector form first the expressions of currents should be in the form of $I_m \sin(\omega t + \phi)$. Thus converting i_3 and i_4 to standard form.

$$i_3 = 5 \cos(\omega t - 30^\circ) = 5 \sin(\omega t - 30^\circ + 90^\circ)$$
$$\therefore \; i_3 = 5 \sin(\omega t + 60^\circ)$$

Similarly, $i_4 = -10 \sin(\omega t + 45^\circ) = 10 \sin(\omega t + 45^\circ + 180^\circ)$

$$\therefore \; i_4 = 10 \sin(\omega t + 225^\circ)$$

$$\therefore \; \overline{I_1} = \frac{5}{\sqrt{2}} \angle 0^\circ = 3.53 \angle 0^\circ$$

$$\overline{I_2} = \frac{10}{\sqrt{2}} \angle -30^\circ = 7.07 \angle -30^\circ$$

$$\overline{I_3} = \frac{5}{\sqrt{2}} \angle 60^\circ = 3.53 \angle 60^\circ$$

and $\overline{I_4} = \frac{10}{\sqrt{2}} \angle 225^\circ = 7.07 \angle 225^\circ$

$$\overline{I} = \overline{I_1} + \overline{I_2} + \overline{I_3} + \overline{I_4}$$
$$= (3.53 \angle 0^\circ) + (7.07 \angle -30^\circ) + (3.53 \angle 60^\circ) + (7.07 \angle 225^\circ)$$
$$= 6.41 - 5.477\, j$$
$$= 8.44 \angle -40.4^\circ$$
$$= \boxed{11.9 \sin(\omega t - 40.4^\circ)}$$

Unsolved Examples

1. Find rms and average values of the following :

(i)

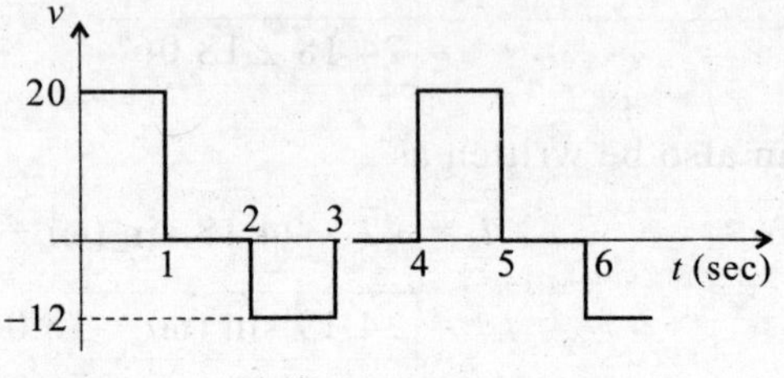

[Ans. V_{av} = 2 V, V_{rms} = 11.66 V**]**

(ii)

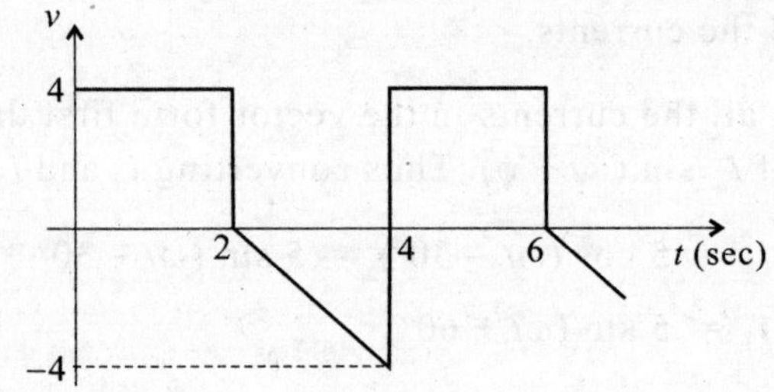

[Ans. V_{av} = 1 V, V_{rms} = 3.26 V**]**

(iii)

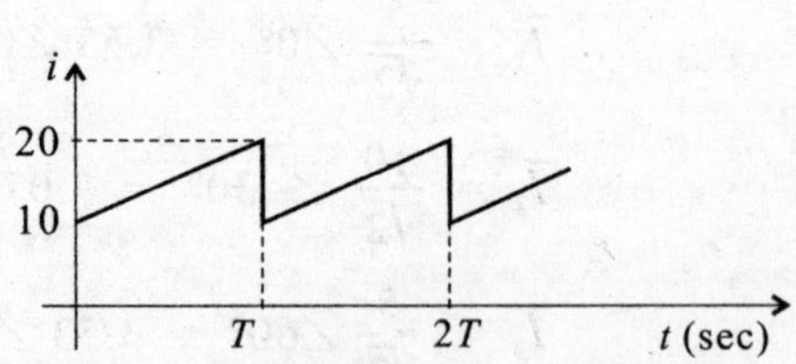

[Ans. I_{av} = 15 A, I_{rms} = 15.27 A**]**

(iv)

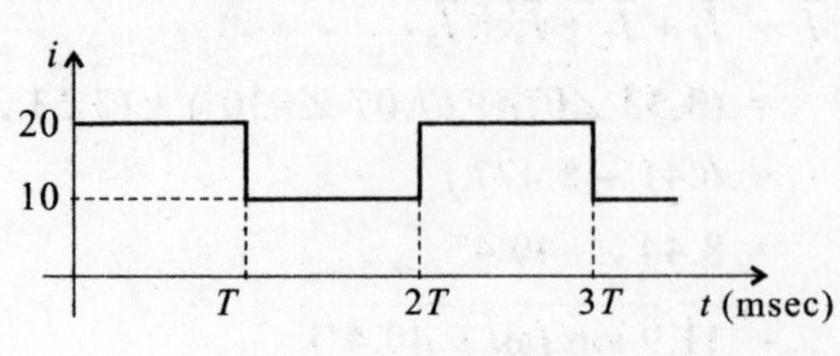

[Ans. I_{av} = 15 A, I_{rms} = 15.81 A**]**

(v)

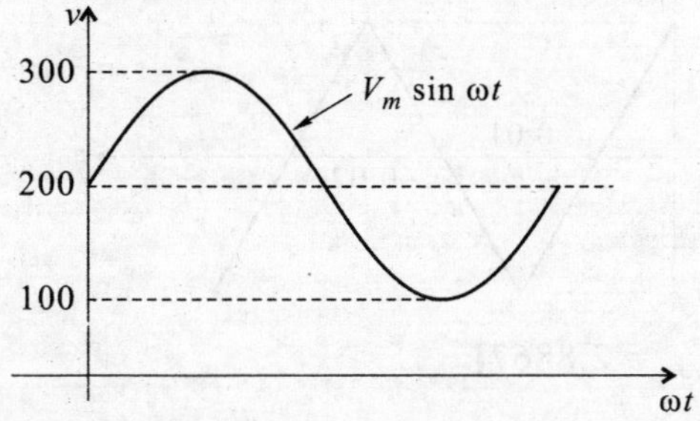

[Ans. $V_{av} = 200$ V, $V_{rms} = 212.13$ V**]**

(vi)

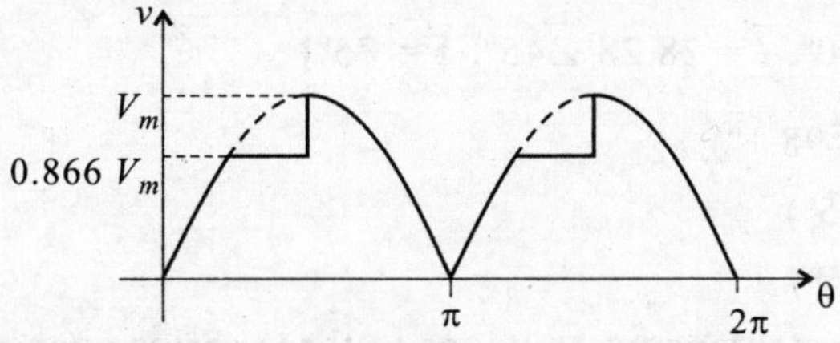

[Ans. $V_{av} = 0.644\ V_m$, $V_{rms} = 0.6875\ V_m$**]**

(vii)

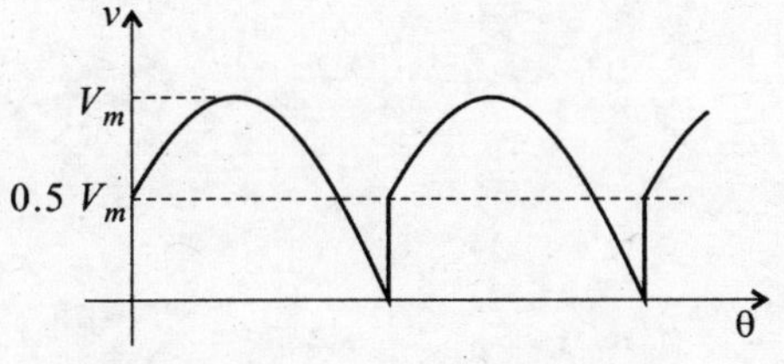

[Ans. $V_{av} = 0.713\ V_m$, $V_{rms} = 0.7633\ V_m$**]**

(viii)

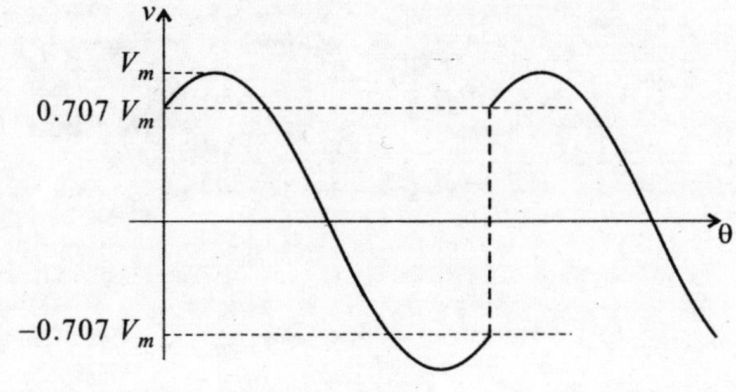

[Ans. $V_{av} = 0.7245\ V_m$, $V_{rms} = 1.1\ V_m$**]**

(ix)

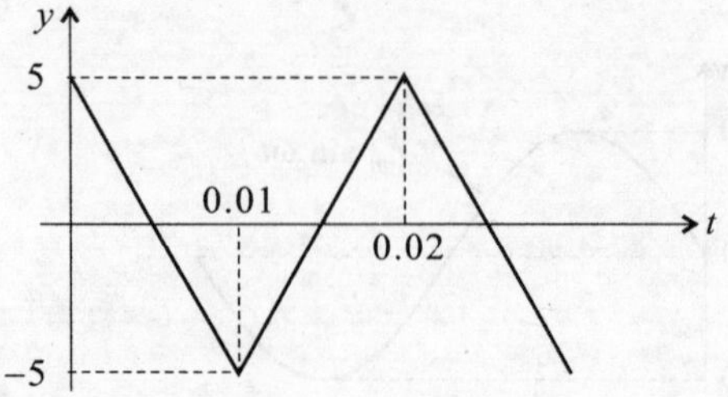

[Ans. $Y_{av} = 2.5$, $Y_{rms} = 2.8867$**]**

2. Two sine waves are represented by the following expression

$$e = 282 \sin(314t - \pi/6) \quad \text{and} \quad i = 40 \sin(314t + \pi/4).$$

Find maximum and rms value of each. Also, find the phase difference between the two showing vector diagram.

[Ans. $\overline{E} = 199.4 \angle -30°$, $\overline{I} = 28.28 \angle 45°$, $\phi = 75°$**]**

3. $v_1 = 147.3 \cos(\omega t + 98.1°)$

$v_2 = 294 \cos(\omega t - 45°)$

$v_3 = 88 \sin(\omega t + 135°)$

v_1, v_2 and v_3 are the instantaneous voltages in three series connected circuit. Find the resultant voltage. Also show all the vectors on vector diagram.

[Ans. $\overline{V}_R = 1176.31 \angle 90°$**]**

CHAPTER

4 A.C. CIRCUITS

In the previous chapter we have studied the various types of alternating signals. Sine-wave is the basic form of alternating signal, hence for all our study, unless otherwise stated, the supply a.c. signal is a pure sine wave. We shall now study the steady-state response of the basic circuit parameters (R, L and C) to a sinusoidal signal. Steady-state means the signal is continuously applied for a reasonably long time.

When electric energy is supplied to a circuit element or elements, it will respond in one or more of the following three ways

i) If energy is consumed, the circuit element is a pure resistor.

ii) If energy is stored in magnetic field, the circuit element is pure inductor

iii) If energy is stored in electric field, the circuit element is pure capacitor.

A practical circuit (device) will exhibit more than one of the above properties or perhaps all three at the same time, but one may be predominant. Let us first consider the circuit assuming them to be purely resistive, inductive or capacitive. Then the various combinations of these elements are taken later. We will first establish the phase angle relationship between the current through and the voltage across each of the circuit parameters. These relationships remain the same for a given parameter irrespective of the manner in which these parameters are connected in the circuit.

4.1 A.C. Through Pure Resistance

The potential difference across the terminals of a pure resistance is directly proportional to the current through it (ohms law), the constant of proportionality being R, the resistance.

$$\text{i.e.} \quad v(t) = R\, i(t) \qquad \text{..... (4.1)}$$

$$\therefore \quad i(t) = \frac{v(t)}{R} \qquad \text{..... (4.2)}$$

Let $v(t) = V_m \sin \omega t$ be the supply voltage.

From equation (3.21) rms value of supply voltage

$$V = \frac{V_m}{\sqrt{2}}$$

Vector representation of supply voltage will be

$$\overline{V} = V \angle 0^\circ \quad \text{..... (4.3)}$$

From equation (4.2)

$$i(t) = \frac{v(t)}{R} = \frac{V_m}{R} \sin \omega t$$

$$\text{or } i(t) = I_m \sin \omega t \quad \text{..... (4.4)}$$

$$\text{where } I_m = \frac{V_m}{R}$$

Dividing both sides by $\sqrt{2}$

$$\frac{I_m}{\sqrt{2}} = \frac{V_m}{\sqrt{2}} \frac{1}{R}$$

$$\text{or } I = \frac{V}{R}$$

The vector representation of $i(t)$ from equation (4.4) will be

$$\overline{I} = I \angle 0^\circ \quad \text{..... (4.5)}$$

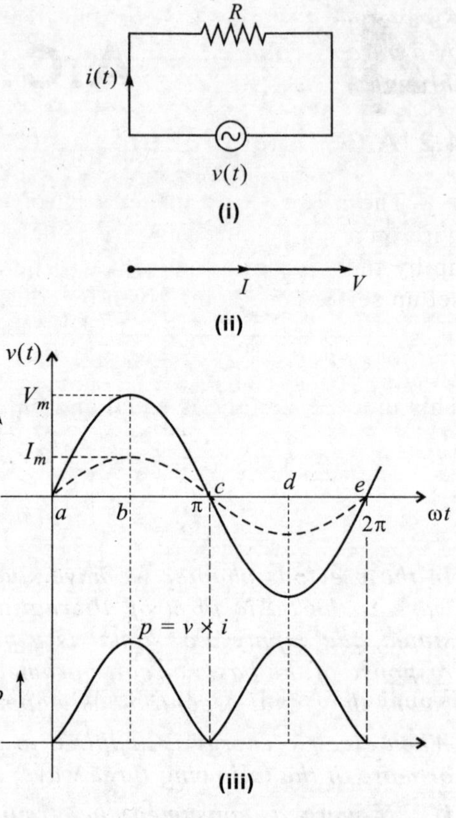

Fig. 4.1 : a.c. through pure resistance.

Drawing vectors $\overline{V}$ and $\overline{I}$ as in Fig. 4.1(ii).

We observe that for pure resistance voltage and current vectors are along the same phase. The instantaneous values of $v(t)$ and $i(t)$ are also drawn. Their zero crossing are same. If we plot instantaneous power p [Fig. 4.1(iii)], we observe that between from a - c i.e. 0 - π, the product of v and i is positive with peak occurring at b (π/2). Now, between c and e both current and voltage are negative hence their product is again positive.

$$\text{The instantaneous power } p = v \times i$$

$$= V_m \sin \omega t \times I_m \sin \omega t \quad \text{... } [\because \sin^2 \omega t = 1 - \cos 2\omega t]$$

$$= 2 \frac{V_m}{\sqrt{2}} \cdot \frac{I_m}{\sqrt{2}} \sin^2 \omega t \quad \text{... [Dividing and multiplying by 2]}$$

$$= 2\, V I \sin^2 \omega t$$

$$= V I (1 - \cos 2\omega t)$$

$$= V I - V I \cos 2\omega t$$

The average power over a complete cycle

$$P = V I \quad \text{..... (4.6)}$$

As average value of $V\,I\cos 2\omega t$ over complete cycle is zero. Thus, the *power consumed by a pure resistance is given by the product of rms values of voltage across it and current through it.*

4.2 A.C. Through Pure Inductance

The nearest way to get a purely (highly) inductive load is to wind a coil of copper wire on a laminated iron core. Such a coil is called a *choke coil*. The magnetic field set up by the alternating current will be alternating; hence this changing magnetic field will set up self induced emf given by equation (2.15), i.e.

$$e = -L\frac{di}{dt}$$

This induced voltage is equal and opposite to the supply voltage v at every instant

$$\therefore\ v = -e = +L\frac{di}{dt} \quad \text{..... (4.7)}$$

$$\text{Let}\quad v(t) = V_m \sin \omega t$$

$$\overline{V} = \frac{V_m}{\sqrt{2}}\angle 0^\circ = V\angle 0^\circ \quad \text{..... (4.8)}$$

$$\text{where } V = \text{rms value of applied voltage.}$$

From equaion (4.7)

$$i = \frac{1}{L}\int v\,dt \quad \text{..... (4.9)}$$

$$= \frac{1}{L}\int V_m \sin \omega t\,dt$$

$$= -\frac{V_m}{\omega L}\cos \omega t$$

$$\therefore\ i = \frac{V_m}{\omega L}\sin\left(\omega t - \frac{\pi}{2}\right)$$

$$\text{or } i = I_m \sin\left(\omega t - \frac{\pi}{2}\right) \quad \text{..... (4.10)}$$

$$\text{where } I_m = \frac{V_m}{\omega L}$$

Divide both sides by $\sqrt{2}$

$$\frac{I_m}{\sqrt{2}} = \frac{V_m}{\sqrt{2}}\frac{1}{\omega L}$$

$$\text{or } I = \frac{V}{\omega L}$$

$$\text{or } \omega L = \frac{V}{I} \quad \text{..... (4.11)}$$

$$\text{or } X_L = \frac{V}{I} \quad \text{where } X_L = \omega L \quad \text{..... (4.12)}$$

X_L is called the *inductive reactance*. As it can be seen from equation (4.11), it is ratio of voltage (rms) by the current (rms) its unit is ohms.

Note : *Unit of inductance L is Hennery where as that of inductive reactance is Ohms.*

Representing equation (4.10) of current in the vector form ($\overline{I}$)

$$\overline{I} = \frac{I_m}{\sqrt{2}} \angle -\pi/2 = I \angle -\pi/2 \qquad ..... (4.13)$$

Let, us draw the vector (phasor) diagram from equations (4.8) and (4.13), the current vector lags behind the voltage by 90º, as shown in Fig. 4.2(ii). Drawing the instantaneous voltage and current waveforms as in Fig. 4.2(iii) the current lags behind voltage by $\pi/2$. Now, plotting instantaneous power p by multiplying v and i observe that in Fig. 4.2(iii), at a, b, c, d, e either voltage is zero (a, c, e) or current is zero (b, d). Thus product of v and i i.e. p instantaneous power is zero at these points, between a-b, voltage is positive but current in negative thus power is negative. Between b-c, both voltage and current are positive, and between d-c both are negative hence between these internals power is positive.

$$p = v \times i$$

$$= V_m \sin \omega t \times I_m \sin\left(\omega t - \frac{\pi}{2}\right)$$

$$= -V_m\, I_m \sin \omega t \cos \omega t$$

$$= -2\, \frac{V_m}{\sqrt{2}} \cdot \frac{I_m}{\sqrt{2}} \sin \omega t \cos \omega t$$

$$p = -\, V I \sin 2\omega t \qquad ..... (4.14)$$

The average power P over complete cycle

$$P = 0 \qquad ..... (4.15)$$

as full cycle average of $\sin 2\omega t$ is zero.

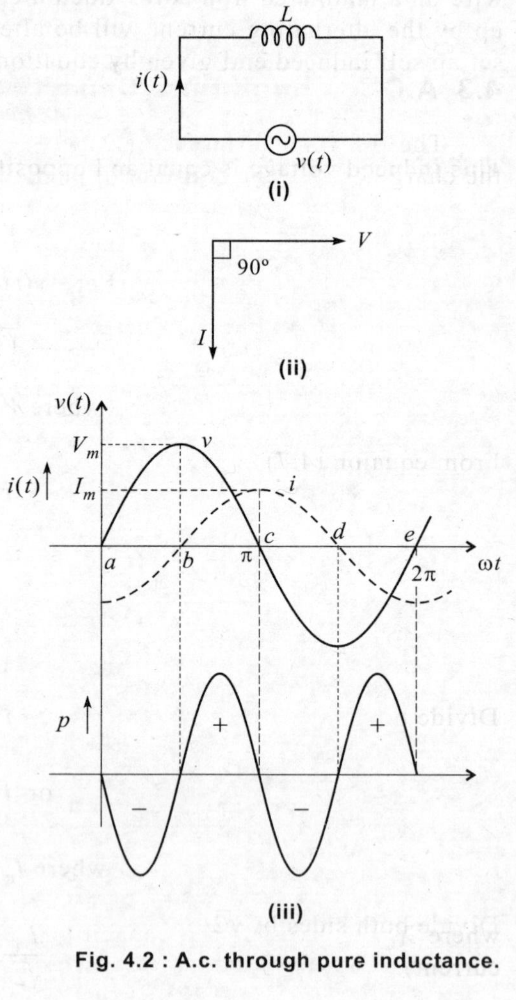

Fig. 4.2 : A.c. through pure inductance.

Thus, "**important observations**" for pure inductance are:

(i) Inductive current lags its own voltage by 90º.

(ii) The average power consumed by inductance is zero as inductance does not consume power. It absorbs power in one half cycle and gives it off in other half.

(iii) In a.c. circuits inductance L is to be replaced by X_L, the inductive reactance.

For d.c. circuits the ratio of voltage to current was called *resistance*, but now we will generalize this term for a.c. circuits as impedance i.e. *the ratio of voltage across a circuit to the current through it*. This impedance is equal to resistance for purely resistive circuit. Now, this impedance is equal to inductive reactance X_L for inductive circuit.

$$\therefore \text{Impedance} = \frac{\overline{V}}{\overline{I}} = \frac{V\angle 0^\circ}{I\angle -90^\circ} = \frac{V}{I}\angle 90^\circ = X_L\angle 90^\circ$$

Converting impedance to rectangular form

$$\text{Impedance} = j\,X_L \qquad \text{..... (4.16)}$$

4.3 A.C. Through Pure Capacitance

The potential difference (v) between the terminals of a capacitor is proportional to the charge q on it, the constant of proportionality is C, with unit as Farads.

$$\text{i.e. } q(t) = C\,v(t)$$

$$\text{but } i = \frac{dq}{dt}$$

$$\text{or } i = C\frac{dv}{dt} \qquad \text{..... (4.17)}$$

$$\text{Let, } v = V_m \sin \omega t$$

$$\therefore i = C\frac{d}{dt}\,V_m \sin \omega t$$

$$= \omega C\,V_m \cos \omega t$$

$$= \omega C\,V_m \sin\left(\omega t + \frac{\pi}{2}\right)$$

$$\therefore i = I_m \sin\left(\omega t + \frac{\pi}{2}\right) \qquad \text{..... (4.18)}$$

$$\text{where } I_m = \omega C\,V_m$$

Divide both sides by $\sqrt{2}$

$$\frac{I_m}{\sqrt{2}} = \omega C\frac{V_m}{\sqrt{2}}$$

$$\text{or } I = \omega C\,V$$

$$\text{or } \frac{V}{I} = \frac{1}{\omega C} = X_C \qquad \text{..... (4.19)}$$

where $X_C = \dfrac{1}{\omega C}$, is the capacitive reactance whose unit is ohms (ratio of voltage to current).

The vector representations for supply voltage is

$$\overline{V} = V\angle 0^\circ$$

and for current from equation (4.18) is $\overline{I} = I\angle 90^\circ$

$$\text{where } I = \frac{I_m}{\sqrt{2}} = \text{rms value of current.}$$

Thus drawing the vector diagram as in Fig. 4.3 (ii), we observe current leads the voltage vector by 90°.

Plotting the instantaneous value of v and i as in Fig. 4.3(iii), i leads by 90°. Finding instantaneous power $p = vi$. At instants a, b, c, d, e either voltage or current in zero, hence the instantaneous power is zero, between ab, cd both voltage and current are either positive or negative hence p is positive, between bc, de voltage and current have apposite polarity hence p is negative.

$$p = v \times i$$

$$= V_m \sin \omega t \times I_m \sin\left(\omega t + \frac{\pi}{2}\right)$$

$$= V_m I_m \sin \omega t \cos \omega t$$

$$= 2 \frac{V_m}{\sqrt{2}} \cdot \frac{I_m}{\sqrt{2}} \sin \omega t \cos \omega t$$

$$p = V I \sin 2\omega t \qquad \text{..... (4.20)}$$

$$\text{Average power } P = 0 \qquad \text{..... (4.21)}$$

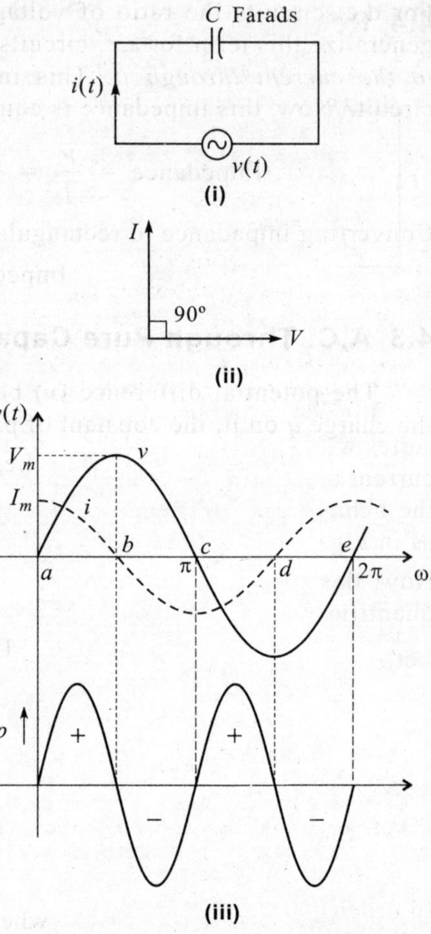

Fig. 4.2 : A.c. through pure capacitance.

Thus important observations for a capacitor.

(i) Capacitive current leads its own voltage by 90°.

(ii) The average power consumed by a capacitor is zero i.e. Capacitor does not consume power its absorbs power in one half cycle (+ve) and gives off power in other half cycle (–ve power).

(iii) In a.c. circuits capacitance C is replaced by $X_C = \dfrac{1}{\omega C}$, the capacitive reactance.

$$\therefore \text{Impedance} = \frac{\overline{V}}{\overline{I}} = \frac{V \angle 0^\circ}{I \angle 90^\circ} = \frac{V}{I} \angle -90^\circ = X_C \angle -90^\circ \qquad \text{..... (4.22)}$$

Converting impedance to rectangular form

$$\text{Impedance} = -j X_C$$

4.4 Resistance and Inductance in Series

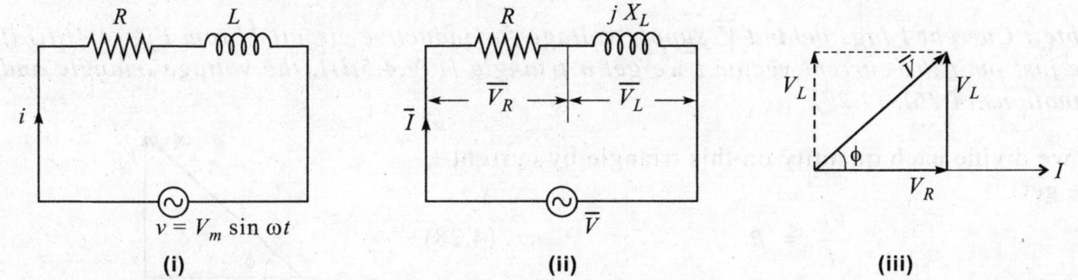

Fig. 4.4 : *R-L* series circuit.

Fig. 4.4(i) shows a.c. voltage $v(t)$ applied to a circuit consisting of resistance R in series with inductance L (Henery). First step here is to convert all the quantities (voltage, current and inductance) to their complex notations (i.e. $\overline{V}, \overline{I}, j X_L$) from d.c. to a.c. circuits the behaviour of resistance does not change (hence R remains same). Redraw the circuit as in Fig. 4.4(ii).

Now, the difference between d.c. circuits and a.c. circuits is that d.c. circuits have scalar quantities where as a.c. circuits have vector quantities.

Let,

$$\text{Supply voltage (vector)} = \overline{V}$$

$$\text{Voltage across resistance} = \overline{V_R} = \overline{I}\,R \quad \text{..... (4.23)}$$

$$\text{where } \overline{I} = \text{Current in the circuit.}$$

$$\text{Voltage across inductance} = \overline{V_L} = \overline{I}\,(j\,X_L) \quad \text{..... (4.24)}$$

$$X_L = 2\pi f L = \omega L$$

In order to draw the vector diagram, let us keep in mind behavior of ac through resistance and inductance (section 4.2 and 4.3). We know that for resistance voltage ($\overline{V_R}$) and current ($\overline{I}$) are in phase and for inductance voltage ($\overline{V_L}$) and current ($\overline{I}$) have a phase difference of 90º i.e. "inductive current lags its own voltage by 90º". Thus, to draw the vector diagram we should take a reference quantity which is common to all components. A careful observation here shows that current $\overline{I}$, is same through source, resistance and inductance.

- So assume $\overline{I}$ as the reference vector [Fig. 4.4(iii)]
- Now, draw $\overline{V_R}$ along $\overline{I}$
- $\overline{V_L}$ leads $\overline{I}$ by 90º (or $\overline{I}$ lags behind $\overline{V_L}$) so at the tip of $\overline{V_R}$ draw $\overline{V_L}$
- Observing the circuit of Fig. 4.4(ii)

$$\overline{V} = \overline{V_R} + \overline{V_L} \quad \text{..... (4.25)}$$

∴ Vector sum of $\overline{V_R}$ and $\overline{V_L}$ indicates supply voltage $\overline{V}$.

From Fig. 4.4(iii),

$$V^2 = V_R^{\,2} + V_L^{\,2} \quad \text{..... (4.26)}$$

$$\phi = \tan^{-1}\frac{V_L}{V_R} \quad ..... (4.27)$$

Note : *Current $\overline{I}$ lags behind $\overline{V}$, supply voltage for inductive circuit. From Fig. 4.4(iii) if we just omit the current vector $\overline{I}$ we get a triangle [Fig.4.5(i)], the voltage triangle and equations (4.26), (4.27)*

If we divide each quantity on this triangle by current I, we get

$$\frac{V_R}{I} = R \quad ..... (4.28)$$

$$\frac{V_L}{I} = X_L \quad ..... (4.29)$$

$$\text{and } \frac{V}{I} = Z = \text{Impedance} \quad ..... (4.30)$$

In complex plane $\overline{Z} = R + j\,X_L$ ..... (4.31)

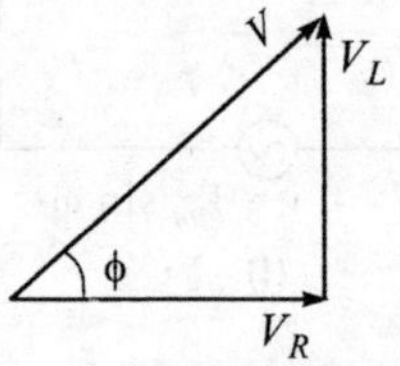

Fig. 4.5(i) : Voltage triangle.

This is called the *impedance triangle* [Fig. 4.5(ii)]. From this figure

$$Z = \sqrt{R^2 + X_L^{\,2}} \quad ..... (4.32)$$

$$\phi = \tan^{-1}\frac{X_L}{R} \quad ..... (4.33)$$

$$\cos\phi = \frac{R}{Z} \quad ..... (4.34)$$

$$\sin\phi = \frac{X_L}{Z} \quad ..... (4.35)$$

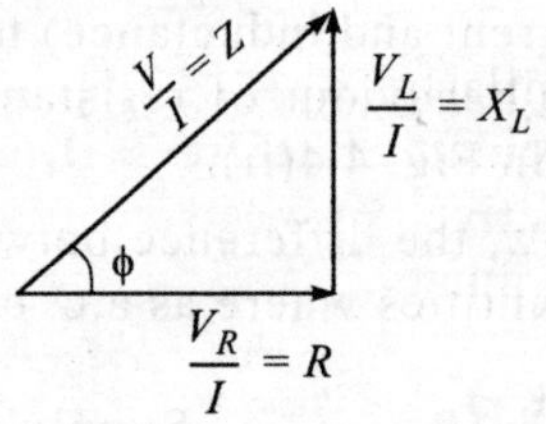

Fig. 4.5(ii) : Impedance triangle.

If each quantity of Fig. 4.5(i) is multiplied by I, we get the *power triangle*. From this triangle, apparently the power fed to the circuit is VI or

$$\text{Apparent power} = VI \quad ..... (4.36)$$

But inductance does not consume power (section 4.2), the element which consumes power is the resistance R.

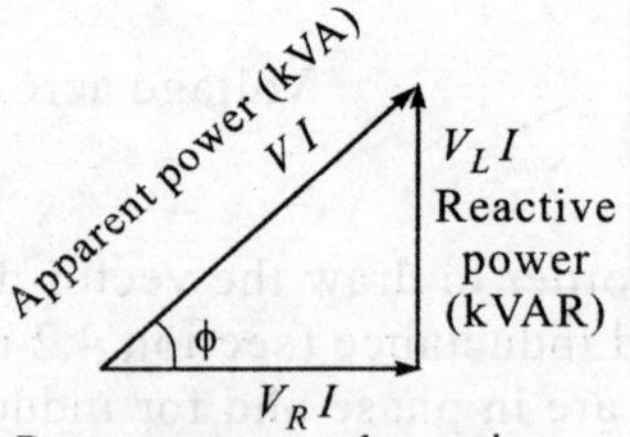

Fig. 4.5(iii) : Power triangle.

$$\therefore \text{Power consumed} = V_R I \quad ..... (4.37)$$

$$= V I \cos\phi \quad ..... (4.38)$$

Thus cos ϕ is the '*factor*' to be multiplied to '*apparent power*' to get the actual power consumed. Hence,

$$\text{Power factor} = \cos\phi \text{ (lagging)} \quad ..... (4.39)$$

It is lagging power factor as current lags the supply voltage and $V_L I$ is called the *reactive power*.

$$\text{Reactive power} = V_L I \quad ..... (4.40)$$

$$= V I \sin\phi \quad ..... (4.41)$$

The units of various powers are

Apparent power	$\Rightarrow$	volt-ampere (VA) or kVA (kilo volt-ampere)
Actual power consumed	$\Rightarrow$	watts (W) or kW (kilo watts)
Reactive power	$\Rightarrow$	volt-ampere-reactive VAR or kVAR

Note : *Observe that all these triangle (voltage impedance or power) here are right angled triangles. Knowing any two quantities on a particular triangle remaining quantities can be calculated.*

Ex.: If R, power factor ($\cos\phi$) are known, ϕ can be calculated. Then

$$R = Z\cos\phi \quad \Rightarrow \quad Z = \frac{R}{\cos\phi}$$

$$X = Z\sin\phi$$

Similarly if two voltages are known i.e. $\overline{V}$ and $\overline{V}_R$, then ϕ can be calculated, $\overline{V}_L$ can be calculated. Similarly if power factor and apparent power are known, power consumed and reactive power also can be obtained. These observations are very important while solving the numericals later.

4.5 Resistance and Capacitance in Series

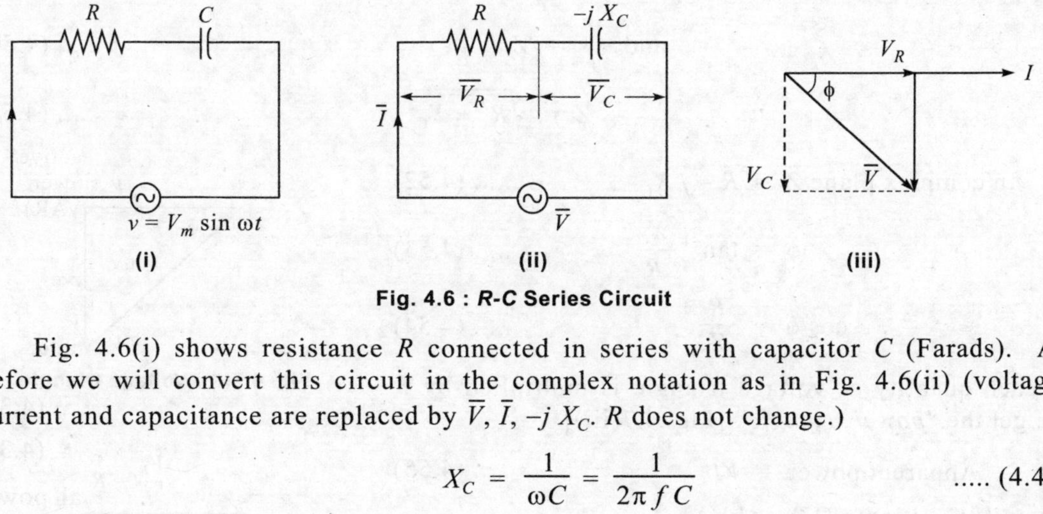

Fig. 4.6 : *R-C* Series Circuit

Fig. 4.6(i) shows resistance R connected in series with capacitor C (Farads). As before we will convert this circuit in the complex notation as in Fig. 4.6(ii) (voltage, current and capacitance are replaced by $\overline{V}$, $\overline{I}$, $-j\,X_C$. R does not change.)

$$X_C = \frac{1}{\omega C} = \frac{1}{2\pi f C} \qquad \text{..... (4.42)}$$

The voltage across supply is $\overline{V}$, resistance $\overline{V}_R$ and that across capacitance is $\overline{V}_C$ the current in circuit is $\overline{I}$.

$$\text{Then,} \quad \overline{V}_R = \overline{I}\,R \qquad \text{..... (4.43)}$$

$$\overline{V}_C = \overline{I}\,(-j\,X_C) \qquad \text{..... (4.44)}$$

$$\text{The supply voltage} \quad \overline{V} = \overline{V}_R + \overline{V}_C \qquad \text{..... (4.45)}$$

To draw the vector diagram [Fig. 4.6(iii)], the common quantity $\overline{I}$ is taken as reference. Then draw $\overline{V_R}$ along $\overline{I}$ (as voltage across resistance and its current are in phase). Now, as capacitive current leads its voltage as in other wards capacitive voltage will lag behind its current then draw $\overline{V_C}$ behind $\overline{I}$ by 90º.

Adding $\overline{V_R}$ and $\overline{V_C}$ we get supply voltage $\overline{V}$ at an angle ϕ with respect to $\overline{I}$. As $\overline{V}$, $\overline{V_R}$ and $\overline{V_C}$ form a right angle triangle,

$$V = \sqrt{V_R^{\,2} + V_C^{\,2}} \qquad ..... (4.46)$$

$$\phi = \tan^{-1}\frac{V_C}{V_R} \qquad ..... (4.47)$$

Note : *The current I leads the voltage supply in a capacitive circuit.*

From Fig 4.6(iii), if we just omit the current vector, we get the "*voltage triangle*" [Fig 4.7(i)].

If we divide each quantity on voltage by current | *I* | we get the "*impedance triangle*". [Fig 4.7(ii)].

$$\frac{V_R}{I} = R \qquad ..... (4.48)$$

$$\frac{V_C}{I} = X_C \qquad ..... (4.49)$$

$$\text{and } \frac{V}{I} = Z \qquad ..... (4.50)$$

$$Z = \sqrt{R^2 + X_C^{\,2}} \qquad ..... (4.51)$$

In complex plane $\overline{Z} = R - j\,X_C$ ..... (4.52)

$$\phi = \tan^{-1}\frac{X_C}{R} \qquad ..... (4.53)$$

$$\cos\phi = \frac{R}{Z} \qquad ..... (4.54)$$

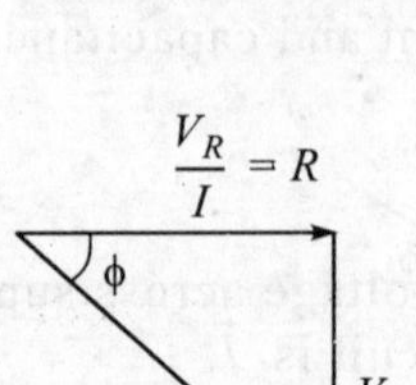

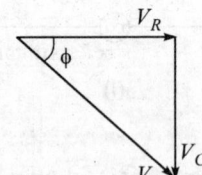

Fig. 4.7(i) : Voltage triangle.

If each quantity of voltage triangle is multiplied by *I* we get the "*power triangle*".[Fig. 4.7(iii)]

Apparent power $= VI$ ..... (4.55)

its unit is volt-amp (VA or kVA)

The power consuming element is only resistance, the capacitance does not consume power.

$\therefore$ Power consumed $= V_R I$ ..... (4.56)

$= V I \cos\phi$ ..... (4.57)

(watt or kW)

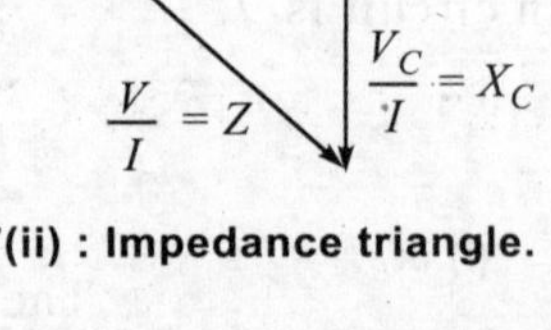

Fig. 4.7(ii) : Impedance triangle.

$$\text{Reactive power} = V_C I \quad ..... (4.58)$$

$$= V I \sin \phi \quad ..... (4.59)$$

(VAR or kVAR)

$$\text{Power factor} = \cos \phi \text{ (leading)} \quad ..... (4.60)$$

It is called '*power factor*' because it is the factor which apparent power is multiplied to get the active or actual power consumed. This power factor (*pf*) is a leading power factor as circuit current $\overline{I}$ leads the supply voltage.

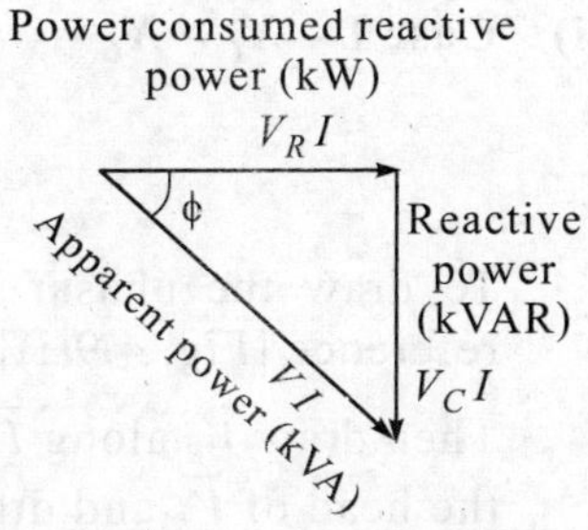

Fig. 4.7(iii) : Power triangle.

4.6 *R-L-C* Series Circuit

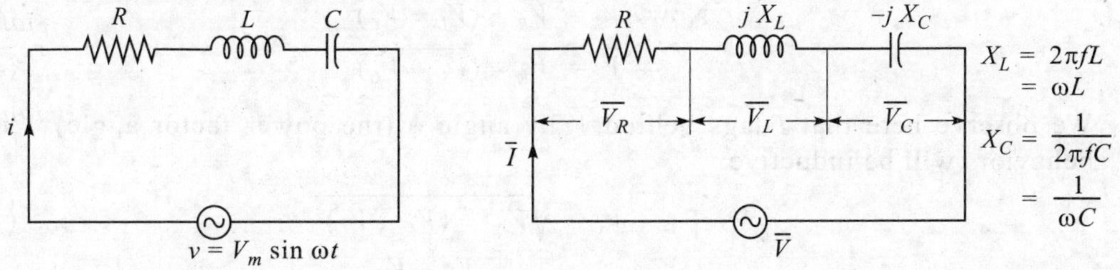

(i) (ii)

Fig. 4.8 : *R-L-C* series circuit.

Fig. 4.8(i) shows a series circuit containing *R*, *L* and *C* with source *v*(*t*). Let us obtain the circuit of Fig. 4.8(ii) by replacing each component and quantity by vector notation. The circuit impedance $\overline{Z}$ can be given by

$$\overline{Z} = R + j X_L - j X_C \quad ..... (4.61)$$

$$= R + j(X_L - X_C) \quad ..... (4.62)$$

$$| Z | = \sqrt{R^2 + (X_L - X_C)^2} \quad ..... (4.63)$$

Let us now analyze the circuit for the following cases

(i) $X_L > X_C$, **(ii)** $X_L < X_C$ and **(iii)** $X_L = X_C$

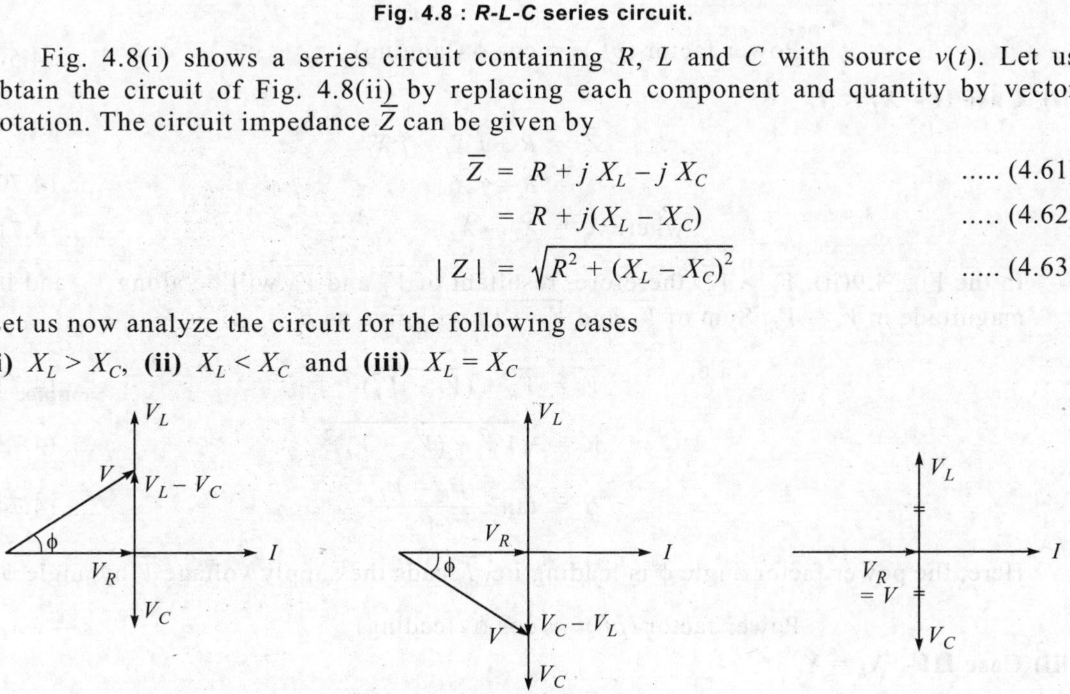

(i) $X_L > X_C$ lagging *pf* **(ii) $X_L < X_C$ leading *pf*** **(iii) $X_L = X_C$ unity *pf***

Fig. 4.9 : Vector diagram for *R-L-C* series circuit.

(i) Case I - $X_L > X_C$

$$\overline{Z} = R + jX \quad \text{..... (4.64)}$$

$$\text{where } X = X_L - X_C \quad \text{..... (4.65)}$$

To draw the phasar diagram (vector diagram), as it is a series circuit, take $\overline{I}$ as reference [Fig. 4.9(i)]

Then draw $\overline{V_R}$ along $\overline{I}$ as it is resistive voltage drop. Then draw $\overline{V_L}$ leading $\overline{I}$ by 90º at the head of $\overline{V_R}$ and draw $\overline{V_C}$ behind $\overline{I}$ by 90º at the head of $\overline{V_R}$. $|\overline{V_L}| > |\overline{V_C}|$ as $X_L > X_C$ and both carry same current I.

We first find $\overline{V_L} + \overline{V_C}$, as they are opposite to each other $(V_L - V_C)$ will be obtained along $\overline{V_L}$.

$$\text{Now, } \overline{V} = \overline{V_R} + (\overline{V_L} + \overline{V_C}) \quad \text{..... (4.66)}$$

$$\overline{V} = \overline{V_R} + (\overline{V_L - V_C}) \quad \text{..... (4.67)}$$

We observe here that $\overline{I}$ lags behind $\overline{V}$ by angle ϕ (the power factor angle). Circuit behaviors will be inductive.

$$V = \sqrt{V_R^2 + (V_L - V_C)^2} \quad \text{..... (4.68)}$$

$$\phi = \tan^{-1} \frac{V_L - V_C}{V_R} \quad \text{..... (4.69)}$$

$$\text{Power factor } (pf) = \cos\phi \text{ (lagging)}$$

(ii) Case II - $X_L < X_C$

$$\overline{Z} = R + jX_L - jX_C$$

$$= R - jX \quad \text{..... (4.70)}$$

$$\text{where } X = X_C - X_L \quad \text{..... (4.71)}$$

In the Fig. 4.9(ii), $\overline{V_C} > \overline{V_L}$ therefore, resultant of $\overline{V_L}$ and $\overline{V_C}$ will be along V_C and its magnitude in $V_C - V_L$. Sum of $\overline{V_R}$ and $\overline{V_C - V_L}$ will give us $\overline{V}$

i.e.

$$\overline{V} = \overline{V_R} + (\overline{V_C - V_L}) \quad \text{..... (4.72)}$$

$$V = \sqrt{V_R^2 + (V_C - V_L)^2} \quad \text{..... (4.73)}$$

$$\phi = \tan^{-1} \frac{V_C - V_L}{V_R} \quad \text{..... (4.74)}$$

Here, the power factor angle ϕ is leading i.e. $\overline{I}$ leads the supply voltage $\overline{V}$ by angle ϕ

$$\text{Power factor } (pf) = \cos\phi \text{ (leading)}$$

(iii) Case III - $X_L = X_C$

$$\overline{Z} = R + jX_L - jX_L \quad \text{... (as } X_L = X_C)$$

$$\overline{Z} = R \quad \text{..... (4.75)}$$

In Fig. 4.9(iii)
$$I X_L = I X_C$$
$$\therefore V_L = V_C$$

$\therefore$ Resultant of $\overline{V_L}$ and $\overline{V_C}$ is zero and
$$\overline{V} = \overline{V_R}$$
$$\phi = 0$$
$$\text{Power factor } (pf) = \cos 0 = 1 \text{ i.e. unity } pf \ (upf)$$

Note : *It is important to note down that while doing calculations, the currents and voltages should be calculated in the polar form always and the impedance should be written in both rectangular and polar form. In the rectangular form the real part indicated the resistance while the imaginary part indicates the reactance. If imaginary part is positive, the reactance is inductive and if it has a negative sign than the reactance is capacitive effectively.*

Ex. 4.1 : A coil of inductance 0.08 H and negligible resistance is connected in series with a 15 resistance. The combined circuit is energized from a 240 V, 50 Hz supply. Calculate **(i)** Reactance of coil **(ii)** Impedance of circuit **(iii)** Current in the circuit **(iv)** Voltage across resistance **(v)** Voltage across coil **(vi)** Power observed by the circuit **(vii)** Power factor **(viii)** Draw the vector diagram.

Solution : Given : $R = 15\ \Omega$

$L = 0.08$ H, $V = 240$ volts

$\therefore \overline{V} = 240 \angle 0°$ (assume)

$f = 50$ Hz

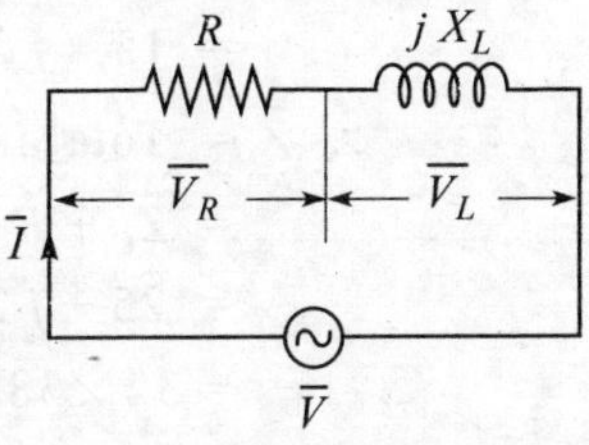

Fig. 4.10

(i) $X_L = 2\pi f L = 2\pi \times 50 \times 0.08 = 25.13\ \Omega$

(ii) $\overline{Z} = R + j X_L = 15 + j\,25.13 = 29.26 \angle 59.16°$

(iii) $\overline{I} = \dfrac{\overline{V}}{\overline{Z}} = \dfrac{240 \angle 0°}{29.26 \angle 59.16°} = 8.2 \angle -59.16°$ amp

(iv) Voltage across resistance $= \overline{V_R} = \overline{I} R = (8.2 \angle -59.16°) \times 15 = 123.04 \angle -59.16°$

(v) Voltage across coil $= \overline{V_L} = \overline{I}(j X_L) = (8.2 \angle -59.16°)(j\,25.13) = 206.14 \angle 30.84°$

(vi) Power observed by the circuit $= I^2 R = 8.2^2 \times 15 = 1008.6$ watts

(vii) Power factor $= \cos\phi$

where ϕ is the angle between supply voltage $\overline{V}$ and current $\overline{I}$.
$$\therefore \phi = -59.16°$$
$$\text{thus } \cos\phi = 0.513 \text{ (lagging)}$$

(viii) To draw the phasor diagram, take $\overline{I}$ as the reference (Fig. 4.11) as in series circuits same current is flowing through all the components.

Then, $\overline{V_R}$ is in phase with $\overline{I}$. $\overline{V_L}$ leads $\overline{I}$ by 90°.

(Inductive current lags its own voltage). So draw $\overline{V_L}$.

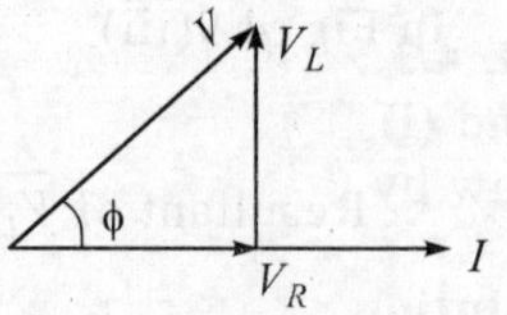

Fig. 4.11

Phasor sum of $\overline{V_R}$ and $\overline{V_L}$ is the supply voltage $\overline{V}$. Angle between $\overline{V}$ and $\overline{I}$ is ϕ, the power factor angle. As current lags behind voltage ($\overline{V}$) it is a lagging power factor.

Ex. 4.2 : A choke coil having a resistance of 15 Ω and an inductance of 63.7 mH is connected in series with a non-inductive resistance of 10 Ω. The circuit has been connected to 200 V, 50 Hz mains. Calculate **(i)** current **(ii)** power factor **(iii)** voltage across coil **(iv)** voltage across non-inductive resistance. Draw the phasor diagram

Solution : Given : R_C = Resistance of coil = 15 Ω

L_C = Inductance of coil = 63.7×10^{-3} H

$R = 10\ \Omega,\ f = 50\ \text{Hz},\ V = 200\ \text{V}$

$X_L = 2\pi f L_C = 2\pi \times 50 \times 63.7 \times 10^{-3}$

$= 20\ \Omega$

$\therefore\ \overline{Z_C}$ = Impedance of coil = $R_C + j X_L$

$= 15 + j\,20$

$\therefore\ \overline{Z}$ = Total impedance of the circuit

$= \overline{Z_C} + R = 15 + j\,20 + 10$

$= 25 + j\,20$

$= 32\ \angle 38.6^\circ$

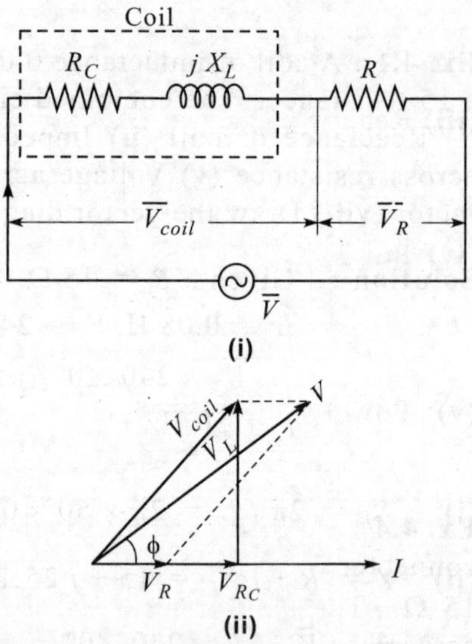

Fig. 4.12

(i) $\overline{I} = \dfrac{\overline{V}}{\overline{Z}} = \dfrac{200\ \angle 0^\circ}{32\ \angle 38.6^\circ} = \boxed{6.25\ \angle -38.6^\circ\ \text{amp}}$

(ii) Power factor = $\cos\phi = \cos(-38.6^\circ) = \boxed{0.78\ \text{(lagging)}}$

(iii) $\overline{V}_{coil} = \overline{I}\,\overline{Z_C} = (6.25\ \angle -38.6^\circ)(15 + j\,20) = \boxed{156.25\ \angle 14.53^\circ}$

(iv) $\overline{V_R} = \overline{I}\,R = (6.25\ \angle -38.6^\circ)\ 10 = \boxed{62.5\ \angle -38.6^\circ}$

To draw the phasor (vector) diagram take current as reference vector (as series circuit) Fig. 4.12(ii). Now V_{RC} will be in phase with I (resistive drop). $\overline{V_L}$, the voltage across inductance will lead I by 90°. Vector sum of $\overline{V_{RC}}$ and $\overline{V_L}$ will be $\overline{V}_{coil}$. Then draw $\overline{V_R}$ in phase with $\overline{I}$ smaller that $\overline{V_{RC}}$ as $R_C > R$. Parallelogram between $\overline{V_R}$ and $\overline{V}_{coil}$ will give the resultant vector $\overline{V}$ the supply voltage. The power factor angle ϕ is the angle between applied voltage and current $\overline{I}$.

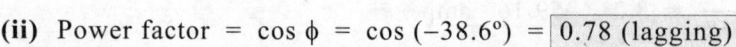

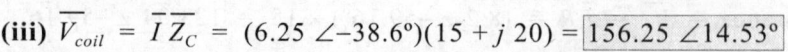

Ex. 4.3 : In a series *R-L* circuit $i(t) = 5 \sin(314\,t + 2\pi/3)$ and $v(t) = 20 \sin(314\,t + 5\pi/6)$. Find **(i)** Impedance **(ii)** Resistance **(iii)** Inductance **(iv)** Power factor **(v)** Average power draw by the circuit. Draw vector diagram.

Solution :

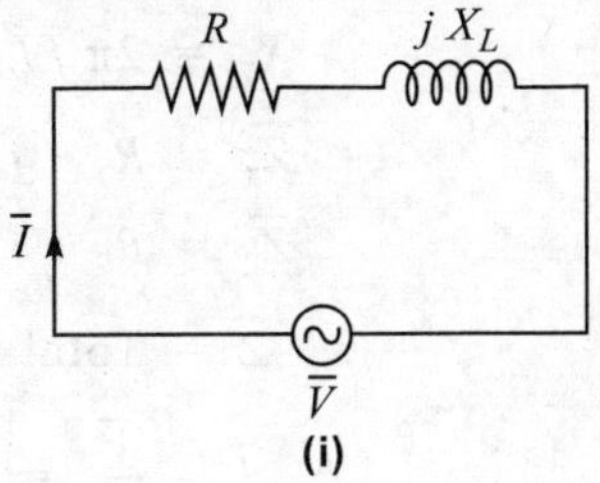

$$v(t) = 20 \sin(314\,t + 5\pi/6)$$

$$i(t) = 5 \sin(314\,t + 2\pi/3)$$

$$V_m = 20,\ I_m = 5,\ \omega = 314$$

$$\therefore\ \overline{V} = \frac{V_m}{\sqrt{2}} \angle 5\pi/6 = 14.14 \angle 150^\circ \text{ volts}$$

$$\text{and } \overline{I} = \frac{I_m}{\sqrt{2}} \angle 2\pi/3 = 3.53 \angle 120^\circ \text{ amp}$$

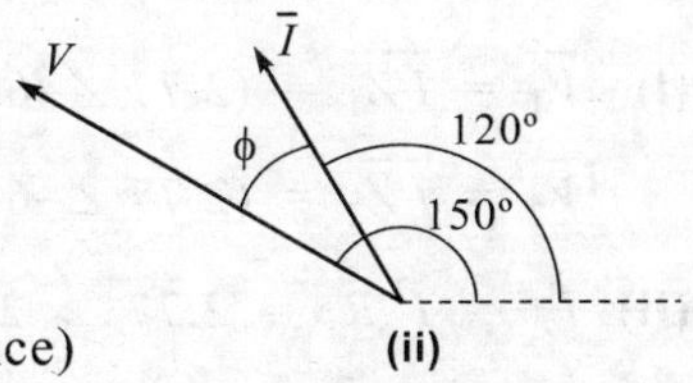

Fig. 4.13

(i) $\overline{Z} = \dfrac{\overline{V}}{\overline{I}} = \dfrac{14.14 \angle 150^\circ}{3.53 \angle 120^\circ} = 3.47 + j\,2 = \boxed{4 \angle 30^\circ}$ ohms

(ii) Resistance = $\boxed{3.47\ \Omega}$ (Real part of impedance)

(iii) Reactance = $X_L = \omega L = 2$ (Imaginary part of impedance)

$$\therefore\ L = \frac{2}{\omega} = \frac{2}{314} = \boxed{6.37 \times 10^{-3} \text{ H}}$$

(iv) Power factor = $\cos \phi$

where $\phi = 150^\circ - 120^\circ = 30^\circ$

$$\therefore\ pf = \cos 30^\circ = \boxed{0.866 \text{ (lagging)}}$$

(v) Power drawn = $V I \cos \phi$

$$= 14.14 \times 3.53 \times \cos 30^\circ = \boxed{43.22 \text{ watts}}$$

Ex. 4.4 : An inductive coil having a resistance of 25 Ω and inductance of 0.04 H has been connected in series with another inductive coil of inductance 0.2 H and resistance of 15 Ω. The whole circuit is energized from 230 V, 50 Hz mains. Calculate **(i)** Voltage across each coil **(ii)** Power dissipated in each coil **(iii)** Total power observed **(iv)** Power factor of the circuit. Draw the vector diagram.

Solution :

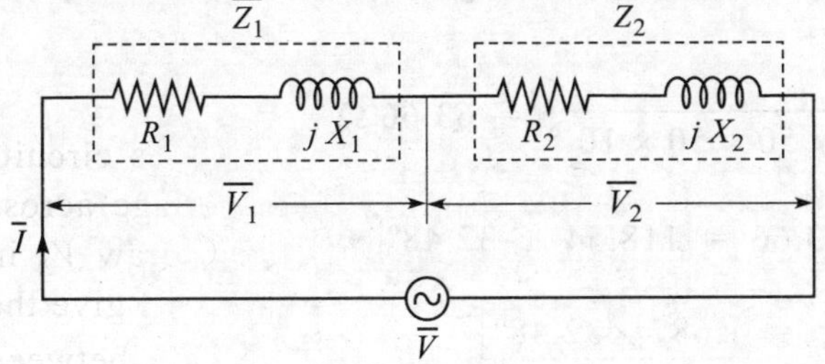

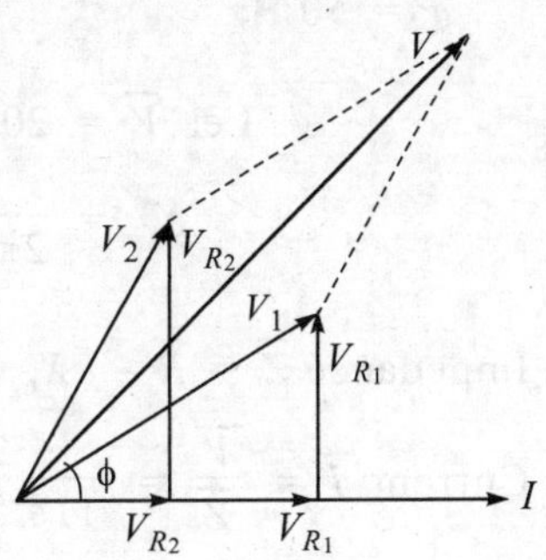

Fig. 4.14

Given : $R_1 = 25\ \Omega$, $L_1 = 0.04$ H, $R_2 = 15\ \Omega$, $L_2 = 0.2$ H, $V = 230$ V, $f = 50$ Hz

$$\text{Let } \overline{V} = 230\ \angle 0^\circ$$

$$\therefore\ X_1 = 2\pi f L_1 = 2\pi \times 50 \times 0.04 = 12.57$$

$$X_2 = 2\pi f L_2 = 2\pi \times 50 \times 0.2 = 62.83$$

$$\therefore\ \overline{Z_1} = R_1 + j X_1 = 25 + j\,12.57 = 27.98\ \angle 26.69^\circ$$

$$\overline{Z_2} = R_2 + j X_2 = 15 + j\,62.87 = 64.6\ \angle 76.57^\circ$$

$$\therefore\ \overline{Z} = \text{Total impedance} = \overline{Z_1} + \overline{Z_2} = 40 + j\,75.40 = 83.13\ \angle 65.1^\circ$$

$$\overline{I} = \frac{\overline{V}}{\overline{Z}} = \frac{230\ \angle 0^\circ}{83.13\ \angle 65.1^\circ} = 2.77\ \angle -65.1^\circ$$

(i) $\overline{V_1} = \overline{I}\,\overline{Z_1} = (2.77\ \angle -65.1^\circ)(25 + j\,12.57) = \boxed{75.26\ \angle -35.37^\circ}$

$\overline{V_2} = \overline{I}\,\overline{Z_2} = (2.77\ \angle -65.1^\circ)(15 + j\,62.87) = \boxed{173\ \angle 14.52^\circ}$

(ii) $P_1 = I^2 R_1 = 2.77^2 \times 25 = \boxed{191.82 \text{ watts}}$

$P_2 = I^2 R_2 = 2.77^2 \times 15 = \boxed{115.09 \text{ watts}}$

(iii) $P = P_1 + P_2 = \boxed{306.91 \text{ watts}}$

(iv) Power factor $= \cos\phi = \cos(-65.1^\circ) = \boxed{0.42 \text{ (lagging)}}$

Ex. 4.5 : A series circuit consisting of resistance of 100 Ω and a capacitance of 50 μf in energized from 200 V, 50 Hz mains. Find **(i)** Impedance **(ii)** Current **(iii)** Power factor **(iv)** Phase angle **(v)** Voltage across resistance **(vi)** Voltage across capacitance.

Solution :

Given : $R = 100\ \Omega$

$C = 50\ \mu f = 50 \times 10^{-6}$ f

$V = 200$ V

$f = 50$ Hz

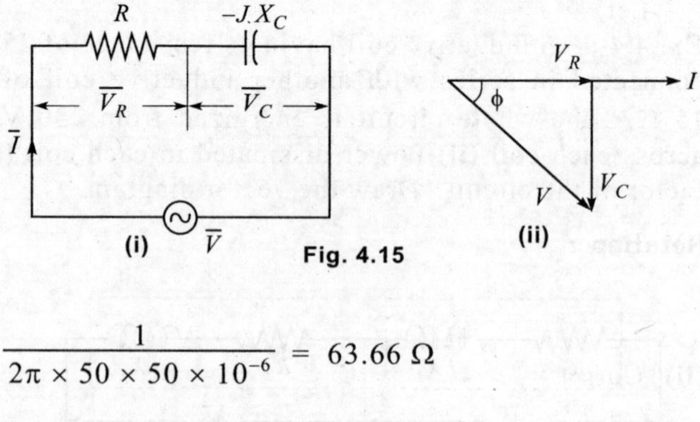

Fig. 4.15

$$\text{Let } \overline{V} = 200\ \angle 0^\circ$$

$$X_C = \frac{1}{2\pi f C} = \frac{1}{2\pi \times 50 \times 50 \times 10^{-6}} = 63.66\ \Omega$$

(i) Impedance $\overline{Z} = R - j X_C = 100 - j\,63.66 = \boxed{118.54\ \angle -32.48^\circ}$

(ii) Current $\overline{I} = \frac{\overline{V}}{\overline{Z}} = \frac{200\ \angle 0^\circ}{118.54\ \angle -32.48^\circ} = \boxed{1.687\ \angle 32.48^\circ}$

(iii) Power factor $= \cos\phi = \cos 32.48^\circ = \boxed{0.843 \text{ (leading)}}$

(iv) Phase angle ϕ = $\boxed{32.48^\circ}$ (ϕ is the angle between applied voltage $\overline{V}$ and $\overline{I}$)

(v) Voltage across resistance $\overline{V_R} = \overline{I}\,R = (1.687 \angle 32.48^\circ) \times 100$

$= \boxed{168.7 \angle 32.48^\circ \text{ volts}}$

(vi) Voltage across capacitance $\overline{V_C} = \overline{I}\,(-j X_C) = (1.687 \angle 32.48^\circ)(-j\, 63.66)$

$= \boxed{107.39 \angle -57.52^\circ}$

To draw the vector diagram use following steps

(i) As it is a series circuit, take $\overline{I}$ as reference [refer Fig 4.15(ii)].

(ii) $\overline{V_R}$ is in phase with $\overline{I}$.

(iii) As capacitive current leads, thus $\overline{V_C}$ lags behind its current $\overline{I}$, by 90°.

(iv) Vector sum of $\overline{V_R}$ and $\overline{V_C}$ gives $\overline{V}$, the supply voltage.

Ex. 4.6 : A choke coil having resistance of 10 Ω and inductance of 0.05 H is connected in series with a condenser of 100 μf. The circuit in energized from 200 V, 50 Hz supply. Calculate **(i)** Impedance **(ii)** Current **(iii)** Power factor **(iv)** Power absorbed by the circuit.

Solution :

Given : $R = 10\ \Omega$

$L = 0.05$ H

$C = 100 \times 10^{-6}$ f

$V = 200$ V

$f = 50$ Hz

Let $\overline{V} = 200 \angle 0^\circ$

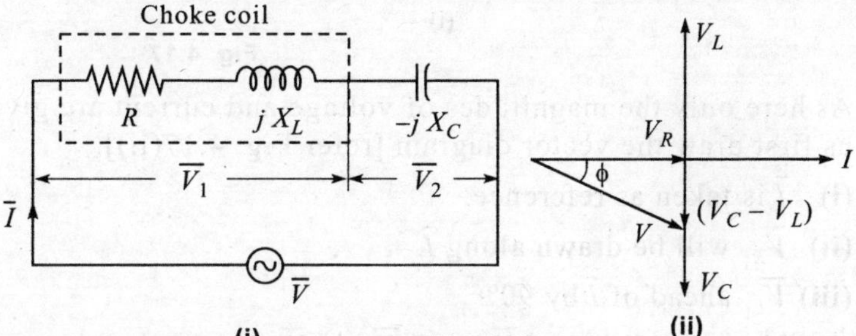

Fig. 4.16

$$X_L = 2\pi f C = 2\pi \times 50 \times 0.05 = 15.71\ \Omega$$

$$X_C = \frac{1}{2\pi f C} = \frac{1}{2\pi \times 50 \times 100 \times 10^{-6}} = 31.83\ \Omega$$

(i) Impedance $\overline{Z} = R + j X_L - j X_C = 10 + j\,15.71 - j\,31.83 = 10 - j\,16.12$

$= \boxed{18.97 \angle -58.19^\circ}$

(ii) Current $\overline{I} = \dfrac{\overline{V}}{\overline{Z}} = \dfrac{200 \angle 0^\circ}{18.97 \angle -58.19^\circ} = \boxed{10.54 \angle 58.19^\circ}$

(iii) Power factor = $\cos\phi = \cos 58.19^\circ = \boxed{0.5271}$ (leading as angle of $\overline{I}$ is positive)

(iv) Power absorbed = $V I \cos\phi = 200 \times 10.54 \cos 58.19^\circ$

$= \boxed{1111.13 \text{ watts}}$

Ex. 4.7 : A choke coil is connected in series with non-inductive resistance. The combination is connected across 250 V, 50 Hz mains and draws a current of 5 A from the line. The voltage across choke coil and non inductive resistance are 200 V and 125 V respectively. Calculate

(i) Impedance, resistance and reactance of coil.

(ii) Power absorbed by the coil.

(iii) Power absorbed by non-inductive resistance.

(iv) Total power absorbed.

Solution :

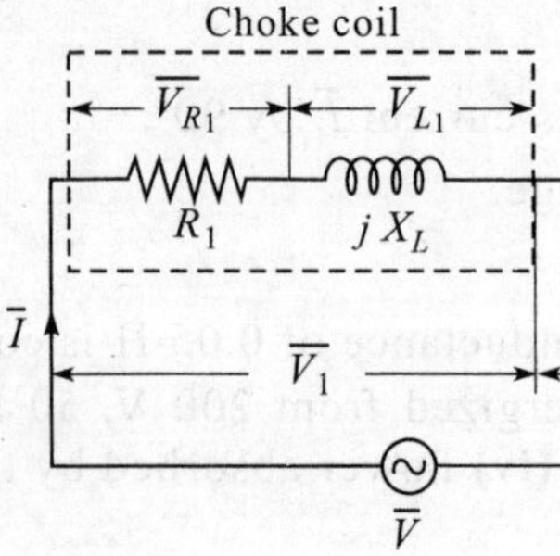

(i)

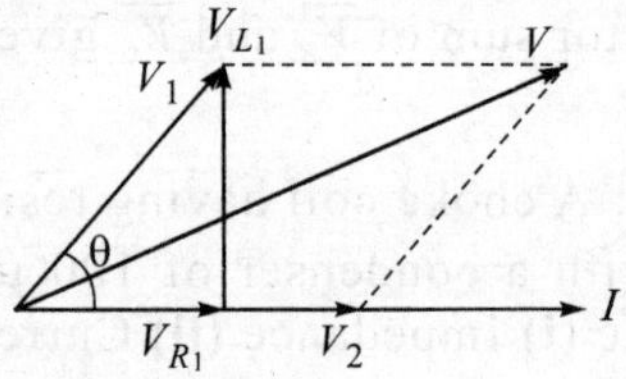

(ii)

Fig. 4.17

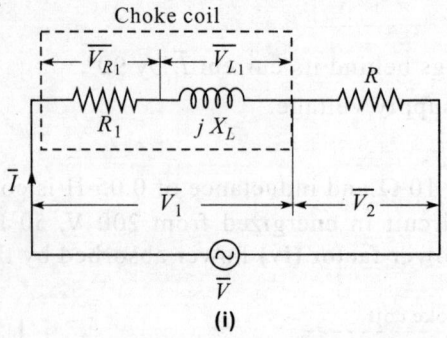

As here only the magnitudes of voltage and current are give, the angles are not known, let us first draw the vector diagram [refer Fig. 4.17(ii)].

(i) $\overline{I}$ is taken as reference.

(ii) $\overline{V}_{R_1}$ will be drawn along $\overline{I}$.

(iii) $\overline{V}_{L_1}$ ahead of $\overline{I}$ by 90°.

(iv) Vector addition of $\overline{V}_{R_1}$ and $\overline{V}_{L_1}$ is $\overline{V}_1$.

(v) $\overline{V}_2$ is the resistive drop so draw $\overline{V}_2$ is phase with $\overline{I}$.

(vi) Parallelogram of $\overline{V}_1$ and $\overline{V}_2$ will give us the resultant $\overline{V}$ (the diagonal)

Now, recollect the vector addition theorem given below.

$$V^2 = V_1^{\ 2} + V_2^{\ 2} + 2\, V_1\, V_2 \cos\theta$$

Given : $V = 250$ V, $V_1 = 200$ V, $V_2 = 125$ V, $I = 5$ A

$$\therefore\ 250^2 = 200^2 + 125^2 + 2 \times 200 \times 125 \cos\theta$$

$$\therefore\ \cos\theta = 0.1375$$

$$\text{or } \theta = 82.09^\circ$$

Now from the vector diagram [Fig. 4.17(ii)]

$$V_{R_1} = V_1 \cos\theta = 200 \cos 82.09^\circ = 27.5$$

$$V_{L_1} = V_1 \sin\theta = 200 \sin 82.09^\circ = 198.09$$

(i) Resistance of coil $R_1 = \dfrac{V_{R_1}}{I} = \dfrac{27.5}{5} = \boxed{5.5\ \Omega}$

Resistance of coil $X = \dfrac{V_{L_1}}{I} = \dfrac{198.09}{5} = \boxed{39.62\ \Omega}$

Impedance of coil $= R_1 + jX = 5.5 + j\,39.62 = \boxed{40\ \angle 82.09^\circ}$

Non-inductive resistance of coil $R = \dfrac{V_2}{I} = \dfrac{125}{5} = \boxed{25\ \Omega}$

(ii) Power absorbed by coil $P_1 = I^2 R_1 = 5^2 \times 5.5 = \boxed{137.5 \text{ watts}}$

(iii) Power absorbed by non-inductive resistance, $P_2 = I^2 R = 5^2 \times 25 = \boxed{625 \text{ watts}}$

(iv) Total power absorbed $= P_1 + P_2 = 137.5 + 625 = \boxed{762.5 \text{ watts}}$

Ex. 4.8 : An impedance A consists of a resistance 5 Ω in series with an inductive reactance of 9.42 Ω. This is connected in series with another impedance B consisting of resistance 10 Ω and a capacitive reactance of 31.8 Ω. The whole circuit is energized from 100 V a.c. supply. Calculate **(i)** Current taken by the circuit **(ii)** p.f. of circuit. Draw the phaser diagram.

Solution :

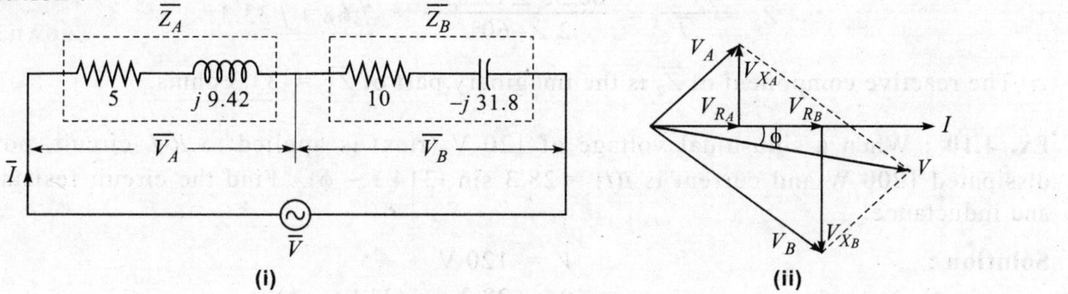

Fig. 4.18

Let $\overline{V} = V\angle 0^\circ = 100\angle 0^\circ$

$$\overline{Z_A} = R_A + jX_A = 5 + j\,9.42$$

$$\overline{Z_B} = R_B - jX_B = 10 - j\,31.8$$

$$\therefore\ \overline{Z} = \text{Total impedance} = \overline{Z_A} + \overline{Z_B}$$

$$= 5 + j\,9.42 + 10 - j\,31.8 = 15 - j\,22.38$$

$$= 26.94\ \angle -56.17^\circ$$

(i) Current $\overline{I} = \dfrac{\overline{V}}{\overline{Z}} = \dfrac{100\ \angle 0^\circ}{26.94\ \angle -56.17^\circ} = \boxed{3.71\ \angle 56.17^\circ}$

(ii) Power factor of the circuit $pf = \cos 56.17 = \boxed{0.5567 \text{ (leading)}}$

Ex. 4.9 : An rms voltage of 100 ∠0° V is applied to a series combination of $\overline{Z}_1$ and $\overline{Z}_2$. When $\overline{Z}_1$ is 20 ∠30°, the effective voltage drop across $\overline{Z}_1$ is found to be 40∠–30°. Find the reactive component of $\overline{Z}_2$.

Solution :

Given : $\overline{Z}_1 = 20\angle 30^\circ$,

$\overline{V}_1 = 40\angle -30^\circ$,

$\overline{V} = 100\angle 0^\circ$

$$\overline{I} = \frac{\overline{V}_1}{\overline{Z}_1} = \frac{40\angle -30^\circ}{20\angle 30^\circ} = 2\angle -60^\circ$$

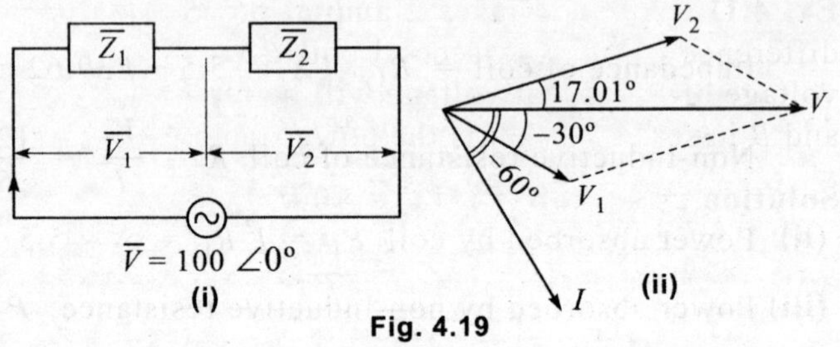

Fig. 4.19

From Fig. 4.19

$$\overline{V} = \overline{V}_1 + \overline{V}_2$$

$$\therefore\ 100\angle 0^\circ = 40\angle -30^\circ + \overline{V}_2$$

$$\therefore\ \overline{V}_2 = 100\angle 0^\circ + 40\angle -30^\circ$$

$$= 68.35\angle 17.01^\circ$$

(This calculation can be done directly in the complex mode of calculator)

$$\overline{Z}_2 = \frac{\overline{V}_2}{\overline{I}} = \frac{68.35\angle 17.01^\circ}{2\angle -60^\circ} = \boxed{7.68 + j\,33.3}$$

∴ The reactive component of $\overline{Z}_2$ is the imaginary part of $\overline{Z}_2$ = $\boxed{33.3 \text{ ohms.}}$

Ex. 4.10 : When a sinusoidal voltage of 120 V (rms) is applied to *R-L* circuit, power dissipated 1200 W and current is $i(t) = 28.3 \sin (314\,t - \phi)$. Find the circuit resistance and inductance.

Solution :

$$V = 120 \text{ V}$$

$$i(t) = 28.3 \sin (314\,t - \phi)$$

$$\therefore \text{ rms current } I = \frac{28.3}{\sqrt{2}} = 20 \text{ amp}$$

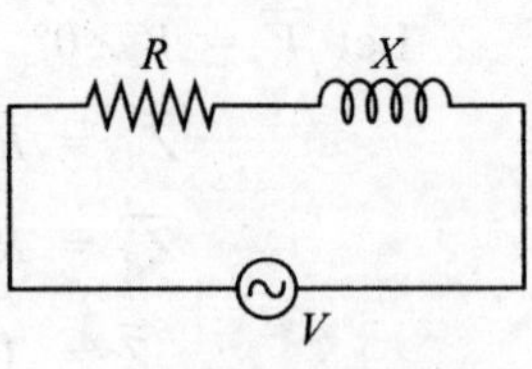

Fig. 4.20

$$\text{Power} = I^2 R$$

$$\therefore\ 1200 = 20^2 \times R$$

$$\therefore\ \boxed{R = 3\ \Omega}$$

$$Z = \frac{V}{I} = \frac{120}{20} = 6\ \Omega$$

$$Z = \sqrt{R^2 + X^2}$$

$$\therefore\ 6^2 = 3^2 \times X^2$$

$$\text{or } X = 5.196\ \Omega$$

$$\text{But } X = \omega L$$

From expression for $i(t)$, $\omega = 314$

$\therefore\ 5.196 = 314\,L$ thus $\boxed{L = 0.0165 \text{ H}}$

Ex. 4.11 : A coil *A* takes 2 amp at power factor of 0.8 lagging with an applied potential difference of 10 V. A second coil *B* takes a 2 A with p.f of 0.7 lagging with an applied voltage of 5 V. What voltage will be required to produce a total current of 2 A with coil *A* and *B* in series ? What is the power factor in this case?

Solution : For Coil *A* : $V_1 = 10$ V, $I_1 = 2$ A, $p.f. = \cos\phi_1 = 0.8$ lagging

$$\therefore\ Z_1 = \frac{V_1}{I_1} = \frac{10}{2} = 5\ \Omega$$

$$\phi_1 = \cos^{-1} 0.8 = 36.87^\circ$$

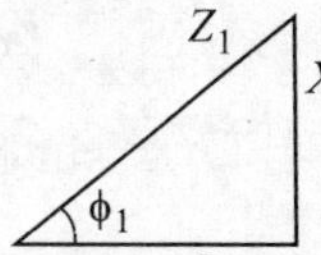

Fig. 4.21

From Fig. 4.21 triangle, the impedance

$$R_1 = Z_1 \cos\phi_1 = 5 \times 0.8 = 4\ \Omega$$

$$X_1 = Z_1 \sin\phi_1 = 5 \times 0.6 = 3\ \Omega$$

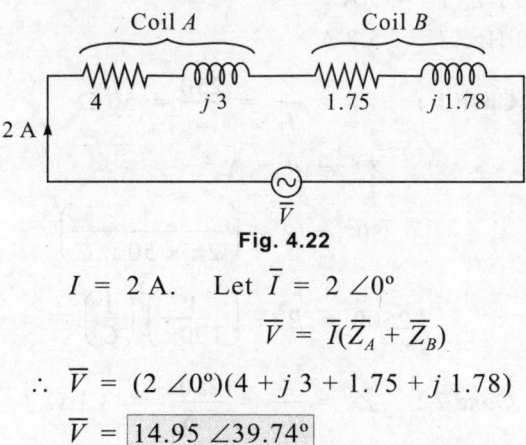

For Coil *B* : $V_2 = 5$ V, $I_2 = 2$ A, $p.f. = \cos\phi_2 = 0.7$ lagging

$$\therefore\ Z_2 = \frac{V_2}{I_2} = \frac{5}{2} = 2.5\ \Omega$$

$$\phi_2 = \cos^{-1} 0.7 = 45.57^\circ$$

From impedance triangle (similar to Fig. 4.21)

$$R_2 = Z_2 \cos\phi_2 = 2.5 \times 0.7 = \boxed{1.75\ \Omega}$$

$$X_2 = Z_2 \sin\phi_2 = 2.5 \times 0.71 = \boxed{1.78\ \Omega}$$

When coil *A* and *B* are in series (Fig. 4.22)

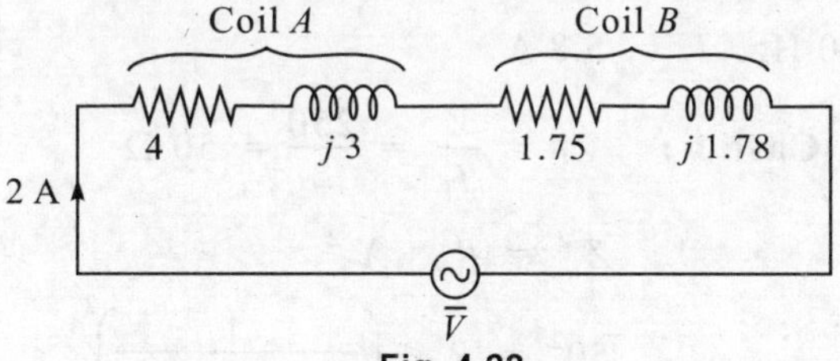

Fig. 4.22

$$I = 2\text{ A.} \quad \text{Let } \bar{I} = 2\angle 0^\circ$$

$$\bar{V} = \bar{I}(\bar{Z}_A + \bar{Z}_B)$$

$$\therefore\ \bar{V} = (2\angle 0^\circ)(4 + j\,3 + 1.75 + j\,1.78)$$

$$\bar{V} = \boxed{14.95 \angle 39.74^\circ}$$

The power factor angle is 39.74° with current lagging behind the applied voltage.

$$\therefore\ p.f. = \cos 39.74^\circ = \boxed{0.7689 \text{ lagging}}$$

Ex. 4.12 : A capacitor of 35 μf is connected in series with a variable resistance. The circuit is connected across 50 Hz supply. Find the resistance for a condition when voltage across capacitor is half the supply voltage.

Solution : Given : $C = 35\ \mu f$, $f = 50$ Hz

$$X_C = \frac{1}{2\pi f C} = \frac{1}{2\pi \times 50 \times 35 \times 10^{-6}} = 90.94\ \Omega$$

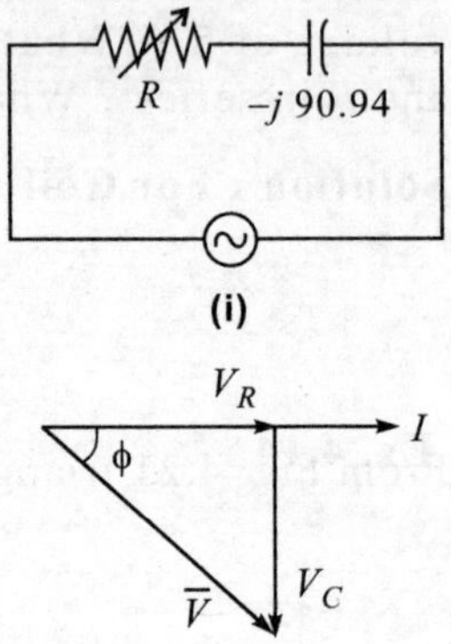

(i) (ii)

Fig. 4.23

From [Fig 4.23(ii)]

$$V_C = \frac{1}{2} V = V \sin \phi$$

$$\therefore \sin \phi = \frac{1}{2} \quad \therefore \phi = 30^\circ$$

$$\frac{V_C}{V_R} = \tan \phi$$

But $V_C = I X_C$ and $V_R = I R$

$$\therefore \frac{X_C}{R} = \tan 30^\circ$$

$$\therefore R = \frac{X_C}{\tan 30^\circ} = \frac{90.94}{0.577} = \boxed{157.51\ \Omega}$$

Ex. 4.13 : A resistance and capacitance are connected across 250 V supply. When supply frequency is 50 Hz, current is 5 A. When supply frequency increases to 60 Hz it draws 5.8 A. Find *R*, *C* and power drawn in second case.

Solution : Given : $V = 250$ V

Case 1 : $f_1 = 50$ Hz, $I_1 = 5$ A

Case 2 : $f_2 = 60$ Hz, $I_2 = 5.8$ A

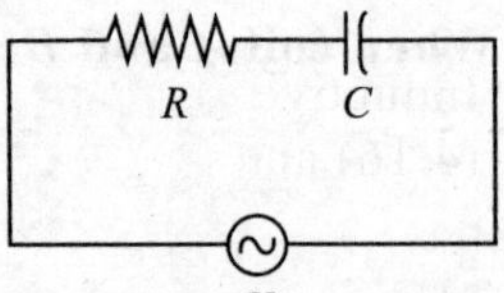

Fig. 4.24

Case 1 : $$Z_1 = \frac{V}{I_1} = \frac{250}{2} = 50\ \Omega$$

$$Z_1^2 = R^2 + X_1^2$$

$$50^2 = R^2 + \left(\frac{1}{2\pi \times 50 \times C}\right)^2$$

$$2500 = R^2 + \left(\frac{1}{100\pi}\right)^2 \left(\frac{1}{C}\right)^2 \quad \text{..... (i)}$$

Case 2 : $$Z_2 = \frac{V}{I_2} = \frac{250}{5.8} = 43.1\ \Omega$$

$$Z_2^2 = R^2 + X_2^2$$

$$43.1^2 = R^2 + \left(\frac{1}{2\pi \times 60 \times C}\right)^2$$

$$1857.61 = R^2 + \left(\frac{1}{120\pi}\right)^2 \left(\frac{1}{C}\right)^2 \quad \text{..... (ii)}$$

Solving equation (i) and (ii), we get

$$R^2 = 397.63$$

$$\left(\frac{1}{C}\right)^2 = 2.07 \times 10^8$$

$$\therefore \; R = \boxed{19.94 \; \Omega}$$

$$C = \boxed{69.5 \times 10^{-6} \text{ f}}$$

$$\text{Power drawn} = I_2^2 R = 5.8^2 \times 19.94 = \boxed{670.78 \text{ watts}}$$

Ex. 4.14 : In Fig. 4.25 find $\overline{V}_1$, $\overline{V}_2$ and draw the vector diagram.

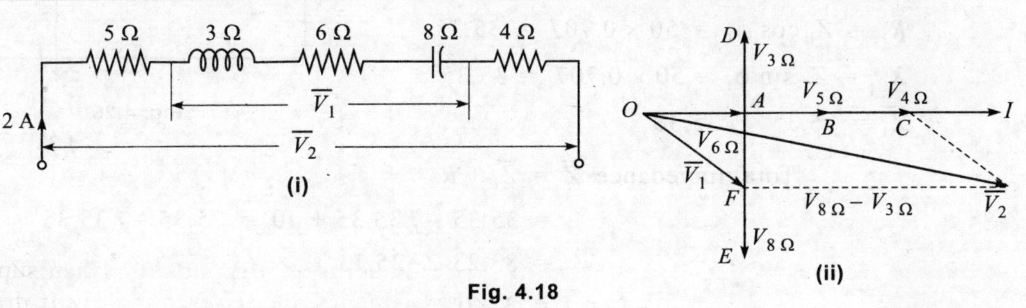

Fig. 4.18

Solution : Let us find the impedance ($\overline{Z}_1$) across which $\overline{V}_1$ is defined.

$$\overline{Z}_1 = j\,3 + 6 - j\,8 = 6 - j\,5$$

Inductive reactance is taken as $+j\,X_L$ and capacitive reactance $(-j\,X_C)$ [refer equation (4.16) and (4.22)]. Similarly, define $\overline{Z}_2$ across which $\overline{V}_2$ is specified.

$$\therefore \; \overline{Z}_2 = 5 + j\,3 + 6 - j\,8 + 4 = 15 - j\,5$$

$$\text{Let } \overline{I} = I \angle 0^\circ = 2 \angle 0^\circ$$

$$\therefore \; \overline{V}_1 = \overline{I}\,\overline{Z}_1 = (2 \angle 0^\circ)(6 - j\,5) = \boxed{15.62 \angle -39.8^\circ}$$

$$\text{and } \overline{V}_2 = \overline{I}\,\overline{Z}_2 = (2 \angle 0^\circ)(15 - j\,5) = \boxed{31.62 \angle -18.43^\circ}$$

For the vector diagram

(i) Take I as reference vector (series circuit).

(ii) $\overline{V}_{6\,\Omega}$ will be in phase with $\overline{I}$ (OA).

(iii) $\overline{V}_{3\,\Omega}$ will lead $\overline{I}$ by 90º (inductive drop) (AD).

(iv) $\overline{V}_{8\,\Omega}$ will lag $\overline{I}$ by 90º (capacitive drop) (AE).

(v) $AF = AE - AD = \overline{V}_{8\,\Omega} - \overline{V}_{3\,\Omega}$.

(vi) $\overline{V}_1 = \overline{V}_{6\,\Omega} + \overline{V}_{3\,\Omega} + \overline{V}_{8\,\Omega}$ i.e. resultant of OA and AF or $OF = \overline{V}_1$.

(vii) $AB = \overline{V}_{5\,\Omega}$ (resistive drop).

(viii) $BC = \overline{V}_{4\,\Omega}$ (resistive drop).

(ix) $\overline{V}_2 = \overline{V}_1 + \overline{V}_{5\,\Omega} + \overline{V}_{4\,\Omega}$ i.e. diagonal of parallel gram drawn between OC and OF.

Ex. 4.15 : A load consisting of a capacitor in series with a resistor, has an impedance of 50 Ω and power factor 0.707 leading. The load is connected in series with 40 Ω resistance across a.c. supply and the resulting current is 3 A. Determine the supply voltage and overall phase angle.

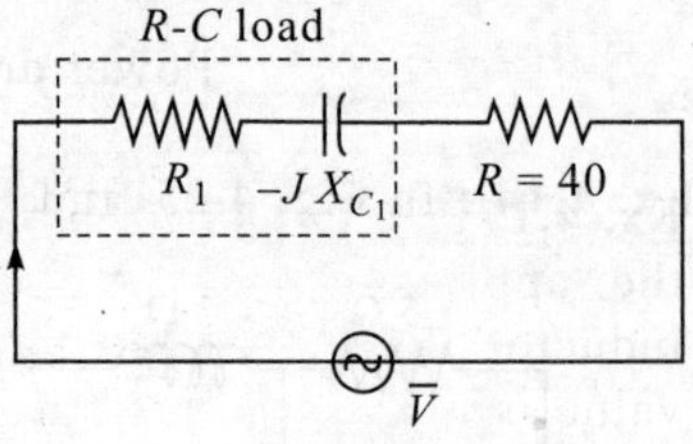

Fig. 4.26

Solution : Impedance of R-C circuit $= 50\ \Omega = Z_1$

$$p.f. = 0.707 \text{ leading} = \cos\phi_1$$

$$\therefore \phi_1 = 45^\circ$$

$$\therefore R_1 = Z_1 \cos\phi_1 = 50 \times 0.707 = 35.35$$

$$X_{C_1} = Z_1 \sin\phi_1 = 50 \times 0.707 = 35.35$$

$$\overline{Z}_1 = 35.35 - j\,35.35$$

$$\text{Total impedance } \overline{Z} = \overline{Z}_1 + R$$

$$= 35.35 - j\,35.35 + 40 = 75.35 - j\,35.35$$

$$= 83.23\ \angle{-25.13^\circ}$$

$$\text{Let } \overline{I} = 3\ \angle 0^\circ$$

$$\therefore \overline{V} = \text{Supply voltage} = \overline{I}\,\overline{Z} = (3\ \angle 0^\circ)(83.23\ \angle{-25.13^\circ}) = \boxed{249.69\ \angle{-25.13^\circ}}$$

Over all phase angle = $\boxed{25.13^\circ \text{ leading}}$ (as current leads the voltage).

Ex. 4.16 : A resistance R, $L = 0.01$ H and C are in series. When a voltage of 400 sin (3000 t – 10°) is applied across it , the current is $10\sqrt{2}$ cos (3000 t – 55°). Find R and C.

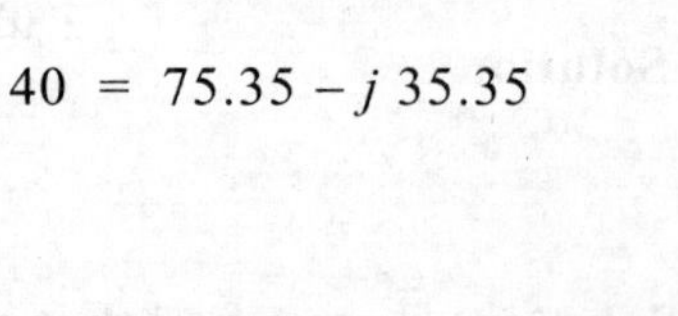

Fig. 4.27

Solution :

$$v(t) = 400 \sin(3000\,t - 10^\circ)$$

$$\therefore \overline{V} = \frac{400}{\sqrt{2}}\ \angle{-10^\circ} = 282.84\ \angle{-10^\circ}$$

$$i(t) = 10\sqrt{2}\cos(3000\,t - 55^\circ) = 10\sqrt{2}\sin(3000\,t - 55^\circ + 90^\circ)$$

$$= 10\sqrt{2}\sin(3000\,t + 35^\circ)$$

$$\therefore \overline{I} = \frac{10\sqrt{2}}{\sqrt{2}}\ \angle 35^\circ = 10\ \angle 35^\circ$$

$$\overline{Z} = \frac{\overline{V}}{\overline{I}} = \frac{282.84\ \angle{-10^\circ}}{10\ \angle 35^\circ} = 28.28\ \angle{-45^\circ} = 20 - j\,20$$

From Fig. 4.27, $\overline{Z} = R + j(X_L - X_C)$

$$\therefore R = \boxed{20\ \Omega}$$

$$X_L - X_C = 20$$

$$\therefore X_C = X_L - 20$$

$$X_L = \omega L = 3000 \times 0.01 = 30$$

$$\therefore X_C = 30 - 20 = 10$$

$$X_C = \frac{1}{\omega C}$$

$$\text{or } C = \frac{1}{\omega X_C} = \frac{1}{3000 \times 10} = \boxed{33.33 \times 10^{-6}\ \mu f}$$

Ex. 4.17 : A series *R-L-C* circuit has a current which lags the applied voltage by 45°. The voltage across the inductor has maximum value equal to twice maximum value of voltage across the capacitor. The voltage across the inductor is 300 sin ωt and $R = 20\ \Omega$. Find the value of inductance and capacitance if supply frequency is 50 Hz.

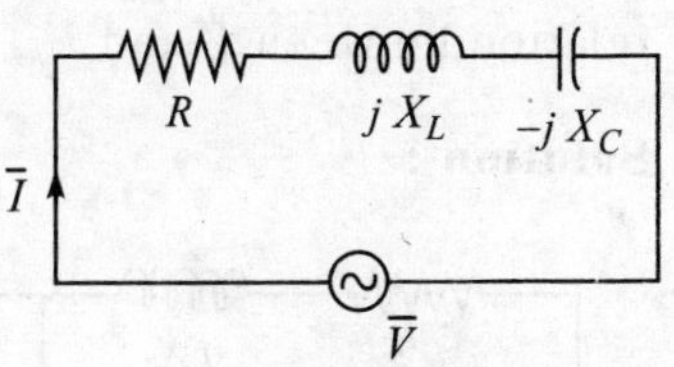

Fig. 4.28

Solution :

$$\overline{Z} = R + j(X_L - X_C)$$

$$\phi = \tan^{-1} \frac{X_L - X_C}{R}$$

$$\therefore R = 20\ \Omega,\ \phi = 45^\circ,\ f = 50 \text{ Hz}$$

$$\therefore \tan 45^\circ = \frac{X_L - X_C}{R}$$

$$\therefore R = X_L - X_C = 20 \qquad \text{..... (1)}$$

$$v_L(t) = 300 \sin \omega t$$

$$\therefore V_{L_{max}} = 300$$

$$\text{Given that } V_{L_{max}} = 2 V_{C_{max}}$$

$$\text{or } V_L = 2\ V_C$$

$$\therefore I X_L = 2\ I X_C$$

$$\therefore X_L = 2\ X_C \qquad \text{..... (2)}$$

From equations (1) and (2), we have

$$X_L - X_C = 20$$

$$\text{or } 2\ X_C - X_C = 20$$

$$\therefore X_C = 20 \text{ and } X_L = 40$$

$$\text{i.e. } X_L = 2\pi f L = 40$$

$$L = \frac{40}{2\pi \times 50} = \boxed{0.127 \text{ H}}$$

$$\text{i.e. } X_C = \frac{1}{2\pi f C} = 20$$

$$C = \frac{1}{2\pi \times 50 \times 20} = \boxed{159.15 \times 10^{-6} \text{ f}}$$

Ex. 4.18 :

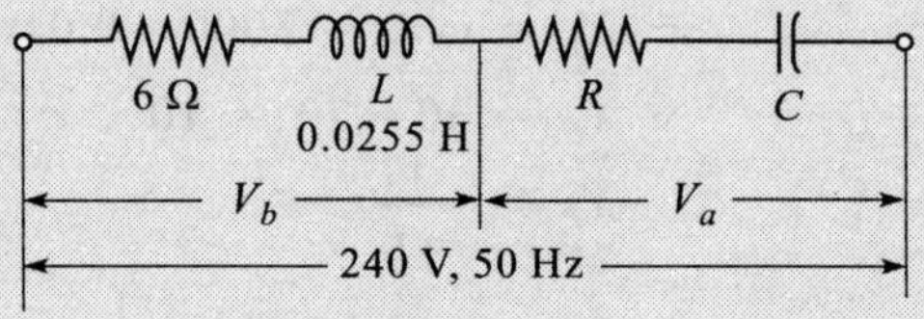

Fig. 4.29

Find R and C so that $V_b = 3V_a$ and V_a and V_b are in quadrature. Find also the phase relation between V and V_b, V_a and I. Draw vector diagram.

Solution :

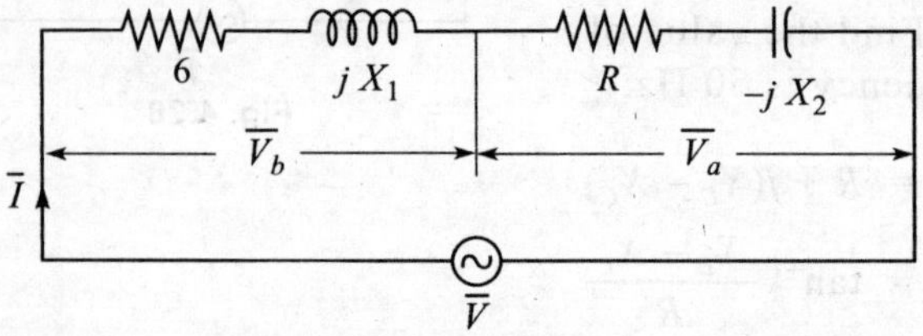

(i)

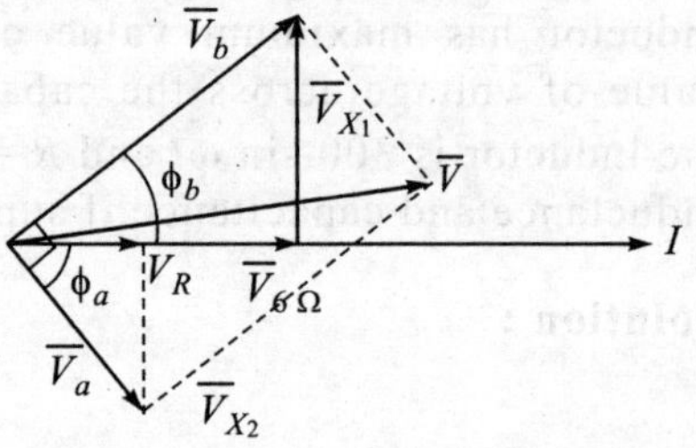

(ii)

Fig. 4.30

Given : $V = 240$ V, $L = 0.0255$ H, $f = 50$ Hz

$$\therefore X_1 = 2\pi f L = 2\pi \times 50 \times 0.0255 = 8$$

Draw the vector diagram as shown in Fig. 4.30(ii)

(i) As it is a series circuit, take I as reference.

(ii) $\overline{V_{6\,\Omega}}$ will be in phase with I (resistance drop).

(iii) $\overline{V_{X_1}}$ will lead I by 90° (inductive drop).

(iv) Sum of $\overline{V_{6\,\Omega}}$ and $\overline{V_{X_1}}$ will be $\overline{V_b}$.

(v) Given that $\overline{V_a}$ and $\overline{V_b}$ are in quadrature and $V_b = 3V_a$, draw V_a $(= \frac{1}{3} V_b)$ and behind V_b by 90°.

(vi) Vector sum of $\overline{V_a}$ and $\overline{V_b}$ will be $\overline{V}$.

$$\therefore \phi_a + \phi_b = 90^\circ$$

$$\phi_b = \tan^{-1} \frac{X_1}{R} = \tan^{-1} \frac{8}{6} = 53.13^\circ$$

$$\therefore \phi_a = 90^\circ - \phi_b = 36.87^\circ$$

$$V_a^2 + V_b^2 = V^2 \qquad [\because V_a \text{ and } V_b \text{ are in quadrature}]$$

$$\text{But } V_b = 3V_a$$

$$\therefore \; V_a^2 + 9V_a^2 = V^2$$

$$10V_a^2 = V^2$$

$$V_a = \sqrt{\frac{240^2}{10}} = \boxed{75.89 \text{ volts}}$$

$$\text{and } V_b = 3V_a = \boxed{227.68 \text{ volts}}$$

$$V_{6\,\Omega} = V_b \cos\phi_b = 227.68 \cos 53.13^\circ = 136.61$$

$$I = \frac{V_{6\,\Omega}}{6\,\Omega} = \frac{136.61}{6} = \boxed{22.77}$$

$$V_R = V_a \cos\phi_a = 75.89 \cos 36.87^\circ = 60.71$$

$$V_{X_2} = V_a \sin\phi_a = 75.89 \cos 36.87^\circ = 45.53$$

$$\therefore \; R = \frac{V_R}{I} = \frac{60.71}{22.77} = \boxed{2.66\ \Omega}$$

$$X_2 = \frac{V_{X_2}}{I} = \frac{45.53}{22.77} = 2$$

$$X_2 = \frac{1}{2\pi f C} = 2$$

$$\therefore \; C = \boxed{1.591 \times 10^{-3} \text{ f}}$$

4.7 A.C. Parallel Circuits

So far we have seen impedances connected in series. Now let us assume two impedances $\overline{Z}_1$, $\overline{Z}_2$ connected in parallel to each other (Fig. 4.31). When we say impedance, it means the circuit element may be either pure R, L, C or a combination of two or more elements.

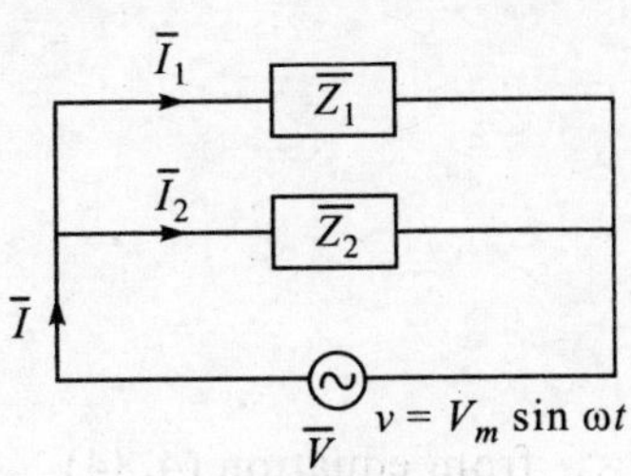

Fig. 4.31

A careful observation of Fig. 4.31 says that voltage across each branch is same i.e. $\overline{V}$.

$$\therefore \; \overline{I}_1 = \frac{\overline{V}}{\overline{Z}_1} \quad \ldots\ldots (4.76)$$

$$\text{and } \overline{I}_2 = \frac{\overline{V}}{\overline{Z}_2} \quad \ldots\ldots (4.77)$$

$$\overline{I} = \overline{I}_1 + \overline{I}_2 \quad \ldots\ldots (4.78)$$

$$\overline{I} = \frac{\overline{V}}{\overline{Z}_1} + \frac{\overline{V}}{\overline{Z}_2} \quad \ldots\ldots (4.79)$$

$$\overline{I} = \overline{V}\left(\frac{1}{\overline{Z}_1} + \frac{1}{\overline{Z}_2}\right) \quad \ldots\ldots (4.80)$$

$$\therefore \ \bar{I} = \frac{\bar{V}}{\bar{Z}} \qquad \text{..... (4.81)}$$

$$\text{where} \ \frac{1}{\bar{Z}} = \frac{1}{\bar{Z}_1} + \frac{1}{\bar{Z}_2} \qquad \text{..... (4.82)}$$

***Note :** This equation (4.82) is similar to equivalent resistance of two parallel branches except for here impedance are vectors.*

The reciprocal of impedance is called '*admittance*' $\bar{Y}$

$$\therefore \ \bar{Y} = \bar{Y}_1 + \bar{Y}_2 \qquad \text{..... (4.83)}$$

Similarly for many parallel admittances

$$\bar{Y} = \bar{Y}_1 + \bar{Y}_2 + \bar{Y}_3 + \bar{Y}_4 + \text{......} \qquad \text{..... (4.84)}$$

Just as impedance has two parts resistance (the real part) and reactance (the imaginary part), the admittance also has two parts i.e. *conductance* G (real part of Y) and '*susceptance*' B (imaginary part of Y).

The unit of admittance is mho '℧'.

Ex. 4.19 : Find $\bar{Z}_{eq}$ and $\bar{Y}_{eq}$ for the circuit in Fig. 4.32 across terminal AB.

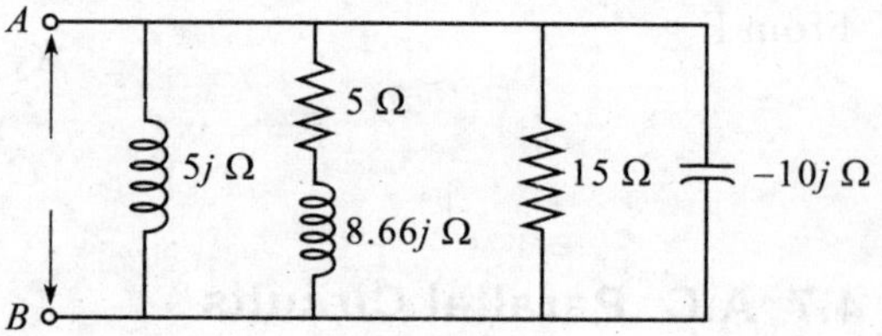

Fig. 4.32

Solution : Let

$$\bar{Z}_1 = 5j$$
$$\bar{Z}_2 = 5 + 8.66j$$
$$\bar{Z}_3 = 15$$
$$\bar{Z}_4 = -10j$$

$$\therefore \ \bar{Y}_1 = \frac{1}{\bar{Z}_1} = \frac{1}{5j} = -0.2j$$

$$\bar{Y}_2 = \frac{1}{5 + 8.66j} = 0.05 - 0.0866j$$

$$\bar{Y}_3 = \frac{1}{15} = 0.067$$

$$\bar{Y}_4 = \frac{1}{-10j} = 0.1j$$

$\therefore$ from equation (4.84)

$$\bar{Y}_{eq} = \bar{Y}_1 + \bar{Y}_2 + \bar{Y}_3 + \bar{Y}_4 + \text{......}$$
$$= -0.2j + 0.05 - 0.0866j + 0.067 + 0.1j$$
$$= 0.117 - 0.186j = \boxed{0.219 \angle -57.83^\circ \text{ mho}}$$

$$\text{and} \ \bar{Z}_{eq} = \frac{1}{\bar{Y}_{eq}} = 2.42 + 3.85j$$
$$= \boxed{4.55 \angle 57.83^\circ \text{ ohms}}$$

Ex. 4.20 : Find the total impedance between AB in Fig. 4.33. Also the phase angle between applied voltage and total current.

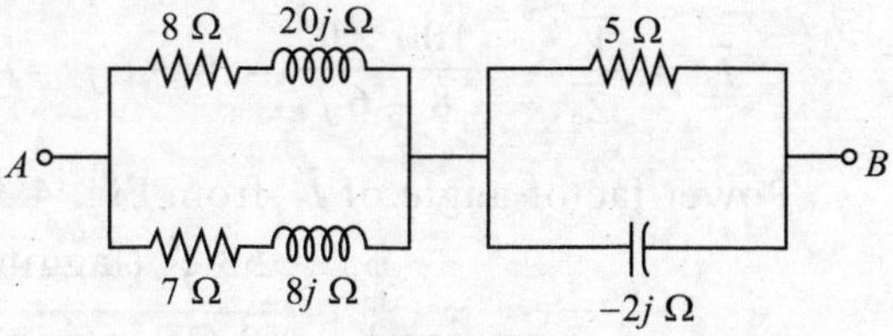

Fig. 4.33

Fig. 4.33 reduces to Fig. 4.33(i)

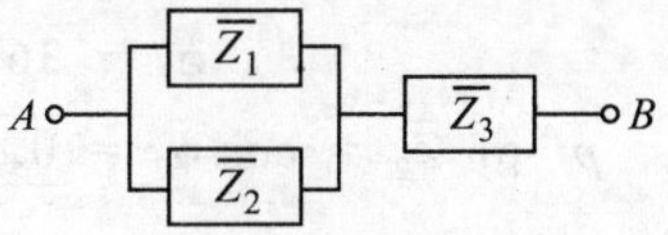

Fig. 4.33(i)

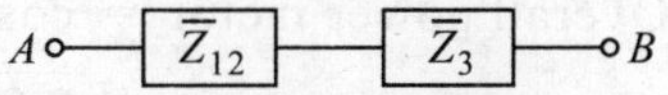

Fig. 4.33(ii)

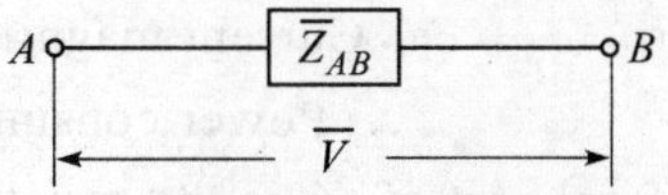

Fig. 4.33(iii)

Solution : Let

$$\overline{Z}_1 = 8 + 20\,j$$

$$\overline{Z}_2 = 7 + 8\,j$$

$$\overline{Z}_3 = 5 \parallel (-2\,j)$$

$$= \frac{5(-2\,j)}{5 + (-2\,j)} = 0.69 - 1.72\,j$$

From Fig. 4.33(ii)

$$\overline{Z}_{12} = \overline{Z}_1 \parallel \overline{Z}_2 = \frac{\overline{Z}_1 \parallel \overline{Z}_2}{\overline{Z}_1 + \overline{Z}_2}$$

$$= \frac{(8 + 20\,j)(7 + 8\,j)}{(8 + 20\,j) + (7 + 8\,j)}$$

$$= 4.11 + 5.92\,j$$

From Fig. 4.33(iii)

$$\therefore\ \overline{Z}_{AB} = \overline{Z}_{12} + \overline{Z}_3$$

$$= 4.11 + 5.92\,j + 0.69 - 1.72\,j$$

$$= 4.80 + 4.19\,j = 6.38\ \angle 41.15^\circ$$

If supply voltage $\overline{V} = V\angle 0^\circ$

$$\text{then } \overline{I} = \frac{\overline{V}}{\overline{Z}_{AB}} = \frac{V\angle 0^\circ}{6.38\ \angle 41.15^\circ} = \boxed{\frac{V}{6.38}\ \angle -41.15^\circ}$$

$\therefore$ the current lags behind supply voltage by $\boxed{41.15^\circ}$.

Ex. 4.21 : Two circuit impedance $(6 + 8j)$ Ω and $(8 - 6j)$ Ω are connected in parallel. A voltage of 100 V is applied across it. Find **(i)** current and power factor of each **(ii)** over all current and power factor **(iii)** power consumed by each impedance and **(iv)** total power consumed.

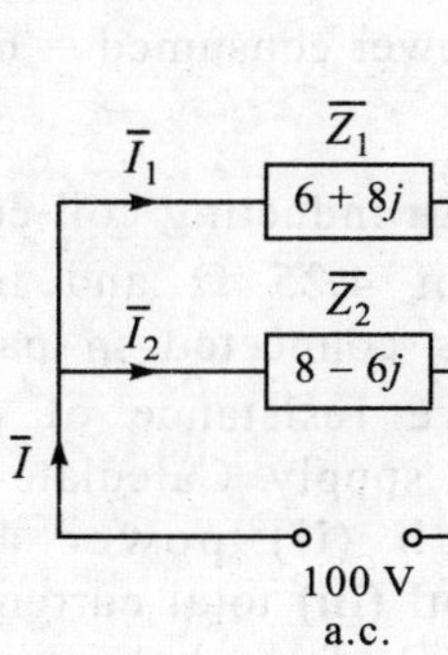

(i)

Solution : Let

$$\overline{V} = 100\ \angle 0^\circ$$

$$\overline{Z}_1 = 6 + 8\,j$$

$$\overline{Z}_2 = 8 - 6\,j$$

(i) $\therefore\ \overline{I}_1 = \dfrac{\overline{V}}{\overline{Z}_1} = \dfrac{100\ \angle 0^\circ}{6 + 8\,j} = 6 - 8\,j = \boxed{10\ \angle -53.1^\circ}$

$$\overline{I}_2 = \frac{\overline{V}}{\overline{Z}_2} = \frac{100\angle 0^\circ}{8-6j} = 8+6j = \boxed{10\angle 36.87^\circ}$$

Power factor angle of $\overline{I}_1$ from Fig. 4.34(ii)

$$\phi_1 = 53.1^\circ \text{ (lagging)}$$

$$\therefore\ pf \text{ of } \overline{Z}_1 = \cos\phi_1 = \boxed{0.6 \text{ (lagging)}}$$

Power factor angle of $\overline{I}_2$ from Fig. 4.34(ii)

$$\phi_2 = 36.87^\circ \text{ (leading)}$$

$$\therefore\ pf \text{ of } \overline{Z}_2 = \cos\phi_2 = \boxed{0.8 \text{ (leading)}}$$

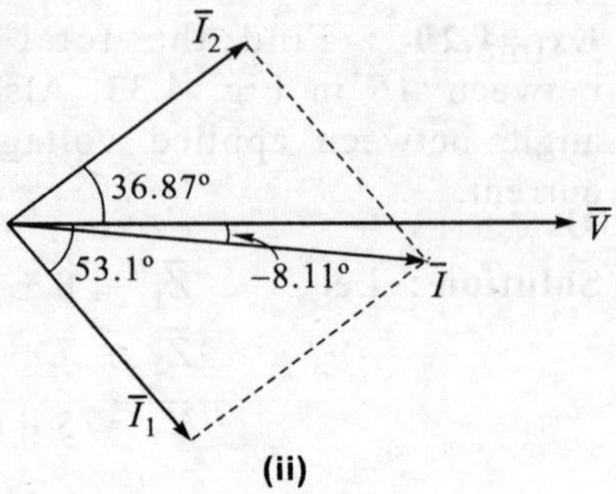

Fig. 4.34

(ii) $\overline{I} = \overline{I}_1 + \overline{I}_2 = 10\angle -53.1^\circ + 10\angle 36.87^\circ = \boxed{14.14\angle -8.115^\circ}$

Overall power factor $= \cos 8.115^\circ$ (lagging) [as –ve value of angle]

$= \boxed{0.99 \text{ (lagging)}}$

(iii) Real part of $\overline{Z}_1$ is the resistive component

i.e. $R_1 = 6\ \Omega$

Current magnitude of $I_1 = 10$ A

$\therefore$ Power consumed in $Z_1 = I_1^2 R_1 = 600$ watts

Real part of $\overline{Z}_2$ is the resistive component (the power consuming component)

i.e. $R_2 = \boxed{8\ \Omega}$

Current magnitude of $I_2 = \boxed{10 \text{ A}}$

$\therefore$ Power consumed in $Z_2 = I_2^2 R_2 = \boxed{800 \text{ watts}}$

(iv) Total power consumed $= 600 + 800 = \boxed{1400 \text{ watts}}$

Ex. 4.22 : An inducting coil consisting of a resistance of 4.25 Ω and inductance of 0.0375 H is connected in parallel with a non-inductive resistance of 20 Ω across 54 V, 50 Hz supply. Calculate **(i)** current in each branch **(ii)** power absorbed by inductive coil **(iii)** total current drawn from the supply **(iv)** pf of whole circuit.

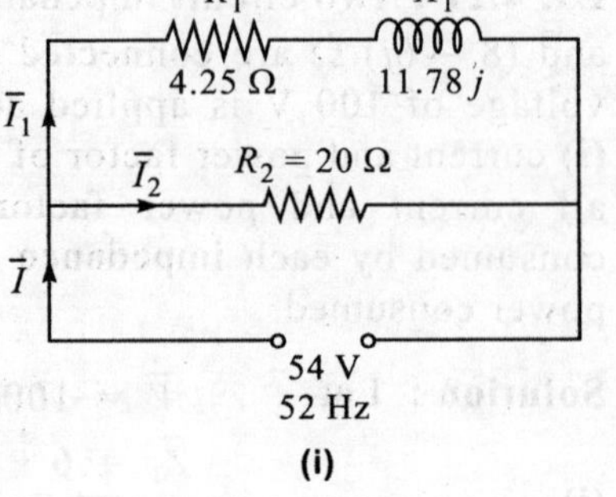

Solution : $R_1 = 4.25\ \Omega$ = Resistance of coil

$L_1 = 0.0375$ H = Inductance of coil

$\therefore\ X_1 = 2\pi f L = 2\pi \times 50 \times 0.0375 = 11.78\ \Omega$

$\therefore$ Impedance of coil $\overline{Z}_1 = R_1 + X_1 j = 4.25 + 11.78j$

Let $\overline{V} = 54\angle 0^\circ$

(i) $\overline{I}_1 = \dfrac{\overline{V}}{\overline{Z}_1} = \dfrac{54\angle 0^\circ}{4.25 + 11.78j} = 1.46 - 4.05j$

$= 4.31\angle -70.16^\circ$

$\overline{I}_2 = \dfrac{\overline{V}}{R_2} = \dfrac{54\angle 0^\circ}{20} = \boxed{2.7\angle 0^\circ}$

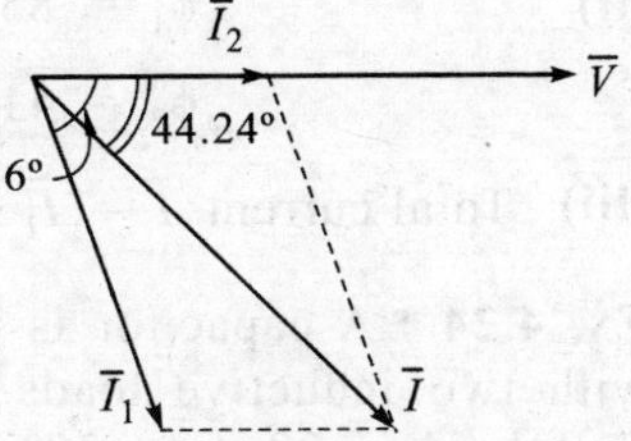

(ii)
Fig. 4.35

(ii) Power absorbed by coil $= I_1^2 R_1 = 4.31^2 \times 4.25$ [remember in power $= I^2 R$ I is not vector]

$= \boxed{78.95 \text{ watts}}$

(iii) Total current $\overline{I} = \overline{I}_1 + \overline{I}_2 = 4.31\angle -70.16^\circ + 2.7\angle 0^\circ = \boxed{5.81\angle -44.24^\circ}$

(iv) Power factor of whole circuit $= \cos 44.24^\circ$ (lagging) [as –ve value of angle]

$= \boxed{0.716 \text{ (lagging)}}$

Ex. 4.23 : An inductive circuit having a resistance of 5 Ω and inductance of 0.019 H and a capacitive circuit with a resistance of 8 Ω and a capacitance of 454.7 µf are connected parallel across 100 V, 50 Hz supply. Calculate **(i)** current in each branch **(ii)** phase angle of each current **(iii)** total current drawn.

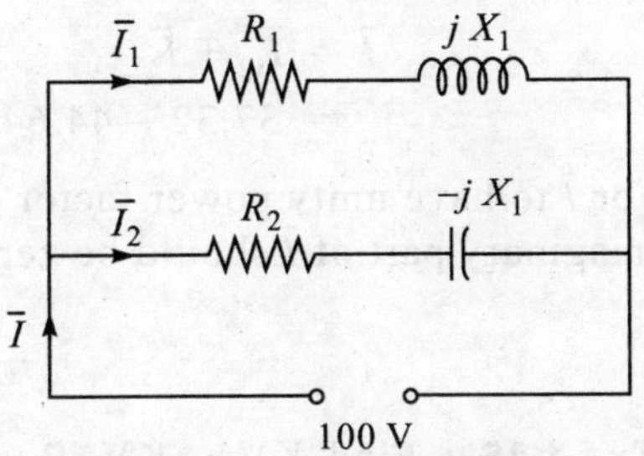

(i)

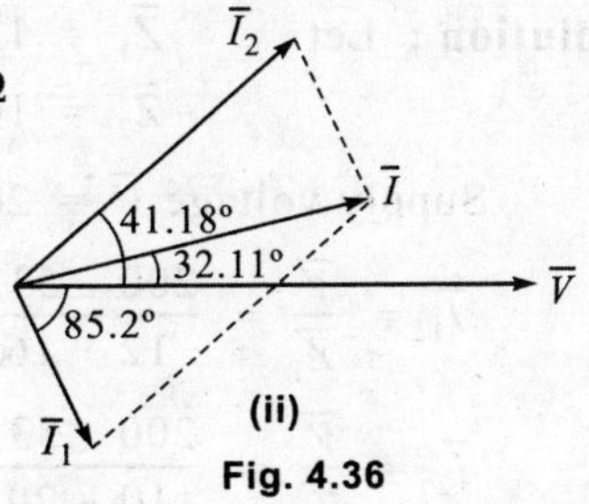

(ii)
Fig. 4.36

Solution : Given : $V = 100$ V, $f = 50$ Hz

$R_1 = 5\ \Omega$

$L_1 = 0.19$ H

$\therefore X_1 = 2\pi f L = 2\pi \times 50 \times 0.19 = 59.69\ \Omega$

$R_2 = 8\ \Omega$

$C = 454.7\ \mu f = 454.7 \times 10^{-6}$ f

$X_2 = \dfrac{1}{2\pi f C} = 7\ \Omega$

$\therefore \overline{Z}_1 = 5 + 59.69j$

$\overline{Z}_2 = 8 - 7j$

(i) $\overline{I}_1 = \dfrac{\overline{V}}{\overline{Z}_1} = \dfrac{100\angle 0^\circ}{5 + 59.69j} = \boxed{1.67\angle -85.21^\circ}$

$\overline{I}_2 = \dfrac{\overline{V}}{\overline{Z}_2} = \dfrac{100\angle 0^\circ}{8 - 7j} = \boxed{9.41\angle 41.18^\circ}$

(ii) $\phi_1 = \boxed{85.21^\circ \text{ (lagging)}}$

$\phi_2 = \boxed{41.18^\circ \text{ (leading)}}$

(iii) Total current $\overline{I} = \overline{I}_1 + \overline{I}_2 = 1.67 \angle -85.21^\circ + 9.41 \angle 41.18^\circ = \boxed{8.53 \angle 32.11^\circ}$

Ex. 4.24 : A capacitor is placed in parallel with two inductive loads. Current through first load is 20 A at 30° and in second is 40 A at 60° lag. What must be the current in the capacitor so that the current in the external circuit is of unity power factor?

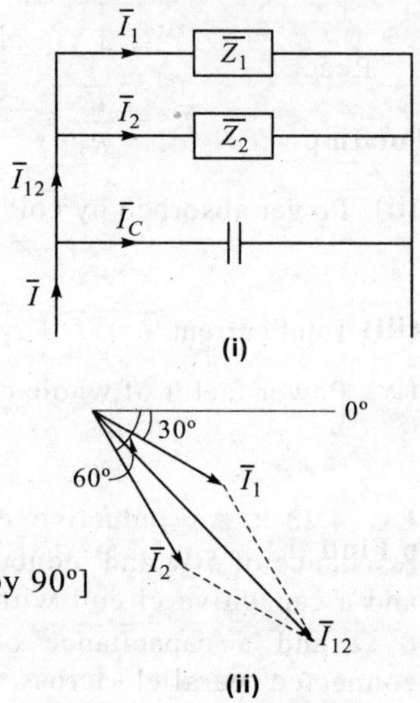

Fig. 4.37

Solution : Refer Fig. 4.37 (given)

$$\overline{I}_1 = 20 \angle -30^\circ \text{ Amp}$$

$$\overline{I}_2 = 40 \angle -60^\circ \text{ Amp}$$

$$\therefore \overline{I}_{12} = \overline{I}_1 + \overline{I}_2$$

$$= 20 \angle -30^\circ + 40 \angle -60^\circ = 37.32 - 44.64\,j$$

$$\overline{I} = \overline{I}_{12} + \overline{I}_C$$

$$= 37.32 - 44.64\,j + I_C\,j \quad [\text{as } \overline{I}_C \text{ will lead } \overline{V} \text{ by } 90^\circ]$$

For $\overline{I}$ to have unity power factor ($\phi = 0^\circ$) imaginary part of $\overline{I}$ should be zero

$$\therefore \overline{I}_C = \boxed{44.64 \text{ Amp}}$$

Ex. 4.25 : Find KVA, KVAR and KW for each branch and power factor of the whole circuit is Fig. 4.38(i).

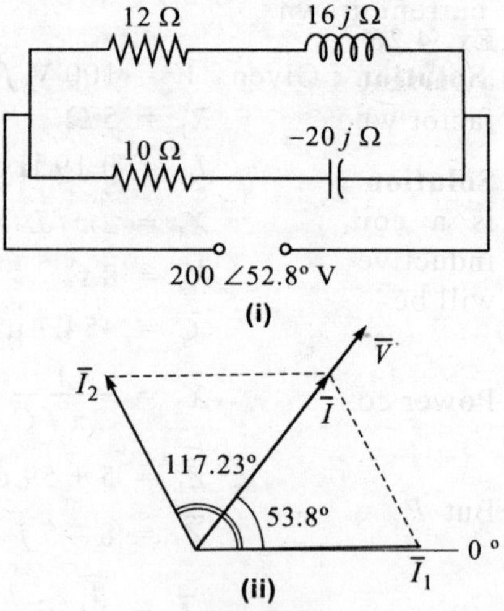

Fig. 4.38

Solution : Let $\overline{Z}_1 = 12 + 16\,j$

$$\overline{Z}_2 = 10 - 20\,j$$

Supply voltage $\overline{V} = 200 \angle 53.8^\circ$

$$\therefore \overline{I}_1 = \frac{\overline{V}}{\overline{Z}_1} = \frac{200 \angle 53.8^\circ}{12 + 16\,j} = 10 \angle 0.67^\circ$$

$$\overline{I}_2 = \frac{\overline{V}}{\overline{Z}_2} = \frac{200 \angle 53.8^\circ}{10 - 20\,j} = -4.09 + 7.95\,j$$

$$= 8.94 \angle 117.23^\circ$$

For Impedance Z_1

$$\phi_1 = \text{The angle between } \overline{V} \text{ and } \overline{I}_1 \text{ from Fig. 438(ii)}$$

$$= 53.8 - 0.67 = 53.13^\circ$$

$$\therefore \; KVA_1 = \frac{V \times I_1}{1000} = \frac{200 \times 10}{1000} = \boxed{2}$$

[Refer Fig. 4.5(iii) and equations (4.36), (4.38) and (4.41)]

$$\text{Power consumed } (KW_1) = \frac{V I_1 \cos \phi_1}{1000} = \frac{200 \times 10 \times \cos 53.13^\circ}{1000} = \boxed{1.2 \text{ KW}}$$

$$\text{Reactive power } (KVAR_1) = \frac{V I_1 \sin \phi_1}{1000} = \frac{200 \times 10 \times \sin 53.13^\circ}{1000} = \boxed{1.2 \text{ KVAR}}$$

For Impedance $\overline{Z}_2$

$$\phi_2 = \text{Angle between } \overline{V} \text{ and } \overline{I}_2 = 117.23 - 53.8$$

$$\phi_2 = 53.13^\circ$$

$$\therefore \; KVA_2 = \frac{V \times I_2}{1000} = \frac{200 \times 8.94}{1000} = \boxed{1.788 \text{ KVA}}$$

$$KW_2 = \frac{V I_2 \cos \phi_2}{1000} = \frac{200 \times 8.94 \times \cos 63.43^\circ}{1000} = \boxed{0.799 \text{ KW}}$$

$$KVAR_2 = \frac{V I_1 \sin \phi_2}{1000} = \frac{200 \times 8.94 \times \sin 63.43^\circ}{1000} = \boxed{1.6 \text{ KVAR}}$$

To Find the Total Current $\overline{I}$

$$\overline{I} = \overline{I}_1 + \overline{I}_2 = 10 \angle 0.67^\circ + 8.94 \angle 117.23^\circ = \boxed{10 \angle 53.78^\circ}$$

$$\therefore \; \phi_2 = \text{Angle between } V \text{ and } I \approx 0^\circ$$

$$\therefore \; \text{Power factor of whole circuit} = \cos \phi$$

$$= \boxed{1 \text{ i.e. unity power factor.}}$$

Ex. 4.26 : The power dissipated is coil A is 300 W and in B is 400 watts. Each coil takes a current of 5 A when connected to 110 V, 50 Hz supply. Find current drawn and power factor when the coils are in **(i)** series **(ii)** parallel.

Solution : Let us first consider coil A. As it is a coil it will have resistance R_A and inductive reactance X_A and its impedance $\overline{Z}_A$ will be

$$\overline{Z}_A = R_A + X_A j \qquad \text{..... (1)}$$

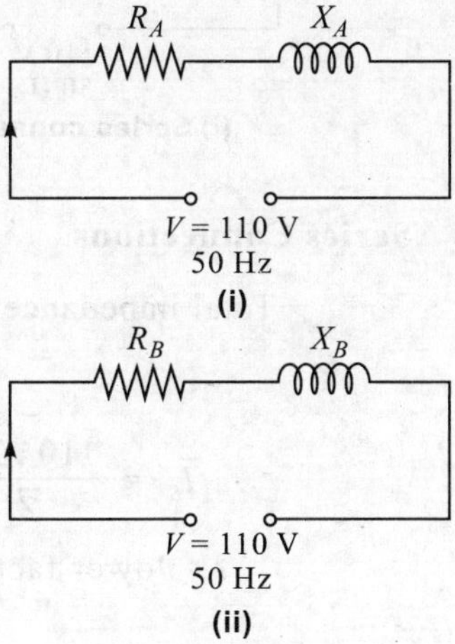

Fig. 4.39

Power consumed in $\overline{Z}_A$ is P_A

$$P_A = 300 \text{ watts (given)}$$

But $P_A = I_A^2 R_A$ and $I_A = 5$ A (given)

$$\therefore \; 300 = 5^2 R_A$$

$$\text{or } R_A = 12 \, \Omega$$

$$\frac{V}{I_A} = Z_A$$

$$\therefore\ Z_A = \frac{110}{5} = 22\ \Omega$$

From equation (1) above

$$Z_A^{\ 2} = R_A^{\ 2} + X_A^{\ 2}$$

$$\therefore\ 22^2 = 12^2 + X_A^{\ 2}$$

$$\text{or } X_A = 18.43$$

Similarly for coil B

$$\overline{Z}_B = R_B + X_B j$$

$$P_B = 400 \text{ watts} \qquad \text{(given)}$$

$$P_B = I_B^{\ 2} R_B$$

$$\therefore\ 400 = 5^2 R_B$$

$$\therefore\ R_B = 16\ \Omega$$

$$Z_B = \frac{V}{I_B} = \frac{110}{5} = 22\ \Omega$$

$$Z_B^{\ 2} = R_B^{\ 2} + X_B^{\ 2}$$

$$\therefore\ X_B = \sqrt{22^2 - 16^2} \quad \text{or } X_B = 15.09$$

$$\therefore\ \overline{Z}_A = 12 + 18.43j \text{ and } \overline{Z}_B = 16 + 15.09\,j$$

Now Fig. 4.40(i) shows $\overline{Z}_A$ and $\overline{Z}_B$ in series and Fig. 4.40(ii) shows parallel connection.

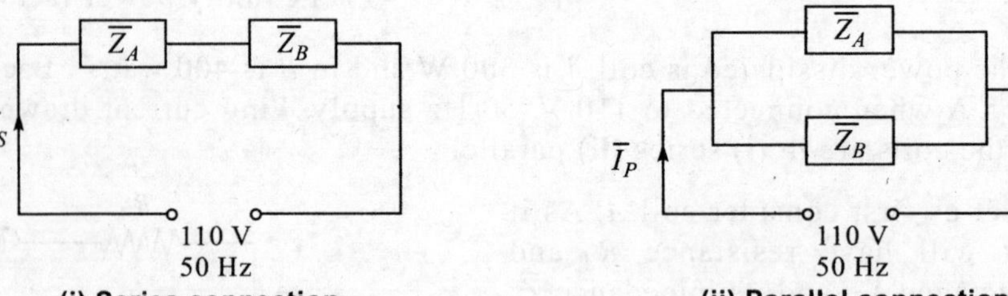

(i) Series connection. **(ii) Parallel connection.**

Fig. 4.40

(i) Series Connections

$$\text{Total impedance } \overline{Z} = \overline{Z}_A + \overline{Z}_B = 12 + 18.43\,j + 16 + 15.09\,j$$

$$= 28 + 33.52\,j$$

$$\therefore\ \overline{I}_S = \frac{110\ \angle 0^\circ}{\overline{Z}} = \frac{110\ \angle 0^\circ}{28 + 33.52\,j} = \boxed{2.52\ \angle{-50.13^\circ}\ \text{Amp}}$$

$$\therefore\ \text{Power factor} = \cos 50.13^\circ \text{ (lagging) [as –ve value of angle]}$$

$$= \boxed{0.64 \text{ (lagging)}}$$

(ii) Parallel Connections

$$\overline{I}_A = \frac{110 \angle 0^\circ}{\overline{Z}_A} = \frac{110 \angle 0^\circ}{12 + 18.43\,j} = 5 \angle -56.93^\circ \text{ Amp}$$

$$\overline{I}_B = \frac{110 \angle 0^\circ}{\overline{Z}_B} = \frac{110 \angle 0^\circ}{16 + 15.09\,j} = 5 \angle -43.32^\circ \text{ Amp}$$

$$\therefore\ \overline{I}_P = \overline{I}_A + \overline{I}_B = 5 \angle -56.93^\circ + 5 \angle -43.32^\circ$$

$$= \boxed{9.93 \angle -50.125^\circ}$$

$$\therefore \text{ Power factor} = \cos 50.125^\circ \text{ (lagging) [as -ve value of angle]}$$

$$= \boxed{0.64 \text{ (lagging)}}$$

Ex. 4.27 : In a series parallel circuit two parallel branches A and B are in series with C. Their impedances are $\overline{Z}_A = 10 + 8\,j$, $\overline{Z}_B = 9 - 6\,j$ and $\overline{Z}_C = 3 + 2\,j$. If voltage across $\overline{Z}_C$ is $100 \angle 0^\circ$, find $\overline{I}_A$ and $\overline{I}_B$.

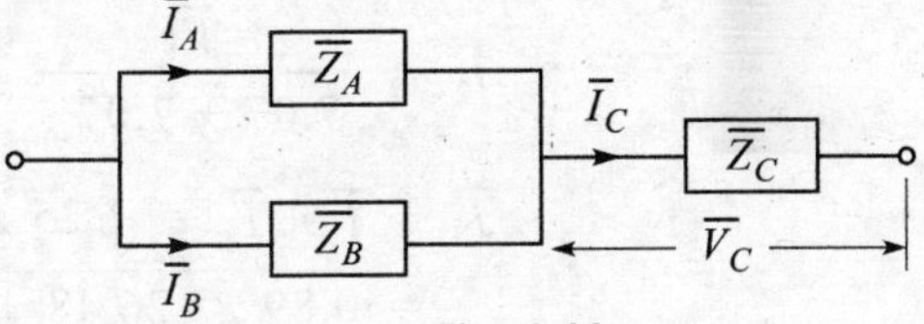

Fig. 4.41

Solution : Given : $\overline{Z}_A = 10 + 8\,j$, $\overline{Z}_B = 9 - 6\,j$ and $\overline{Z}_C = 3 + 2\,j$

$$\overline{V}_C = 100 \angle 0^\circ$$

Refer Fig. 4.41,

$$\overline{I}_C = \frac{\overline{V}_C}{\overline{Z}_C} = \frac{100 \angle 0^\circ}{3 + 2\,j} = \boxed{27.73 \angle -33.69^\circ}$$

Using current division rule for parallel branches

$$\overline{I}_A = \frac{\overline{I}_C\,\overline{Z}_B}{\overline{Z}_A + \overline{Z}_B} = \frac{(27.73 \angle -33.69^\circ)(9 - 6\,j)}{10 + 8\,j + 9 - 6\,j} = \boxed{15.7 \angle -73.39^\circ}$$

$$\overline{I}_B = \overline{I}_C - \overline{I}_A = (27.73 \angle -33.69^\circ) - (15.7 \angle -73.39^\circ)$$

$$= \boxed{18.59 \angle -1.04^\circ}$$

Ex. 4.28 : In the circuit of Fig. 4.42(i), the source frequency is 500 rad/sec, $\overline{I}_1$ is $1.25 \angle 26^\circ$ A. Find $\overline{I}_2$ and $\overline{I}_3$ source voltage and power factor.

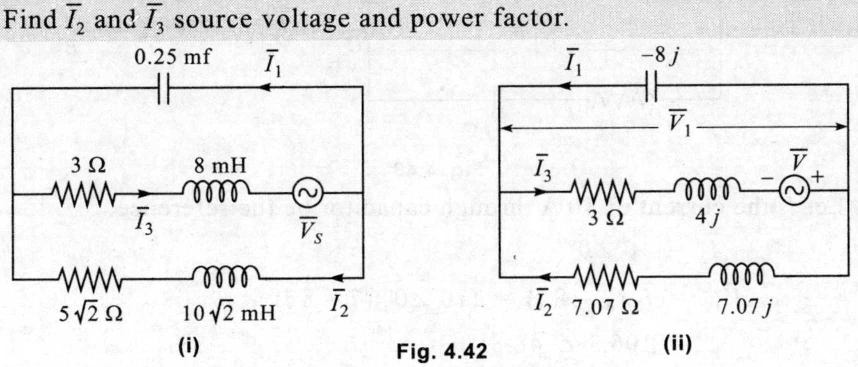

Fig. 4.42

Solution : Given : $\omega = 500$ rad/sec.

$$\bar{I}_1 = 1.25 \angle 26^\circ \text{ A}$$

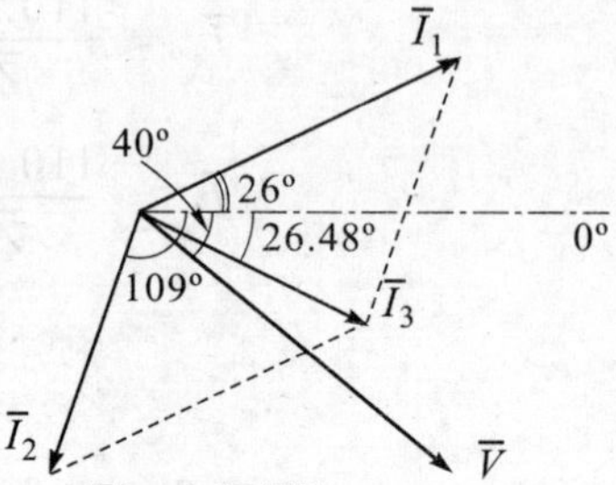

Fig. 4.42(iii)

Converting L and C to reactance, we get Fig. 4.42(ii)

$$X_1 = \frac{1}{\omega C} = \frac{1}{500 \times 0.25 \times 10^{-3}} = 8$$

$$X_2 = \omega L_2 = 500 \times 10\sqrt{2} \times 10^{-3} = 7.07$$

$$X_3 = \omega L = 500 \times 8 \times 10^{-3} = 4$$

From Fig. 4.42(ii) $\bar{V}_1 = \bar{I}_1 (-8j) = (1.25 \angle 26^\circ)(-8j)$

$$= 10 \angle -64^\circ$$

$$\therefore \quad \bar{I}_2 = \frac{\bar{V}_1}{7.07 + 7.07j} = \frac{10 \angle -64^\circ}{7.07 + 7.07j} = \boxed{1 \angle -109^\circ}$$

$$\bar{I}_3 = \bar{I}_1 + \bar{I}_2 = 1.25 \angle 26^\circ + 1 \angle -109^\circ$$

$$= \boxed{0.89 \angle -26.48^\circ}$$

Applying KVL to upper closed loop in Fig. 4.42(ii)

$$\bar{V} = \bar{I}_1 (-8j) + \bar{I}_3 (3 + 4j)$$

$$= (1.25 \angle 26^\circ)(-8j) + (0.89 \angle -26.48^\circ)(3 + 4j)$$

$$= 10.89 \angle -40^\circ$$

$\therefore$ Angle between $\bar{V}$ and $\bar{I}_3 = 40^\circ - 26.48^\circ = \boxed{13.52^\circ \text{ (leading)}}$

as $\bar{I}_3$ leads $\bar{V}$ [Fig. 4.42(iii)]

$\therefore$ Power factor $= \cos 13.52^\circ = \boxed{0.9722 \text{ (leading)}}$

Ex. 4.29 : Find $\bar{V}_{AB}$ in Fig. 4.43 so that 10 A current may flow through the capacitor.

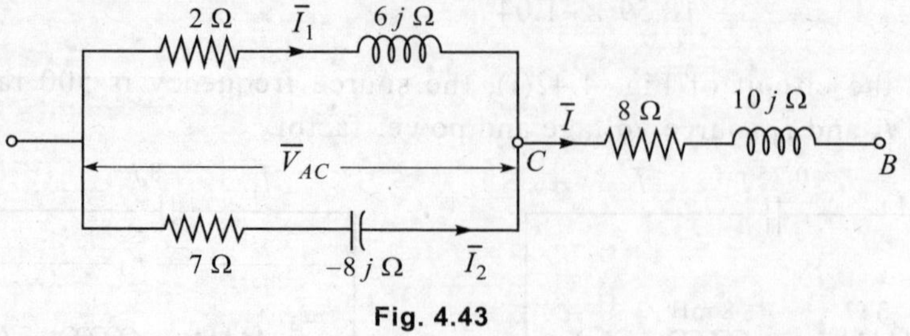

Fig. 4.43

Solution : Let $\bar{I}_2$ the current of 10 A through capacitor be the reference.

$$\bar{I}_2 = 10 \angle 0^\circ$$

$$\bar{V}_{AC} = \bar{I}_2 (7 - 8j) = (10 \angle 0^\circ)(7 - 8j)$$

$$= 106.3 \angle -48.81^\circ$$

$$\therefore\ \overline{I}_1 = \frac{\overline{V}_{AC}}{2+6j} = 16.81\ \angle{-120.38^\circ}$$

$$\overline{I} = \overline{I}_1 + \overline{I}_2 = 16.81\ \angle{-120.38^\circ} + 10\ \angle 0^\circ$$

$$= 14.57\ \angle{-84.09^\circ}$$

$$\overline{V}_{CB} = \overline{I}\,(8+10j) = (14.57\ \angle{-84.09^\circ})(8+10j)$$

$$= 186.59\ \angle{-32.75^\circ}$$

$$\overline{V}_{AB} = \overline{V}_{AC} + \overline{V}_{CB} = 106.3\ \angle{-48.81^\circ} + 186.59\ \angle{-32.75^\circ}$$

$$= \boxed{290.3\ \angle{-38.56^\circ}}$$

Ex. 4.30 : An inductive coil draws a current of 10 A and dissipates 1400 watts when it is energized from 200 V, 50 Hz supply. When another coil is connected in series with it, the circuit takes 5.35 A at 0.85 lagging power factor, the supply being same. Determine the total current taken from the supply and its power factor when the two coils are connected in parallel across the same supply.

Solution : Let $I_1 = 10$ A

$$P_1 = 1400 \text{ watts}$$

$$\overline{V} = 200\ \angle 0^\circ \text{ volts}$$

$$f = 50 \text{ Hz}$$

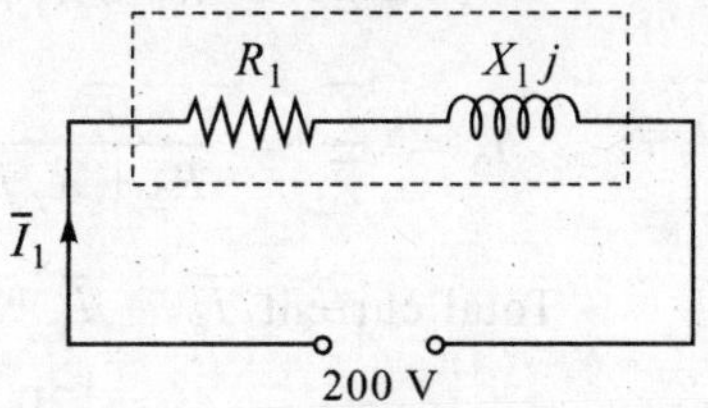

Fig. 4.44(i)

From Fig. 4.44(i)

$$P_1 = I_1^2 R_1$$

$$\therefore\ 1400 = 10^2 R_1$$

$$\text{or } R_1 = 14\ \Omega$$

$$\overline{Z}_1 = \text{Impedance of coil 1}$$

$$\frac{V}{I_1} = Z_1$$

$$\therefore\ Z_1 = \frac{200}{10} = 20\ \Omega$$

$$Z_1^{\,2} = R_1^{\,2} + X_1^{\,2}$$

$$\therefore\ X_1 = \sqrt{20^2 - 14^2} = 14.28$$

$$\therefore\ \overline{Z}_1 = R_1 + X_1 j = 14 + 14.28j$$

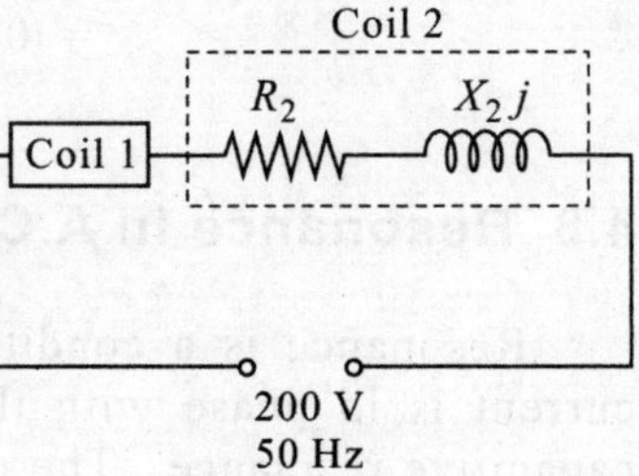

Fig. 4.44(ii)

From Fig. 4.44(ii), let the total impedance in series be $\overline{Z}$

where $\overline{Z} = R + Xj$; $R = R_1 + R_2$ and $X = X_1 + X_2$

$I_S = 5.35$ A and its power factor $= 0.85$ (lagging)

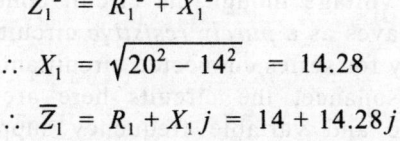

$$\therefore\ \phi_S = \cos^{-1} 0.85 = 31.79^\circ$$

$$Z = \frac{V}{I_S} = \frac{200}{5.35} = 37.38$$

∴ From Fig. 4.44(iii)

$$R = Z\cos\phi_S = 37.38 \times 0.85 = 31.77$$

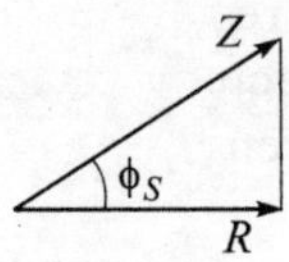

Fig. 4.44(iii)

$$\text{But } R = R_1 + R_2$$

$$\therefore R_2 = R - R_1$$

$$\text{or } R_2 = 31.77 - 14 = 17.77$$

$$X = Z\sin\phi_S = 37.38 \sin 31.79^\circ$$

$$\therefore X = 19.69$$

$$\therefore X_2 = X - X_1$$

$$\text{or } X_2 = 19.69 - 14.28 = 5.41$$

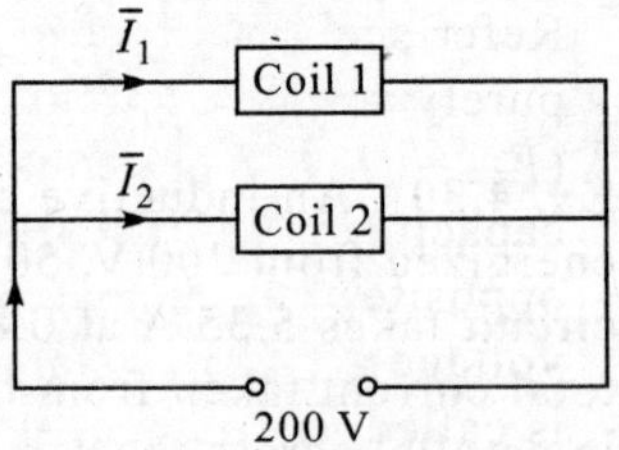

Fig. 4.44(iv)

Refer Fig. 4.44(iv) for parallel connection of two coils.

$$\bar{I}_1 = \frac{\bar{V}}{\bar{Z}_1} = \frac{\bar{V}}{R_1 + X_1 j} = \frac{200\angle 0^\circ}{14 + 14.28j} = 10\angle{-45^\circ}$$

$$\bar{I}_2 = \frac{\bar{V}}{\bar{Z}_2} = \frac{\bar{V}}{R_2 + X_2 j} = \frac{200\angle 0^\circ}{17.77 + 5.41j} = 10.76\angle{-16.9^\circ}$$

$$\text{Total current } \bar{I}_P = \bar{I}_1 + \bar{I}_2 = 10\angle{-45^\circ} + 10.76\angle{-16.9^\circ}$$

$$= \boxed{20.1\angle{-30.4^\circ}}$$

$$\therefore \text{Power factor of } \bar{I}_P = \cos 30.4^\circ \text{ (lagging) [as } \bar{I} \text{ lags behind } \bar{V} \text{ by } 30.4^\circ]$$

$$= \boxed{0.8625 \text{ (lagging)}}$$

4.8 Resonance in A.C. Circuits

Resonance is a condition in a.c. circuits under steady condition wherein the load current is in phase with the supply voltage though the circuit contains inductive and capacitive reactance. The circuit behaves as a *purely resistive* circuit. This phenomenon of resonance is studied here separately for series connected circuit and parallel connected circuit. In order the understand resonance, the circuits here are considered to be connected across a constant voltage and variable frequency supply. As the supply frequency changes the inductive and capacitive reactances change ($X_L = 2\pi f L$ and $X_L = 1/2\pi f C$) where as the circuit resistance does not depend upon frequency ($R = \rho l/A$). hence, the impedance of the circuit will also change thus changing the current and power factor of the circuit. Note that at resonance as circuit impedance will be only resistive and power factor (cos ϕ) of the circuit will be unity.

4.8.1 Series Resonant Circuit

Consider Fig. 4.45(i), it consists of a pure resistance inductance and capacitance connected in series. The circuit impedance is given by

$$\overline{Z} = R + j X_L - j X_C$$

If in this circuit $X_L = X_C$ then $\overline{Z} = R$

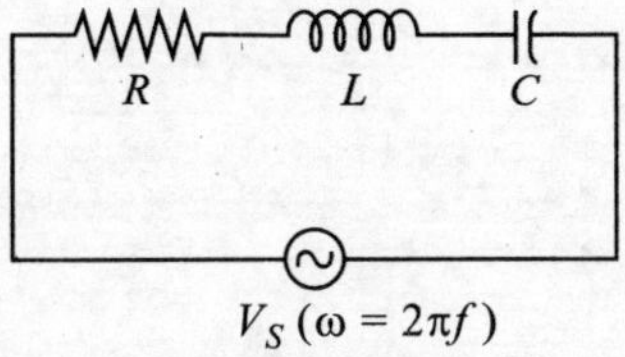

Fig. 4.45(i) : *R-L-C* series circuit.

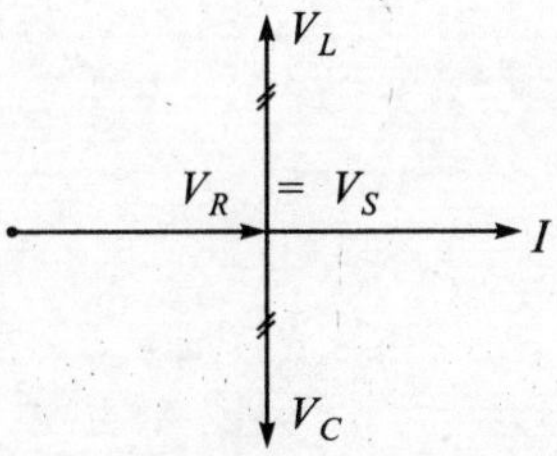

Fig. 4.45(ii) : Vector diagram when $X_L = X_C$

Refer section 4.6 case III, i.e. the circuit behaves as purely resistive circuit. The voltage across inductor ($V_L = I\ X_L$) is equal to the voltage across the capacitor ($V_C = I\ X_C$) as these vectors are equal and opposite they cancel each other and $V_R = V_S$ i.e. voltage across resistance is equal to supply voltage it is called *Resonance*.

Let us express this condition with subscript '*o*' i.e. $\omega_o = 2\pi f_o$, Z_o, X_{Co}, X_{Lo}, etc.

$$\therefore \text{ at resonance } X_{Lo} = X_{Co} \qquad \text{..... (4.85)}$$

$$\text{or } \omega_o L = \frac{1}{\omega_o C} \qquad \text{..... (4.86)}$$

$$\therefore \omega_o = \frac{1}{\sqrt{L C}} \qquad \text{..... (4.87)}$$

$$\therefore f_o = \frac{1}{2\pi \sqrt{L C}} \qquad (\because \omega_o = 2\pi f_o) \qquad \text{..... (4.88)}$$

$$\text{At resonance, } Z_o = R + j\,0 = R$$

$$I_o = \frac{V}{Z_o} = \frac{V}{R}$$

(a) Effect of Variation of Frequency

In this circuit of Fig. 4.45 (i) R, L, C and V_S are kept fixed and the supply frequency ω (= $2\pi f$) is varied from 0 to ∞.

As resistance R does not depend on frequency the plot of R v/s ω is as shown in Fig. 4.46. $X_L = \omega L$ i.e. X_L is directly proportional to ω and remember $+j$ is associated with X_L, the variation of X_L with ω is a straight line. $X_C = 1/\omega C$ i.e. X_C varies inversely proportional to ω and $-j$ is associated with X_C thus variation of X_C (rectangular hyperbola) is plotted along negative imaginary axis.

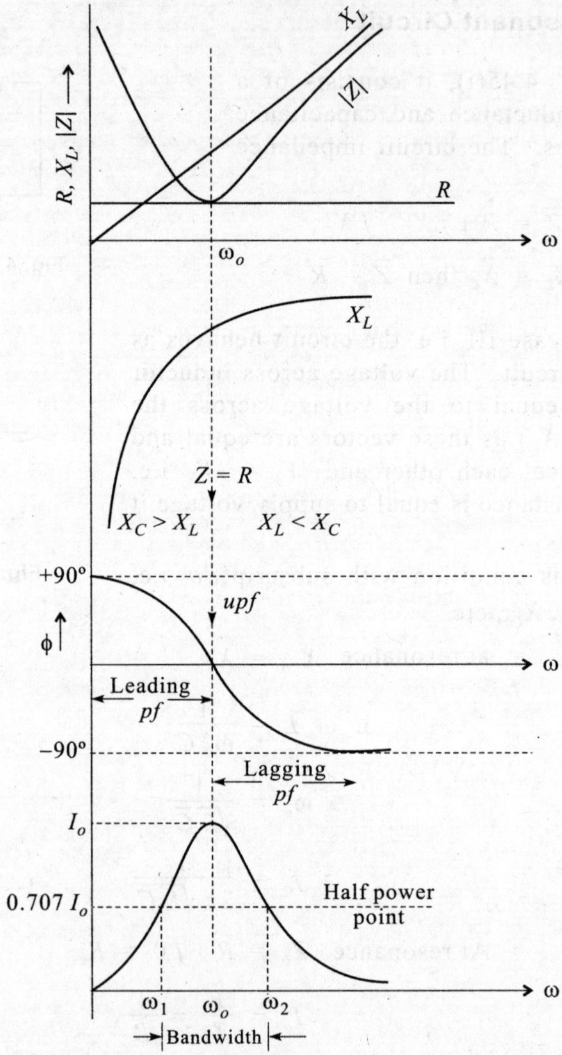

Fig. 4.46

Observe the variations of X_L and X_C with ω. X_L increases from a low value (0 Ω) to a large value, whereas X_C reduces from a large value to a very low value as ω increases from '0' to '∞'.

$$\text{At } \omega_o, \; X_L = X_C$$

$$\therefore \omega_o = \frac{1}{\sqrt{L\,C}}$$

$$\text{or } f_o = \frac{1}{2\pi\sqrt{L\,C}}$$

$$\bar{Z} = R + j(X_L - X_C)$$

$$|Z| = \sqrt{R^2 + (X_L - X_C)^2}$$

At resonance (ω_o) ; $Z = R$ (as $X_L = X_C$)

Power factor is unity ($\phi = 0°$)

For $\omega < \omega_o$ (observe Fig. 4.46) $\quad X_C > X_L$

$$\therefore \; \overline{Z} = R - jX \quad \text{where } X = X_L - X_C$$

$$Z = \sqrt{R^2 + X^2}$$

Circuit behaves as capacitive circuit, power factor is leading.

For $\omega > \omega_o$

$$X_L > X_C$$

$$\therefore \; \overline{Z} = R + jX$$

Circuit behaves as inductive circuit, power factor is lagging.

Observe the impedance Z from $\omega = 0$ to $\omega = \infty$ (Fig. 4.46). We observe that at resonance (ω_o) $Z = R$ and this is the minimum value of impedance. Hence, if we plot the variation of current as the frequency changes we see that at ω_o, the resonant current I_o has its maximum value given by

$$I_o = \frac{V_S}{R} \qquad \text{..... (4.89)}$$

The voltage across inductance V_{Lo} is given by

$$V_{Lo} = I_o X_{Lo} = I_o \omega_o L$$

$$= \frac{V_S}{R} \frac{1}{\sqrt{LC}} L$$

$$V_{Lo} = \frac{V_S}{R} \sqrt{\frac{L}{C}} \qquad \text{..... (4.90)}$$

$$\text{Also, } V_{Co} = V_{Lo}$$

$$\therefore \; V_{Co} = \frac{V_S}{R} \sqrt{\frac{L}{C}} \qquad \text{..... (4.91)}$$

It may be seen that V_{Lo} and V_{Co} may be many times greater than the supply voltage.

(b) Band Width

At resonance, the circuit impedance is minimum and the resonant current $I_o (= V_S / R)$ is maximum. This peak value of current depends upon the value of R, the circuit resistance. It is observed that larger the value of R, lower is the value of I_o (Fig. 4.47). Circuits with smaller values of R give rise to a larger resonant current and this rise of current is sharper with respect to small R circuits.

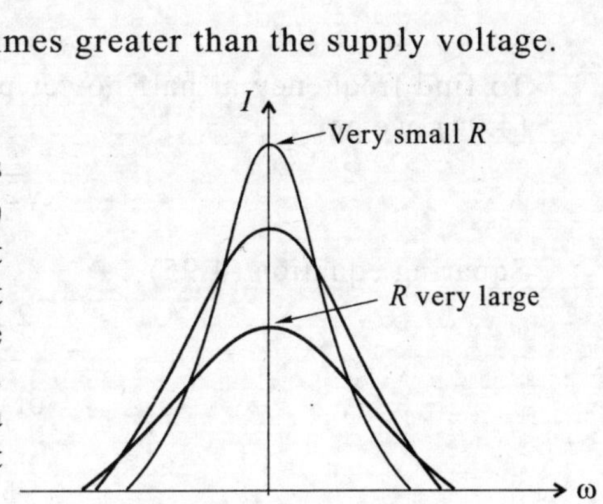

Fig. 4.47 : Resonance curve.

Circuits with sharper curve for current have sharp-resonance or high selectivity and hence a better quality as explained later.

The current versus frequency curve is called "*Resonance Curve*" (Fig. 4.47) The frequencies at which the power dissipated is half of the power dissipated at resonance (P_o) are called *half power points* i.e.

At half power frequencies, power $P_h = \frac{1}{2} P_o$

$$= \frac{1}{2} I_o^2 R$$

$$\text{or } P_h = \left(\frac{I_o}{\sqrt{2}}\right)^2 R$$

In other words, we can say, when current in the circuit is $I_o/\sqrt{2}$ the power dissipated in the circuit is half the power dissipated at resonance or at half power point.

$$\text{or at half power point, } I_h = \frac{I_o}{\sqrt{2}} = 0.707\, I_o \qquad \text{..... (4.91)}$$

Now, refer to the resonance curve of Fig. 4.48. Draw a horizontal line at 0.707 I_o (the half power points).

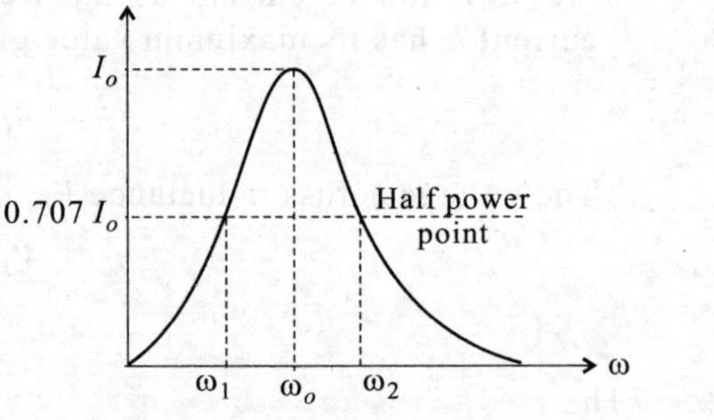

Fig. 4.48

At half power current, I_h can be given by

$$I_h = \frac{I_o}{\sqrt{2}} = \frac{V_o}{\sqrt{2}\, R} \qquad \text{..... (4.92)}$$

Or the circuit impedance from equation (4.92) can be given by Z_h

$$Z_h = \sqrt{2}\, R \qquad \text{..... (4.93)}$$

From *R-L-C* series circuit, the circuit impedance at any frequency ω can be given by

$$Z = \sqrt{R^2 + \left(\omega L - \frac{1}{\omega C}\right)^2} \qquad \text{..... (4.94)}$$

To find frequency at half power point equate impedances from equations (4.93) and (4.94), we get

$$\sqrt{2}\, R = \sqrt{R^2 + \left(\omega L - \frac{1}{\omega C}\right)^2} \qquad \text{..... (4.95)}$$

Squaring equation (4.95)

$$2 R^2 = R^2 + \left(\omega L - \frac{1}{\omega C}\right)^2$$

$$\text{or } R^2 = \left(\omega L - \frac{1}{\omega C}\right)^2$$

$$\therefore \pm R = \omega L - \frac{1}{\omega C}$$

Re-arranging this equation we get

$$\pm R\omega C = \omega^2 LC - 1$$

$$\text{or } \omega^2 LC \pm R\omega C - 1 = 0 \qquad \text{..... (4.96)}$$

To find value of ω at half power we find root of equation (4.96)

$$\omega_1, \omega_2 = \frac{\pm RC \pm \sqrt{R^2C^2 + 4LC}}{2LC}$$

$$= \pm \frac{RC}{2LC} \pm \sqrt{\frac{R^2C^2}{4L^2C^2} + \frac{4LC}{4L^2C^2}}$$

$$\omega_1, \omega_2 = \pm \frac{R}{2L} \pm \sqrt{\frac{R^2}{4L^2} + \frac{1}{LC}} \qquad \text{..... (4.97)}$$

In this equation if $R^2 << 4L^2$, $\frac{R^2}{4L^2}$ becomes negligible, then

$$\omega_1, \omega_2 = \pm \frac{R}{2L} \pm \sqrt{\frac{1}{LC}}$$

$$\text{But } \sqrt{\frac{1}{LC}} = \omega_o$$

$$\omega_1, \omega_2 = \pm \frac{R}{2L} \pm \omega_o \qquad \text{..... (4.98)}$$

The negative sign with ω_o in equation (4.98) indicate negative resonant frequencies which is not possible hence dropping the negative sign with ω_o, we get

$$\omega_1, \omega_2 = \pm \frac{R}{2L} + \omega_o \qquad \text{..... (4.99)}$$

$$\text{or } \omega_1 = \omega_o - \frac{R}{2L} \qquad \text{..... (4.100)}$$

$$\text{and } \omega_2 = \omega_o + \frac{R}{2L} \qquad \text{..... (4.101)}$$

ω_1 and ω_2 are called the "*lower and upper cut-off frequencies*".

$$\text{Band width} = \omega_2 - \omega_1 \qquad \text{..... (4.102)}$$

From equations (4.100) and (4.101), by subtracting and adding equations, we get

$$\omega_2 - \omega_1 = \frac{R}{L} \qquad \text{..... (4.103)}$$

$$\omega_2 + \omega_1 = 2\omega_o$$

$$\text{or } \omega_o = \frac{\omega_2 + \omega_1}{2} \qquad \text{..... (4.104)}$$

(c) Quality Factor

The quality factor is defined as *the voltage magnification in the circuit.*

$$\therefore \text{ Voltage magnification } = \frac{V_L \text{ or } V_C}{V_S}$$

At resonance $V_L = I_o X_L$, $V_C = I_o X_C$ and $V_S = I_o R$

$$\therefore Q\text{-factor} = \frac{V_L}{V_S} = \frac{V_C}{V_S}$$

$$= \frac{I_o X_L}{I_o R} = \frac{I_o X_C}{I_o R}$$

$$= \frac{X_L}{R} = \frac{X_C}{R}$$

$$= \frac{\omega_o L}{R} = \frac{1}{\omega_o C R}$$

$$= \frac{1}{\sqrt{LC}} \frac{L}{R} = \frac{\sqrt{LC}}{CR}$$

$$\therefore Q\text{-factor} = \frac{1}{R}\sqrt{\frac{L}{C}} \qquad \text{..... (4.105)}$$

$$\text{Now, } Q\text{-factor} = \omega_o \frac{L}{R} = \frac{\omega_o}{R/L}$$

From equation (4.103) $\quad \frac{R}{L} = \omega_2 - \omega_1$

$$\therefore Q = \frac{\omega_o}{\omega_2 - \omega_1} \qquad \text{..... (4.106)}$$

$$\therefore Q = \frac{\omega_o}{\textit{Band width}} \qquad \text{..... (4.107)}$$

i.e. larger the band width poor is the quality factor and vice-versa.

Problems on Resonance

Ex. 4.31 : A series circuit with resistance of 5 Ω inductance of 20 mH and a variable capacitance has an applied voltage with frequency of 1000 rad/sec. Find value of capacitance for resonance.

Solution : The conditions for resonance is

$$X_L = X_C$$

$$\text{or } \omega_o = \frac{1}{\sqrt{LC}}$$

Given : $\omega_o = 1000$ rad/sec and $L = 20 \times 10^{-3}$ H

$$\therefore\ 1000 = \frac{1}{\sqrt{20 \times 10^{-3} \times C}}$$

$$\therefore\ C = \boxed{50 \times 10^{-6}\ \text{f}}$$

Ex. 4.32 : A series circuit with resistance of 10 Ω, capacitance of 20 μf and a variable inductance has an applied voltage of 10 ∠0° with a frequency of 1000 rad/sec. The inductance is adjusted until the voltage across resistance is maximum. Find voltage across each element under this condition.

Solution : Given :

$$R = 10\ \Omega,\ C = 20 \times 10^{-6}\ \text{f}$$

$$\omega = 1000\ \text{rad/s and}\ \overline{V} = 10\ \angle 0^\circ$$

$$\therefore\ X_C = \frac{1}{\omega C} = \frac{1}{1000 \times 20 \times 10^{-6}}$$

$$= 50\ \Omega$$

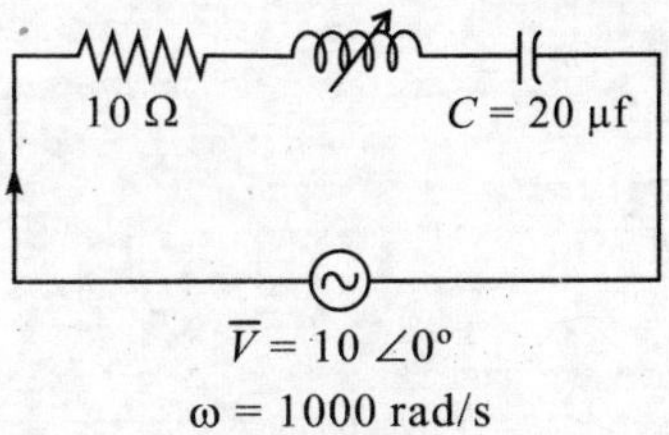

Fig. 4.49

At resonance, voltage across resistance is maximum and

$$\overline{V}_R = \overline{V} = \boxed{10\ \angle 0^\circ}$$

$$\therefore\ \overline{I} = \frac{\overline{V}_R}{R} = \frac{10\ \angle 0^\circ}{10} = 1\ \text{Amp}$$

$$X_L = X_C = 50\ \Omega$$

$$\overline{V}_R = 10\ \angle 0^\circ$$

$$\overline{V}_L = \overline{I}\,(j\,X_L) = (10\ \angle 0^\circ)(j\,50)$$

$$= \boxed{500\ \angle 90^\circ}$$

$$\overline{V}_C = \overline{I}\,(-j\,X_C) = (10\ \angle 0^\circ)(-j\,50)$$

$$= \boxed{500\ \angle -90^\circ}$$

Ex. 4.33 : A coil having resistance of 10 Ω and inductance of 0.05 H is connected in series with a capacitance of 50 μf. The series circuit is connected across an a.c. supply of 100 V. The frequency of supply is varied to achieve resonance. Find the resonant frequency. Find current and voltage across capacitor under this condition.

Solution : Refer Fig. 4.50.

Given : $R = 10\ \Omega,\ C = 50 \times 10^{-6}\ \text{f}$

$L = 0.05\ \text{H and}\ V = 100\ \text{V}$

At resonance, resonant frequency ω_o is given by

$$\omega_o = \frac{1}{\sqrt{L\,C}}$$

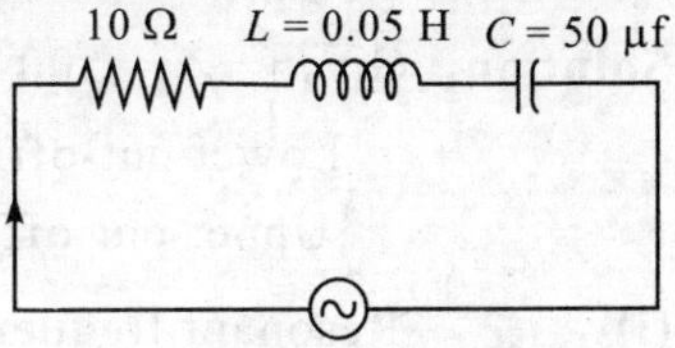

Fig. 4.50

$$= \frac{1}{\sqrt{0.05 \times 50 \times 10^{-6}}}$$

$$= \boxed{632.4 \text{ rad/s}}$$

$$\omega_o = 2\pi f_o$$

$$\therefore f_o = \boxed{100.6 \text{ Hz}}$$

At resonance

$$V_R = V = 100 \text{ V}$$

$$\therefore I = \frac{V_R}{R} = \frac{100}{10} = \boxed{10 \text{ amp}}$$

$$X_C = \frac{1}{2\pi f_o C} = \frac{1}{2\pi \times 100.6 \times 50 \times 10^{-6}} = 31.62 \ \Omega$$

$$\therefore \overline{V}_C = \overline{I}(-j X_C) = (10 \angle 0^\circ)(-j\, 31.62)$$

$$= \boxed{316.2 \angle -90^\circ \text{ volts}}$$

Ex. 4.34 : A series *R-L-C* circuit has $R = 100\ \Omega$, $L = 0.5$ H and $C = 40\ \mu$f. Find resonant frequency, lower and upper half power frequencies.

Solution:

$$\omega_o = \frac{1}{\sqrt{LC}} = \frac{1}{\sqrt{0.5 \times 40 \times 10^{-6}}}$$

$$= \boxed{223.61 \text{ rad/s}}$$

$$\text{Lower half power frequency} = \omega_o - \frac{R}{2L}$$

$$= 223.61 - \frac{100}{2 \times 0.5} = \boxed{123.61 \text{ rad/s}}$$

$$\text{Upper half power frequency} = \omega_o + \frac{R}{2L}$$

$$= 223.61 + \frac{100}{2 \times 0.5} = \boxed{323.61 \text{ rad/s}}$$

Ex. 4.35 : A series resonant circuit has an impedance of 500 Ω at resonant frequency. The cut off frequencies are 10 kHz and 100 Hz.

Determine : **(i)** Resonant frequency **(ii)** Band width

(iii) Values of *R*, *L* and *C* **(iv)** *Q*-factor.

Solution : Given : $Z = 500\ \Omega$ at resonance.

Lower cut-off frequency, $f_1 = 100$ Hz

Upper cut-off frequency, $f_2 = 10000$ Hz

(i) Resonant frequency

$$f_0 = \frac{f_1 + f_2}{2} = \frac{100 + 10000}{2} = \boxed{5050 \text{ Hz}}$$

(ii) Band width $\omega_2 - \omega_1 = 2\pi(f_2 - f_1) = 2\pi(10000 - 100) = \boxed{62203.53 \text{ rad/s}}$

(iii) At resonance, $Z = R$

$$\therefore R = 500\ \Omega$$

$$\text{Band width} = \frac{R}{L}$$

$$\therefore 62203.53 = \frac{500}{L}$$

$$\therefore L = 8.04 \times 10^{-3} \text{ H}$$

$$f_o = \frac{1}{2\pi\sqrt{LC}}$$

$$\therefore 5050 = \frac{1}{2\pi\sqrt{8.04 \times 10^{-3} \times C}}$$

$$\therefore C = \boxed{0.12 \times 10^{-6} \text{ f}}$$

(iv) $Q\text{-factor} = \frac{\omega_o}{\omega_2 - \omega_1} = \frac{f_o}{f_2 - f_1} = \frac{5050}{10000 - 100}$

$$= \boxed{0.51}$$

Ex. 4.36 : A constant voltage at a frequency of 1 MHz is applied to an inductor in series with a variable capacitor. When the capacitor is set to 500 pf, the current has its maximum value while the current is reduced to half when the capacitor is 600 pf. Find resistance, inductance and *Q*-factor of the inductor.

Solution : Given : $f = 1 \times 10^6$ f

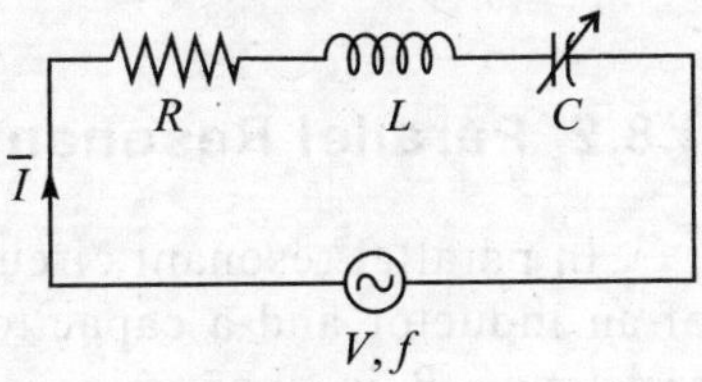

Fig. 4.51

Case 1 : When $C = 500 \times 10^{-12}$ f, current has its maximum value i.e. it is resonant condition.

$$f = \frac{1}{2\pi\sqrt{LC}}$$

$$\therefore 1 \times 10^6 = \frac{1}{2\pi\sqrt{L \times 500 \times 10^{-12}}}$$

$$\therefore L = 5.07 \times 10^{-5} \text{ H} = 0.05 \text{ mH}$$

At resonance, maximum value of current is

$$I = \frac{V}{R}$$

Case 2 : When $C = 600 \times 10^{-12}$ f, current is half of Case 1

$$\text{i.e. } I_1 = \frac{I}{2} = \frac{V}{2R} \qquad \text{..... (i)}$$

$$Z_1 = \sqrt{R^2 + (X_L - X_C)^2}$$

$$\therefore\ I_1 = \frac{V}{Z_1} = \frac{V}{\sqrt{R^2 + (X_L - X_C)^2}} \qquad \text{..... (ii)}$$

From equations (i) and (ii), we get

$$\frac{V}{2R} = \frac{V}{\sqrt{R^2 + (X_L - X_C)^2}}$$

$$\therefore\ 4R^2 = R^2 + (X_L - X_C)^2$$

$$\text{or } 3R^2 = (X_L - X_C)^2$$

$$\text{or } R = \frac{X_L - X_C}{\sqrt{3}} \qquad \text{..... (iii)}$$

$$X_L = 2\pi f L = 2\pi \times 1 \times 10^6 \times 0.05 \times 10^{-3} = \boxed{314.16\ \Omega}$$

$$X_C = \frac{1}{2\pi f C} = \frac{1}{2\pi \times 1 \times 10^6 \times 600 \times 10^{-12}}$$

$$= \boxed{265.26\ \Omega}$$

From equations (iii), we get

$$R = \frac{314.16 - 265.26}{\sqrt{3}} = \boxed{28.23\ \Omega}$$

$$Q\text{-factor} = \frac{\omega L}{R} = \frac{314.16}{28.23} = \boxed{11.13}$$

4.8.2 Parallel Resonant Circuit

In parallel resonant circuit, the a.c. supply is connected across a parallel combination of an inductor and a capacitor. In general the inductor will have some loss, i.e. a small resistance R is shown in series with inductor L (Fig. 4.52) where as capacitor with negligible resistance are easily available. From circuit of Fig. 4.52 at any frequency ω.

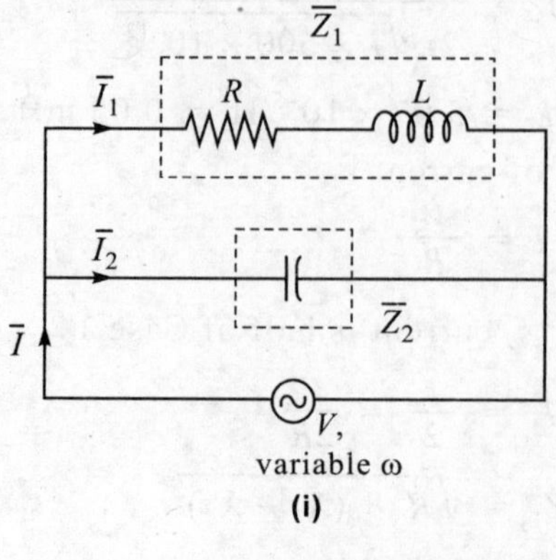

(i)

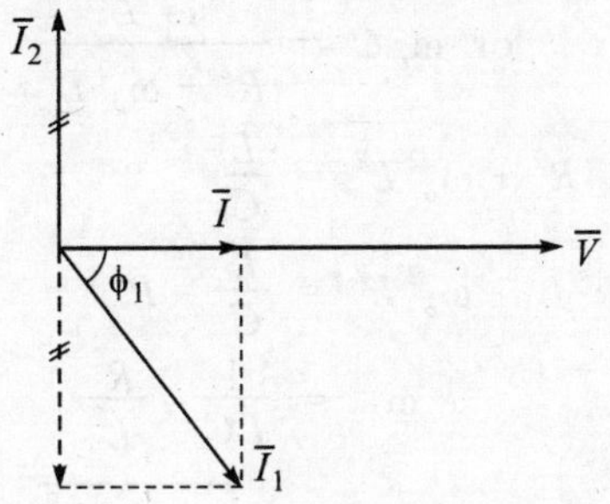

(ii)

Fig. 4.52 : Parallel resonant circuit.

$$\overline{Z}_1 = R + j\,X_L$$

$$\overline{Z}_1 = R + j\,\omega\,L \qquad \text{..... (4.108)}$$

$$\text{and } \overline{Z}_2 = -\,j\,X_C$$

$$\overline{Z}_2 = \frac{-j}{\omega\,C} \qquad \text{..... (4.109)}$$

Thus admittances $\overline{Y}_1$ and $\overline{Y}_2$ are given by

$$\overline{Y}_1 = \frac{1}{\overline{Z}_1} = \frac{1}{R + j\,\omega\,L}$$

$$= \frac{R - j\,\omega\,L}{(R + j\,\omega\,L)(R - j\,\omega\,L)}$$

$$\overline{Y}_1 = \frac{R - j\,\omega\,L}{R^2 + \omega^2\,L^2} \qquad \text{..... (4.110)}$$

$$\text{and } \overline{Y}_2 = -\frac{\omega\,C}{j} = j\,\omega\,C \qquad \text{..... (4.111)}$$

$\therefore$ The total admittance of circuit $\overline{Y} = \overline{Y}_1 + \overline{Y}_2$

$$\overline{Y} = \frac{R - j\,\omega\,L}{R^2 + \omega^2\,L^2} + j\,\omega\,C$$

$$\overline{Y} = \frac{R}{R^2 + \omega^2\,L^2} + j\left[\omega\,C - \frac{\omega\,L}{R^2 + \omega^2\,L^2}\right] \qquad \text{..... (4.112)}$$

The necessary condition for resonance to occur is that the circuit behaves as purely resistive i.e. the imaginary part of equation (4.112) is zero.

Let that frequency be ω_o i.e.

$$\omega_o\,C - \frac{\omega_o\,L}{R^2 + \omega_o^{\,2}\,L^2} = 0$$

$$\text{or } \omega_o C = \frac{\omega_o L}{R^2 + \omega_o^2 L^2}$$

$$\text{i.e. } R^2 + \omega_o^2 L^2 = \frac{L}{C}$$

$$\omega_o^2 L^2 = \frac{L}{C} - R^2$$

$$\omega_o^2 = \frac{1}{LC} - \frac{R^2}{L^2}$$

$$\omega_o = \sqrt{\frac{1}{LC} - \frac{R^2}{L^2}} \qquad \text{..... (4.113)}$$

If $R < L$ than $R^2 << L^2$, neglect $\frac{R^2}{L^2}$

$$\omega_o = \sqrt{\frac{1}{LC}} \qquad \text{..... (4.114)}$$

$$\therefore f_o = \frac{1}{2\pi\sqrt{LC}} \qquad \text{..... (4.115)}$$

The admittance Y_o at resonance from equation (4.112) will be

$$Y_o = \frac{R}{R^2 + \omega_o^2 L^2} \qquad \text{..... (4.116)}$$

This admittance will have minimum value at ω_o. For all other values of ω the admittance will have higher value as equation (4.112) will have some imaginary part for all values of ω, except $\omega = \omega_o$.

Thus, in other words at resonance admittance is minimum or impedance (= 1/*admittance*) will be maximum at resonance. Hence, in case of parallel circuits, the circuit current will be minimum at resonant frequency.

$$Z_o = \frac{1}{Y_o} = \frac{R^2 + \omega_o^2 L^2}{R}$$

$$\text{Now, } \omega L > R \quad \therefore \omega^2 L^2 >> R^2$$

$$\therefore Z_o = \frac{\omega_o^2 L^2}{R}$$

Substituting for ω_o from equation (4.114), we get

$$Z_o = \frac{1}{LC}\frac{L^2}{R}$$

$$Z_o = \frac{L}{CR} \qquad \text{..... (4.117)}$$

$$I_o = \frac{V}{Z_o}$$

$$\therefore I_o = \frac{V}{L/CR} = \frac{VCR}{L} \qquad \text{..... (4.118)}$$

(a) Band Width : As shown in Fig. 4.53, the half power frequencies ω_1 and ω_2 are defined where the impedance reduces to $Z_o/\sqrt{2}$ (= 0.707 Z_o).

$$\text{Band width} = \omega_2 - \omega_1$$

Let us write equation (4.112) as

$$\overline{Y} = G + j\,(B_C - B_L)$$

where $G = \dfrac{R}{R^2 + \omega^2 L^2}$

is the conductance and $B_C = \omega C$ the susceptance of capacitive branch and

$$B_L = \frac{\omega L}{R^2 + \omega^2 L^2}$$

the inductive susceptance.

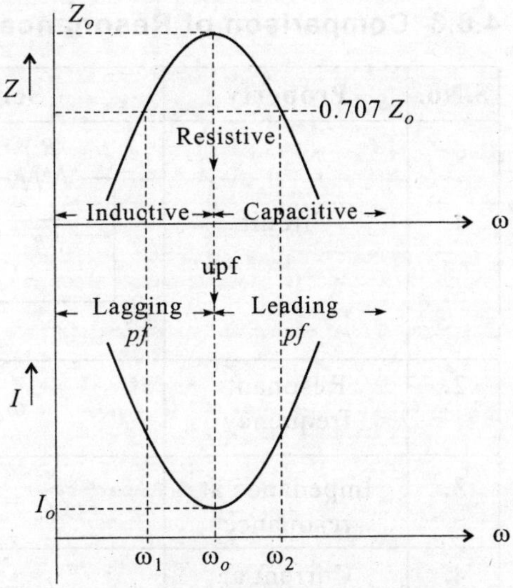

Fig. 4.53 : Impedance and current versus frequency for parallel resonance.

$$\overline{Z} = \frac{1}{\overline{Y}} = \frac{1}{G + j\,(B_C - B_L)}$$

$$\overline{Z} = \frac{G}{G^2 + (B_C - B_L)^2} - j\,\frac{(B_C - B_L)}{G^2 + (B_C - B_L)^2} \qquad \text{..... (4.119)}$$

Let us examine this impedance [equation (4.119)] for various values of ω.

At $\omega = \omega_o$, $(B_C - B_L) = 0$, circuit is purely resistive and power factor is unity.

For $\omega < \omega_o$, $B_C < B_L$, the imaginary part of $\overline{Z}$ equation (4.119) will be positive, the circuit is inductive and power factor is lagging. For $\omega > \omega_o$, $B_C > B_L$, the imaginary part of $\overline{Z}$ equation (4.119) will be negative, the circuit is capacitive and power factor will be leading

(b) Quality Factor : It can be seen from the vector diagram of Fig. 4.52(ii) both branch currents I_1 and I_2 are much larger than I. This shown that in parallel circuits at resonance, the current drawn from the source is greatly magnified.

The amount by which the line current is magnified in parallel circuit is called the *Q-factor*. At resonance, the reactive components of the two branch currents are equal and opposite. From Fig. 4.52(ii)

$$I_2 = I_1 \sin\phi_1 \qquad \text{..... (4.120)}$$

$$Q = \frac{\textit{Current through capacitor}}{\textit{Line current}} = \frac{I_2}{I} = \frac{I_1 \sin\phi_1}{I_1 \cos\phi_1} = \tan\phi_1$$

$$\therefore\ Q = \tan\phi_1 = \frac{\omega_o L}{R} \qquad \text{..... (4.121)}$$

4.8.3 Comparison of Resonance in Series and Parallel Circuits

S.No.	Property	Series Circuit	Parallel Circuit
1.	Circuit	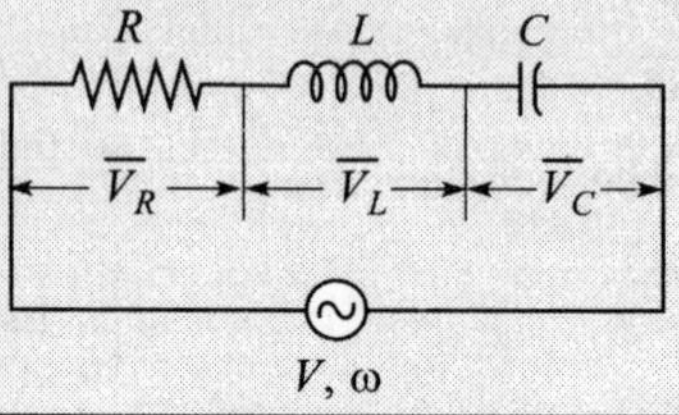	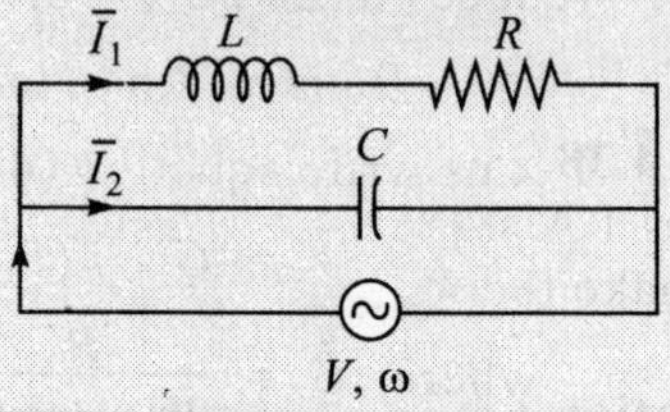
2.	Resonant frequency	$\omega_o = \frac{1}{\sqrt{LC}}$	$\omega_o = \frac{1}{\sqrt{LC}}$ if $R^2 << L^2$
3.	Impedance at resonance	$Z = R$, minimum	$Z_o = \frac{L}{CR}$, maximum
4.	Current at resonance	$I_o = \frac{V}{R}$, maximum	$I_o = \frac{V}{L/CR}$, minimum
5.	Magnifications	Voltage	Current
6.	Nature of circuit below ω_o	Capacitive	Inductive
7.	Nature of circuit above ω_o	Inductive	Capacitive
8.	Power factor at resonance	Unity	Unity

Ex. 4.37 : An inductive coil of resistance 20 Ω and inductance of 0.2 H is connected in parallel with 200 μf capacitor with variable frequency 230 V supply. Find resonant frequency and current at resonance.

Solution : Given : $R = 20\ \Omega$, $L = 0.2$ H, $C = 200$ μf

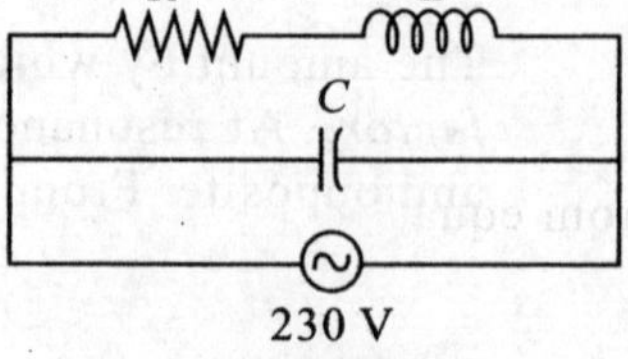

Fig. 4.54

From equation (4.113), resonant frequency ω_o is given by

$$\omega_o = \sqrt{\frac{1}{LC} - \frac{R^2}{L^2}}$$

$$= \sqrt{\frac{1}{0.2 \times 200 \times 10^{-6}} - \frac{20^2}{0.2^2}}$$

$$\omega_o = \boxed{122.47 \text{ rad/s}}$$

$$\text{or } f_o = \frac{\omega_o}{2\pi} = \boxed{19.5 \text{ Hz}}$$

Current at resonance I_o is given by equation (4.118)

$$I_o = \frac{VCR}{L} = \frac{230 \times 200 \times 10^{-6} \times 20}{0.2}$$

$$\therefore \; I_o = \boxed{4.6 \text{ Amp}}$$

Ex. 4.38 : A choke coil of negligible resistance connected across a 500 V, 50 Hz supply takes 1 A at 0.8 power factor. What capacitance must be placed in parallel with it in order to make the power factor of the combination equal to unity.

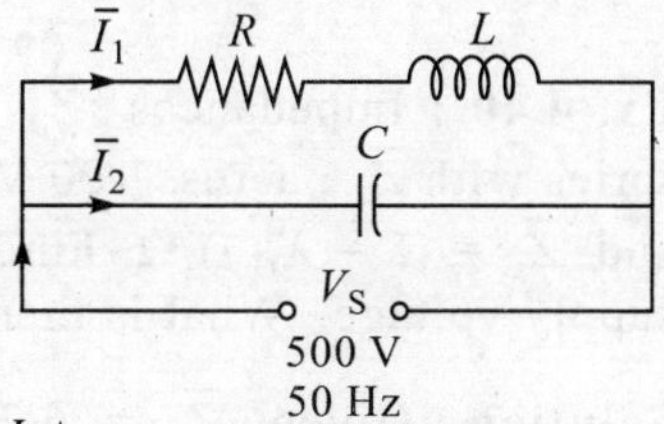

Fig. 4.55(i)

Solution : Given : $I_1 = 1$ A, $\cos \phi_1 = 0.8$

$$\therefore \; \phi_1 = 36.87°$$

For unity power factor of I, from Fig. 4.55(ii), we get

$$I_2 = I_1 \sin \phi_1 = 1 \sin 36.87°$$

$$I_2 = \boxed{0.6 \text{ A}}$$

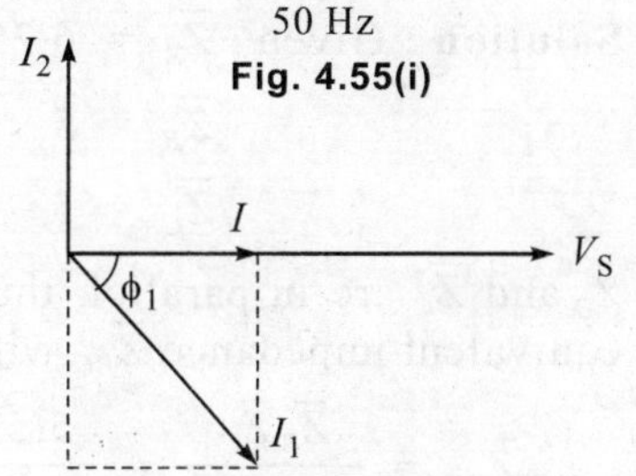

Fig. 4.55(ii)

From Fig. 4.55(i),

$$I_2 = \frac{V}{X_C} = \omega C V$$

$$\therefore \; 0.6 = (2\pi \times 50) \times C \times 500$$

$$\therefore \; C = \frac{0.6}{100\pi \times 500} = 3.82 \times 10^{-6} \text{ f}$$

$$C = \boxed{3.82 \; \mu\text{f}}$$

Ex. 4.39 : An inductive circuit of resistance 2 Ω and inductance of 0.01 H is connected to a 250 V, 50 Hz supply. What capacitance placed in parallel will produce resonance? Find the total current taken from the supply and the current in each branch of the circuit.

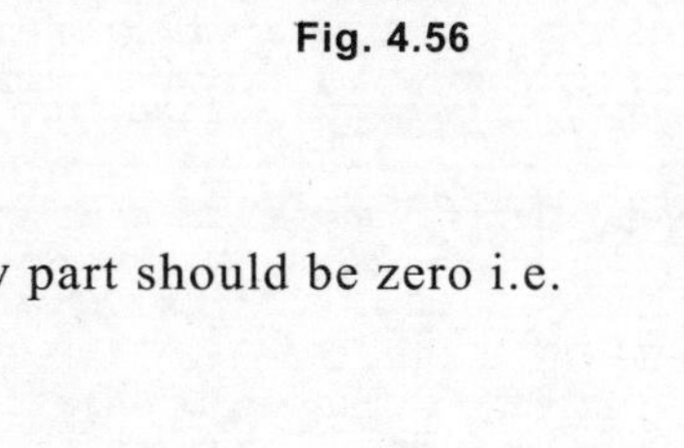

Fig. 4.56

Solution : Given : $R = 2 \; \Omega$, $L = 0.01$ H, $V_S = 250$ V

$f = 50$ Hz

$$\therefore \; \omega = 2\pi f = 100\pi$$

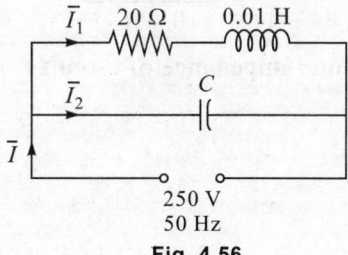

$$X_L = \omega L = 3.14$$

From equation (4.112), for resonance to occur the imaginary part should be zero i.e.

$$C = \frac{L}{R^2 + \omega^2 L^2}$$

$$\therefore \; C = \frac{0.01}{2^2 + (100\pi \times 0.01)^2}$$

$$C = \boxed{7.215 \; \mu\text{f}}$$

$$\overline{I}_1 = \frac{250}{20 + 3.14\,j} = 67.15\ \angle -57.5^\circ$$

$$\overline{I}_2 = \frac{250}{-j\,X_C} = 250\,j\,\omega\,C$$

$$= 56.834\ \angle 90^\circ$$

$$\overline{I} = \overline{I}_1 + \overline{I}_2 = 67.15\ \angle -57.5^\circ + 56.834\ \angle 90^\circ$$

$$\overline{I} = \boxed{36.07\ \angle 0^\circ \text{ Amp}}$$

Ex. 4.40 : Impedances $\overline{Z}_B$ and $\overline{Z}_C$ are in parallel to each other and this is connected in series with $\overline{Z}_A$, across 100 V, 50 Hz a.c. supply. If $\overline{Z}_A = (6.25 + 1.25j)\ \Omega$; $\overline{Z}_B = (5 + 0j)\ \Omega$ and $\overline{Z}_C = (5 - X_C\,j)\ \Omega$. Find X_C such that total current of the circuit will be in phase with supply voltage. What is then the circuit current and power?

Solution : Given : $\overline{Z}_A = 6.25 + 1.25\,j$

$\overline{Z}_B = 5$

$\overline{Z}_C = 5 - X_C\,j$

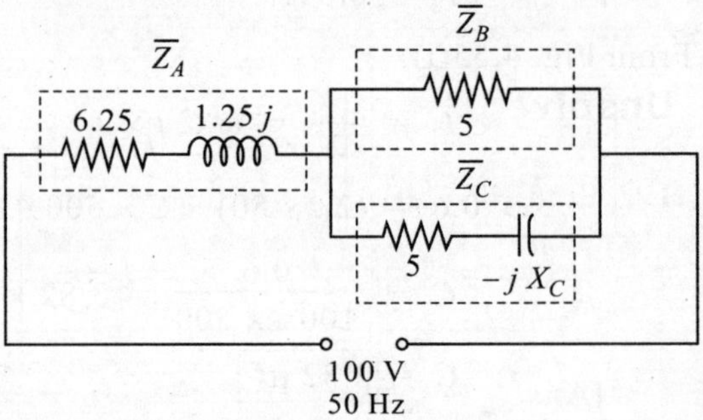

Fig. 4.57

$\overline{Z}_B$ and $\overline{Z}_C$ are in parallel, thus their equivalent impedance $\overline{Z}_{BC}$ will be

$$\overline{Z}_{BC} = \frac{\overline{Z}_B\,\overline{Z}_C}{\overline{Z}_B + \overline{Z}_C} = \frac{5(5 - X_C\,j)}{5 + 5 - X_C\,j}$$

$$= \frac{25 - 5\,X_C\,j}{10 - X_C\,j}$$

Total impedance of circuit $\overline{Z} = \overline{Z}_A + \overline{Z}_{BC}$

$$\therefore\ \overline{Z} = 6.25 + 1.25\,j + \frac{25 - 5\,X_C\,j}{10 - X_C\,j}$$

$$= 6.25 + 1.25\,j + \frac{(25 - 5\,X_C\,j)(10 + X_C\,j)}{(10 - X_C\,j)(10 + X_C\,j)}$$

$$= 6.25 + 1.25\,j + \frac{250 - 50\,X_C\,j + 25\,X_C\,j + 5\,X_C^2}{100 + X_C^2}$$

$$= 6.25 + 1.25\,j + \frac{250 + 5\,X_C^2}{100 + X_C^2} - \frac{25\,X_C\,j}{100 + X_C^2}$$

$$= 6.25 + \frac{250 + 5\,X_C^2}{100 + X_C^2} + j\left[1.25 - \frac{25\,X_C}{100 + X_C^2}\right]$$

For total current to be in phase with voltage the reactive (imaginary) part of $\overline{Z}$ should be zero.

$$\therefore\ 1.25 - \frac{25\,X_C}{100 + X_C^{\,2}} = 0$$

$$125 + 1.25\,X_C^{\,2} - 25\,X_C = 0$$

$$X_C = \frac{25 \pm \sqrt{25^2 - 625}}{2.5}$$

$$X_C = 10$$

$$\therefore\ \overline{Z} = \boxed{10 + j\,0}$$

$$\therefore\ I = \frac{V}{Z} = \frac{100}{10} = \boxed{10\text{ A}}$$

$$\text{Power} = 10^2 \times 10$$

$$= \boxed{1000\text{ watts}}$$

Unsolved Problems

1. Find the impedance of the circuit shown in Fig. 4.58.

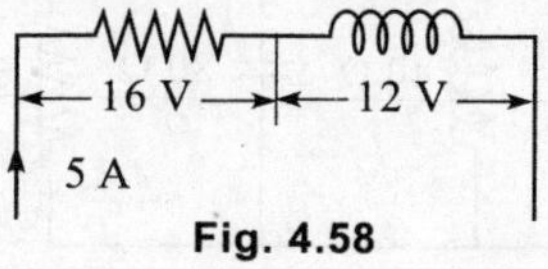

Fig. 4.58

[Ans. 4 Ω**]**

2. Find the applied voltage of the circuit shown in Fig. 4.59.

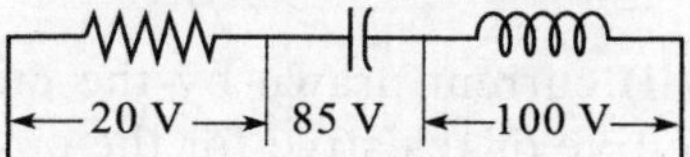

Fig. 4.59

[Ans. 25 V**]**

3. Find the power factor of the circuit given in Fig. 4.60.

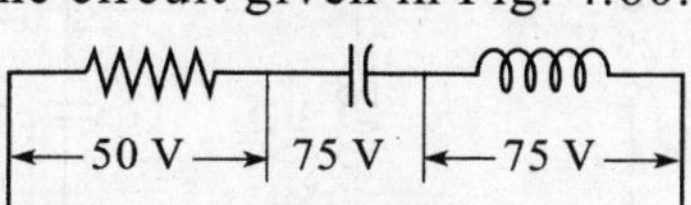

Fig. 4.60

[Ans. Unity**]**

4. Find the ammeter and the voltmeter reading in the circuit (Fig. 4.61).

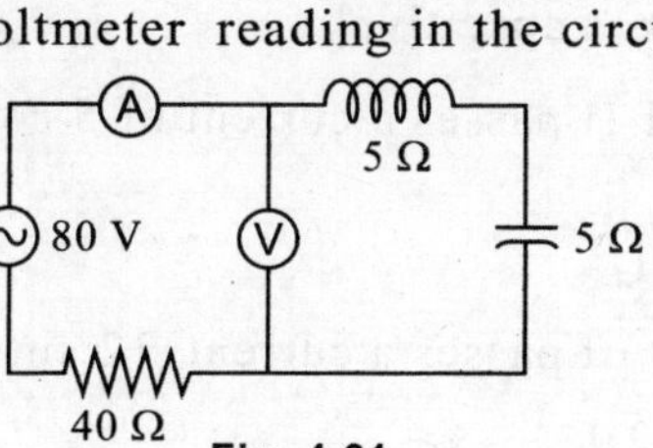

Fig. 4.61

[Ans. 2 A, 0 V**]**

5. In a series *R-L-C* circuit, the capacitance is changed from *C* to 4*C*. For the same resonating frequency, the inductor should be charged from *L* to ______.

[Ans. $L/4$**]**

6. Find **(i)** power consumed by the circuit **(ii)** active component of line current **(iii)** p.f of circuit and **(iv)** total current for the circuit shown in Fig. 4.62.

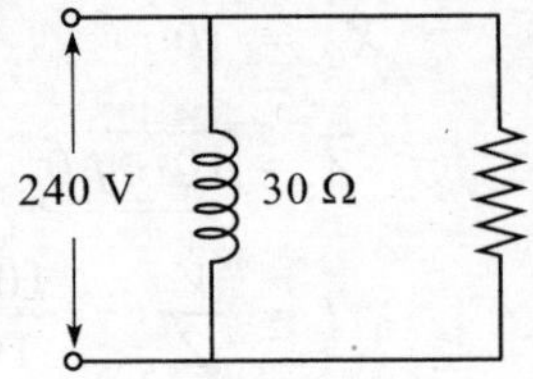

Fig. 4.62

[Ans. 1920 W, 8 A, 0.707 lag, $8\sqrt{2}$ A**]**

7. For the circuit shown in Fig. 4.63, find **(i)** power consumed **(ii)** active component of current **(iii)** line current **(iv)** p.f. **(v)** impedance of circuit and say whether the circuit is inductive, resistive or capacitive.

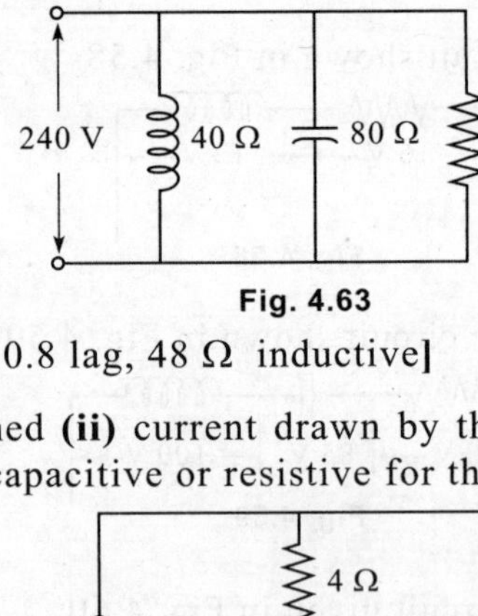

Fig. 4.63

[Ans. 960 W, 4 A, 5 A, 0.8 lag, 48 Ω inductive**]**

8. Find **(i)** power consumed **(ii)** current drawn by the circuit and **(iii)** say whether the circuit is inductive or capacitive or resistive for the circuit shown in Fig. 4.64.

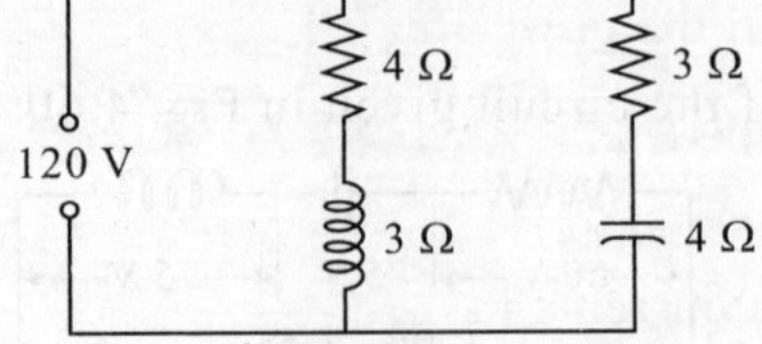

Fig. 4.64

[Ans. 4032 watts, 33.94 A, Capacitive**]**

9. A pure inductance of 0.01 H passes a current of 5 cos 2000*t* amp. What is the voltage across it ?

[Ans. $100 \sin (2000t + \pi)$**]**

10. A pure capacitance of 30 μf passes a current 12 sin 2000 *t*. Find the voltage.

[Ans. $200 \sin (2000t - \pi/2)$**]**

11. A voltage of 125 V at 50 Hz is applied across a non-inductive resistance connected in series with a capacitance. The current is 2.2 A. The power loss in resistance is 96.8 watts. Find R and C.

[Ans. 20 Ω, 59.85 μf]

12. A coil of pf 0.5 in series with 79.57 μf capacitance is connected across 50 Hz supply. The potential difference across the coil is equal to the potential difference across the capacitance. Find the resistance and inductance of the coil.

[Ans. 20 Ω, 0.11 H]

13. Find $\bar{I}$, $\bar{V}_1$, $\bar{V}_2$ and power factor of the circuit in Fig. 4.65.

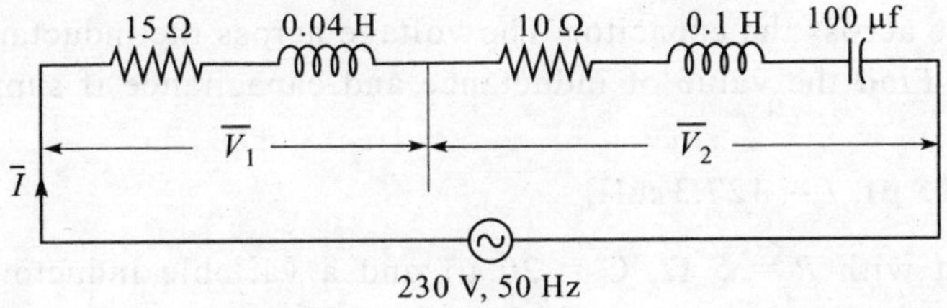

Fig. 4.65

[Ans. $\bar{I}$ = 8.27 ∠–25.92° amp, $\bar{V}_1$ = 161.94∠14° volts, $\bar{V}_2$ = 82.77∠–28.32 volts]

14. A current of 5 A flows through a non inductive resistance in series with a choke coil (choke is impure and has some resistance). When supplied by 250 V, 50 Hz supply. If the voltage across resistance is 125 V cross coil is 200 V. Calculate **(i)** Impedence, reactance resistance of coil **(ii)** power absorbed by the coil **(iii)** total power and **(iv)** draw the phasor diagram.

[Ans. Z_{coil} = 40, R_C = 5.5 Ω, X_L = 39.62 Ω, 137.5 watts, 762.5 watts]

15. A resistance in series with a capacitance connected across a 250 V supply draw 5 A current at a frequency of 50 Hz. When the frequency is increased to 60 Hz, it draws 5.8 A. Find R and C and the power drawn by the circuit in the second case.

[Ans. R = 19.94 Ω and C = 69.4 × 10^{-6} f]

16. A voltage of 200 ∠25° volts is supplied to a circuit composed of two parallel branches. If the branch currents are 10 ∠40° A and 20 ∠–30° A, determine the KVA, KVAR and KW in each branch. Also the power factor of the combined circuit.

[Ans. KVA_1 = 2, KW_1 = 1.93, $KVAR_1$ = 0.52, KVA_2 = 4, KW_2 = 2.29, $KVAR_2$ = 3.28 p.f. = 0.8374 lagging]

17. In a series circuit of R = 5 and L = 0.06 H, V_L = 15 sin 200 t. Find total voltage, current and the angle by which the current lags the supply voltage and the magnitude of the impedance.

[Ans. $\bar{I}$ = 0.88 ∠–90°, $\bar{V}$ = 11.49 ∠–22.62°, ϕ = 67.38 lag, Z = 13 Ω]

18. Two coils *A* and *B* have resistances of 12 Ω and 6 Ω respectively and inductance of 0.02 H and 0.03 H respectively. These coil are connected in parallel and a voltage of 200 V and 50 Hz is applied to their common terminals. Find **(i)** current in each coil **(ii)** total current and power factor of combination **(iii)** if a resistance of 15 Ω in series with a condenser of 120 μf is connected in parallel with the above combination. Find the total current and p.f.

[Ans. (i) $\overline{I}_A = 14.77 \angle -27.62°$, $\overline{I}_B = 17.91 \angle -57.50°$ **(ii)** $\overline{I}_1 = 31.58 \angle -44.03°$, p.f. = 0.72 (lag) **(iii)** $\overline{I} = 30.6 \angle -32.05°$, p.f. = 0.847 (lag)]

19. An *R-L-C* series circuit has a current which lags behind the applied voltage by 45°. The voltage across the inductor has maximum value equal to twice the maximum value of voltage across the capacitor. The voltage across the inductance is 300 sin ωt and R = 20 Ω. Find the value of inductance and capacitance if supply frequency is 50 Hz.

[Ans. C = 159.15 μf, L = 127.3 mH]

20. A series circuit with R = 5 Ω, C = 20 μf and a variable inductor has an applied voltage of 10 ∠0°, with frequency of 1000 rad/s. The inductance is adjusted until the voltage across resistance is maximum. Find the voltage across each element.

[Ans. $\overline{V}_R = 10 \angle 0°$, $\overline{V}_L = 100 \angle 90°$, $\overline{V}_C = 100 \angle -90°$]

CHAPTER 5

THREE-PHASE CIRCUITS

So far in the previous chapters on Alternating Current System, we have considered only one electrical circuit with two supply wires called the ***single-phase a.c. system****. In a.c. systems, however, it is possible to use two, three or more individual circuits in the same apparatus or machine. The voltages and frequencies are the same but they have a definite phase difference. The actual phase difference between these circuits depends upon the number of circuits or "****phases****".*

5.1 Generation of 3-Phase A.C. System

Consider Fig. 3.2 (a.c. dynamo) where there was a single coil which was rotated in the field. This a.c. so generated was called as *single-phase a.c. supply*. If this dynamo has two coils x and y separated by 90° as in Fig. 5.1(a) then the voltages V_x and V_y will have a phase difference of 90°, as seen in Fig. 5.1(b).

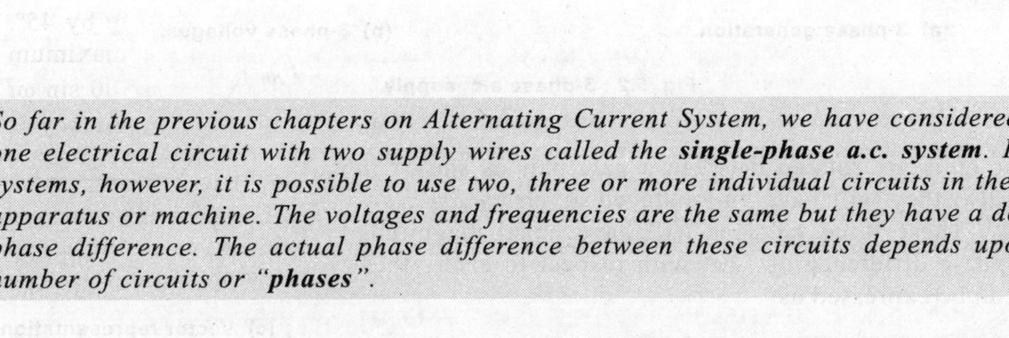

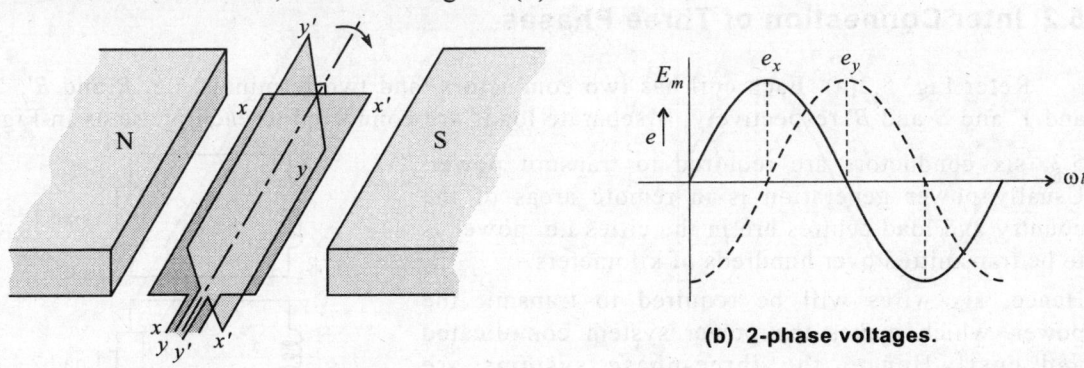

(a) Dynamic with two coils. **(b) 2-phase voltages.**

Fig. 5.1 : Generation of 2-phase a.c.

Such a supply may be connected to the load by 4 wires or three wires, the voltage of each phase will have same magnitude but a phase difference of 90° will be present.

Now let us consider Fig. 5.2(a) where there are three similar coils namely RR', YY' and BB' such that they are placed at equal angles to each other i.e. 360/3 = 120° with respect to each other.

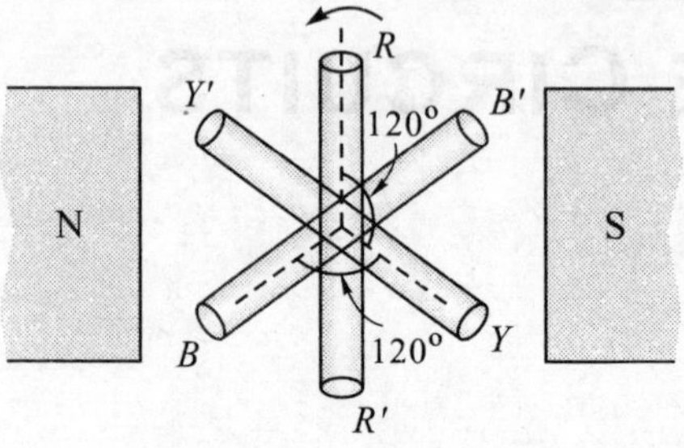

(a) 3-phase generation.

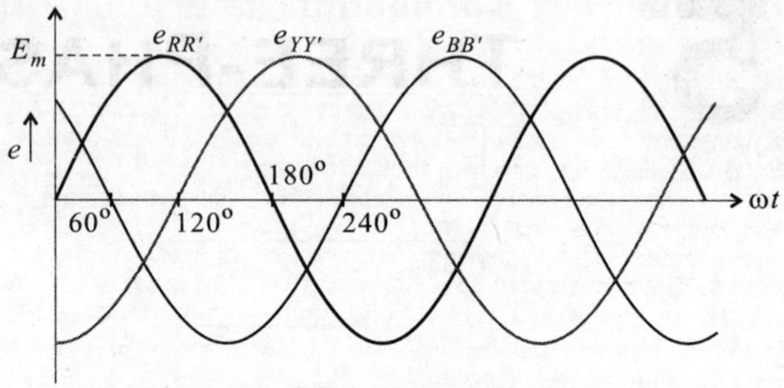

(b) 3-phase voltages.

Fig. 5.2 : 3-phase a.c. supply.

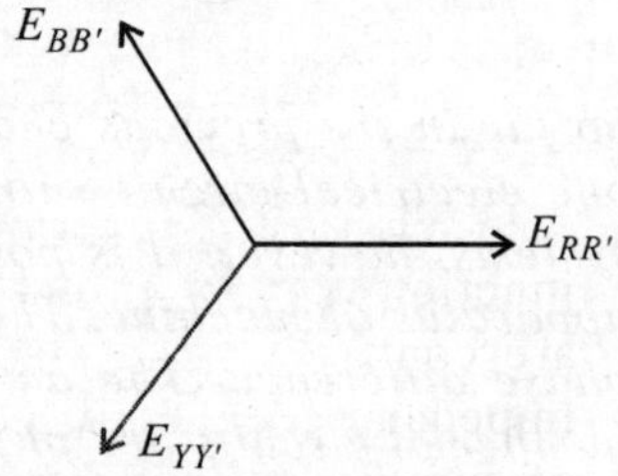

(c) Vector representation.

If these coils are rotated between a pale pair as shown in Fig. 5.2(a) they will have emf induced given by $e_{RR'}$, $e_{YY'}$ and e_{BB}'. These three voltages will have equal magnitude and a phase difference of 120° with respect to each other. They can be expressed as

$$e_{RR}' = E_m \sin \omega t \qquad ..... (5.1)$$

$$e_{yy}' = E_m \sin (\omega t - 120°) \qquad ..... (5.2)$$

$$e_{BB}' = E_m \sin (\omega t - 240°) \qquad ..... (5.3)$$

5.2 Inter Connection of Three Phases

Refer Fig. 5.2(a). Each coil has two conductors, and two terminals, i.e. R and R', Y and Y' and B and B' respectively. If separate loads are connected to each phase as in Fig. 5.3, six conductors are required to transmit power. Usually power generation is in remote areas of the country and load centres are in the cities i.e. power is to be transmitted over hundreds of kilometers.

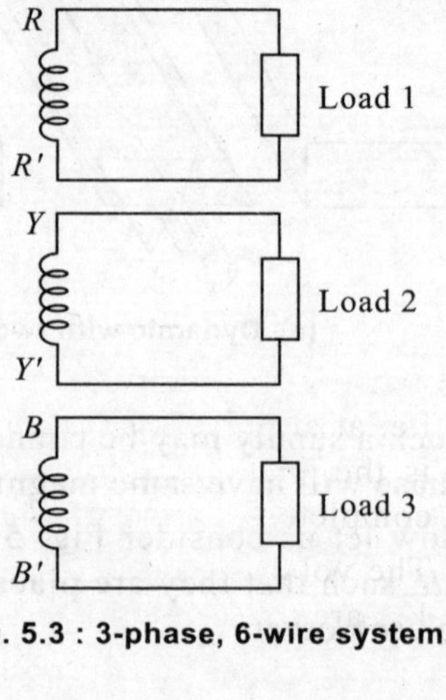

Fig. 5.3 : 3-phase, 6-wire system.

Hence, six wires will be required to transmit the power, which makes the power system complicated and costly.Hence, the three-phase systems are interconnected. This results in saving of wire material over hundreds of kilometers. The general methods of interconnection are

(i) Star or Y-connection

(ii) Delta (Δ) connection

5.3 Star or Y Connection

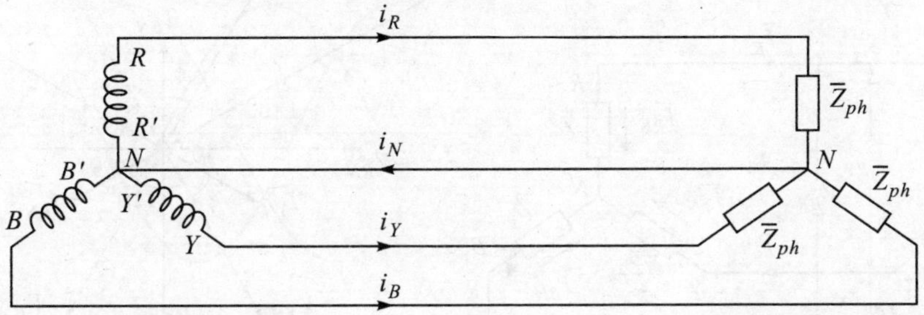

3-phase star connected generator. **3-phase star connected load.**

Fig. 5.4 : 3-Phase, 4-wire, star connected system.

When similar terminals (R', Y' and B') of the three phases are connected together at junction N, it is called a "*star connection*". The remaining three terminals (R, Y and B) are connected to a star connected load (Fig. 5.4) where all the three loads have equal impedance Z_{ph}. As all voltages are equal and all impedances are also same the magnitudes of currents in each impedance will also be same and will have a phase difference of 120° each. Thus, the three currents can be given by

$$i_R = I_m \sin \omega t \quad ..... (5.4)$$

$$i_Y = I_m \sin (\omega t - 120°) \quad ..... (5.5)$$

$$i_B = I_m \sin (\omega t - 240°) \quad ..... (5.6)$$

Applying KCL at N, we get

$$\begin{aligned} i_N &= i_R + i_Y + i_B \\ &= I_m \sin \omega t + I_m \sin (\omega t - 120°) + I_m \sin (\omega t - 240°) \\ &= I_m \sin \omega t + I_m \left[2 \sin \frac{\omega t - 120° + \omega t - 240°}{2} . \cos \frac{\omega t - 120° - \omega t + 240°}{2} \right] \\ &= I_m \sin \omega t + I_m \left[2 \sin (\omega t - 180°) . \cos 60° \right] \\ &= I_m \sin \omega t + I_m \left[2 (-\sin \omega t) . \frac{1}{2} \right] \\ &= I_m \sin \omega t - I_m \sin \omega t \\ &= 0 \end{aligned}$$

i.e. at any instant the current in the wire connected to both the N terminals is zero or 'N' is the "*neutral*" terminal. As there is no current in the neutral wire, it can be omitted completely in case of "*balanced load and balanced supply*", as in Fig. 5.5(a).

The voltage between two supply lines is called the "*line voltage*". The voltages $\overline{V}_{RY}$, $\overline{V}_{YB}$, $\overline{V}_{BR}$ are the line voltages.

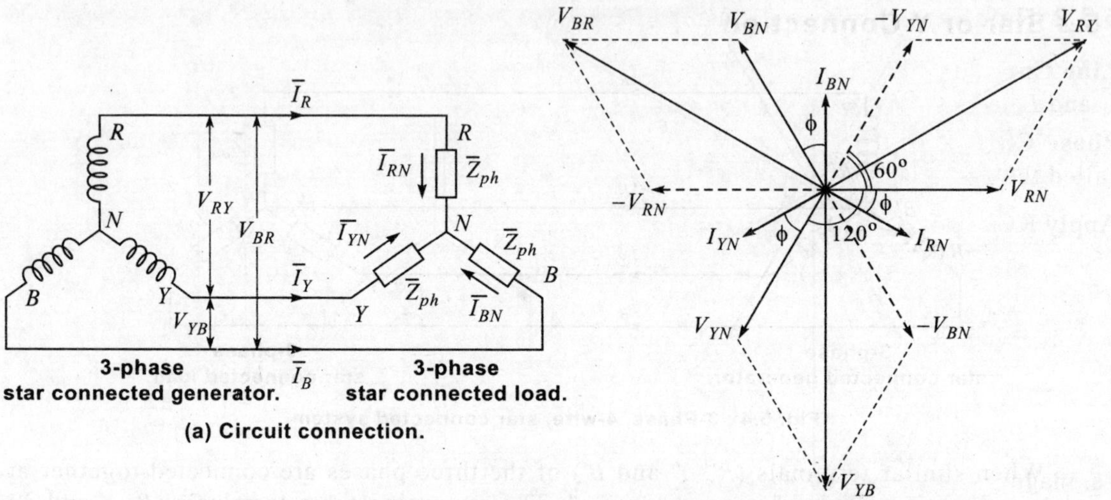

Fig. 5.5 : 3-phase, 3-wire system.

The voltages between the supply line and the neutral point N of the load is called the "*phase voltage*". Voltages $\overline{V}_{RN}$, $\overline{V}_{yN}$, and $\overline{V}_{BN}$ are the phase voltages.

5.3.1 Relation Between Phase and Line Voltages (Star Connection)

From Fig. 5.5(a) voltage $\overline{V}_{RY}$ can be given by

$$\overline{V}_{RY} = \overline{V}_{RN} + \overline{V}_{NY} \qquad \text{..... (5.7)}$$

$$\text{i.e.} \quad \overline{V}_{RY} = \overline{V}_{RN} - \overline{V}_{YN} \qquad \text{..... (5.8)}$$

From Fig. 5.5(b) observe $\overline{V}_{RN}$, $\overline{V}_{YN}$, $-\overline{V}_{YN}$ and $\overline{V}_{RY}$. Magnitude of $\overline{V}_{RN}$ and $\overline{V}_{YN}$ are equal.

$$|\overline{V}_{RN}| = |-\overline{V}_{YN}| = V_{ph}$$

The angle between $\overline{V}_{RN}$ and $-\overline{V}_{YN}$ is 60°.

$\therefore$ Resultant of $\overline{V}_{RN}$ and $-\overline{V}_{YN}$ is given by

$$|V_{RY}| = \sqrt{V_{ph}^{\ 2} + V_{ph}^{\ 2} + 2V_{ph}\,V_{ph}\cos 60°} \qquad \text{..... (5.9)}$$

$$\text{or } |V_{RY}| = \sqrt{V_{ph}^{\ 2} + V_{ph}^{\ 2} + 2V_{ph}^{\ 2} \times \frac{1}{2}}$$

$$\text{but } |V_{RY}| = V_{line}$$

$$\therefore \quad V_{line} = \sqrt{3}\,V_{ph} \qquad \text{..... (5.10)}$$

Similarly for other line voltages can be drawn as follows

$$\overline{V}_{YB} = \overline{V}_{YN} - \overline{V}_{BN} \qquad \text{..... (5.11)}$$

$$\overline{V}_{BR} = \overline{V}_{BN} - \overline{V}_{RN} \qquad \text{..... (5.12)}$$

5.3.2 Relation Between Line and Phase Currents (Star Connection)

Line Currents : The current in the supply lines is called the line current. The currents $\overline{I_R}$, $\overline{I_Y}$ and $\overline{I_B}$ in Fig. 5.5(a) are the line currents.

Phase Currents : The currents in each phase (i.e. between line and neutral of load) is called the phase current. Currents $\overline{I_{RN}}$, $\overline{I_{YN}}$ and $\overline{I_{BN}}$ are the phase currents.

Apply KCL at node R of load. We find that

$$\overline{I_R} = \overline{I_{RN}} \quad \text{..... (5.14)}$$

$$\text{and } \overline{I_B} = \overline{I_{BN}} \quad \text{..... (5.15)}$$

$$\text{i.e } \overline{I_{line}} = \overline{I_{ph}} \quad \text{..... (5.16)}$$

$$\text{or } \boxed{I_{line} = I_{ph}} \quad \text{..... (5.17)}$$

i.e. magnitudes as well as phase of line and phase currents are equal in star connection. If the phase impedance has lagging power factor ϕ, than phase currents will lag behind phase voltages by an angle ϕ as shown in Fig. 5.5.

5.5.3 Power Consumed in Star Connected Load

If V_{ph} is the phase voltage, I_{ph} is the current in each phase and ϕ is the angle of impedance then power consumed per phase $= V_{ph} I_{ph} \cos \phi$.

There are three-phases, all phase impedances are equal, thus the load is "*balanced*".

$$\therefore \text{ Total power consumed } \boxed{P = 3V_{ph} I_{ph} \cos \phi} \quad \text{..... (5.18)}$$

For star connected load

$$V_{ph} = \frac{V_l}{\sqrt{3}} \quad \text{[refer equation (5.10), } V_l = \sqrt{3}\, V_{ph}\text{]}$$

$$\text{and } I_{ph} = I_l$$

$$\therefore \quad P = 3\,\frac{V_l}{\sqrt{3}}\, I_l \cos \phi$$

$$\text{or } \boxed{P = \sqrt{3}\, V_l I_l \cos \phi} \quad \text{..... (5.19)}$$

where V_l is the supply voltage (line voltage) I_l is the line current and remember that ϕ is the angle of impedance or the angle between phase voltages and phase current.

5.3.4 Volt-Ampere and Reactive Volt-Ampere Relation in Star Connected Load

For balanced load

$$\text{Volt-amp per phase} = V_{ph} I_{ph}$$

$$\therefore \text{ Total volt-amp} = 3V_{ph} I_{ph}$$

$$\therefore \text{ 3-phase KVA (kilo volt-amp)} = \frac{3V_{ph} I_{ph}}{1000} \quad \text{..... (5.20)}$$

$$\text{Total KVA} = \frac{\sqrt{3}\, V_l\, I_l}{1000} \quad \text{as } V_l = \sqrt{3}\, V_{ph} \qquad \text{..... (5.21)}$$

Similarly, Reactive volt-amp per phase $= V_{ph}\, I_{ph} \sin\phi$

$$\text{Reactive volt-amp (VAR)} = 3V_{ph}\, I_{ph} \sin\phi \qquad \text{..... (5.22)}$$

$$\therefore\ \text{KVAR} = \frac{3V_{ph}\, I_{ph} \sin\phi}{1000} \qquad \text{..... (5.23)}$$

$$\text{also KVAR} = \frac{\sqrt{3}\, V_l\, I_l \sin\phi}{1000} \qquad \text{..... (5.24)}$$

5.4 Delta or Δ Connection

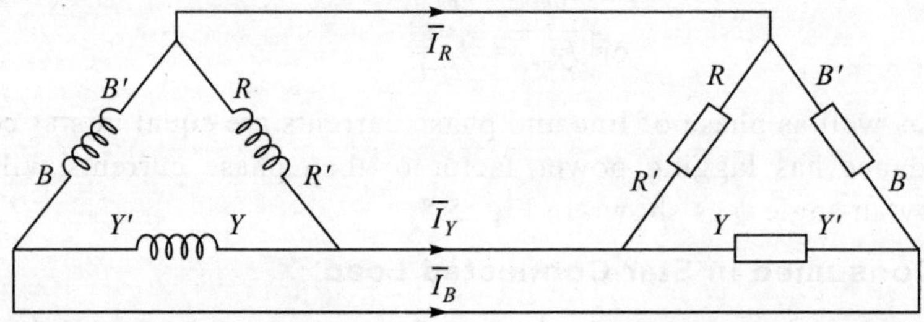

Delta connected generator. **Delta connected load.**

Fig. 5.6 : 3-phase, 3-wire delta connected load.

When the dissimilar ends of loads in Fig. 5.3 are connected i.e. *R'Y*, *Y'B* and *B'R* as shown in Fig. 5.6 it is called *delta connection*.

Let us inspect the load voltages $V_{RR'}$, $V_{YY'}$, $V_{BB'}$.

It is seen from Fig. 5.7 the line voltage (V_l) i.e. voltage between any two supply lines is same as V_{ph}. (i.e. voltage across *RR'* here).

5.4.1 Relation Between Phase and Line Voltages in Delta Connected Load

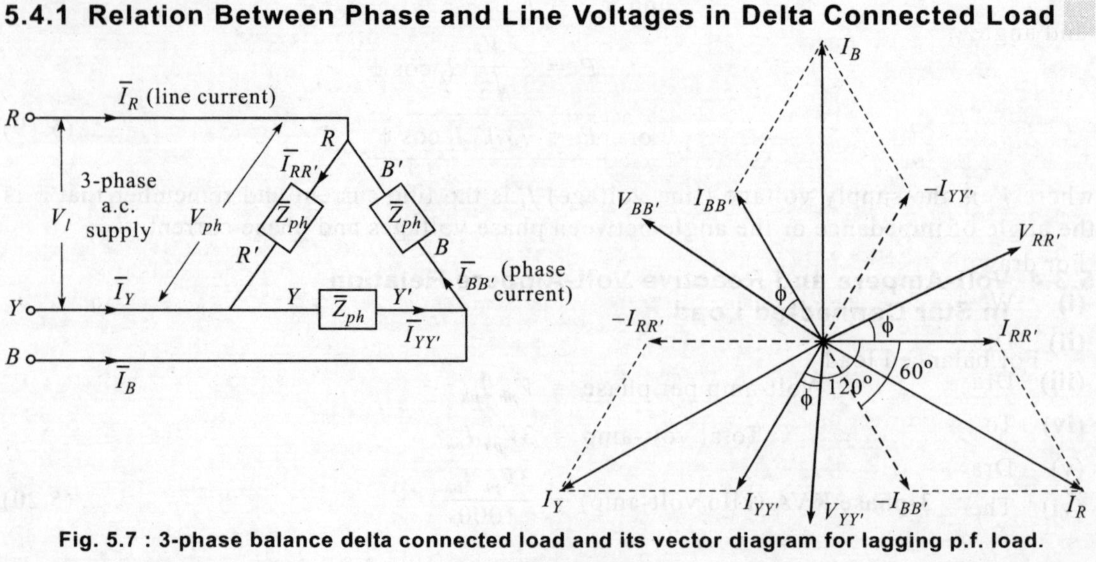

Fig. 5.7 : 3-phase balance delta connected load and its vector diagram for lagging p.f. load.

From the above discussion

$$\boxed{V_l = V_{ph}} \qquad \text{..... (5.25)}$$

Let

$$V_{RR'} = V_m \sin \omega t$$

$$V_{YY'} = V_m \sin (\omega t - 120°)$$

and $V_{BB'} = V_m \sin (\omega t - 240°)$

Then

$$V_{RR'} + V_{YY'} + V_{BB'} = 0$$

i.e. at any instant sum of the three voltage is zero. This indicates that the three-phase connected in delta will not have circulating currents within the delta connection.

5.4.2 Relation Between Line and Phase Currents

As the three impedances of the load are equal (i.e. balanced load) and the three voltages of supply are also equal in magnitude and have a phase difference of 120° between them (i.e. balanced supply) the three-phase currents ($\bar{I}_{RR'}$, $\bar{I}_{YY'}$ and $\bar{I}_{BB'}$) will have equal magnitudes and will differ in phase by 120° each.

Refer Fig. 5.7. From the figure it is seen that (apply KCL at each junction)

$$\bar{I}_R = \bar{I}_{RR'} - \bar{I}_{BB'}$$

$$\bar{I}_Y = \bar{I}_{YY'} - \bar{I}_{RR'}$$

$$\bar{I}_B = \bar{I}_{BB'} - \bar{I}_{YY'}$$

Thus, $\bar{I}_R$ is the vector sum of $\bar{I}_{RR'}$ and $-\bar{I}_{BB'}$ (equal and opposite to $I_{BB'}$).

The magnitude of $|\bar{I}_{RR'}| = |-\bar{I}_{YY'}| = I_{ph}$

and angle between $\bar{I}_{RR'}$ and $\bar{I}_{YY'}$ is 60°.

If $|\bar{I}_R| = I_l$

then $I_l = \sqrt{I_{ph}^2 + I_{ph}^2 + 2 I_{ph} I_{ph} \cos 60°}$

$$\boxed{\therefore\ I_l = \sqrt{3}\, I_{ph}} \qquad \text{..... (5.26)}$$

For drawing the phases (vector) diagram

(i) We have taken $I_{RR'}$ as the reference.

(ii) Draw $I_{YY'}$ of equal magnitude as $I_{RR'}$ and lagging behind it by 120°.

(iii) Draw $I_{BB'}$ at an angle of 120° to $I_{YY'}$ and equal in magnitude to $I_{YY'}$.

(iv) To find I_R (which is $I_{RR'} - I_{YY'}$) draw $-I_{YY'}$ equal and opposite to $I_{YY'}$.

(v) Draw parallelogram between $I_{RR'}$ and $-I_{YY'}$.

(vi) The diagonal is I_R.

(vii) Similarly, draw I_Y (vector sum of $I_{YY'}$ and $-I_{RR'}$) and I_B (vector sum of $I_{BB'}$ and $-I_{YY'}$).

(viii) To draw the phase voltages (which are same as line voltages) ahead of phase currents if load is lagging power factor. (As for lagging power factor load current lags the voltage). Thus, draw $V_{RR'}$, $V_{YY'}$ and $V_{BB'}$ as in Fig. 5.7.

5.4.3 Power Consumed in Delta Connected Load

Power consumed per phase = $V_{ph}\, I_{ph} \cos\phi$ when the load is balance, the power consumed in three-phases P is given as

$$\text{Total power consumed} \quad \boxed{P = 3V_{ph}\, I_{ph} \cos\phi} \qquad \text{..... (5.27)}$$

where, ϕ = angle between phase voltage and phase current or the angle of phase impedance.

But, for delta connection

$$V_{ph} = V_l$$

$$\text{and } I_{ph} = \frac{I_l}{\sqrt{3}}$$

$$\therefore \quad \boxed{P = \sqrt{3}\, V_l\, I_l \cos\phi} \qquad \text{..... (5.28)}$$

5.4.4 Volt-Ampere and Reactive Volt-Ampere Relation in Delta Connected Load

$$\text{Total 3-phase volt-ampere} = 3V_{ph}\, I_{ph}$$

$$\therefore \text{ KVA} = \frac{3V_{ph}\, I_{ph}}{1000} = \frac{\sqrt{3}\, V_l\, I_l}{1000} \qquad \text{..... (5.29)}$$

$$\text{Total 3-phase reactive volt-ampere} = 3V_{ph}\, I_{ph} \sin\phi$$

$$\therefore \text{ KVAR} = \frac{3V_{ph}\, I_{ph} \sin\phi}{1000} = \frac{\sqrt{3}\, V_l\, I_l \sin\phi}{1000} \qquad \text{..... (5.30)}$$

Ex. 5.1 : Each of the star connected load consists of an impedance of 5 + 20 *j*. The line voltages are 400 V. Find the various line currents, phase voltages, phase currents, power consumed.

Solution : Given : $\bar{Z}_{ph} = 5 + 20\,j$

$$V_l = 400 \text{ V}$$

For Star Connection :

$$V_{ph} = \frac{V_l}{\sqrt{3}}$$

$$\therefore \quad V_{ph} = \frac{400}{\sqrt{3}} = \boxed{230.94 \text{ V}}$$

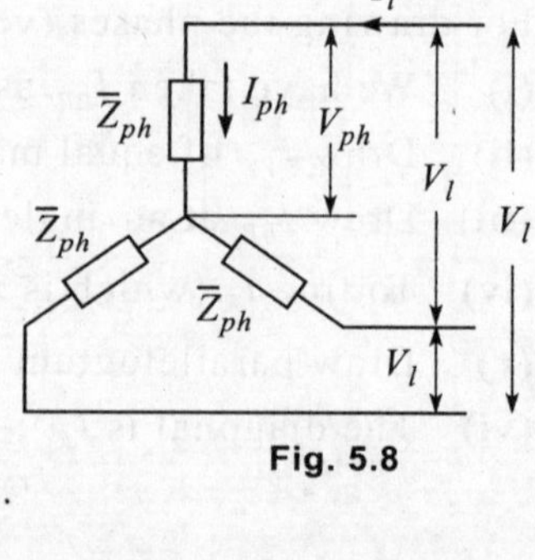

Fig. 5.8

$$\therefore \quad \overline{I}_{ph} = \frac{V_{ph}}{\overline{Z}_{ph}} = \frac{230.94}{5 + 20j} = 11.2 \angle -75.96^\circ$$

$$\therefore \quad |I_{ph}| = 11.2 \text{ A} \; ; \; \phi = -75.96^\circ$$

$$\boxed{I_l = I_{ph} = 11.2 \text{ A}}$$

$$\text{Power consumed} \quad P = 3 V_{ph} \, I_{ph} \cos \phi$$

$$= 3 \times 230.94 \times 11.2 \times \cos 75.96^\circ$$

$$\boxed{P = 1882.47 \text{ watts}}$$

Ex. 5.2 : Each of the delta connected load consists of a 50 Ω resistance in series with 50 μf capacitor. The supply is 440 V, 3-phase, 50 Hz. Calculate **(i)** phase current **(ii)** line current **(iii)** power factor **(iv)** and draw the vector diagram showing currents and voltages.

Solution :

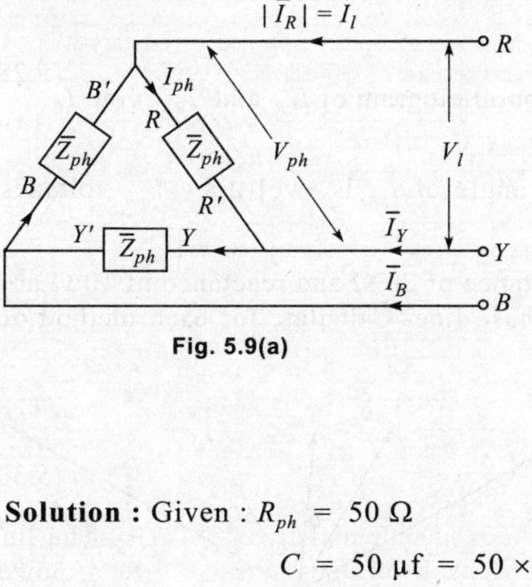

Fig. 5.9(a)

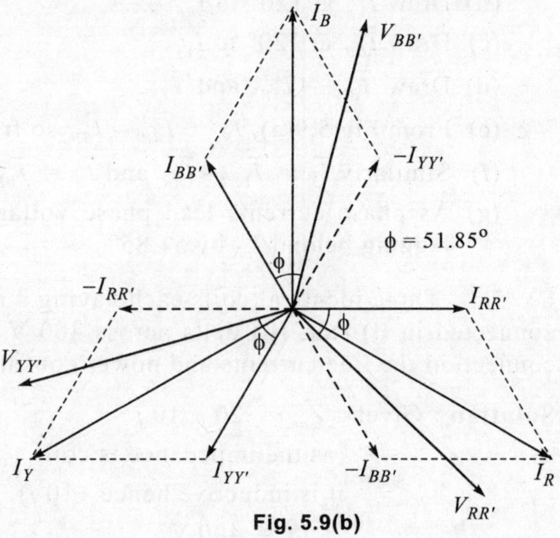

Fig. 5.9(b)

Solution : Given : $R_{ph} = 50 \, \Omega$

$$C = 50 \, \mu\text{f} = 50 \times 10^{-6} \text{ f}$$

$$f = 50 \text{ Hz}$$

$$V_l = \text{supply voltage} = 440 \text{ V}$$

$$\therefore \quad X_{ph} = \frac{1}{2\pi f C} = \frac{1}{2\pi \times 50 \times 50 \times 10^{-6}} = 63.66 \, \Omega$$

$$\therefore \quad \overline{Z}_{ph} = R_{ph} - j X_{ph} = 50 - 63.66 j$$

[–ve sign as capacitive reactance]

$$V_{ph} = V_l \quad \text{for delta connections}$$

$$\therefore \quad V_{ph} = 440 \text{ V}$$

(i) $$\overline{I}_{ph} = \frac{V_{ph}}{\overline{Z}_{ph}} = \frac{440}{50 - 63.66\,j} = 5.43 \angle 51.85^{\circ}$$

$$\therefore \; I_{ph} = \boxed{5.43 \text{ A}}\;;\; \phi = 51.85^{\circ} \text{ (leading)}$$

(ii) $$I_l = \sqrt{3}\, I_{ph} \quad \text{for delta connection}$$

$$\therefore \; I_l = \sqrt{3} \times 5.43$$

$$I_l = \boxed{9.4 \text{ A}}$$

(iii) $$\text{Power factor} = \cos\phi = \cos 51.85^{\circ}$$

$$\text{p.f.} = \boxed{0.6177} \text{ (leading)}$$

(iv) Refer Fig. 5.9(b)

- **(a)** Take phase current $\overline{I}_{RR'}$ as reference.
- **(b)** Draw $\overline{I}_{YY'}$ at 120° to $\overline{I}_{RR'}$.
- **(c)** Draw $\overline{I}_{BB'}$ at 120° to $\overline{I}_{YY'}$.
- **(d)** Draw $\overline{I}_{BB'}$, $-\overline{I}_{RR'}$, and $\overline{I}_{YY'}$.
- **(e)** From Fig 5.9(a), $\overline{I}_R = \overline{I}_{RR'} - \overline{I}_{BB'}$ so from parallelogram of $\overline{I}_{RR'}$ and $\overline{I}_{BB'}$, find $\overline{I}_R$.
- **(f)** Similarly $\overline{I}_Y = \overline{I}_{YY'} - \overline{I}_{RR'}$ and $\overline{I}_B = \overline{I}_{BB'} - \overline{I}_{YY'}$.
- **(g)** As phase currents lead phase voltages [angle of I_{ph} is +ve] draw V_{ph} voltages lagging behind I_{ph} by 51.85°.

Ex. 5.3 : Three identical coils each having a resistance of 20 Ω and reactance of 10 Ω are connected in **(i)** star, **(ii)** delta across 400 V, 3-phase line. Calculate for each method of connection the line currents and power consumed.

Solution : Given : $\overline{Z}_{ph} = 20 + 10\,j$

(as the impedance is coil, it is inductive hence $+10\,j$)

$$V_l = 400 \text{ V}$$

(i) Star Connection :

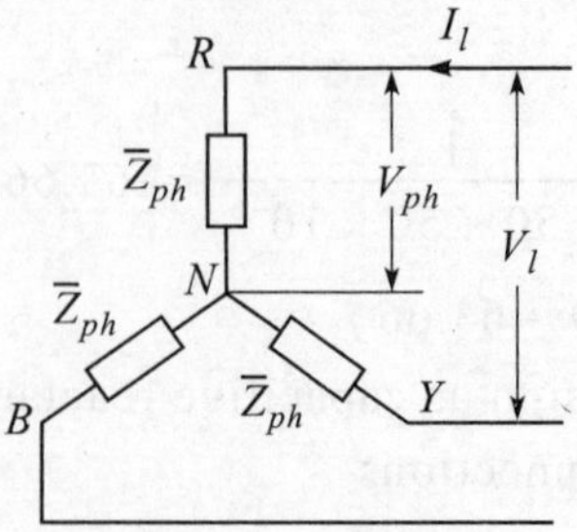

Fig. 5.10(a)

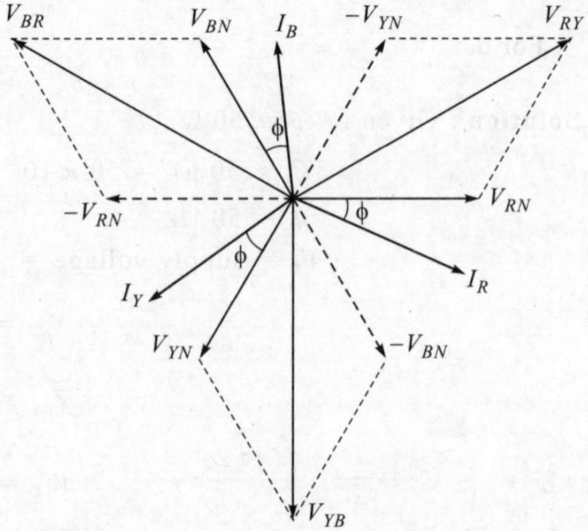

Fig. 5.10(b)

For star connection :

$$V_l = \sqrt{3}\, V_{ph} \quad \text{and} \quad I_l = I_{ph}$$

$$\therefore \; V_{ph} = \frac{V_l}{\sqrt{3}} = \frac{400}{\sqrt{3}} = \boxed{230.94 \text{ V}}$$

$$\therefore \; \bar{I}_{ph} = \frac{V_{ph}}{\bar{Z}_{ph}} = \frac{230.94}{20 + 10j} = 10.33 \angle{-26.56^\circ}$$

$$\therefore \; I_{ph} = 10.33 \text{ A} \; ; \; \phi = -26.56^\circ$$

$$\boxed{I_l = I_{ph} = 10.33 \text{ A}}$$

$$\text{Power consumed} \quad P = 3 V_{ph} I_{ph} \cos\phi$$

$$= 3 \times 230.94 \times 10.33 \times \cos 26.56^\circ$$

$$\boxed{P = 6401.55 \text{ watts}}$$

(ii) Delta Connection :

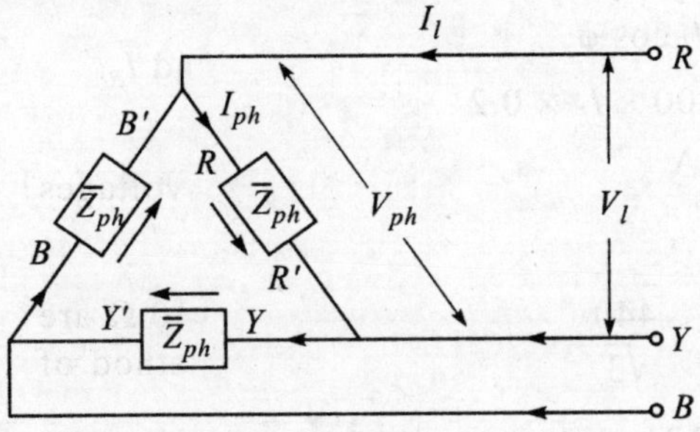

Fig. 5.10(c)

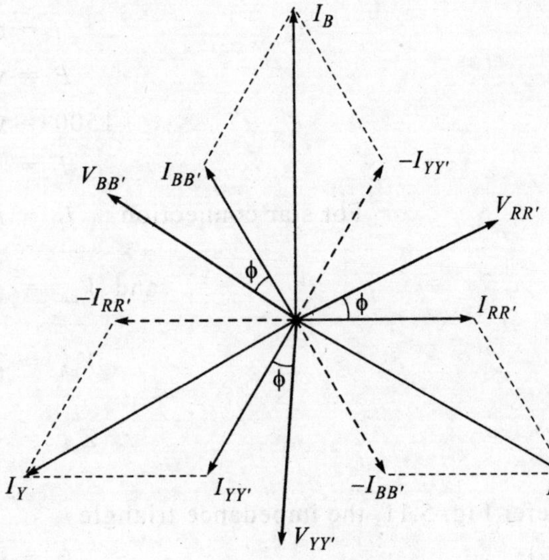

Fig. 5.10(d)

For delta connection :

$$V_{ph} = V_l$$

$$\therefore \; V_{ph} = 440 \text{ V}$$

$$\bar{I}_{ph} = \frac{V_{ph}}{\bar{Z}_{ph}} = \frac{440}{20 + 10j}$$

$$= 17.86 \angle{-26.56^\circ}$$

$$\therefore \; I_{ph} = \boxed{17.86 \text{ A}} \; ; \; \phi = -26.56^\circ$$

$$I_l = \sqrt{3}\, I_{ph}$$

$$\therefore \; I_l = \sqrt{3} \times 17.86$$

$$I_l = \boxed{30.99 \text{ A}}$$

Power consumed $P = 3V_{ph} I_{ph} \cos\phi$

$= 3 \times 400 \times 17.86 \times \cos 26.56°$

$P = \boxed{19202.41 \text{ watts}}$

Note : *From the above calculations, it is seen that power consumed in delta connected load is more than power consumed in star connected load of same impedance and*

$$\boxed{P_{Delta} = 3\,P_{Star}}$$

Ex 5.4 : Three similar coils connected in star take total power of 1.5 kW at a p.f. of 0.2 lagging from a 3-phase 440 V, 50 Hz supply. Calculate the resistance and inductance of the phase impedance.

Solution : Given : Load is star connected

$$P = 1.5 \text{ kW} = 1500 \text{ watts}$$

$$\text{p.f.} = \cos\phi = 0.2 \text{ (lagging)}$$

$$V_l = 440 \text{ V}$$

$$f = 50 \text{ Hz}$$

$$P = \sqrt{3}\, V_l I_l \cos\phi$$

$$\therefore 1500 = \sqrt{3} \times 400 \times I_l \times 0.2$$

$$\therefore I_l = 9.84 \text{ A}$$

For star connection : $I_l = I_{ph}$

and $V_{ph} = \dfrac{V_l}{\sqrt{3}} = \dfrac{440}{\sqrt{3}}$

$$\therefore V_{ph} = 254.03 \text{ V}$$

$$\therefore Z_{ph} = \frac{V_{ph}}{I_{ph}} = 25.82\ \Omega$$

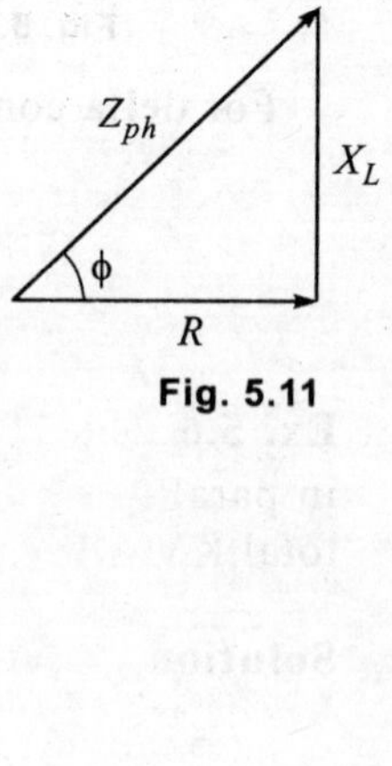

Fig. 5.11

Refer Fig. 5.11, the impedance triangle

$$\phi = \cos^{-1} 0.2 = 78.46°$$

$$\therefore R = Z\cos\phi = 25.82 \times 0.2$$

$$R = \boxed{5.104\ \Omega}$$

$$\therefore X_L = Z\sin\phi = 25.3\ \Omega$$

But $X_L = 2\pi f L$

$$\therefore L = \frac{X_L}{2\pi f} = \frac{25.3}{2\pi \times 50}$$

$$L = \boxed{0.08 \text{ H}}$$

Ex. 5.5 : A balanced 3-phase star connected load of 100 kW, takes a leading current of 80 A. When connected across 3-phase 1100 V, 50 Hz supply. Find the circuit constants of the load per phase.

Solution : Given : Star connected load

$$P = 100 \text{ kW} = 100 \times 1000 \text{ watts}$$

$$I_l = I_{ph} = 80 \text{ A}$$

p.f. is leading thus impedance is capacitive.

$$V_l = 1100 \text{ V}$$

$$f = 50 \text{ Hz}$$

$$P = 3 V_l I_l \cos\phi$$

$$100 \times 1000 = 3 \times 1100 \times 80 \times \cos\phi$$

$$\therefore \cos\phi = 0.3788$$

$$\therefore \phi = 67.74^\circ$$

$$Z_{ph} = \frac{V_{ph}}{I_{ph}} = \frac{V_l/\sqrt{3}}{I_{ph}} = \frac{1100}{\sqrt{3} \times 80} = 7.94 \ \Omega$$

From the impedance triangle (Fig. 5.12),

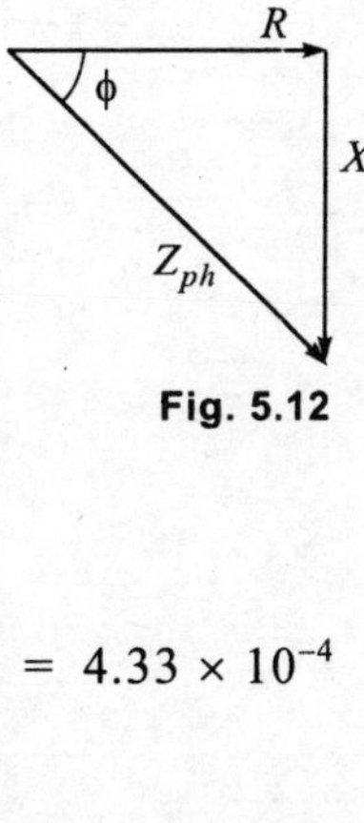

Fig. 5.12

$$R = Z_{ph} \cos\phi = 7.94 \times 0.3788$$

$$\therefore R = \boxed{3 \ \Omega}$$

$$X_C = Z_{ph} \sin\phi = 7.94 \sin 67.74^\circ$$

$$X_C = 7.35 \ \Omega$$

$$X_C = \frac{1}{2\pi f C}$$

$$\therefore C = \frac{1}{2\pi f X_C} = \frac{1}{2\pi \times 50 \times 7.35} = 4.33 \times 10^{-4}$$

$$\therefore C = \boxed{433 \ \mu f}$$

Ex. 5.6 : Each of the delta connected load consists of a non-reactive resistance of 100 Ω in parallel with a capacitance of 31.8 μf. Calculate, the line current, power absorbed, the total KVA, KVAR and power factor when connected to 416 V, 3-phase, 50 Hz supply.

Solution : Given : Z_{ph} is R in parallel with C

$$R = 100 \ \Omega$$

$$C = 31.8 \ \mu f = 31.8 \times 10^{-6} \text{ f}$$

$$V_l = 416 \text{ V}$$

$$f = 50 \text{ Hz}$$

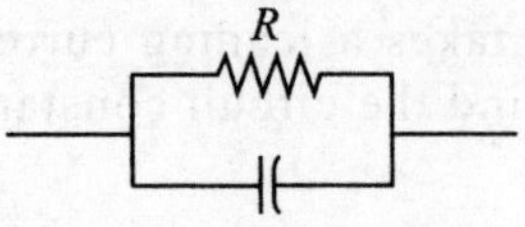

Fig. 5.13

$$X_C = \frac{1}{2\pi f C} = \frac{1}{2\pi \times 50 \times 31.8 \times 10^{-6}}$$

$$= 100.97\ \Omega$$

$$\therefore \bar{Z}_{ph} = \frac{R(-X_C j)}{R - X_C j} = \frac{100(-100.97 j)}{100 - 100.97 j}$$

$$= 71.05 \angle -44.72^\circ$$

For Delta Connected Load :

$$V_l = V_{ph} \quad \text{and} \quad I_l = \sqrt{3}\, I_{ph}$$

$$\therefore V_{ph} = 416 \text{ V}$$

$$\therefore \bar{I}_{ph} = \frac{V_{ph}}{\bar{Z}_{ph}} = \frac{416}{71.05 \angle -44.72^\circ} = 5.85 \angle 44.72^\circ$$

$$\therefore I_{ph} = 44.72 \text{ A} \;;\; \phi = 44.72^\circ$$

$$\therefore I_l = \sqrt{3}\, I_{ph} = \sqrt{3} \times 5.85$$

$$I_l = \boxed{10.13 \text{ A}}$$

$$\text{Power consumed } P = 3 V_{ph} I_{ph} \cos \phi$$

$$= 3 \times 416 \times 5.85 \times \cos 44.72^\circ$$

$$P = \boxed{5187.6 \text{ watts}}$$

$$\text{Total KVA} = \frac{3 V_{ph} I_{ph}}{1000} = \frac{3 \times 416 \times 5.85}{1000}$$

$$\therefore \text{KVA} = \boxed{7.3}$$

$$\text{Total KVAR} = \frac{3 V_{ph} I_{ph} \sin \phi}{1000} = \text{KVA} \sin \phi$$

$$\therefore \text{KVAR} = \boxed{5.137}$$

$$\text{Power factor} = \cos \phi = \cos 44.72^\circ$$

$$\text{p.f.} = \boxed{0.71} \text{ (leading)}$$

Ex. 5.7 : Each phase of a delta connected load contains a 50 mH inductor in series with the parallel combination of 50 Ω and 50 μf. The supply 550 V, 800 rad/s. Find the line and phase currents and the total power drawn by the load.

Solution : Given :

$$R = 100\ \Omega$$

$$L = 50 \text{ mH} = 50 \times 10^{-3} \text{ H}$$

$$\omega = 800 \text{ rad/s}, \; C = 50\ \mu\text{f}$$

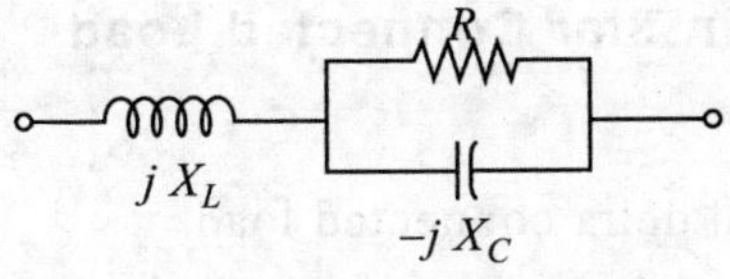

Fig. 5.14(a) : Phase impedance.

$$X_C = \frac{1}{\omega C} = 25\ \Omega$$

$$\therefore \bar{Z}_{ph} = j X_L + \frac{R(-j X_C)}{R - j X_C} = 40 j + \frac{50(-25 j)}{50 - 25 j}$$

$$= 10 + 20 j$$

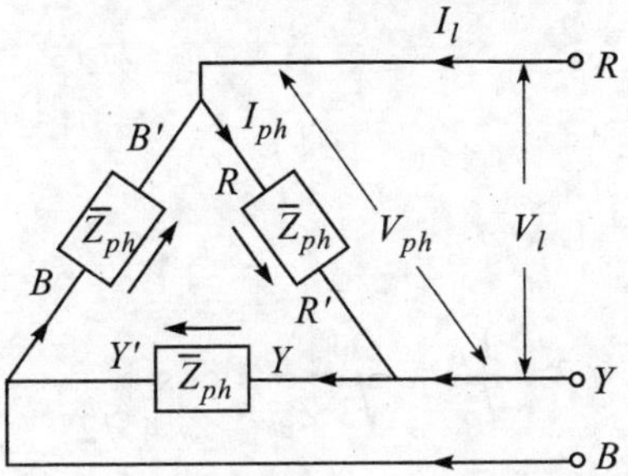

Fig. 5.14(b)

For Delta Connected Load :

$$V_{ph} = V_l = 550\text{ V}$$

$$\therefore \bar{I}_{ph} = \frac{V_{ph}}{\bar{Z}_{ph}} = \frac{550}{10 + 20 j} = 24.6 \angle -63.43^{\circ}$$

$$\therefore I_{ph} = \boxed{24.6\text{ A}}\ ;\ \phi = -63.43^{\circ}$$

$$\therefore I_l = \sqrt{3}\, I_{ph} = \sqrt{3} \times 24.6 = \boxed{42.6\text{ A}}$$

Power consumed $P = 3 V_{ph} I_{ph} \cos\phi$

$$= 3 \times 550 \times 24.6 \times \cos 63.43^{\circ}$$

$$P = 18155.53\text{ watts} = \boxed{18.155\text{ kW}}$$

5.5 Comparisons

5.5.1 Comparison Between Star and Delta Connected Loads

Sr. No.	Star Connection	Delta Connection
1.	Similar terminals of the load are connected together and 3-phase supply is connected to the other terminals to form star connected load.	Dissimilar ends of the load are connected together to form the three load terminals to form delta connected load.
2.	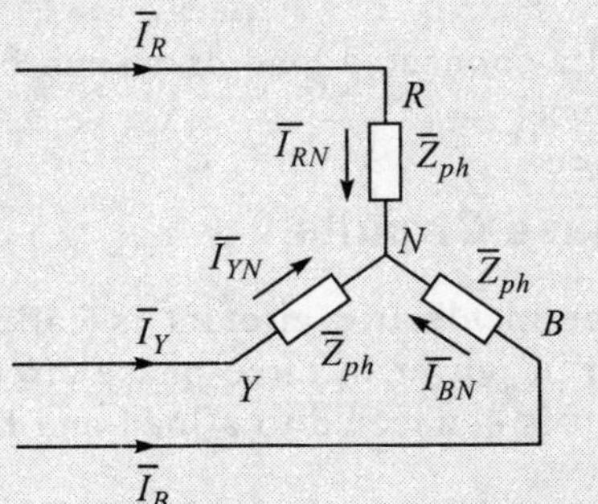	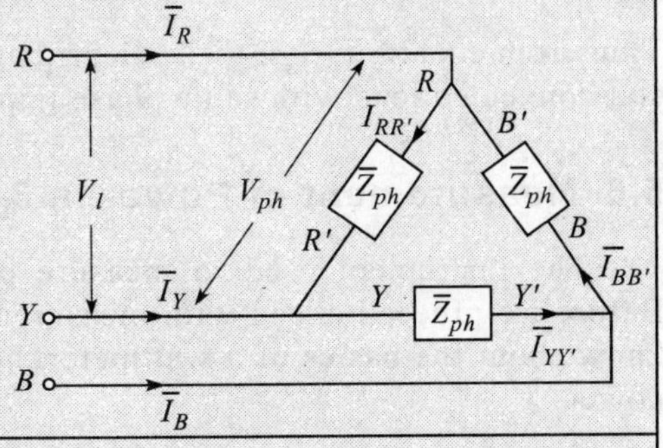
3.	$V_l = \sqrt{3}\, V_{ph}$	$V_l = V_{ph}$
4.	$I_l = I_{ph}$	$I_l = \sqrt{3}\, I_{ph}$
5.	$P = 3 V_{ph} I_{ph} \cos\phi$ $= \sqrt{3}\, V_l I_l \cos\phi$	$P = 3 V_{ph} I_{ph} \cos\phi$ $= \sqrt{3}\, V_l I_l \cos\phi$

5.5.2 Comparison Between the Power Consumed in Star Connected Load and Delta Connected Load

Let, $\bar{Z}_{ph}$ = Per phase impedance in star and delta connected load.

V_l = Supply line voltage.

For Star Connection :

$$V_{ph} = \frac{V_l}{\sqrt{3}}$$

$$\text{and } I_{ph} = \frac{V_{ph}}{Z_{ph}} = \frac{V_l}{\sqrt{3}\, Z_{ph}}$$

$$\therefore\ P_{star} = 3\, V_{ph}\, I_{ph} \cos\phi = 3 \cdot \frac{V_l}{\sqrt{3}} \cdot \frac{V_l}{\sqrt{3}\, Z_{ph}} \cdot \cos\phi$$

$$P_{star} = \frac{V_l^2}{Z_{ph}} \cos\phi \qquad \text{..... (5.31)}$$

For Delta Connection :

$$V_{ph} = V_l$$

$$\text{and } I_{ph} = \frac{V_{ph}}{Z_{ph}} = \frac{V_l}{Z_{ph}}$$

$$\therefore\ P_{delta} = 3\, V_{ph} \,.\, I_{ph} \cos\phi = 3.\, V_l \,.\, \frac{V_l}{Z_{ph}} \cos\phi$$

$$P_{delta} = 3\, \frac{V_l^2}{Z_{ph}} \cos\phi \qquad \text{..... (5.31)}$$

From equations (5.31) and (5.32) we get,

$$\boxed{P_{delta} = 3P_{star}} \qquad \text{..... (5.33)}$$

Thus from equation (5.33) it is clear that delta connected load draws more power than the star connected load with same phase impedance.

5.6 Measurement of Power in 3-Phase Circuits

The instrument used to measure power in electric circuits is called "*wattmeter*". Before we proceed ahead with measurement of power in three-phase circuits, let us first know about the basics of a wattmeter, how it is connected to a load and how it measures power.

As we know, power in a.c. circuits is given by

$$P = V\, I \cos\phi$$

The wattmeter has a voltage coil and a current coil. The deflection produced by the wattmeter is proportional to the product of voltage (across its voltage coil) current (through its current coil) and cosine of the angle between the two. This can be well understood from Fig. 5.15.

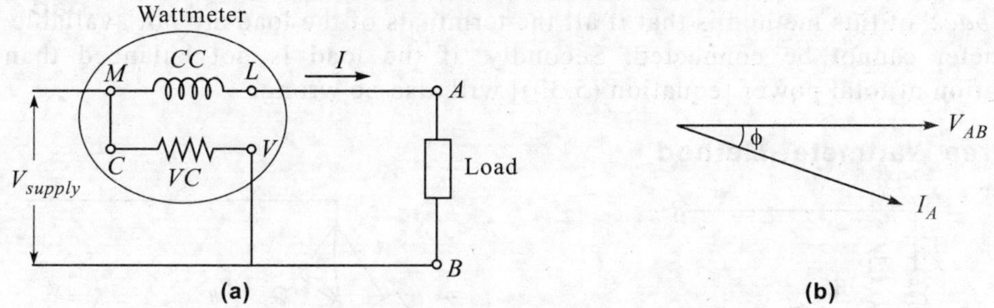

Fig. 5.15 : Measurement of 1-phase power by wattmeter.

In the wattmeter, *CC* is the current coil with terminals *M* and *L*, where '*M*' stands for '*mains*' i.e. *M* has to be connected to supply mains. *L* stands for '*load*' i.e. *L* has to be connected to the ''*load*'. *VC* is the voltage coil which is connected in parallel to the load. Terminals *C* (common) is the common terminal to be connected to *M* and *V* (voltage) terminal is to be connected to the other end of load. Here, the power measured by wattmeter is *P* given by

$$P = V_{AB}\, I \cos \phi \qquad \text{..... (5.34)}$$

where ϕ is the power factor angle of load [Fig. 5.15(b)]. The instantaneous power measured is *p*, where

$$p = v_{AB}\, i \qquad \text{..... (5.35)}$$

If the supply is d.c., ϕ will be zero and wattmeter will give *VI* as the power.

5.6.1 One Wattmeter Method

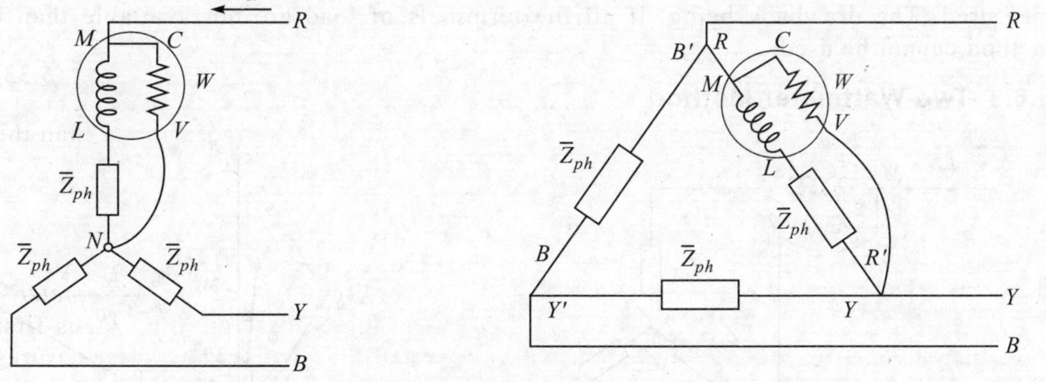

Fig. 5.16 : Measurement of 1-phase power - 1 wattmeter method.

For a balance load where all the terminals (*RR*' *YY*' and *BB*') of the load are available single wattmeter can indicate the total power measured. In star as well as delta connected load the wattmeter (Fig. 5.16) has been connected to *R*-phase

$$\text{i.e.} \quad W = V_{RN}\, I_R \cos \phi \qquad \text{..... (5.36)}$$

which is also the power per phase

$$\therefore \quad W_{total} = 3\, W \qquad \text{..... (5.37)}$$

The '*drawback*' of this method is that if all the terminals of the load are not available than the wattmeter cannot be connected. Secondly, if the load is not balanced than the approximation of total power [equation (5.37)] will also be wrong.

5.6.2 Three Wattmeter Method

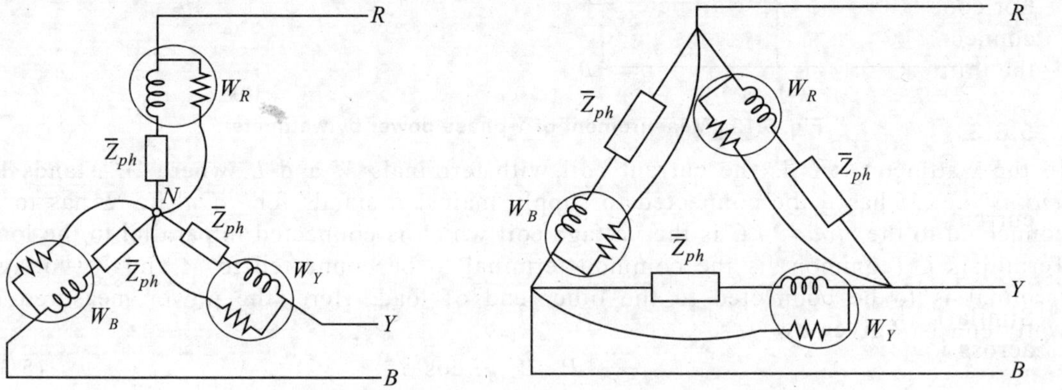

Fig. 5.17 : Measurement of power - 3 wattmeter method.

If the load is unbalance (unequal impedances) and all the terminals of the load are available, then one wattmeter is connected in each phase i.e. W_R, W_Y and W_B as shown in Fig. 5.17. The total power measured will be,

$$W_{total} = W_R + W_Y + W_B \quad ..... (5.38)$$

The advantage of this method is that the total power for unbalanced load can be measured. The drawback being, if all the terminals of load are not available than this method cannot be used.

5.6.3 Two Wattmeter Method

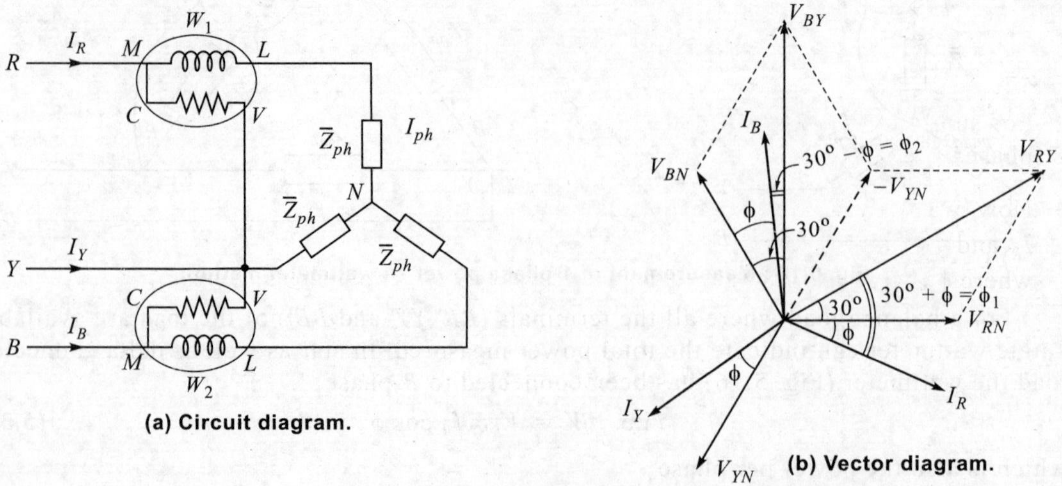

(a) Circuit diagram. **(b) Vector diagram.**

Fig. 5.18 : Two wattmeter method for star-connected load.

Two wattmeter method has advantage over the previous two methods of measuring power this method an be used even when all the terminals of individual phases of load are not available. Secondly, it not only measures power it also measurers the power factor of the circuit. The author wishes to deal with star and delta connected loads separately for a clear understanding.

For connecting the two wattmeters to the load, the current coils of the two wattmeters are connected to two supply lines and the voltage coils are connected between these lines and the third supply line as shown in Fig. 5.18 and 5.19.

5.6.3.1 Star connected load

Refer Fig. 5.18, wattmeter W_1 and W_2 are as shown, current coil (*ML*) of W_1 carries current $\overline{I}_R$ and voltage coil (*CV*) is connected across $\overline{V}_{RY}$.

$$\therefore \quad w_1 = i_R \, v_{RY} \qquad \text{..... (5.39)}$$

Similarly, current coil (*ML*) of W_2 carries current I_B and voltage coil (*CV*) is connected across $\overline{V}_{BY}$.

$$\therefore \quad w_2 = i_B \, v_{BY} \qquad \text{..... (5.40)}$$

$$\text{Instantaneous power, } w = w_1 + w_2$$

$$\therefore \quad w = i_R \, v_{RY} + i_B \, v_{BY} \qquad \text{..... (5.41)}$$

$$= i_R (v_{RN} - v_{YN}) + i_B (v_{BN} - v_{YN})$$

$$= i_R \, v_{RN} - i_R \, v_{YN} + i_B \, v_{BN} - i_B \, v_{YN}$$

$$= i_R \, v_{RN} + i_B \, v_{BN} - v_{YN} (i_R + i_B)$$

$$\text{But} \quad i_R + i_Y + i_B = 0$$

$$= i_R + i_B = i_Y$$

$$\therefore \quad w = i_R \, v_{RN} + i_B \, v_{BN} + i_Y \, v_{YN} \qquad \text{..... (5.42)}$$

$$w = w_R + w_Y + w_B \qquad \text{..... (5.43)}$$

i.e. sum of the two wattmeter readings gives the total power consumed in the three-phases.

Now, wattmeter W_1 indicates product of $\overline{I}_R$, $\overline{V}_{RY}$ and cos ϕ_1, where ϕ_1 is the angle between $\overline{I}_R$ and $\overline{V}_{RY}$ (= $\overline{V}_{RN}$ – $\overline{V}_{YN}$). Fig. 5.18 (b) shows $\overline{I}_R$, $\overline{V}_{RN}$, $-\overline{V}_{RN}$ and $\overline{V}_{RY}$. Here $\phi_1 = 30 + \phi$ where ϕ_1 is the phase angle of impedance per phase.

$$\therefore \quad W_1 = I_R \, V_{RY} \cos (30 + \phi) \qquad \text{..... (5.44)}$$

$$\text{But} \quad I_R = I_L, \quad \text{the line current and}$$

$$V_{RY} = V_L, \quad \text{the line voltage}$$

$$\therefore \quad W_1 = I_L \, V_L \cos (30 + \phi) \qquad \text{..... (5.45)}$$

Similarly, wattmeter W_2 indicates product of I_B, V_{BY} and cos ϕ_2, where ϕ_2 is the angle between I_B and V_{BY}. Fig. 5.18(b) shows I_B, V_{BN}, $-V_{YN}$, V_{BY} and $\phi_2 = 30 + \phi$

$$\therefore \quad W_2 = I_B\, V_{BY} \cos(30 - \phi)$$

$$\therefore \quad W_2 = I_L\, V_L \cos(30 - \phi) \qquad \text{..... (5.46)}$$

In order to find power factor angle ϕ from equation (5.45) and equation (5.46),

$$W_1 + W_2 = V_L I_L \cos(30 + \phi) + V_L I_L \cos(30 - \phi)$$

$$= V_L I_L [\cos(30 + \phi) + \cos(30 - \phi)]$$

$$= V_L I_L \left[2 \cos \frac{30 + \phi + 30 - \phi}{2} \cdot \cos \frac{30 + \phi - 30 + \phi}{2}\right]$$

$$= V_L I_L\ [2 \cos 30.\cos \phi] = V_L I_L \left[2.\frac{\sqrt{3}}{2} \cos \phi\right]$$

$$W_1 + W_2 = \sqrt{3}\ V_L I_L \cos \phi \qquad \text{..... (5.47)}$$

Similarly,

$$W_2 - W_1 = V_L I_L \cos(30 - \phi) - V_L I_L \cos(30 + \phi)$$

$$= V_L I_L [\cos(30 - \phi) - \cos(30 + \phi)]$$

$$= V_L I_L \left[2 \sin \frac{30 - \phi + 30 + \phi}{2} \cdot \sin \frac{30 + \phi - 30 + \phi}{2}\right]$$

$$= V_L I_L\ [2 \sin 30 \sin \phi]$$

$$= V_L I_L \left[2\ \frac{1}{2} \sin \phi\right]$$

$$W_2 - W_1 = V_L I_L \sin \phi \qquad \text{..... (5.48)}$$

Dividing equation 5.48 by equation 5.47 we get,

$$\frac{W_2 - W_1}{W_2 + W_1} = \frac{\sin \phi}{\sqrt{3} \cos \phi} \qquad \text{..... (5.49)}$$

$$\text{or} \quad \tan \phi = \sqrt{3}\ \frac{W_2 - W_1}{W_2 + W_1} \qquad \text{..... (5.50)}$$

$$\text{or} \quad \phi = \tan^{-1}\left\{\sqrt{3}\ \frac{W_2 - W_1}{W_2 + W_1}\right\} \qquad \text{..... (5.51)}$$

Thus, the two wattmeter readings will not only give the total power ($W = W_1 + W_2$), they will also give the power factor angle ϕ (equation 5.51).

5.6.3.2 Delta Connected Load

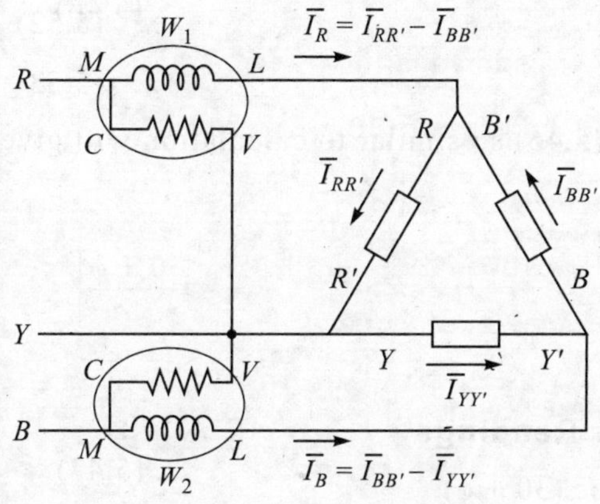

(a) Circuit diagram.

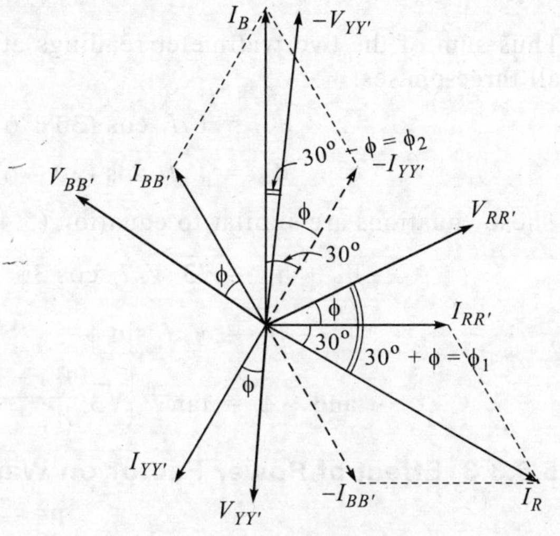

(b) Vector diagram.

Fig. 5.19 : Two wattmeter method for delta connected load.

Fig. 5.19 (a) shows delta connected load with two wattmeters. Wattmeter reading W_1 indicates product of $\overline{I}_R$, $\overline{V}_{RY}$ and $\cos\phi_1$. In delta connection

$$\overline{I}_R = \overline{I}_{RR'} - \overline{I}_{BB} \quad \text{[KCL at node } R]$$

$$\overline{I}_R = \text{line current} = \overline{I}_l$$

$$\overline{V}_{RY} = \overline{V}_{RR'} = \overline{V}_l = \text{line voltage}$$

$$\phi_1 = 30 + \phi = \text{angle between } \overline{I}_R \text{ and } \overline{V}_{RR}\text{, Fig. 3.19(b).}$$

Wattmeter reading W_2 indicates product of $\overline{I}_B$

$\overline{V}_{BY}$ $(= \overline{V}_{Y'Y} = -\overline{V}_{YY'})$ and $\cos\phi_2$. where ϕ_2 is the angle between $\overline{I}_B$ and $-\overline{V}_{YY'}$

$$\overline{I}_B = \overline{I}_{BB'} - \overline{I}_{YY'}$$

$$\overline{I}_B = I_l$$

$$\overline{V}_{BY} = -\overline{V}_{YY'} = V_l$$

$$\text{and} \quad \phi_2 = 30 - \phi$$

Instantaneous power,
$$w = w_1 + w_2$$
$$= i_R v_{RR'} + i_B v_{Y'Y} = i_R v_{RR'} - i_B v_{YY'}$$
$$= (i_{RR'} - i_{BB'})v_{RR'} - (i_{BB'} - i_{YY'})v_{YY'}$$
$$= i_{RR'} v_{RR'} - i_{BB'} v_{RR'} - i_{BB'} v_{YY'} + i_{YY'} v_{YY'}$$
$$= i_{RR'} v_{RR'} + i_{YY'} v_{YY'} - i_{BB'} (v_{RR'} + i_{BB'} v_{YY'})$$

$$= i_{RR'} v_{RR'} + i_{YY'} v_{YY'} + i_{BB'} v_{BB'} \quad \left\{ \begin{array}{r} \because v_{RR'} + v_{YY'} + v_{BB'} = 0 \\ \text{or } v_{RR'} + v_{YY'} = -v_{BB'} \end{array} \right\}$$

Thus sum of the two wattmeter readings at any instant is the sum of power consumed in all three-phases.

$$\therefore \quad W_1 = V_l I_l \cos (30 + \phi) \qquad ..... (5.52)$$

$$W_2 = V_l I_l \cos (30 - \phi) \qquad ..... (5.53)$$

These equations are similar to equation (5.45) and (5.46) so similar to calculation will give

$$W_1 + W_2 = \sqrt{3}\ V_l\ I_l\ \cos 3\phi$$

$$W_2 - W_1 = V_l\ I_l \sin \phi$$

$$\text{and} \quad \phi = \tan^{-1} \left\{ \sqrt{3}\ \frac{W_2 - W_1}{W_1 + W_2} \right\}$$

5.6.3.3 Effect of Power Factor on Wattmeter Readings

$$W_1 = V_l I_l \cos (30 + \phi)$$

$$W_2 = V_l I_l \cos (30 - \phi)$$

The change in the readings of the two wattmeters is expressed in tabular form here.

p.f. angle ϕ	Power factor $\cos \phi$	W_1 (watts) $= V_l I_l \cos (30 + \phi)$	W_2 (watts) $= V_l I_l \cos (30 - \phi)$
60°	0.5	0 watts (cos 90°)	+ve reading
< 60°	>0.5	$30° + \phi < 90°$ $\therefore W_1$ = +ve reading	$30° - \phi$ = −ve $\therefore W_2$ = +ve reading
> 60°	< 0.5	$30° + \phi > 90°$ $\therefore W_1$ = −ve reading*	$30° - \phi$ = −ve $\therefore W_2$ = +ve reading

* *A negative reading means the wattmeter tends to deflect in opposite directions. To get the reading on wattmeter interchange either connection to current coil (M and L) or the voltage coil (C and V).*

Ex. 5.8 : A 3-phase motor load has a power factor of 0.397 lagging. Two wattmeters connected to measure power show the input as 30 kW. Find reading of each wattmeter.

Solution : Given : $\cos \phi = 0.397 \quad \therefore \phi = 66.6°$

$$W = 30 \text{ kW} = 30000 \text{ watts}$$

$$\text{Total power, } W = W_1 + W_2 = 30000 \text{ watts} \qquad ..... (i)$$

$$\tan \phi = \sqrt{3}\ \frac{W_2 - W_1}{W_1 + W_2}$$

$$\therefore \tan 66.6° = \frac{\sqrt{3}\,(W_2 - W_1)}{30000}$$

$$\therefore W_2 - W_1 = 40043.03 \text{ watts} \qquad \text{..... (ii)}$$

Solving equations (i) and (ii), we get

$$W_1 + W_2 = 30000 \text{ watts}$$

$$W_2 - W_1 = 40043.03 \text{ watts}$$

$$\therefore W_2 = 35021.5 \text{ watts and } W_1 = -5021.5 \text{ watts}$$

$$\text{or } W_2 = \boxed{35 \text{ kW}} \text{ and } W_1 = \boxed{-5 \text{ kW}}$$

Ex. 5.9 : A 3-phase *RYB* system has effective line voltage of 173.2 V. Wattmeters in line *R* and *Y* read 301 watts and 1327 watts. Find the impedance of balanced star connected load.

Solution : Given : Star connected load :

$$V_l = 173.2 \text{ V}$$

$$\therefore V_{ph} = \frac{V_l}{\sqrt{3}} = \frac{173.2}{\sqrt{3}} = 100 \text{ V}$$

$$W_1 = 301 \text{ watts and } W_2 = 1327 \text{ watts}$$

$$\text{Total power, } W = W_1 + W_2 = 301 + 1327$$

$$\therefore W = 1628 \text{ watts}$$

$$\phi = \tan^{-1}\left\{\sqrt{3}\,\frac{W_2 - W_1}{W_1 + W_2}\right\} = \tan^{-1}\left\{\sqrt{3}\,\frac{1327 - 301}{301 + 1327}\right\}$$

$$\therefore \phi = 47.5°$$

$$W = 3 V_{ph} I_{ph} \cos\phi$$

$$1628 = 3 \times 100 \times I_{ph} \times \cos 47.5°$$

$$\therefore I_{ph} = 8.03 \text{ A}$$

$$Z_{ph} = \frac{V_{ph}}{I_{ph}} = \frac{100}{8.03}$$

$$Z_{ph} = \boxed{12.45\ \Omega}$$

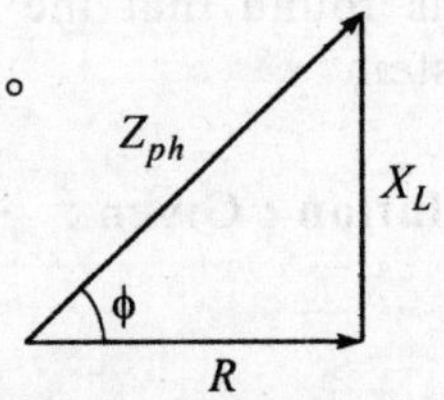

Fig. 5.20 : Impedance triangle.

$$R = Z\cos\phi = 12.45 \cos 47.5°$$

$$\therefore R = \boxed{8.41\ \Omega}$$

$$X_L = Z\sin\phi = 12.45 \sin 47.5°$$

$$\therefore X_L = \boxed{9.18\ \Omega}$$

Ex. 5.10 : Calculate the total power and readings of two wattmeters connected to measure power in three-phase balanced load, if the reactive power is 15 KVAR and the load power factor is 0.8 lagging.

Solution : Given : $\cos\phi = 0.8$ (lagging)

$$\therefore \phi = \cos^{-1} 0.8 = 36.87°$$

$$\text{KVAR} = 15$$

$$\text{Now, KVAR} = \text{KVA} \sin\phi$$

$$\therefore \text{KVA} = \frac{\text{KVAR}}{\sin 36.87°} = 25 \text{ KVA}$$

$$\text{KW} = \text{KVA} \cos\phi = 10 \times 50 = 20 \text{ kW}$$

$$\text{or } W_1 + W_2 = 20 \text{ kW} \quad .... \text{(i)}$$

$$\phi = \tan^{-1}\left\{\sqrt{3}\,\frac{W_2 - W_1}{W_1 + W_2}\right\}$$

$$36.87° = \tan^{-1}\left\{\sqrt{3}\,\frac{W_2 - W_1}{20}\right\}$$

$$\therefore W_2 - W_1 = 8.62 \text{ kW} \quad .... \text{(i)}$$

Solving (i) and (ii), we get

$$W_1 = \boxed{5.69 \text{ kW}}$$

$$\text{and } W_2 = \boxed{14.31 \text{ kW}}$$

Ex. 5.11 : Power in a balanced 3-phase system is measured by two wattmeter method and it is found that the ratio of the two readings is 3:1. What is the power factor of the system?

Solution : Given : $\frac{W_2}{W_1} = \frac{3}{1} \quad \therefore W_2 = 3W_1$

$$\phi = \tan^{-1}\left\{\sqrt{3}\,\frac{W_2 - W_1}{W_1 + W_2}\right\}$$

$$= \tan^{-1}\left\{\sqrt{3}\,\frac{3W_1 - W_1}{W_1 + 3W_1}\right\}$$

$$\phi = \tan^{-1}\frac{2\sqrt{3}}{4}$$

$$\therefore \phi = 40.89°$$

$$\text{Power factor} = \cos\phi = \boxed{0.7559}$$

Ex. 5.12 : A balanced star connected load consists of a resistance in series with capacitance in each phase. The supply is 416 V at 50 Hz, 3-phase. Readings of two wattmeters connected to measure power is 780 watts and 1980 watts. Calculate **(i)** powerfactor of the circuit **(ii)** the line current **(iii)** capacitance of each phase.

Solution : Given :

$$V_l = 416 \text{ V}$$

$$f = 50 \text{ Hz}$$

Star connected load :

$$W_1 = 780 \text{ watts and } W_2 = 1980 \text{ watts}$$

$$\phi = \tan^{-1}\left\{\sqrt{3}\,\frac{W_2 - W_1}{W_1 + W_2}\right\}$$

$$= \tan^{-1}\left\{\sqrt{3}\,\frac{1980 - 780}{1980 + 780}\right\}$$

$$\therefore \phi = 36.98°$$

$$\text{Power factor} = \cos\phi = \cos 36.98° = \boxed{0.7988} \text{ (leading)}$$

{∵ capacitive impedance}

$$\text{Total power, } W = W_1 + W_2 = 780 + 1980$$

$$\therefore W = 2760 \text{ watts}$$

$$W = \sqrt{3}\, V_l I_l \cos\phi$$

$$2760 = \sqrt{3} \times 416 \times I_l \times 0.7988$$

$$\therefore I_l = \boxed{4.79 \text{ A}}$$

For Star Connection :

$$V_{ph} = \frac{V_l}{\sqrt{3}} = \frac{416}{\sqrt{3}} = 240.18 \text{ volts}$$

$$I_{ph} = I_l = 4.79 \text{ A}$$

$$\therefore Z_{ph} = \frac{V_{ph}}{I_{ph}} = \frac{240.18}{4.79} = 50.14\ \Omega$$

$$X_C = Z_{ph} \sin\phi = 50.14 \sin 36.98°$$

$$X_C = 30.16\ \Omega$$

$$X_C = \frac{1}{2\pi f C}$$

$$C = \frac{1}{2\pi f X_C} = \frac{1}{2\pi \times 50 \times 30.16} = 105.5 \times 10^{-6} \text{ f}$$

$$\therefore C = \boxed{105.5\ \mu\text{f}}$$

Ex. 5.13 : Calculate the active and reactive current components in each phase of a star connected 10000 V, 3-phase alternator supplying 5000 kW at a power factor of 0.8. If the total current remains the same when load power factor is raised to 0.9. Find the new output.

Solution : Given : $V_l = 10000$ V

Power factor, $\text{p.f.}_1 = \cos\phi_1 = 0.8 \quad \therefore \phi_1 = 36.87°$

$W = 5000$ kW

$\text{p.f.}_2 = \cos\phi_2 = 0.9$

Star connection load : $W = \sqrt{3}\, V_l I_l \cos\phi$

$$50000 \times 10^3 = \sqrt{3} \times 10000 \times I_l \times 0.8$$

$$\therefore I_l = \boxed{360.84 \text{ A}}$$

Active component of current $= I_l \cos\phi_1 = 360.84 \times 0.8$

$$\therefore I_{active} = \boxed{288.67 \text{ A}}$$

Reactive component of current $= I_l \sin\phi_1 = 360.84 \sin 36.87°$

$$\therefore I_{reactive} = \boxed{216.54 \text{ A}}$$

Now, if $I_l = 360.84$ A and $\text{p.f.}_2 = 0.9$

$$W_2 = \sqrt{3}\, V_l I_l \cos\phi_2 = \sqrt{3} \times 10000 \times 360.84 \times 0.9$$

$$W_2 = \boxed{5624.94 \text{ kW}}$$

Ex. 5.14 : Three identical impedances of 10 ∠53.1° ohms are connected in delta to a three-phase 240 volt supply. Find the line and phase currents and the total power consumed.

Solution : Given : $\bar{Z}_{ph} = 10\angle 53.1°$

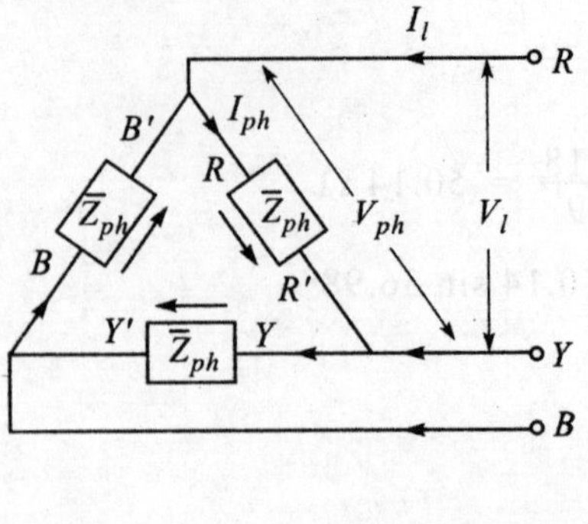

Delta connected load :

$V_l = 240$ V

For Delta Connection :

$V_l = V_{ph} = 240$ V

$$\therefore \bar{I}_{ph} = \frac{V_{ph}}{\bar{Z}_{ph}} = \frac{240}{10\angle 53.1°} = 24\angle -53.1°$$

$$\therefore I_{ph} = \boxed{24 \text{ A}};\ \phi = -53.1°$$

$$\therefore I_l = \sqrt{3}\, I_{ph} = \sqrt{3} \times 24 = \boxed{41.57 \text{ A}}$$

Power consumed $P = 3 V_{ph} I_{ph} \cos\phi$

$$= 3 \times 240 \times 24 \times \cos 53.1°$$

$$P = 10375.3 \text{ watts} = \boxed{10.37 \text{ kW}}$$

Ex. 5.15 : Two wattmeters in line *R* and *Y* of 173.2 volts *RYB* system read 301 and 1327 watts respectively. Find the impedances of a balanced star connected load.

Solution : Given : $W_1 = -301$ watts, $W_2 = 1327$ watts

$V_l = 173.2$ volts

Star connected load :

To find : Impedance in each phase

$$\phi = \tan^{-1}\left\{\sqrt{3}\,\frac{W_2 - W_1}{W_1 + W_2}\right\} = \tan^{-1}\left\{\sqrt{3}\,\frac{1327-(-301)}{1327-301}\right\}$$

$$\therefore \phi = 70.01°$$

$$W_l = V_l I_l \cos(30° + \phi)$$

$$-301 = 173.2 \times I_l \times \cos(30° + 70.01°)$$

$$\therefore I_l = \boxed{10 \text{ A}}$$

$$V_{ph} = \frac{V_l}{\sqrt{3}} = \frac{173.2}{\sqrt{3}} = 100 \text{ volts}$$

$$\therefore Z_{ph} = \frac{V_{ph}}{I_{ph}} = \frac{100}{10} = 10\ \Omega$$

$$\therefore \bar{Z}_{ph} = \boxed{10\angle 70.01°\ \Omega}$$

Unsolved Problems

(1) A balanced star-connected load of 8 + *j*6 Ω per phase is connected to a 3-phase 230 V supply. Find the line current, power factor, power, reactive volt-ampers and total volt-amperes.

[Ans. 13.28 A, 0.8 lag, 4232.28 watts, 3174.22 VAR, 5290.35 VA]

(2) A balanced 3-phase, star connected load of 150 kW takes a leading current of 100 A with a line voltage of 1100 V, 50 Hz. Find the circuit constants of the load per phase. **[Ans.** 5 Ω, 813.11 μf]

(3) A balanced star connected load is supplied from a symmetrical 3-phase 400 V system. The current in each phase is 30 A and lags 30° behind the phase voltage. Find **(a)** Phase voltage **(b)** the total power. Draw the vector diagram showing the currents and voltages.

[Ans. 230.94 V, 18 kW]

(4) A symmetrical 3-phase 400 V system supplies a balanced delta connected load. The current in each branch circuit is 20 A and phase angle is 40° lagging. Find **(a)** the line current and **(b)** the total power. Draw the vector diagram showing all voltages and currents.

[Ans. 34.64 A, 18.385 kW]

(5) The power input to a 2000 V, 50 Hz, 3-phase motor running on full load at an efficiency of 90% is measured by two wattmeters which indicate 300 kW and 100 kW respectively. Calculate **(a)** input **(b)** power factor **(c)** line current.

[**Ans.** 444.44 kW, 0.7559; 152.76 A]

(6) The power taken by a 3-phase 400 V motor is measured by the two wattmeter method and the readings of the two wattmeters are 460 watts and 780 watts. Estimate the power factor of the motor and the line current.

[**Ans.** 0.9129 lagging, 1.96 A]

(7) Three similar chokes, each having a resistance of 5 Ω and a reactance of 12 Ω are connected in delta across a 3-phase 440 V supply. Determine **(i)** Total power taken by this load **(ii)** Readings of the two wattmeters connected to measure the total power consumed.

[**Ans.** 17.185 kW, 20.5 kW, –3.31 kW]

(8) Two wattmeters connected to measure the power input to a 3-phase circuit indicate 8 kW and 0.8 kW, the latter reading obtained after reversing the current coil connections. Find the power and power factor of the load.

[**Ans.** 7.2 kW, 0.4271]

(9) A 7460 watts induction motor runs from 3-phase, 400 V supply. On no-load, the motor takes a line current of 4 A at a power factor of 0.208 lagging. On full load, it operates at a power factor of 0.88 lagging, and an efficiency of 89%. Determine the readings on each of the two wattmeters connected to read total power on **(a)** no load and **(b)** full load.

[**Ans. (a)** –494.43 W, 1070.61 W **(b)** 2885.19 W, 5497.75 W]

(10) For a certain balanced 3-phase load, one wattmeter reads 20 kW land the other 5 kW after the voltage circuit of this wattmeter has been reversed. Calculate the power and power factor of the load.

[**Ans.** 15 kW, 0.3273]

(11) A three-phase three wire 110 V system supplies a delta connected load with equal impedance of 5 $\angle 45^{\circ}$ ohms. Determine the line currents, phase currents and draw the vector diagram.

[**Ans.** 38.1 A, 22 A]

(12) A three 3-phase 208 volt supply is connected to star connected impedances of 20 $\angle -30^{\circ}$. Find line and phase currents and voltages. Draw the vector diagram.

[**Ans.** 6 A, 6 A, 208 V, 120 V]

(13) A three-phase, 100 V supplied is connected to a balanced delta connected load with impedance of 20 $\angle 45^{\circ}$. Determine the line currents and power consumed by the circuit. Also if two wattmeters were used to measure power, indicate the readings of the two wattmeters.

[**Ans.** 5 A, 8.66 A, 1060.63 W, 836.49 W, 224.14 W]

(14) Three identical impedances are connected in star to a 150 V, 3-phase supply. If the per phase impedance is 5 $\angle -30°$. Find the readings of the two wattmeters connected to measure power. What is the total power consumed.

[Ans. 1299 W, 2598 W, 3897 W**]**

(15) The phasor diagram below shows line currents and line voltages of a three-phase 346 volt supply. If the magnitudes of line current is 10 A. Find the impedance of star connected load per phase.

[Ans. 20 Ω**]**

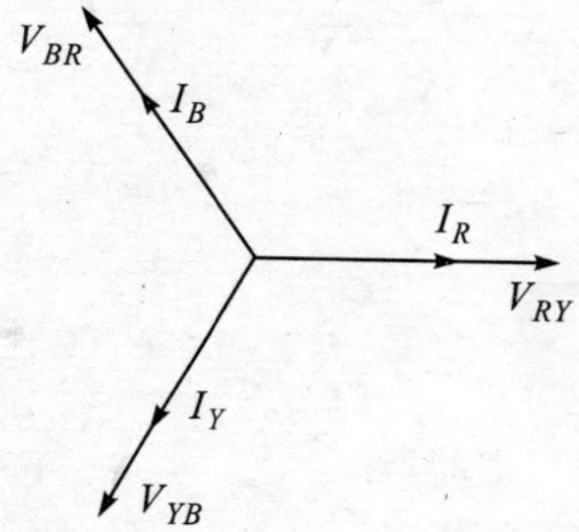

CHAPTER 6

TRANSFORMER

*A transformer is a device that transforms electrical energy from one circuit to another through a medium of magnetic field and **without a change in frequency**.*

*The circuit which receives energy from supply mains is called the **primary winding** and the one which delivers electric energy to the load is called the **secondary winding**. If the secondary winding has more turns as compared to primary winding it is called **a step-up transformer**. If the secondary winding has less turns as compared to primary winding it is called a **step down transformer**. Same transformer can be made to work as a step up or step-down transformer depending upon whether the low voltage or high voltage winding is connected to the supply.*

As a transformer does not have any moving parts hence it is an electric machine with highest possible efficiency and requires minimum amount of maintenance and supervision.

6.1 Need of Transformer

Insulation conditions pose a restriction on generation of alternating voltage from about 11 kV to 22 kV, but transmission of power at this voltage is not economical. Hence, with the help of transformer this voltage is stepped up to 400 kV and higher values to reduce the transmission losses.

Whenever this electrical energy is required it is stepped down to the suitable required voltage. Therefore, use of transformer is wide spread in a.c. transmission and its study is important in electrical transmission systems.

6.2 Transformer Construction

There are two types of transformer constructions namely *core type* and the *shell type*. The two types of transformer differ from each other by the manner in which their windings are wound around the core. The core is a stack of laminated sheets of special steel as shown in Fig. 6.1 and Fig. 6.2.These sheets are insulated from each other by thin varnish. The top and bottom part of the core are called the yoke while the vertical part of yoke is called the *limb or the leg*. In core type, the windings surround the major part of the steel core. Half the primary winding (made of copper wire) is wound over one leg and remaining half is wound on the other leg as shown in Fig. 6.1. The secondary winding is also divided into parts, one half over the primary winding of leg and the other over the primary winding of the other leg. The division of the windings is done to increase the insulation and reduce the leakage of flux between the two windings. Low voltage winding is placed inside the high voltage winding to reduce the amount of insulation required.

In the shell type transformer, the steel core surrounds a major part of the winding as shown in Fig. 6.2. The low voltage (l.v.) winding and the high voltage (h.v.) windings are wound over the central leg and they are sandwiched as shown in figure.

For a given output and voltage rating, core type transformer requires less iron and more copper, the winding conductor material, as compared to the shell type transformer. In core type transformer the flux has a single path around the yoke or legs, where as in shell type the flux of the central limb divides equally in the outer legs.

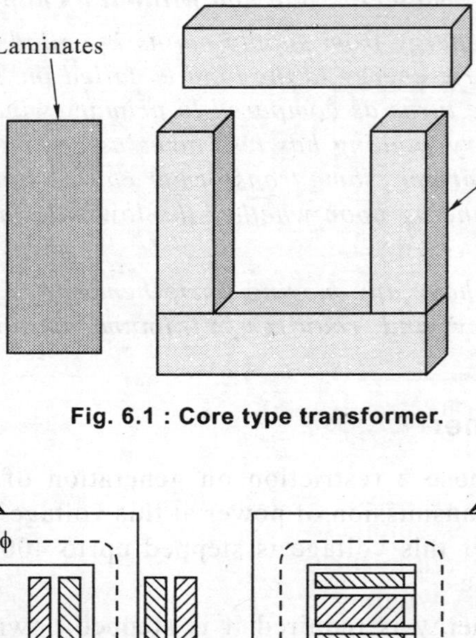

Fig. 6.1 : Core type transformer.

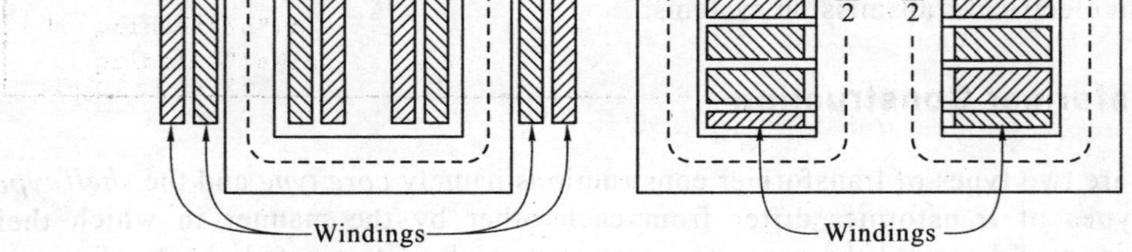

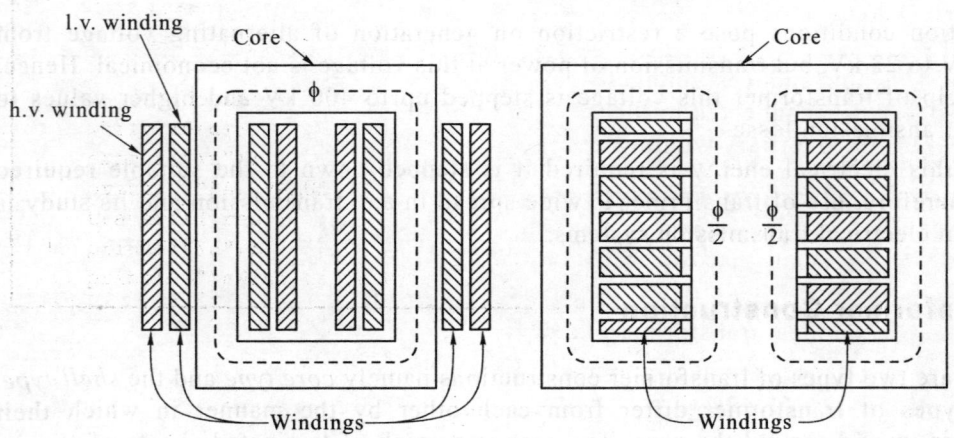

Fig. 6.2 : Shell type transformer.

However, for both types of transformers, the schematic diagram is as shown in Fig. 6.3. If the number of turns in the primary winding i.e. the winding to which supply is connected, is N_1 and the number of turns in the secondary winding i.e. the winding to which load is connected is N_2, then if $N_1 < N_2$ it is called as a *step-up transformer.* While if $N_1 > N_2$ then the transformer is a *step down transformer*. A transformer with $N_1 = N_2$ is called a *1:1 transformer* or the *isolation transformer.*

However it is worth noting here that the same transformer can be made to work as a step up or step down transformer, depending upon which winding N_1 or N_2 is connected to the supply and load. The choice of transformer construction usually depends upon the cost as similar characteristics can be obtained for both.

6.3 Principle of Transformer

It works on the principle of electromagnetic induction. i.e. an emf is induced in a coil if it links with a changing flux. The primary winding P is connected to an alternating voltage source (Fig. 6.3), therefore an alternating current I_0 flows through N_1 turns and hence an alternating mmf (magneto motive force) sets up an alternating flux ϕ which is confined to high permeability iron core.

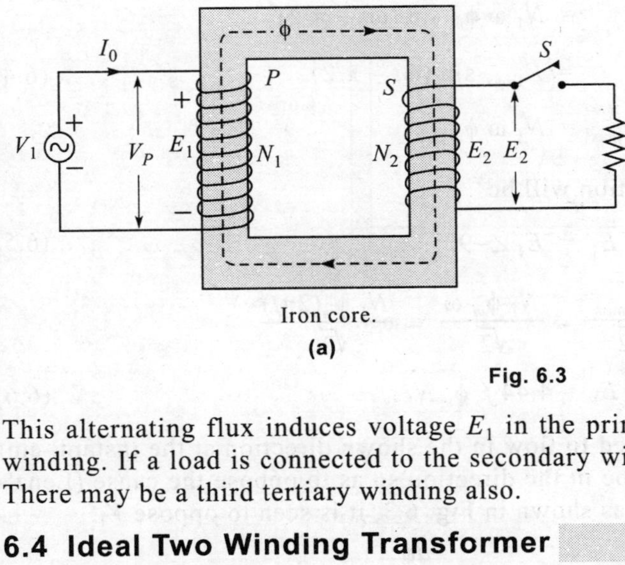

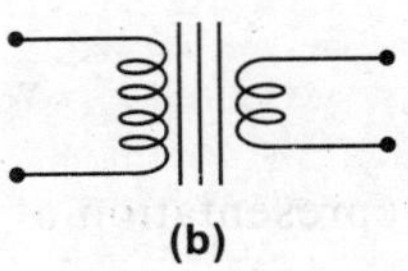

Fig. 6.3

This alternating flux induces voltage E_1 in the primary winding and E_2 in the secondary winding. If a load is connected to the secondary winding, current flows through the load. There may be a third tertiary winding also.

6.4 Ideal Two Winding Transformer

Initially we assume that the transformer is ideal and then the various factors are considered one by one.

Assumptions for an ideal transformer are :

(1) Winding resistances are negligible, and the windings are purely inductive.

(2) All the flux set up by the primary completely links with the secondary winding i.e. there is no leakage flux.

(3) The core losses are negligible i.e. the hysteresis and eddy current losses are absent.

(4) The core has constant permeability i.e. the magnetization curve is linear and there is no saturation of the core.

Let a voltage $\overline{V}_1$ be applied to the primary winding (sinusoidal supply). Then the current $\overline{I}_\phi$ will also be sinusoidal. The mmf and the flux ϕ will closely follow variations of flux i.e. ϕ is in time phase with $\overline{I}_0$ and varies sinusoidally. If $\overline{I}_0$ is zero, ϕ will also be zero and if $\overline{I}_0$ is maximum the flux (ϕ) will also be maximum and so on.

Let the sinusoidal variation in ϕ be given by

$$\phi = \phi_m \sin \omega t \quad \text{..... (6.1)}$$

$$\therefore \quad \overline{\phi} = \phi \angle 0^\circ \quad \text{..... (6.2)}$$

The emf e_1 volts induced in the primary N_1 turns by the alternating flux is given by

$$e_1 = -N_1 \frac{d\phi}{dt} \quad \text{..... (6.3)}$$

Substituting the value of ϕ from equation 6.1 we get,

$$e_1 = -N_1 \, \omega \, \phi_m \cos \omega t$$

$$= N_1 \, \omega \, \phi_m \sin (\omega t - \pi/2)$$

$$= E_{1max} \sin (\omega t - \pi/2) \quad \text{..... (6.4)}$$

$$\text{where,} \quad E_{1max} = N_1 \, \omega \, \phi_m$$

The vector representation of this equation will be

$$\overline{E}_1 = E_1 \angle -90^\circ \quad \text{..... (6.5)}$$

$$\text{And, rms value} \quad E_1 = \frac{E_{1max}}{\sqrt{2}} = \frac{N_1 \, \phi_m \, \omega}{\sqrt{2}} = \frac{N_1 \, \phi_m (2\pi f)}{\sqrt{2}}$$

$$E_1 = 4.44 \, f \, \phi_m N_1 \quad \text{..... (6.6)}$$

Refer Fig. 6.3, the current $\overline{I}_0$ is assumed to flow in the shown direction at the instant, emf induced in the primary turns N_1 must be in the direction so as to oppose the cause (Lenz's law). Therefore, the direction of E_1 is as shown in Fig. 6.3, it is seen to oppose V_1.

$$v_1 = -e_1 = N_1 \frac{d\phi}{dt}$$

$$\overline{V}_1 = -\overline{E}_1 \quad \text{..... (6.7)}$$

Emf in the secondary

$$e_2 = N_2 \frac{d\phi}{dt} = -N_2 \, \omega \, \phi_m \cos \omega t$$

$$= N_2 \, \omega \, \phi_m \sin (\omega t - \pi/2) \quad \text{..... (6.8)}$$

$$\overline{E}_2 = E_2 \angle -90^\circ \quad \text{..... (6.9)}$$

$$\text{where } E_2 = \frac{E_{2max}}{\sqrt{2}}$$

$$= 4.44 \text{ f } N_2 \phi_m \quad \text{..... (6.10)}$$

If V_1 = rms value of supply voltage

E_1 = rms value of primary induced voltage

then, $E_1 = V_1$ (transformer being ideal)

Similarly,

If V_2 = rms value of secondary terminal voltage

E_2 = rms value of secondary induced voltage

then, $E_2 = V_2$

where, V_2 is the secondary terminal voltage. Then from equation (6.4) and (6.8) we get

$$\frac{E_1}{E_2} = \frac{V_1}{V_2} = \frac{N_1}{N_2} \quad \text{..... (6.11)}$$

$$\frac{E_1}{N_1} = \frac{E_2}{N_2} = \sqrt{2}\, \pi \text{f } \phi_m = \text{emf per turn} \quad \text{..... (6.12)}$$

For an ideal transformer

$$\text{input } VA = \text{output } VA$$

$$V_1 \times I_1 = V_2 \times I_2 \quad \text{..... (6.13)}$$

$$\frac{V_1}{V_2} = \frac{I_2}{I_1} = \frac{N_1}{N_2} = \frac{1}{K} \quad \text{..... (6.14)}$$

where, K is the turns ratio or transformation ratio.

If $N_2 > N_1$ then $K > 1$ and it is a step-up transformation.

If $N_2 < N_1$ then $K < 1$ and it is a step-down transformation.

Solved Examples

Ex. 6.1 : The number of primary and secondary turns in a single phase transformer 450 and 45 respectively. If primary is connected to 2.2 kV, 50 Hz supply. Find the secondary voltage on no load.

Solution : Given : N_1 = primary turns = 450, N_2 = secondary turns = 45,

V_1 = primary voltage = 2.2 kV = 2200 volts.

Then,

$$\frac{V_2}{V_1} = \frac{N_2}{N_1}$$

$$\therefore \quad V_2 = \frac{45}{450} \times 2200$$

$$V_2 = \boxed{220 \text{ volts}}$$

Ex. 6.2 : A 3000/200 V, 50 Hz, 1 phase transformer is built on a core having effective cross-sectional area of 150 cm^2 and has 80 turns on low voltage winding.

Find **(a)** Maximum flux density in the care **(b)** Number of high voltage turns.

Solution : Given : $V_1 = 3000$ volts (high voltage), $V_2 = 200$ V (low voltage),

$$N_2 = 80,\ A = 150\ \text{cm}^2 = 0.015\ \text{m}^2,\ f = 50\ \text{Hz.}$$

To find : (a) Maximum flux density $= B_m = \frac{\phi_m}{A}$

$$\textbf{(a)}\quad V_2 = 4.44\ \text{f}\ \phi_m N_2$$

$$200 = 4.44 \times 50 \times \phi_m \times 80$$

$$\therefore\quad \phi_m = 0.011\ \text{wb}$$

$$\text{and}\quad B_m = \frac{\phi_m}{A} = \frac{0.011}{0.015}$$

$$B_m = \boxed{0.75\ \text{wb/m}^2}$$

(b) N_1 = Number of high voltage turns

$$\textbf{(b)}\quad \frac{V_1}{V_2} = \frac{N_1}{N_2}$$

$$\therefore\quad N_1 = \frac{V_1}{V_2} \times N_2 = \frac{3000}{200} \times 80$$

$$N_1 = \boxed{1200\ \text{turns}}$$

Ex. 6.3 : A 2300 volt primary winding of a 50 Hz transformer has 4800 turns. Calculate **(a)** max. value of flux in the core **(b)** the number of turns on the 230 V secondary windings.

Solution : Given : $V_1 = 2300;\ N_1 = 4800, f = 50$ Hz, $V_2 = 230$ V.

To find : ϕ_m and N_2

$$\textbf{(a)}\quad V_1 = 4.44 f \phi_m N_1$$

$$\therefore\quad \phi_m = \frac{2300}{4.44 \times 50 \times 4800}$$

$$\therefore\quad \phi_m = \boxed{2.16\ \text{mwb}}$$

$$\textbf{(b)}\quad \frac{N_2}{N_1} = \frac{V_2}{V_1}$$

$$\therefore\quad N_2 = \frac{230}{2300} \times 4800$$

$$N_2 = \boxed{480\ \text{turns}}$$

Ex. 6.4 : The maximum flux in the core of a 50 Hz transformer that has 1320 primary turns and 46 secondary turns is 45.04 mwb. Calculate the primary and secondary induced voltages.

Solution : Given : $f = 50$ Hz, $\phi_m = 45.04$ mwb $= 6 \times 10^{-3}$ wb $= 45.04 \times 10^{-3}$ wb,

$N_1 = 1320$, $N_2 = 46$.

To find : E_1 and E_2

$$E_1 = 4.44 \times 50 \times 45.04 \times 10^{-3} \times 1320 = \boxed{13198.5 \text{ volts}}$$

$$E_2 = 4.44 \, f \phi_m N_1$$

$$E_2 = 4.44 \times 50 \times 45.04 \times 10^{-3} \times 46 = \boxed{460 \text{ volts}}$$

6.5 Phasor Diagram of Ideal Transformer on No-Load

For drawing the phasor diagram refer equation 6.2, 6.5 and 6.9,

$\overline{\phi} = \phi \angle 0°$ [the reference vector]

$\overline{I_0} = I_0 \angle 0°$ [is in phase with $\overline{\phi}$ hence it will be along $\overline{\phi}$]

$\overline{E_1} = E_1 \angle -90°$ [will lag behind reference by 90°]

$\overline{E_2} = E_2 \angle -90°$ [will lag behind reference by 90°]

$\overline{V_1} = -\overline{E_1}$ [will be equal and opposite to $\overline{E_1}$]

All these vectors are drawn as in Fig. 6.4. Magnitudes of E_1 and E_2 will depend upon their turns ratio N_1/N_2.

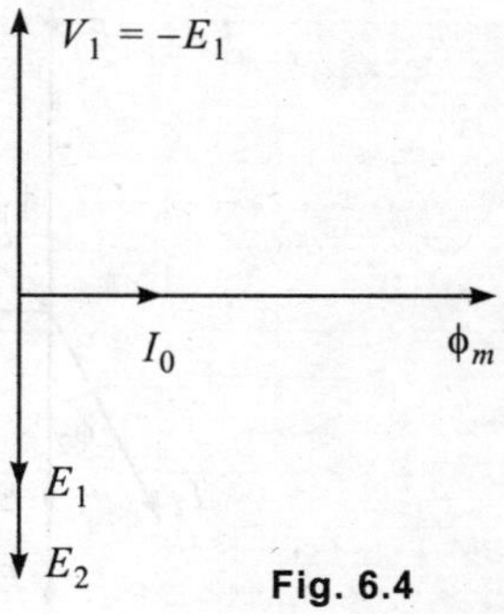

Fig. 6.4

6.6 Phasor Diagram of Ideal Transformer on Load

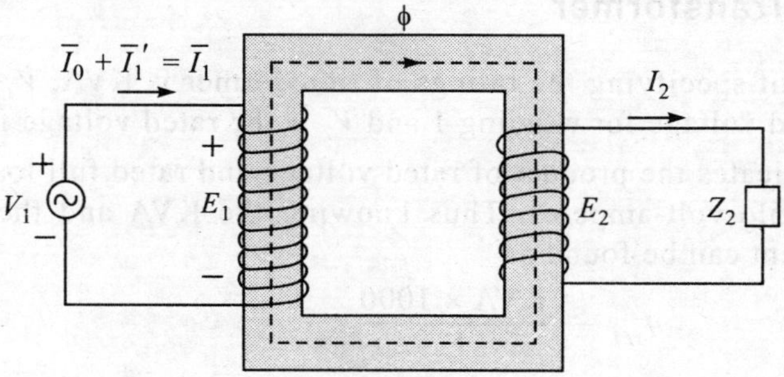

Fig. 6.5

If a load impedance of $\overline{Z_2}$ is connected across the secondary windings (Fig. 6.5).

Let ϕ_2 be the power factor angle of $\overline{Z}_2$. In the following case we have assumed the load power factor to be lagging. Hence $\overline{I}_2$ is drawn lagging behind $\overline{E}_2$ by angle ϕ_2 (Fig. 6.6). considering secondary winding resistance to be zero $\overline{E}_2 = \overline{V}_2$, a current $\overline{I}_2$ flows in the secondary. This current $\overline{I}_2$, according to Lenz's law, will oppose its cause. The cause here is the flux ϕ_m, hence $\overline{I}_2$ tries to reduce ϕ_m, as a result $\overline{E}_1$ also reduces. But, for an ideal transformer

$$\overline{V}_1 = -\overline{E}_1$$

If applied voltage is constant, E_1 will also be constant, hence, ϕ_m will also remain constant. This happens only if the primary draws more current $\overline{I}_1{}'$ from the source, in order to neutralize the demagnetizing effect of $\overline{I}_2$ i.e. compensating ampere-turns are drawn from the primary.

In this $\overline{I}_2$ manner causes the primary to draw more current $\overline{I}_1$ in addition to $\overline{I}_\phi$, such that

$$N_1\overline{I}_1 = -N_2\overline{I}_2 \quad \text{..... (6.15)}$$

$$\overline{I}_1 = -\frac{N_2}{N_1}\overline{I}_2 \quad \text{..... (6.16)}$$

Assuming $\overline{I}_2$ to lag behind $\overline{V}_2$ by a small angle ϕ_2, (Fig. 6.6) $\overline{I}_1{}'$ is drawn opposite to $\overline{I}_2$, such that it follows equation (6.16).

The primary current now is the vector sum of $\overline{I}_1{}'$ and $\overline{I}_0$ as shown in Fig. 6.6.

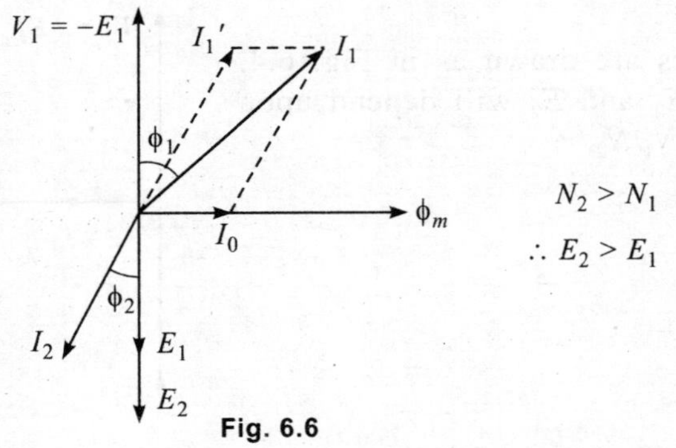

Fig. 6.6

6.7 Ratings of Transformer

A typical way of specifying the ratings of transformer is KVA, V_1/V_2, and frequency, where V_1 is the rated voltage for winding 1 and V_2 is the rated voltage for winding 2.

The KVA rating indicates the product of rated voltage and rated full load current (I_{fl}) of a given winding in kilo-volt-amperes. Thus knowing the KVA and the rated voltage the rated full load current can be found as

$$I_{1fl} = \frac{\text{KVA} \times 1000}{V_1} \quad \text{..... (6.16)}$$

$$I_{2fl} = \frac{\text{KVA} \times 1000}{V_2} \quad \text{..... (6.17)}$$

The rating of the transformer is specified in KVA and not KW. As we have seen above the transformer is subjected to varying loads with varying power factor the output power in kilo watts (kW = KVA × cos ϕ) can not be fixed . The maximum (rated) voltage is given and rated current can be calculated that can be allowed to pass through the transformer without exceeding the losses (heating)

Ex. 6.5 : A 40 KVA, 3300/240V, 50 Hz single phase transformer has 660 turns in the primary. Find **(a)** Secondary turns **(b)** Primary and secondary full load current.

Solution : Given : 40 KVA, $V_1 = 3300$ volts, $V_2 = 240$ V, $F = 50$ Hz, $N_1 = 660$ turns.

(a) N_2 = secondary turns

$$\frac{N_2}{N_1} = \frac{V_2}{V_1}$$

$$\therefore \quad N_2 = \frac{240}{3300} \times 660$$

$$N_2 = \boxed{48 \text{ turns}}$$

(b) I_{1fl} = primary full load current

I_{1fl} = secondary full load current

$$I_{1fl} = \frac{\text{KVA} \times 1000}{V_1} = \frac{40 \times 1000}{3300}$$

$$I_{1fl} = \boxed{12.12 \text{ Amp}}$$

$$I_{2fl} = \frac{\text{KVA} \times 1000}{V_2} = \frac{40 \times 1000}{240}$$

$$I_{2fl} = \boxed{166.67 \text{ Amp}}$$

Ex. 6.6 : A 3300/300 V, single phase 300 KVA transformer has 1100 primary turns. Find

(i) Transformation ratio

(ii) Secondary turns

(iii) Voltage per turn

(iv) Secondary current when it supplies 200 kW at 0.8 power factor lagging.

Solution : Given : $V_1 = 3300$ volts, $V_2 = 300$ volts, Rated KVA = 300 KVA

$$\cos\phi = 0.8 \text{ at } P = 200 \text{ kW} = 200 \times 1000 \text{ W.}$$

(i) Transformation ratio $= K = \frac{V_2}{V_1} = \frac{300}{3300} \quad K = \frac{1}{11}$

(ii) $$\frac{N_2}{N_1} = K$$

$$\therefore \quad N_2 = K.N_1 = \frac{1}{11} \times 1100$$

$$N_2 = \boxed{100 \text{ turns}}$$

(iii) $\quad$ Voltage per turn $= \dfrac{V_1}{N_1} = \dfrac{3300}{100}$

Voltage per turn $= \boxed{33}$

(iv) $\quad P = V_2 I_2 \cos \phi_2$

$$200 \times 10^3 = 300 \times I_2 \times 0.8$$

$$\therefore \quad I_2 = \boxed{833.33 \text{ A}}$$

6.8 Practical Transformer

An ideal transformer never exists, therefore phasor diagram of real transformer with various imperfections are considered one by one.

6.9 No-Load Vector Diagram of Practical Transformer

(a) Effect of Transformer Core Loss

The core loss consists of hysteresis and eddy-current loss. These losses are always present in the ferromagnetic core of the transformer, since transformer is an ac operated device. When the transformer is under no load condition, the primary current I_0 is not purely inductive i.e. it does not lag behind the applied voltage V_1 by 90° but slightly less than 90° (ϕ_0) as the primary current has to supply **(i)** core losses or the iron losses and **(ii)** a very small amount of copper losses.

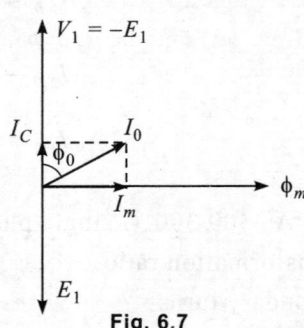

Hence, the no load primary current $\overline{I}_0$ can be resolved into two components (Fig. 6.7) .

In phase with V_1, active or the working component, also called the *core loss component* (I_C) because it mainly supplies the iron loss or the core loss.

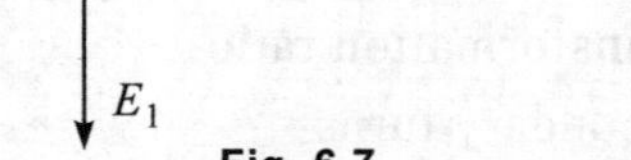

Fig. 6.7

$$I_C = I_0 \cos \phi_0 \qquad \text{..... (6.19)}$$

Other component is in quadrature with V_1, known as the magnetizing component (I_m), as it mainly produces the alternating flux in the core.

$$I_m = I_0 \sin \phi_0 \qquad \text{..... (6.20)}$$

(b) Effect of Transformer Resistance

If the winding resistance is considered then, $\overline{V}_1 \neq -\overline{E}_1$ considering the drop in the resistance. Let $-\overline{E}_1 = \overline{V}_1'$. The winding resistance can now be accounted for by adding $r_1 \overline{I}_0$, drawn parallel to $\overline{I}_0$ at the head of $\overline{V}_1'$ (Fig. 6.8).

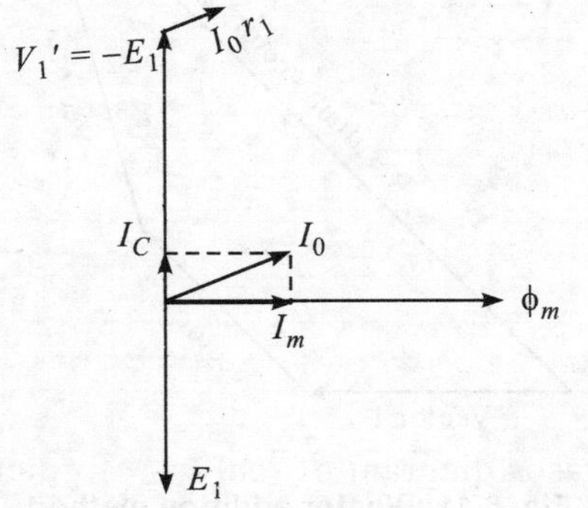

Fig. 6.8

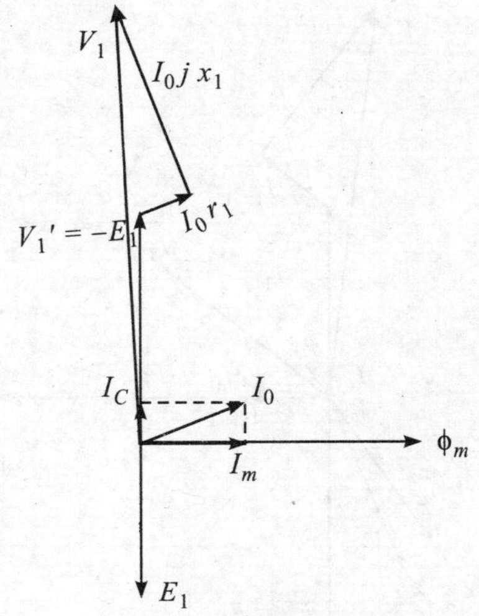

Fig. 6.9

(c) Effect of Leakage Flux

Similar to electric potential difference a magnetic potential difference is necessary for the establishment of flux. This potential difference establishes mutual flux linking with both the windings as well as primary leakage flux which does not link with the secondary winding and exists mainly in the air and it induces emf $E_{x1} = jx_1 I_0$, where x_1 is called as *primary leakage reactance* and E_{x1} leads $I_0 r_1$ by 90° (Fig. 6.9), x_1 is a fictitious quantity merely introduced to represent the effect of primary leakage flux.

The total voltage drop in primary at no load is

$$\overline{I}_0(r_1 + jx_1) = \overline{I}_0 \overline{Z}_1 \qquad ..... (6.21)$$

where, $\overline{Z}_1$ = primary leakage impedance.

The applied voltage is the vector sum of $\overline{V}_1'$ and $\overline{I}_0 \overline{Z}_1$ (i.e. $\overline{I}_0 r_1 + \overline{I}_0 j x_1$).

6.10 Transformer Vector Diagram Under Load Conditions

The vector diagram is considered for the various kinds of load viz: lagging power factor load, unity power factor load and the leading power factor load. In all the cases we start with Fig 6.9 as the reference.

(a) Lagging Power Factor Load

(i) When the load is connected across the secondary (refer Fig. 6.5) current $\overline{I}_2$ starts flowing. Assuming inductive load, the current $\overline{I}_2$ lags behind $\overline{V}_2$ by an angle ϕ_2.

(ii) At first $\overline{V}_2$ is drawn lagging behind $\overline{E}_2$, considering the effect of secondary winding resistance r_2 and the leakage reactance x_2, similar to the primary case.

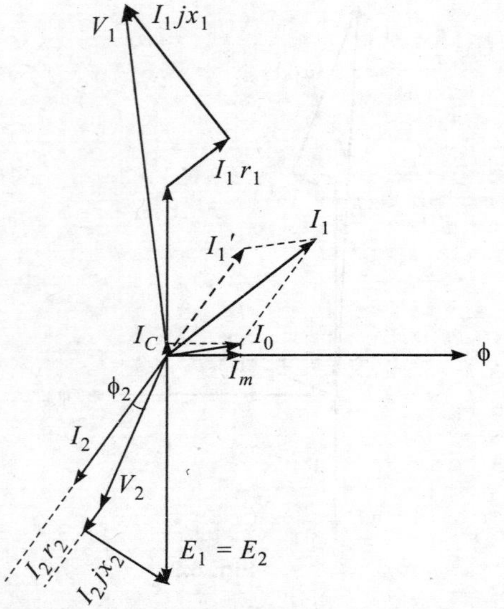

Fig. 6.10 : Vector diagram for lagging p.f. load.

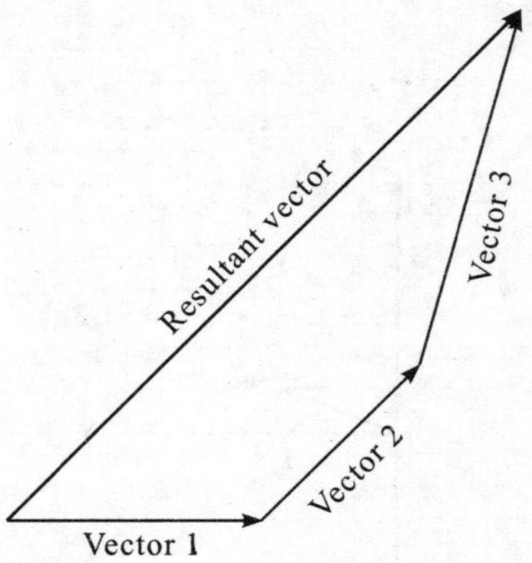

Fig. 6.11 : Vector addition method.

(iii) Refer Fig. 6.10, as discussed earlier, current $\overline{I}_1'$ is drawn from primary (refer Fig. 6.6). Primary current $\overline{I}_1$ is the vector sum of $\overline{I}_0$ and $\overline{I}_1'$.

(iv) Draw $\overline{I}_1 r_1$ parallel to $\overline{I}_1$ and at the head of vector $\overline{V}_1'$.

(v) Perpendicular to this vector $j\overline{I}_1 x_1$ is drawn.

(vi) Vector sum of $\overline{V}_1'$, $\overline{I}_1 r_1$ and $j\overline{I}_1 x_1$ is the applied voltage $\overline{V}_1$ (remember the vector addition method where if there are more than 2 vectors, say 3, then they can be added by drawing the tail of vector 2 at the head of 1, tail of vector 3 at the head of 2, the resultant vector is obtained by joining the tail of vector 1 and head of vector 3 as in Fig. 6.11)

(vii) In order to indicate $\overline{I}_2 r_2$ and $j\overline{I}_2 x_2$, draw a dotted line at the head of $\overline{V}_2$ parallel to $\overline{I}_2$.

(viii) Then drop a perpendicular from $\overline{E}_2$ on this line (at B). The component parallel to $\overline{I}_2$ is $\overline{I}_2 r_2$ and that perpendicular to $\overline{I}_2$ is $j\overline{I}_2\, x_2$.

(b) Unity Power Factor Load

For unity power factor load the current $\overline{I}_2$ is in phase with $\overline{V}_2$ i.e. along $\overline{V}_2$. Following all the above steps from (ii) to (viii) as in the case of lagging power factor load we get the vector diagram as in Fig. 6.12(a).

(c) Leading Power Factor Load

For a leading power factor load $\overline{I}_2$ will lead $\overline{V}_2$ (towards right hand side of $\overline{V}_2$ as in Fig. 6.12(b). Again following steps (ii) to (viii) above we will get the vector diagram for leading power factor load. Here we have considered highly capacitive load.

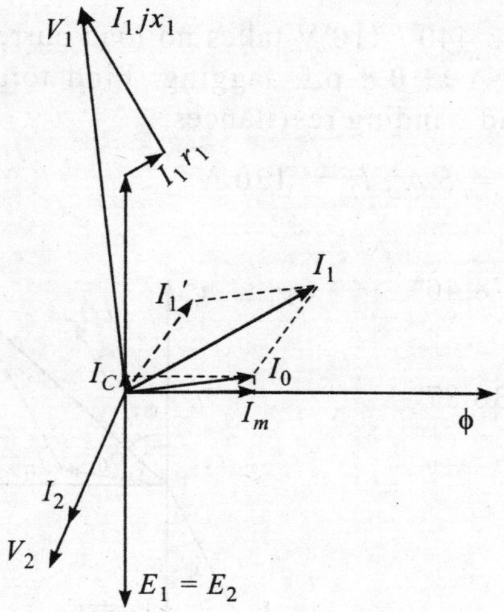

Fig. 6.12(a) : Vector diagram for UPF load.

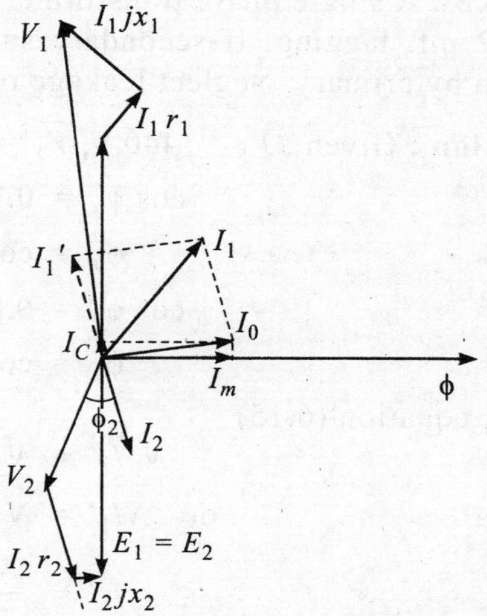

Fig. 6.12(b) : Vector diagram for leading PF load.

Ex. 6.7 : A single phase transformer with 3300/300 V rating gives 0.6 A and 60 W as ammeter and watt meter readings when supply is given to the low voltage winding and high voltage winding is kept open.

Find : **(i)** Power factor of no-load current,

(ii) Magnetizing component and

(iii) Iron loss component.

Solution : Given : $V_{h.v.} = 3300$ V, $V_{l.v.} = 300$ V

On low voltage side ; (with h.v. open)

$$I_0 = 0.6 \text{ A}$$

$$W_0 = 60 \text{ W}$$

(i) $$W_0 = V_0 I_0 \cos \phi_0$$

$$\therefore \quad \cos \phi_0 = \frac{W_0}{V_0 I_0} = \frac{60}{300 \times 0.6} = 0.33$$

p.f. of no load current = 0.33

$$\therefore \quad \phi_0 = \boxed{70.53^\circ}$$

(ii) Magnetizing current $= I_m = I_0 \sin \phi_0$

$$= 0.6 \times \sin 70.53^\circ$$

$$I_m = \boxed{0.56 \text{ A}}$$

(iii) Iron loss component $= I_c = I_0 \cos \phi_0 = 0.6 \times 0.33$

$$I_c = \boxed{0.198 \text{ Amp}}$$

Ex. 6.8 : A single phase transformer with a ratio 440 / 110 V takes no load current of 5 A at 0.2 p.f. lagging. If secondary supplies 120 A at 0.8 p.f. lagging. Find total current drawn by primary. Neglect leakage reactance and winding resistances.

Solution : Given : $V_1 = 440$ V, $V_2 = 110$ V, $I_0 = 5$ A, $I_2 = 120$ A

$$\cos\phi_0 = 0.2 \text{ (lagging)}$$
$$\phi_0 = \cos^{-1} 0.2 = 78.46^\circ$$
$$\cos\phi_2 = 0.8 \text{ (lagging)}$$
$$\phi_2 = \cos^{-1} 0.8 = 36.87^\circ$$

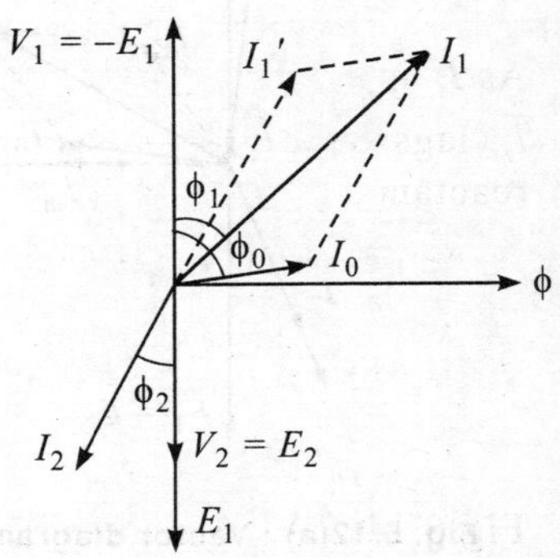

Refer equation (6.15)

$$-N_1 \overline{I_1}' = N_2 \overline{I_2}$$

or $\quad NI_1' = N_2 I_2$

$$\therefore \quad I_1' = \frac{N_2 I_2}{N_1} = \frac{V_2}{V_1} I_1$$

$$I_1' = \frac{110}{440} \times 120 = 30 \text{ A}$$

From Fig. 6.6,

$$\overline{I_1} = \overline{I_0} + \overline{I_1} = I_0 \angle -\phi_0 + I_1' \angle -\phi_2$$
$$= 5 \angle -78.46^\circ + 30 \angle -36.87^\circ$$
$$\overline{I_1} = \boxed{33.9 \angle -42.49^\circ}$$

6.11 Equivalent Circuit of a Transformer

The basic transformer circuit can be resolved into an equivalent circuit in which the resistance and leakage reactance of the transformer are imagined to be external to the winding and whose only function is to transform the voltage.

The equivalent circuit can be drawn if we know the equations describing its behaviour. From the discussion so far, we know that

$$\overline{V_1} = \overline{V_1}' + \overline{I_1}(r_1 + jx_1) \quad ..... (6.22)$$

$$\overline{E_2} = \overline{V_2} + \overline{I_2}(r_2 + jx_2) \quad ..... (6.23)$$

Where, $(r + jx)$ represents the leakage impedances. The winding resistance (r_1 and r_2) and leakage reactances (x_1 and x_2)are usually small.

$\overline{V_1}'$ is treated as voltage drop, the direction of $\overline{I_1}$, magnitude of $\overline{V_1}$ does not change appreciably from no load to full load (Fig. 6.13).

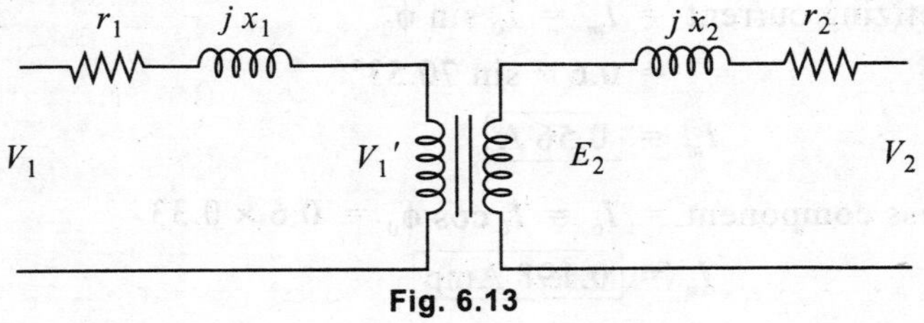

Fig. 6.13

Now, primary current $\overline{I}_1$ consists of two components,

(i) $\overline{I}_1'$ is the load component$_1$ and counteracts the secondary mmf completely.

(ii) $\overline{I}_0$, the exciting current which is further composed of $\overline{I}_C$ and $\overline{I}_m$. $\overline{I}_C$ is in phase with $\overline{V}_1'$.

A resistance R_C in parallel with $\overline{V}_1'$ represents the core loss component,

$$R_C = \frac{V_1'}{I_C} \qquad \text{..... (6.24)}$$

As I_C is small R_C has a large value.

$\overline{I}_m$ lags behind $\overline{V}_1'$ by 90° and therefore can be represented in the equivalent circuit by reactance X_ϕ (this value is also very large as $\overline{I}_m$ is small), such that

$$X_\phi = \frac{V_1'}{I_m} \qquad \text{..... (6.25)}$$

where, R_C = core loss resistance, and

X_ϕ = magnetizing reactance.

Fig 6.14 shows the complete equivalent circuit of a transformer.

Note that, if no load is connected to the secondary terminals of the transformer, I_2 will be zero. Hence, I_1 will also be zero, but I_0 will always be present. Hence, under no load condition a small amount of current (2 - 5% of full load current) will still be drawn from the source and core loss continues to occur.

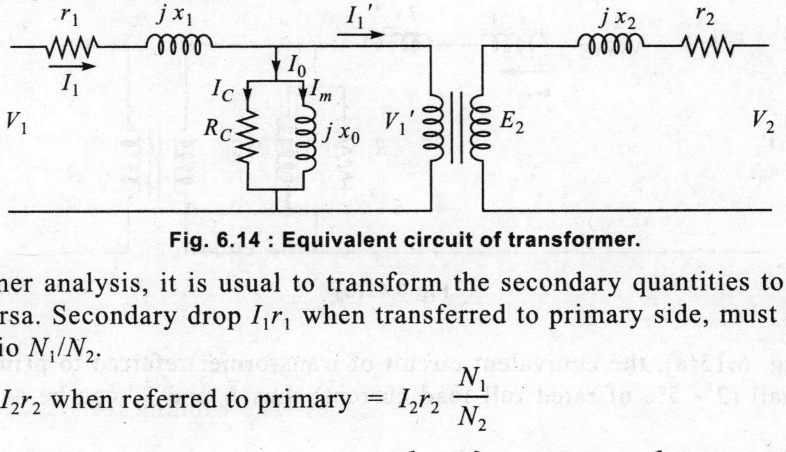

Fig. 6.14 : Equivalent circuit of transformer.

In transformer analysis, it is usual to transform the secondary quantities to primary side and vice-versa. Secondary drop $I_1 r_1$ when transferred to primary side, must be multiplied by turns ratio N_1/N_2.

$$\therefore \quad I_2 r_2 \text{ when referred to primary} = I_2 r_2 \frac{N_1}{N_2}$$

$$= \left(I_1 \frac{N_1}{N_2}\right) r_2 \frac{N_1}{N_2} \quad \text{as} \quad \left(I_2 = I_1 \frac{N_1}{N_2}\right)$$

$$= I_1 r_2 \left[\frac{N_1}{N_2}\right]^2$$

$$= I_1 r_2'$$

$$\text{where} \quad r_2' = r_2 \left[\left(\frac{N_1}{N_2}\right)^2\right] \qquad \text{..... (6.26)}$$

$$\text{Similarly,} \quad I_2 x_2 \frac{N_1}{N_2} = I_1 x_2 \left[\left(\frac{N_1}{N_2}\right)^2\right] = I_1 x_2'$$

$$\text{and} \quad x_2' = x_2 \left[\left(\frac{N_1}{N_2}\right)^2\right] \qquad \text{..... (6.27)}$$

Here, r_2' and x_2' are the secondary resistance and reactance referred to primary refer Fig.6.15(a).

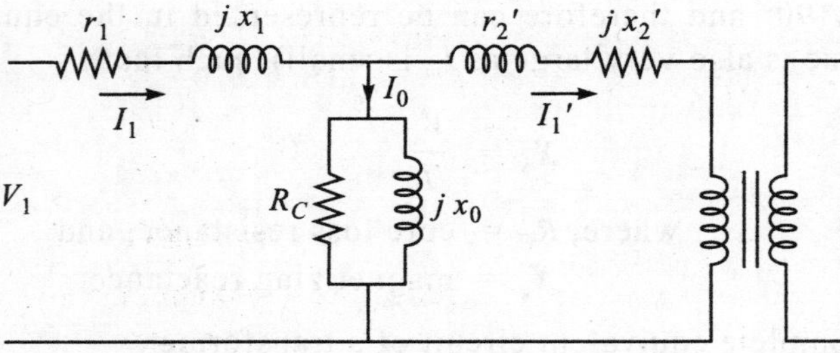

Fig 6.15(a) : E quivalent circuit referred to primary.

6.11.1 Approximate Equivalent Circuit of Transformer

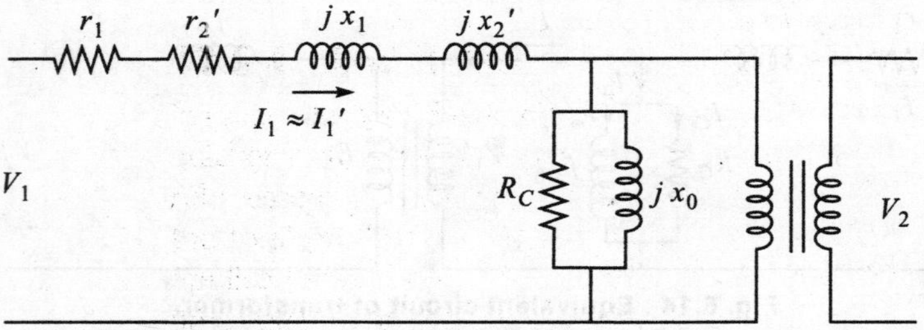

Fig 6.15(b)

Refer Fig. 6.15(a), the equivalent circuit of transformer referred to primary, current $\bar{I}_0$ is very small (2 - 5% of rated full load current) thus $\bar{I}_1$ and $\bar{I}_1'$ can be assumed to be equal.

$$\bar{I}_1 = \bar{I}_1' \qquad \text{..... (6.28)}$$

So, as r_1 and r_2' carry equal currents can be assumed to be on the same side as in Fig. 6.15(b).

$$\text{Now,} \quad r_1 + r_2 = R_1 \qquad \text{..... (6.29)}$$

$$\text{and} \quad x_1 + x_2 = X_1 \qquad \text{..... (6.30)}$$

whereR_1 and X_1 are the total resistance and reactance referred to primary [as shown in fig. 6.15(c)]

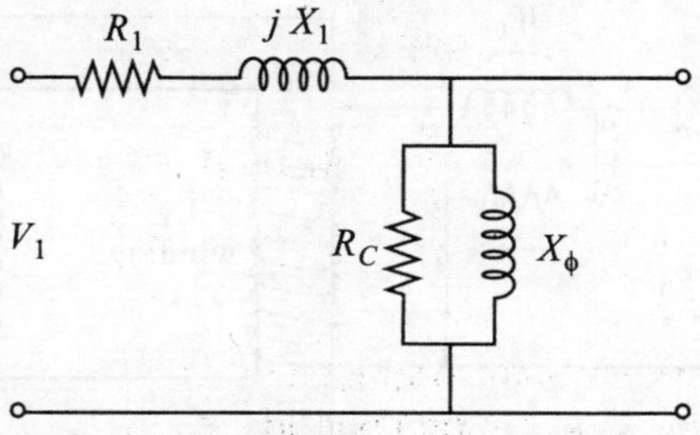

Fig 6.15(c) : Approximate equivalent circuit.

A further approximate equivalent circuit can be obtained by assuming I_0 to be negligible i.e. Fig. 6.15(d). But normally we would consider the approximate equivalent circuit of Fig. 6.15(c) for further reference.

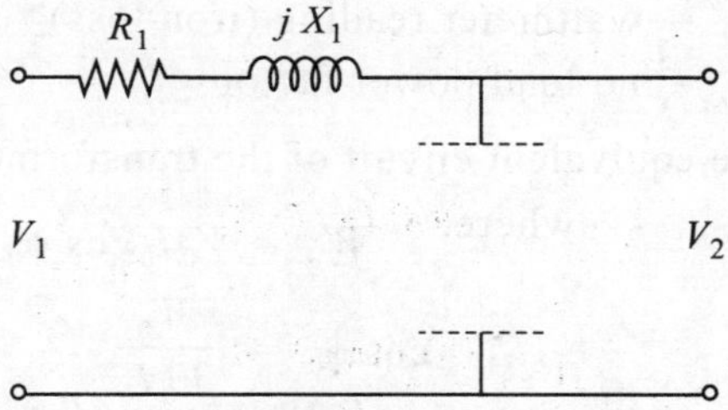

Fig 6.15(d)

6.12 Open Circuit and Short Circuit Test on Transformer

The no load test and the short circuit test help to determine:

(i) the parameters of equivalent circuit,

(ii) voltage regulation, and

(iii) the efficiency of the transformer.

The power required during these tests is equal to the appropriate power loss occurring in the transformer.

(a) Open Circuit (No Load) Test

The high voltage side of the transformer is kept open and rated voltage is applied to the primary winding. The circuit connection is as shown in Fig. 6.16. As the secondary winding is kept open very little current (2 - 5% of full load rated current) is drawn from the source i.e. the no load current $\overline{I_0}$. The ammeter measures this current, The wattmeter measures the losses occurring during the open circuit or no load. As the current is small the copper losses are very small as compared to full load copper losses and hence it can be neglected and the wattmeter thus reads only the iron losses.

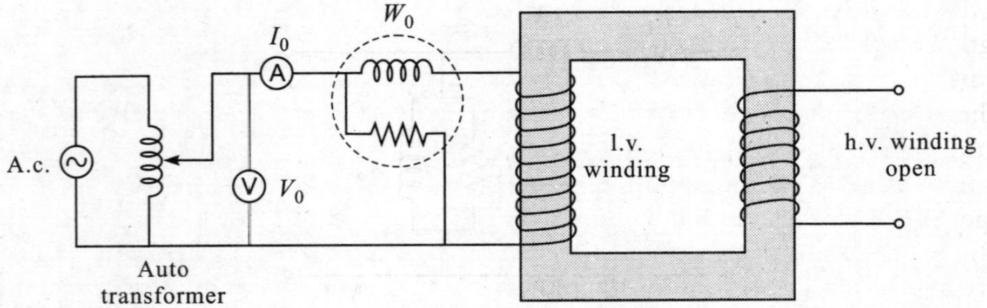

Fig 6.16 : Open circuit test.

Let, V_0 = applied voltage during open circuit test

I_0 = no load current in the primary winding

W_0 = wattmeter reading (iron loss)

ϕ_0 = no load power factor

Then, Fig. 6.17 shows the equivalent circuit of the transformer during open circuit test

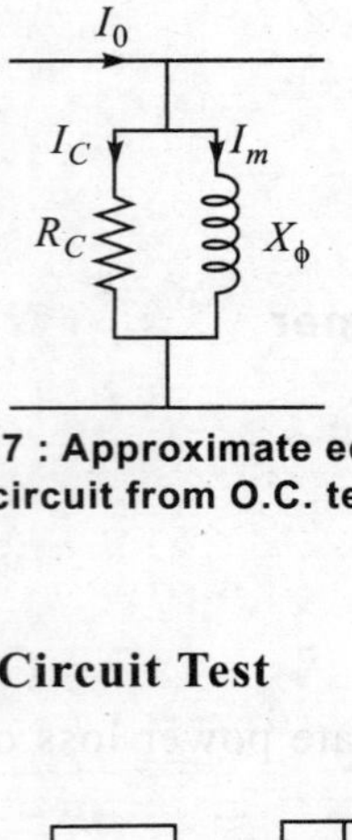

Fig. 6.17 : Approximate equivalent circuit from O.C. test

where, $W_0 = V_0 I_0 \cos \phi_0$

$$\therefore \quad \cos \phi_0 = \frac{W_0}{V_0 I_0} \quad \text{..... (6.31)}$$

$$I_C = I_0 \cos \phi_0 \quad \text{..... (6.32)}$$

$$I_m = I_0 \sin \phi_0 \quad \text{..... (6.33)}$$

$$R_C = \frac{V_0}{I_C} \quad \text{..... (6.34)}$$

and $$X_\phi = \frac{V_0}{I_m} \quad \text{..... (6.35)}$$

(b) Short Circuit Test

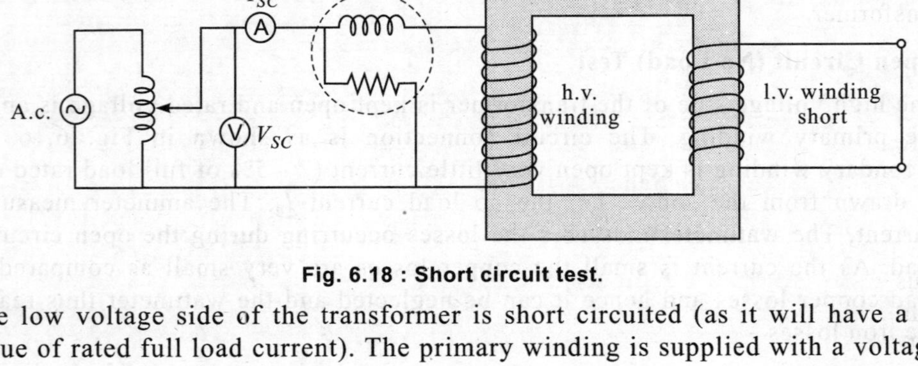

Fig. 6.18 : Short circuit test.

The low voltage side of the transformer is short circuited (as it will have a higher value of rated full load current). The primary winding is supplied with a voltage that will circulate rated current in the primary winding (Fig. 6.18) shows the circuit diagram for short circuit test). During this condition as the secondary is short circuited, very low voltage (5 - 10% of rated value) will give full load rated current in the transformer. The voltmeter measures the applied voltage, ammeter measures the rated current in the winding and the wattmeter measures the losses occurring in the transformer. As the applied voltage is very low, the iron losses which are proportional to the applied voltage, are also low and hence are neglected and the wattmeter measures only the copper losses occurring in both the windings. The equivalent circuit during the short circuit test is as shown in Fig. 6.19. Here, R_2 and X_2 are the total resistance and reactance referred to h.v. side.

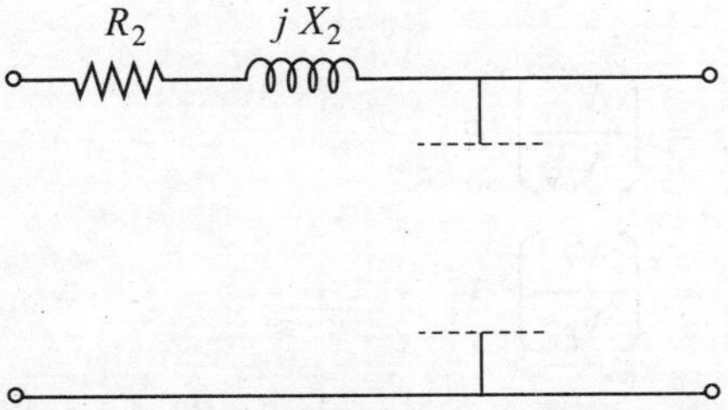

Fig. 6.19 : Approximate equivalent circuit from S.C. test.

Let, V_{SC} = applied voltage during short circuit test

I_{SC} = rated current in the high voltage winding

W_{SC} = wattmeter reading (copper losses)

ϕ_{SC} = power factor of the circuit during short circuit.

Then,

$$R_2 = r_1' + r_2 \quad \text{..... (6.36)}$$

where, r_2 = resistance of h.v. winding

r_1' = resistance of l.v. winding referred to h.v. side

$$R_2 = \frac{W_{SC}}{I_{SC}} \quad \text{..... (6.37)}$$

$$Z_2 = \frac{V_{SC}}{I_{SC}} \quad \text{..... (6.38)}$$

$$X_2 = x_1' + x_2 \quad \text{..... (6.39)}$$

Here, x_2 = leakage reactance of h.v. winding

x_1' = leakage reactance of l.v. winding referred to h.v. side

$$X_2 = \sqrt{Z_1^2 - R_2^2} \quad \text{..... (6.40)}$$

Thus from the open circuit test we get R_c and X_ϕ referred to low voltage side and from the short circuit test we get R_2 and X_2 referred to high voltage side as in Fig. 6.20.

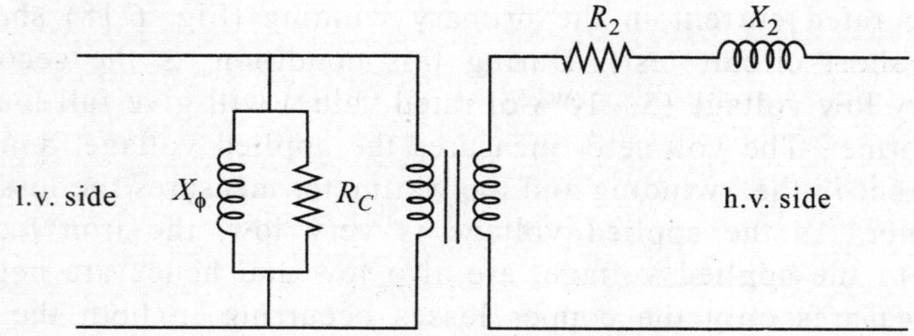

Fig. 6.20 : Equivalent circuit from O.C./S.C. test.

The equivalent circuit can now be calculated referred to h.v. side by the following equations.

$$R_{C2} = \left(\frac{N_{h.v.}}{N_{l.v}}\right)^2 R_C \quad \text{..... (6.41)}$$

$$X_{\phi 2} = \left(\frac{N_{h.v.}}{N_{l.v}}\right)^2 X_\phi \quad \text{..... (6.42)}$$

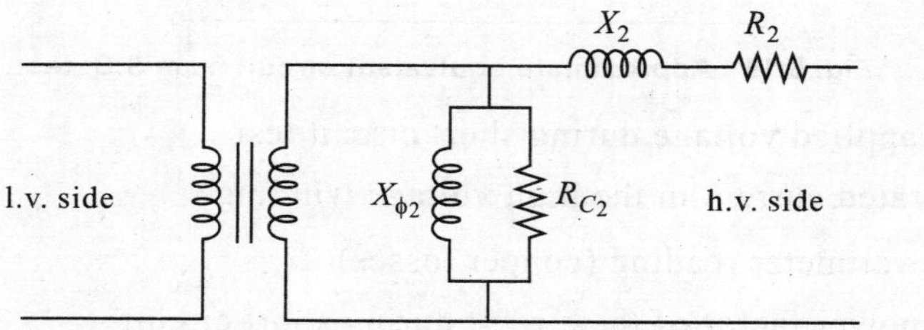

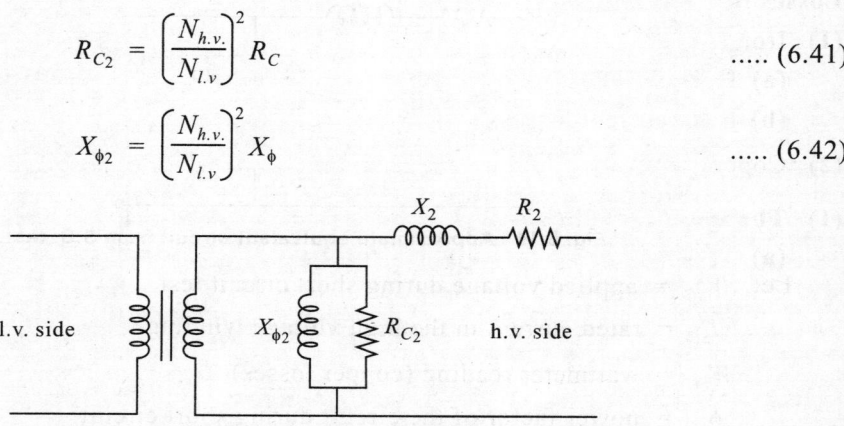

Fig. 6.21 : Equivalent circuit referred to h.v. side.

Similarly, the equivalent circuit referred to l.v. side can de drawn as in Fig. 6.22, where

$$R_1 = \left(\frac{N_{l.v.}}{N_{h.v}}\right)^2 R_2 \quad \text{..... (6.43)}$$

$$R_1 = \left(\frac{N_{l.v.}}{N_{h.v}}\right)^2 X_2 \quad \text{..... (6.44)}$$

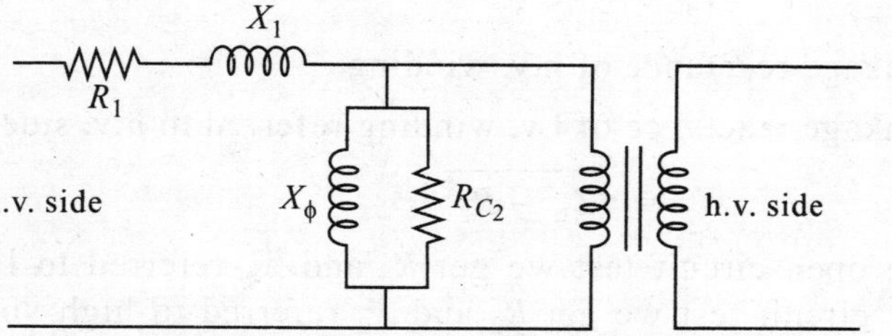

Fig. 6.22 : Equivalent circuit referred to l.v. side.

6.13 Losses and Efficiency of a Transformer

The transformer is a static device, therefore there are no friction and windage losses in it. Therefore, the efficiency of a transformer is very high compared to that of rotating machine. It ranges between 97 - 99% approximately.

The losses taking place in the transformer can be divided into two groups. One is loss due to varying flux which takes place in the iron part of the transformer core. These are dependent the supply frequency and the applied voltage. These losses are the hysteresis loss and the eddy-current loss. These losses are also called the *core loss* or the *iron loss*, as the core losses occur in core made of iron. The other loss is due to current in the windings called the *copper loss*.

Losses in a Transformer

(1) Iron loss

- **(a)** Hysteresis loss
- **(b)** Eddy current loss

(2) Copper loss.

(1) The Iron Losses

(a) The hysteresis loss : Since the flux in the transformer core is alternating, the diapoles of magnetic material are vibrating with the supply frequency *trying to keep up with the direction of flux. This accounts to power loss called hysteresis loss* (W_h). This loss is given by

$$W_h = K_h f B_{max}^{1.6} \quad \text{..... (6.45)}$$

where K_h is a hysteresis constant, f is the supply frequency and B_{max} is the max flux density in the core (which depends upon the supply voltage).

(b) The eddy current loss : If the transformer core was not made of laminations and it was of a solid iron piece, then when this core is subjected to changing flux, emf would be induced in it and as the cross section of this core would be large the resistance ($R = \rho_1/A$) would be negligible. Thus even a small induced voltage would give rise to large circulating currents in the core called the eddy currents. In order to increase the resistance, area of cross-section of core has to be increased. This is done by laminating the core and insulating each lamination by varnish. This reduces the eddy current loss (W_e).This eddy current loss is given

$$W_e = K_e f^2 B_{max}^2 \quad \text{..... (6.46)}$$

where K_e is a constant. These two, the hysteresis and eddy current losses, are voltage dependent.

Note : The input power under no load condition is the total iron loss (W_i) given by

$$W_i = W_h + W_e \quad \text{..... (6.47)}$$

As the transformer works at fixed rated voltage from no load to full load iron losses remain constant. Hence, the iron losses are also called the *constant losses*.

(2) The Copper Loss

The second type of loss takes place due to current flowing in the winding and is known as the copper loss or the I^2R. The total copper losses in the transformer (W_{cu}) can be given by

$$W_{cu} = I_1^2 R_1 \quad ..... (6.48)$$

$$W_{cu} = I_2^2 R_2 \quad ..... (6.49)$$

where, R_1 is the total winding resistance referred to primary and R_2 is the total winding resistance referred to secondary. This loss depends upon the square of the current and the current depends upon the load. As the load varies with the load, copper loss is also called the *variable loss*.

While the iron losses remain constant if the supply voltage and frequency remains constant irrespective of the change in load, the copper losses vary from no load to full load as the current changes. At no load the current is very small as compared to the full load value, the copper losses are assumed to be negligible. The only loss occurring during the no load condition is the iron loss.

$$\text{Efficiency} = \eta = \frac{\text{output}}{\text{input}} \quad ..... (6.50)$$

$$= \frac{\text{output}}{\text{output} + \text{losses}} \quad ..... (6.51)$$

$$= \frac{\text{output}}{\text{output} + \text{iron loss} + \text{cu loss}} \quad ..... (6.52)$$

$$\text{Full load power output} = \text{KVA}_{\text{rated}} \times \cos\phi \times 1000 \quad ..... (6.53)$$

$$\text{Full load copper loss} = W_{cu} = I_2^2 R_2$$

$$\text{At any other load} = \alpha \text{ times full load current } I_2$$

$$\text{Load KVA} = \alpha\ \text{KVA}_{\text{rated}} \quad ..... (6.54)$$

$$\text{Copper loss} = \alpha^2 W_{cu} \quad ..... (6.55)$$

$$\eta = \frac{\alpha\ \text{KVA} \cos\phi_2 \times 1000}{\alpha\ \text{KVA} \cos\phi_2 \times 1000 + W_i + \alpha^2 W_{cu}} \quad ..... (6.56)$$

Note : For full load $\alpha = 1$, and W_{Cu} is as given from equation (6.49).

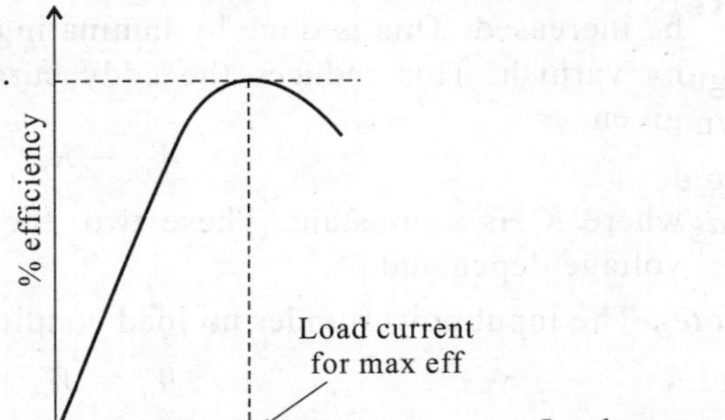

Fig. 6.23 : Efficiency curve.

The efficiency curve of a transformer is as shown in Fig. 6.20. The condition for maximum efficiency can be found. For maximum efficiency the denominator term of equation (6.56) should be minimum, the voltage remaining constant,

$$\frac{d}{dI_2}\left(V_2 \cos\phi_2 + \frac{W_i}{I_2} I_2 + R_2\right) = 0$$

$$\text{or} \quad \frac{-W_i}{I_2^2} + R_2 = 0$$

$$\text{or} \quad I_2^2 R_2 = W_i \qquad \text{..... (6.57)}$$

i.e. for maximum efficiency

Copper loss = Iron loss

6.14 Efficiency Calculation Using O.C./S.C. Test Results

The wattmeter reading in the open circuit test W_0, indicates the no load losses in the transformer. During this test the current in the transformer is very less (I_0 is 2-5% of full load rated current), hence copper losses are considered negligible and the wattmeter indicates only iron losses.

$$W_0 = W_i \qquad \text{..... (6.58)}$$

During the short circuit test, the wattmeter reading is W_{SC}. This test is performed at rated full load current and low voltage. The iron losses are proportional to applied voltage, the iron losses are considered negligible and wattmeter indicates just the full load copper losses.

$$W_{SC} = W_{cu\,fl} \qquad \text{..... (6.59)}$$

The efficiency calculation from O.C./S.C. test results will be

$$\eta = \frac{\alpha \text{ KVA} \cos\phi_2 \times 1000}{\alpha \text{ KVA} \cos\phi_2 \times 1000 + W_0 + \alpha^2 W_{SC}} \qquad \text{..... (6.60)}$$

If the short circuit test is done at full load rated current take $\alpha = 1$ otherwise calculate α.

6.15 Regulation

Regulation is defined as the percentage change in terminal voltage when a given load is thrown off.

It is also defined as *the change in terminal voltage from no load to full load* expressed as *percentage of no load voltage.*

$$\%\ \text{regulation} = \frac{V_{NL} - V_{FL}}{V_{NL}} \times 100 \qquad \text{..... (6.61)}$$

where, V_{NL} = no load terminal voltage

V_{NL} = full load terminal voltage

Refer Fig. 6.21, it is a part of vector diagram at the output. From here regulation can be calculated as follows.

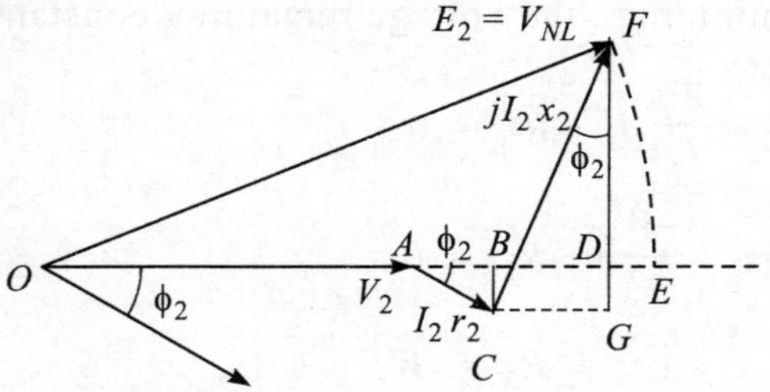

Fig. 6.24 : Vector diagram for lagging pf load.

$OF = E_2 =$ no load secondary terminal voltage

$OA = V_2 =$ secondary terminal voltage at any load

$AC = I_2 R_2$

$CF = I_2 X_2$

Draw an arc with radius OF i.e. FE

Consider $OE \approx OD = E_2$

From Fig. 6.24, we can write

$$AB = AC \cos \phi_2 = I_2 R_2 \cos \phi_2$$

$$BD = CG = CF \sin \phi_2 = I_2 X_2 \sin \phi_2$$

Thus from above equations we get,

$$OD = OA + AB + BD$$

$$E_2 = V_2 + I_2 R_2 \cos \phi_2 + I_2 X_2 \sin \phi_2 \quad \text{..... (6.62)}$$

$$E_2 - V_2 = I_2 R_2 \cos \phi_2 + I_2 X_2 \sin \phi_2 \quad \text{..... (6.63)}$$

$$\therefore \frac{E_2 - V_2}{E_2} \times 100 = \frac{I_2 R_2 \cos \phi_2 + I_2 X_2 \sin \phi_2}{E_2} \times 100 = \text{\% regulation for lagging p.f. load} \quad \text{..... (6.64)}$$

For **leading power factor** load the regulation can be calculated as follows (refer Fig. 6.25)

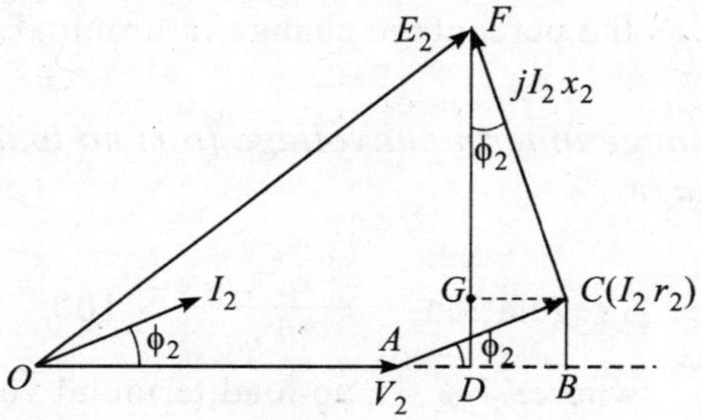

Fig. 6.25 : Vector diagram for leading pf load.

$$OA = V_2$$

I_2 leads V_2 by angle ϕ_2

$$OC = I_2 r_2 \text{ (is parallel to } \bar{I}_2\text{)}$$

$$\therefore AB = AC \cos\phi_2 = I_2 r_2 \cos\phi_2$$

$$CF = I_2 x_2$$

$$\therefore CG = CF \sin\phi_2 = I_2 x_2 \sin\phi_2$$

$$CG = BD$$

$$\therefore OD = OB - BD = OA + AB - BD$$

$$\therefore E_2 = V_2 + I_2 r_2 \cos\phi_2 - I_2 x_2 \sin\phi_2$$

$$E_2 - V_2 = I_2 r_2 \cos\phi_2 - I_2 x_2 \sin\phi_2$$

$$\% \text{ regulation} = \frac{E_2 - V_2}{E_2} \times 100$$

$$\% \text{ regulation for leading p.f. load} = \frac{I_2 R_2 \cos\phi_2 - I_2 X_2 \sin\phi_2}{E_2} \times 100 \quad \text{..... (6.65)}$$

Ex 6.9 : Obtain the approximate equivalent circuit of a 200/2000 V. 1-phase, 30 KVA transformer having following test results referred to l.v. side.

O.C. test (on l.v. side) : 200 V, 6.2 A, 360 watts

S.C. test (on h.v. side) : 75 V, 15A, 600 watts

Solution : Given : Rating: 30 KVA, 200/2000 V, transformer.

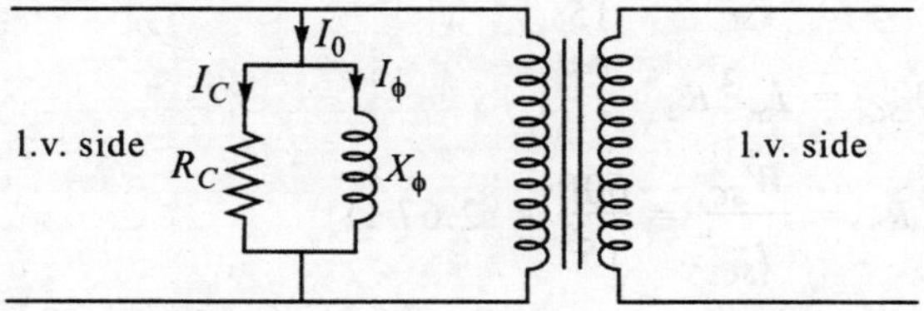

$$\therefore I_{LVfl} = \frac{\text{KVA}}{V_{LV}}$$

$$\frac{30 \times 1000}{2000} = 15 \text{ amp}$$

$$I_{LVfl} = \frac{30 \times 1000}{2000} = 15 \text{ amp}$$

O.C. test (on l.v. side)

$$V_0 = 200 \text{ V}, I_0 = 6.2 \text{ A}, W_0 = 360 \text{ watts}$$

$$W_0 = V_0 I_0 \cos\phi_0$$

$$\therefore \quad \phi_0 = \cos^{-1} \frac{W_0}{V_0 I_0} = \frac{360}{200 \times 6.2} = 73.12^\circ$$

$$I_C = I_0 \cos \phi_0 = 6.2 \times \cos 73.12^\circ$$

$$I_C = 1.8 \text{ amp}$$

$$I_m = I_0 \sin \phi_0 = 6.2 \sin 73.12^\circ = 5.93 \text{ amp}$$

$$R_C = \frac{V_0}{I_C} = \frac{200}{1.8} = 111.11\ \Omega$$

$$R_C = \boxed{111.11\ \Omega}$$

$$X_\phi = \frac{V_C}{I_m} = \frac{200}{5.93} = 33.72\ \Omega$$

$$X_\phi = \boxed{33.72\ \Omega}$$

S.C. test (on h.v. side) : The test is carried out at 15 A which is also the rated tall load current (I_{hvfl} = 15 A)

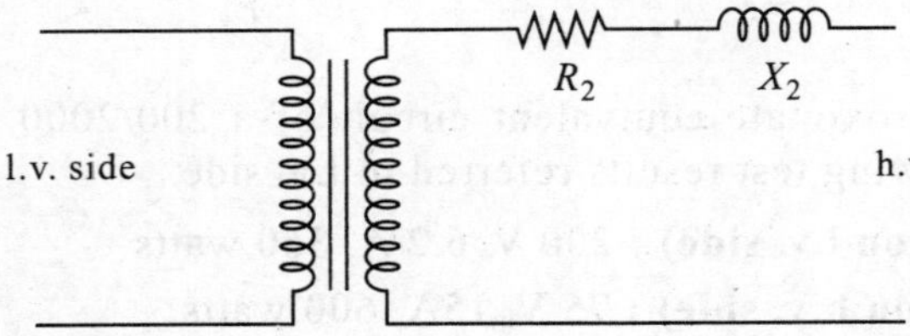

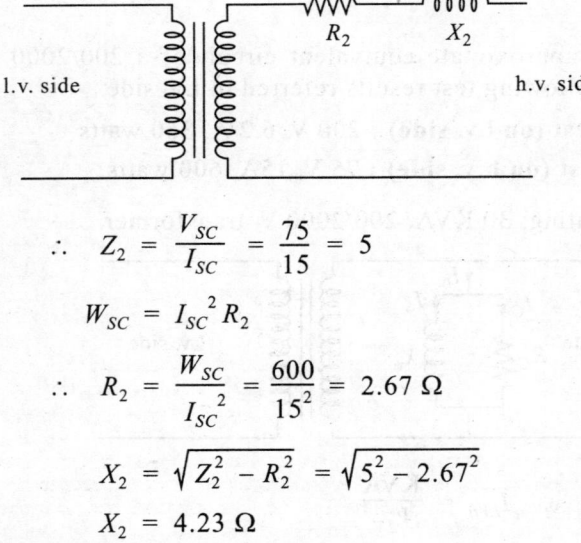

$$\therefore \quad Z_2 = \frac{V_{SC}}{I_{SC}} = \frac{75}{15} = 5$$

$$W_{SC} = I_{SC}^2 R_2$$

$$\therefore \quad R_2 = \frac{W_{SC}}{I_{SC}^2} = \frac{600}{15^2} = 2.67\ \Omega$$

$$X_2 = \sqrt{Z_2^2 - R_2^2} = \sqrt{5^2 - 2.67^2}$$

$$X_2 = 4.23\ \Omega$$

To find equivalent circuit referred to low voltage side.

$$R_1 = \left(\frac{N_{lv}}{N_{hv}}\right)^2 R_2$$

$$R_1 = \left(\frac{200}{2000}\right)^2 \times 2.67 = 0.0267\ \Omega$$

$$R_1 = \boxed{0.0267\ \Omega}$$

$$X_1 = \left(\frac{N_{lv}}{N_{hv}}\right)^2 X_2$$

$$= \left(\frac{200}{2000}\right)^2 \times 4.23 = 0.0423\ \Omega$$

$$X_1 = \boxed{0.0423\ \Omega}$$

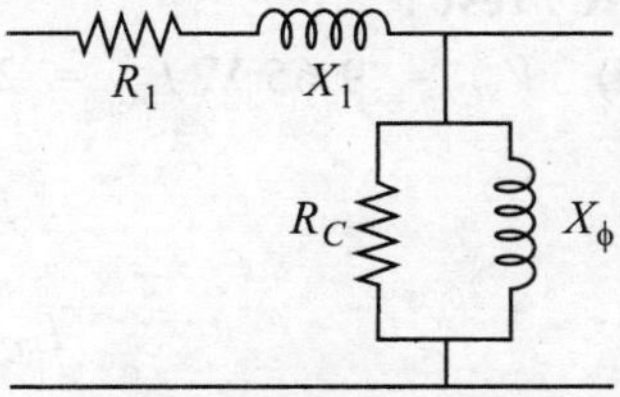

Equivalent circuit referred to l.v. side.

Ex. 6.10 : The following test results were obtained on a 10 KVA, 450/120 V, 50 Hz transformer

O.C. test : 120 V, 4.2 A, 80 W with h.v. side open.

S.C. test : 9.65 V, 22.2 A, 120 W with l.v. winding shorted.

Calculate **(a)** the equivalent circuit (approx) referred to h.v. side, **(b)** efficiency and voltage regulation for 0.8 lagging power factor at full load, **(c)** efficiency at half load 0.8 lagging power factor.

Solution : Given : 10 KVA, $V_1 = 450$ V, $V_2 = 120$ V, $f = 50$ Hz

O.C. test :

$$V_0 = 120\text{ V},\ I_0 = 4.2\text{ A},\ W_0 = 80\text{ watts}$$

$$W_0 = V_0 I_0 \cos\phi_0$$

$$\therefore \quad \phi_0 = \cos^{-1} = \frac{W_0}{V_0 I_0} = \cos^{-1}\frac{80}{120 \times 4.2}$$

$$\phi_0 = 80.87^\circ$$

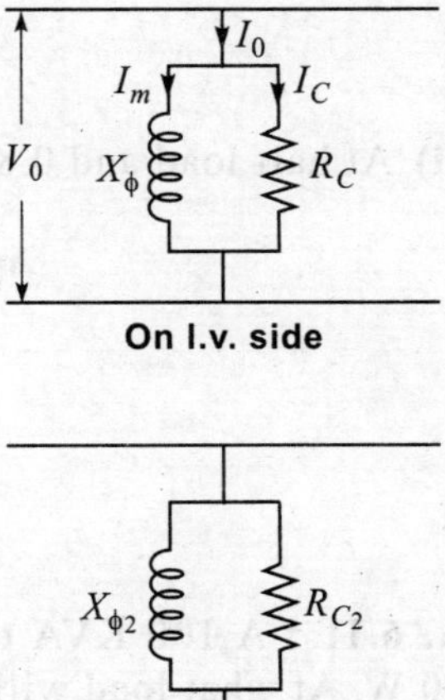

On l.v. side

$$I_m = I_0 \sin\phi_0 = 4.2 \sin 80.87^\circ$$

$$= 4.15$$

$$X_\phi = \frac{V_0}{I_m} = \frac{120}{4.15} = 28.94\ \Omega$$

$$X_{\phi 2} = \text{referred to h.v. side}$$

$$= \left(\frac{N_{hv}}{N_{lv}}\right)^2 \times X_\phi$$

$$= \left(\frac{450}{120}\right)^2 \times 28.94 = 406.97\ \Omega$$

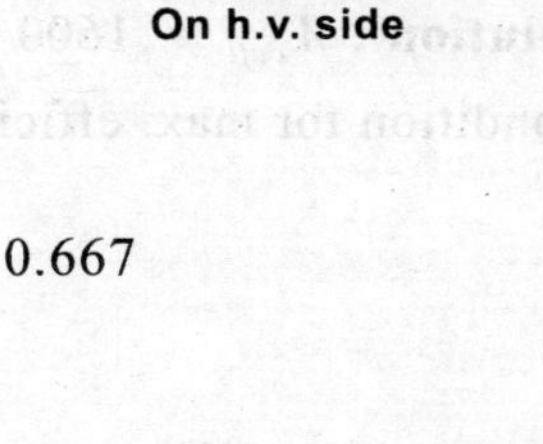

On h.v. side

$$I_C = I_0 \cos\phi_0 = 4.2 \cos 80.87^\circ = 0.667$$

$$R_C = \frac{V_0}{I_C} = \frac{120}{0.67} = 180$$

$$R_{C2} = \text{referred to h.v. side} = \left(\frac{450}{120}\right)^2 \times 180 = \boxed{2532.12\ \Omega}$$

S.C. test :

(i) $V_{SC} = 9.65$ V, $I_{SC} = 22.2$ A, $W_{SC} = 120$ W on h.v. side

$$I_{FC\,hv} = \frac{\text{KVA} \times 1000}{450 \text{ V}} = \frac{1000}{450} = 22.2 \text{ A}$$

$$\therefore \quad I_{SC}^2 R_2 = W_{SC}$$

$$R_2 = \frac{W_{SC}}{I_{SC}^2} = \frac{120}{22.2^2} = \boxed{0.24\ \Omega}$$

$$Z_2 = \frac{V_{SC}}{I_{SC}} = \frac{9.65}{22.2} = \boxed{0.43\ \Omega}$$

$$X_2 = \sqrt{Z_2^2 - R_2^2} = \sqrt{0.43^2 - 0.24^2}$$

$$X_2 = \boxed{0.36\ \Omega}$$

(ii) W_i = iron losses $W_0 = 80$, $W_{cufl} = 120$ W, $\cos\phi = 0.8$

$$\therefore \eta_{fl} = \frac{\text{KVA} \cos\phi \times 1000}{\text{KVA} \cos\phi \times 1000 + W_0 + W_{cufl}} \times 100$$

$$= \frac{10 \times 0.8 \times 1000}{10 \times 0.8 \times 1000 + 80 + 120} \times 100$$

$$= \boxed{97.56\ \%}$$

(iii) At half load and 0.8 pf, $\alpha = 0.5$

$$\eta = \frac{\alpha\ \text{KVA} \cos\phi \times 1000}{\alpha\ \text{KVA} \cos\phi \times 1000 + W_0 + \alpha^2 W_{cufl}} \times 100$$

$$= \frac{0.5 \times 10 \times 0.8 \times 1000}{0.5 \times 10 \times 0.8 \times 1000 + 80 + 0.5^2 \times 120} \times 100$$

$$= \boxed{97.32\ \%}$$

Ex. 6.11 : A 100 KVA transformer has full load copper loss of 1600 W and iron loss of 900 W. At what load will it have maximum efficiency?

Solution : $W_{cufl} = 1600$ W, $W_i = 900$ W

Condition for max. efficiency

$$W_i = W_{cu}$$

$$W_i = \alpha^2 W_{cufl}$$

$$900 = \alpha^2 \times 1600$$

$$\therefore \quad \alpha = \boxed{0.75}$$

i.e. at 0.75 times the full load max. efficiency will occur.

Ex. 6.12 : A 50 KVA, 1-phase transformer of 2300/230 V rating has primary and secondary winding resistances of 2 Ω and 0.02 Ω respectively. The iron loss is 412 watts. Calculate efficiency **(a)** at half of full load and 0.8 lagging pf **(b)** full load and 0.8 pf.

Solution : Given : KVA = 50, V_1 = 2300 V, V_2 = 230 V, r_1 = 2 Ω, r_2 = 0.02 Ω

$$I_1 = \frac{\text{KVA} \times 1000}{V_1} = 21.74 \text{ A}$$

$$I_2 = \frac{\text{KVA} \times 1000}{V_2} = 217.39 \text{ A}$$

$$\text{Total iron loss} = 412 \text{ W}$$

$$\text{Total full load Cu loss} = W_{Cufl} = I_1^2 r_1 + I_2^2 r_2$$

$$= 21.74^2 \times 2 + 217.39^2 \times 0.02 = \boxed{1890.42 \text{ W}}$$

(i) Efficiency at half load, $\alpha = 0.5$

$$\eta = \frac{\alpha \text{ KVA} \cos\phi \times 1000}{\alpha \text{ KVA} \cos\phi \times 1000 + W_0 + \alpha^2 W_{cufl}} \times 100$$

$$= \frac{0.5 \times 50 \times 0.8 \times 1000}{0.5 \times 50 \times 0.8 \times 1000 + 412 + 0.5^2 \times 1890.42} \times 100$$

$$= \boxed{95.76 \%}$$

(ii) Full load efficiency

$$\eta_{fl} = \frac{0.5 \times 0.8 \times 1000}{50 \times 0.8 \times 1000 + 412 + 1890.42} \times 100$$

$$= \boxed{94.55 \%}$$

Ex. 6.13 : A 40 KVA transformer has iron loss of 450 W and full load copper loss of 850 W. If power factor of load is 0.8 lagging, find

(i) Full load efficiency

(ii) Load at which maximum efficiency occurs

(iii) The max. efficiency.

Solution : 40 KVA, W_i = 450 W, W_{cufl} = 850 W,
pf = $\cos\phi$ = 0.8

(i)

$$\eta_{fl} = \frac{\text{KVA} \cos\phi \times 1000}{\text{KVA} \cos\phi \times 1000 + W_i + W_{cufl}} \times 100$$

$$= \frac{40 \times 0.8 \times 1000}{40 \times 0.8 \times 1000 + 450 + 850} \times 100$$

$$= \boxed{96.09 \%}$$

(ii)
$$W_i = \alpha^2 W_{cufl}$$
$$\therefore \quad \alpha = \sqrt{\frac{W_i}{W_{cufl}}} = \sqrt{\frac{450}{850}}$$
$$\alpha = 0.7276$$

i.e. at $\boxed{72.76\ \%}$ of full load max. efficiency will occur.

(iii)
$$\eta_{fl} = \frac{\alpha\ \text{KVA} \cos\phi \times 1000}{\alpha\ \text{KVA} \cos\phi \times 1000 + 2W_i} \times 100 \qquad [\because W_i = W_{cu}]$$
$$= \frac{0.7276 \times 40 \times 0.8 \times 1000}{0.7276 \times 40 \times 0.8 \times 1000 + 2 \times 450} \times 100$$
$$= \boxed{97.26\ \%}$$

Ex. 6.14 : A 1100/220 V transformer has a primary resistance of 0.25 Ω and the secondary resistance of 0.03 Ω. If iron losses amounts to 250 W, determine the secondary current at which maximum efficiency occurs and find the maximum efficiency at 0.8 power factor.

Solution : $V_1 = 1100$, $V_2 = 220$ V, $r_1 = 0.25\ \Omega$, $r_2 = 0.03\ \Omega$, $W_i = 250$ watts

$$r_1' = r_2 \text{ referred to secondary side} = \left(\frac{V_2}{V_1}\right)^2 r_1$$
$$= \left(\frac{220}{1100}\right)^2 \times 0.25 = 0.01\ \Omega$$
$$\therefore \quad R_2 = r_2 + r_1' = 0.03 + 0.01 = 0.04\ \Omega$$
$$= \text{total resistance referred to secondary}$$
$$W_{cu} = I_2^2 R_2$$

For max. efficiency
$$W_{cu} = W_i$$
$$I_2^2 R_2 = W_i$$
$$\text{or} \quad I_2^2 = \frac{250}{0.04} = 6250 \text{ A}$$

i.e. current at max. efficiency is
$$I_2 = \boxed{79.05 \text{ A}}$$
$$\eta_{max} = \frac{V_2 I_2 \cos\phi_2}{V_2 I_2 \cos\phi_2 + 2Wi} \times 100$$
$$= \frac{220 \times 79.05 \times 0.8}{220 \times 79.05 \times 0.8 + 2 \times 250} \times 100$$
$$= \boxed{96.54\ \%}$$

Ex. 6.15 : The efficiency of a 300 KVA, single phase transformer is 97.8% when delivering full load at 0.8 p.f. lagging and 98.4%. When delivering half load at unity power factor. Determine the efficiency at 80% of full load at 0.8 pf lagging.

Solution : KVA = 300, η_{fl} = 97.8 at $\cos\phi_1$ = 0.8 lagging, η_{hl} = 98.4 at $\cos\phi_2 = 1$

To find : η_3 at 80% of full load at $\cos\phi_3 = 0.8$

$$\eta_{fl} = \frac{\text{KVA} \cos\phi_1 \times 1000}{\text{KVA} \cos\phi_1 \times 1000 + W_i + W_{cufl}} \times 100$$

$$\therefore \quad 97.8 = \frac{300 \times 0.8 \times 1000}{300 \times 0.8 \times 1000 + W_i + W_{cufl}} \times 100$$

$$\therefore \quad W_i + W_{cufl} = 5398.77 \text{ watts} \qquad \text{..... (i)}$$

$$\eta_{hl} = \frac{\alpha \text{ KVA} \cos\phi_2 \times 1000}{\alpha \text{ KVA} \cos\phi_2 \times 1000 + W_i + \alpha^2 W_{cufl}} \times 100$$

For $\alpha = 0.5$ $\quad$ [$\because$ half load]

$\cos\phi_2 = 1$

$$\therefore \quad 98.4 = \frac{0.5 \times 300 \times 1000}{0.5 \times 300 \times 1000 + W_i + 0.25\, W_{cufl}} \times 100$$

$$\therefore \quad W_i + 0.25\, W_{cufl} = 2439.02 \text{ watts} \qquad \text{..... (ii)}$$

Solving (i) and (ii),

W_i = 1452.44 watts

W_{cufl} = 3946.33 watts

For $\alpha = 0.8$ $\cos\phi_2 = 0.8$

$$\eta = \frac{0.8 \times 300 \times 0.8 \times 1000}{0.8 \times 300 \times 0.8 \times 1000 + 1452.44 + 0.8^2 \times 3946.33} \times 100$$

$$= \boxed{97.97\ \%}$$

6.16 All Day Efficiency

The distribution transformers are connected to the supply throughout 24 hours a day. During these 24 hours the load demand is changing depending upon the season and time of the day. Hence, all day efficiency is more relevant.

$$\text{All day efficiency} = \frac{\text{o/p in kWhr over 24 hrs}}{\text{o/p in kWhr 24 hrs} + 24 W_i + \text{cu loss in 24 hrs}} \qquad \text{..... (6.66)}$$

Ex. 6.16 : A 120 KVA 3300/300 V single phase transformer has an efficiency of 97 % both on full-load at unity p.f. and on half load at unity power factor. The power factor of the no load current is 0.3 lagging and regulation on full load at 0.8 pf lagging is 2.5 %. Draw equivalent circuit referred to low voltage side.

Solution : KVA = 120, V_1 = voltage on h.v. side = 3300, V_2 = voltage on l.v. side = 300 V

$$\eta = \frac{\alpha \text{ KVA} \times \cos\phi \times 1000}{\alpha \text{ KVA} \times \cos\phi \times 1000 + W_i + \alpha^2 W_{cufl}} \times 100$$

$$\eta = 97\ \% \text{ at full load } \alpha = 1, \text{ pf} = \cos\phi = 1$$

$$97 = \frac{120 \times 1000}{120 \times 1000 + Wi + W_{cufl}} \times 100$$

$$\therefore \quad W_i + W_{cufl} = 3711.34 \qquad \text{..... (i)}$$

$$\eta = 97\ \% \text{ at half load } \alpha = 0.5, \text{ pf} = \cos\phi = 1$$

$$97 = \frac{0.5 \times 120 \times 1000}{0.5 \times 120 \times 1000 + Wi + 0.5^2\, W_{cufl}} \times 100$$

$$\therefore \quad W_i + 0.25 W_{cufl} = 1855.67 \qquad \text{..... (ii)}$$

Solving (i) and (ii),

$$W_i = 1237.11 \text{ watts}$$

$$W_{cufl} = 2474.23 \text{ watts}$$

Referring to l.v. side :

$$W_i = W_0 = V_2 I_0 \cos\phi_0$$

$$\therefore \quad I_0 = \frac{W_0}{V_2 \cos\phi_0}$$

Given $\cos\phi_0 = 0.3$ lagging

$$\therefore \quad I_0 = \frac{1237.11}{300 \times 0.3} = 13.74 \text{ amp}$$

$$I_m = I_0 \sin\phi_0 = 13.11 \text{ A}$$

$$I_C = I_0 \cos\phi_0 = 4.122 \text{ A}$$

$$R_C = \frac{V_0}{I_C} = \frac{300}{4.122} = 72.78\ \Omega$$

$$\therefore \quad R_C = \boxed{72.78\ \Omega}$$

$$X_\phi = \frac{V_C}{I_m} = \frac{300}{13.11} = 22.88\ \Omega$$

$$\therefore \quad X_\phi = \boxed{22.88\ \Omega}$$

When I_2 = full load current in l.v. winding

$$I_2 = \frac{\text{KVA} \times 1000}{V_2} = \frac{120 \times 1000}{300} = 400 \text{ amp}$$

$$W_{cufl} = I_2^2 R_2$$

$$\therefore \quad R_2 = \frac{2474.23}{400^2} = 0.0155\ \Omega$$

$$R_2 = \boxed{0.0155\ \Omega}$$

Regulation for lagging pf load is

$$\%\text{ regulation} = \frac{I_2 R_2 \cos\phi_2 + I_2 X_2 \sin\phi_2}{V_{2\,NL}} \times 100$$

regulation = 2.5% at full load, $\cos\phi = 0.8$

$$2.5 = \frac{400 \times 0.0155 \times 0.8 + 400 \times X_2 \times 0.6}{300} \times 100$$

$$\therefore \quad X_2 = \boxed{0.0106\ \Omega}$$

∴ equivalent circuit referred to l.v. side is

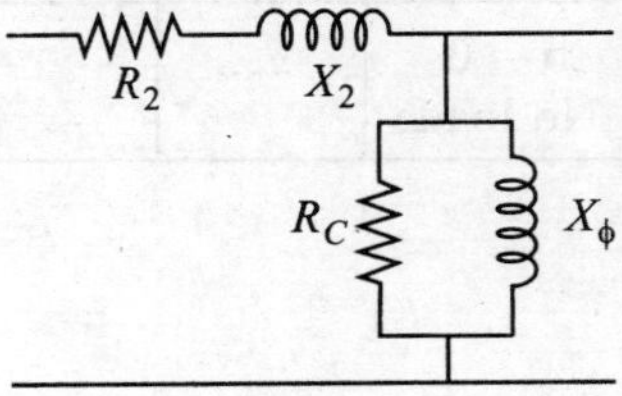

Ex. 6.17 : A 15 KVA, 2000/200 V transformer has an iron loss of 250 W and full load copper loss of 350 W. During the day it is loaded as follows:

No. of hrs	Load	Power factor
9	1/4th load	0.6
7	Full load	0.8
6	3/4th load	1.0
2	No load	—

Find all day efficiency.

Solution : W_i = 250 W,

Iron los per day = 250 × 24 = 6000 Whr = 6 kWhr

W_{cufl} = 350 W

At any load $W_{cu} = \alpha^2 W_{cufl}$

∴ **for 1/4th load** $\alpha = 0.25$

$$\therefore \quad W_{cu} = (0.25)^2 \times 350 = 21.875 \text{ watts}$$

Copper loss for 9 hrs at 1/4th load = 9 × 21.875

= 196.875 Whr

Output in watt hrs for 0.6 pf load being 1/4th load

$$\text{Output} = \alpha \text{ KVA} \cos\phi \times 1000 = 0.25 \times 15 \times 0.6 \times 1000$$
$$= 2250$$

$$\text{O/p in watt hrs for 9 hrs} = 2250 \times 9$$
$$= 20250 \text{ Whr}$$

Making a table for different load, power factor and duration with similar calculation.

Load α	pf $\cos\phi$	o/p in watts $W = \alpha$ KVA $\cos\phi \times 1000$	No. of hrs	o/p in Whr $= W t$	$W_{cu} = \alpha^2 W_{cufl}$	Copper loss in Whr $W_{cu} \times t$
1/4 = 0.25	0.6	2250	9	20250	21.875	196.875
$\alpha = 1$	0.8	12000	7	84000	350	2450
$\alpha = 0.75$	1	11250	6	67500	196.87	1181.25
$\alpha = 0$ No load	---	---	2	---	---	---
		Total :	24 hrs	171750 Whr = 171.75 kWhr		3838.125 Whr = 3.828 kWhr

$$\therefore \eta_{all\ day} = \frac{\text{o/p in kWhr over 24 hrs}}{\text{o/p in kWhr over 24 hrs} + W_i \text{ in 24 hrs} + W_{cu} \text{ loss in 24 hrs}}$$

$$= \frac{171.75}{171.75 + 63.83}$$

$$\therefore \eta_{all\ day} = \boxed{94.59\%}$$

Ex. 6.18 : A 20 KVA, 2000/200 V transformer has an iron loss of 300 W and full load copper loss of 400 W. During the day it is loaded as follows:

No. of hrs	Load	Power factor
8	1/4th load	0.5
6	Full load	0.8
6	3/4th load	1.0
4	No load	—

Find all day efficiency.

Solution : KVA = 20, W_i = 300 W, W_{cuf} = 400

$$\therefore W_i \text{ for 24 hrs} = 300 \times 24 = 7200 \text{ Whr}$$
$$= 7.2 \text{ kWhr.}$$

$$\alpha W_{cufl} = W_{cu} \text{ at any load } \alpha$$

Making a table for different load, power factor and duration with similar calculation.

Load α	pf $\cos\phi$	o/p in watts $W = \alpha$ KVA $\cos\phi \times 1000$	No. of hrs	o/p in Whr $= W t$	$W_{cu} = \alpha^2 W_{cufl}$	Copper loss in Whr $W_{cu} \times t$
0.25	0.6	2500	8	20×10^3	25	200
1	0.8	16000	6	96×10^3	400	2400
0.75	1	15000	6	90×10^3	225	1350
0	---	---	4	---	---	---
		Total :	24 hrs	206×10^3 Whr = 206 kWhr		3950 Whr = 3.95 kWhr

$$\therefore \eta_{all\ day} = \frac{\text{o/p in kWhr over 24 hrs}}{\text{o/p in kWhr 24 hrs} + 24\ W_i \text{ over 24 hrs} + W_{cu} \text{ over 24 hrs}}$$

$$= \frac{206}{206 + 7.2 + 3.95} \times 100$$

$$= \boxed{94.86\%}$$

Ex. 6.19 : A 5 KVA, 230/115 V transformer took 1.2 A and 75 watts when 230 V is applied to h.v. winding and l.v. winding is kept open. If it took 21.75 A and 150 watts when the l.v. winding is short circuited and 17.4 V is applied to the h.v. winding. Find

(i) The no load current as a fraction of full load current

(ii) Percentage regulation on full load at 0.8 pf logging, and

(iii) Load at which maximum efficiency occurs and the max. efficiency.

Solution : KVA = 5, V_1 = voltage of h.v. winding = 230 V,

V_2 = voltage of l.v. winding = 115 V

Open circuit test on h.v. side:

$$V_0 = 230 \text{ V}, I_0 = 1.2 \text{ A}, W_0 = 75 \text{ watts}$$

Short circuit test on h.v. side:

$$V_{sc} = 17.4 \text{ V}, I_{sc} = 21.75 \text{ A}, W_{sc} = 150 \text{ watts.}$$

When I_{1fl} = full load current in h.v. winding

$$I_{1fl} = \frac{\text{KVA} \times 1000}{V_1} = \frac{5 \times 1000}{230}$$

$$I_{1fl} = 21.75 \text{ A}$$

(i)

$$I_0 = \alpha I_{1fl}$$

$$\therefore \quad \alpha = \frac{1.2}{21.75} = 0.0552$$

$$\text{or} \quad \alpha = \boxed{5.52\% \text{ of full load current}}$$

(ii)

$$W_{SC} = I_{SC}^2 R_2$$

$$\therefore \quad R_1 = \frac{W_{SC}}{I_{SC}^2} = \frac{150}{21.75^2} = \boxed{0.3171\ \Omega}$$

$$Z_1 = \frac{V_{SC}}{I_{SC}} = \frac{17.4}{21.75} = 0.8\ \Omega$$

$$X_1 = \sqrt{Z_1^2 - R_1^2} = \sqrt{0.8^2 - 0.3171^2}$$

$$X_1 = 0.7344\ \Omega$$

$$\%\text{ regulation at full load and 0.8 pf} = \frac{I_{1fl} R_1 \cos\phi + I_{1fl} X_1 \cos\phi}{V_1} \times 100$$

$$2.5 = \frac{21.75 \times 0.3171 \times 0.8 + 21.75 \times 0.7344 \times 0.6}{230} \times 100$$

$$\%\text{ regulation} = \boxed{6.566\%}$$

(iii) For maximum efficiency

$$W_i = \alpha^2 W_{cufl}$$

$$W_i = W_0 = 75$$

$$W_{cufl} = W_{SC} = 75$$

$$\therefore \quad 75 = \alpha^2 \times 150$$

$$\therefore \quad \alpha = 0.707$$

At 70.7% of full load current maximum efficiency occurs.

$$\eta_{max} = \frac{\alpha\, KVA \times 1000}{\alpha\, KVA \times 1000 + 2Wi} \times 100$$

$$= \frac{0.707 \times 5 \times 1000}{0.707 \times 5 \times 1000 + 2 \times 75} \times 100$$

$$\eta_{max} = \boxed{95.93\%}$$

Unsolved Examples

1. A 300 KVA, single phase transformer has 300 turns on the primary and 100 turns on the secondary. The primary is connected to 1500 V, 50 Hz supply. Determine:

   (a) The secondary open circuit voltage

   (b) Full load current in both windings

   (c) The max. value of flux

   [**Ans. (a)** 500 V **(b)** 200 A, 600 A **(c)** 0.0225 wb]

2. A 6600/600 V, 1-phase, 50 Hz transformer has maximum value of flux in the core as 0.08 wb. Find the number of turns in each winding.

   [**Ans.** 374 turns, 34 turns]

3. A 300 KVA, 3300/300 V single phase transformer has 1100 primary turns. Find **(a)** transformation ratio **(b)** secondary turns **(c)** voltage per turn **(d)** secondary current it supplies a load of 200 kW at 0.8 power factor logging. Assuming primary and secondary winding resistance and leakage reactance to be negligible.

   [**Ans. (a) 1/11 (b)** 100 turns **(c)** 3 **(d)** 833.33 A]

4. A 4400/400 V single phase transformer gives 0.8 A and 100 W as ammeter and watt meter readings when supply is given to low voltage windings and high voltage winding is kept open. Find **(a)** Power factor of no-load current **(b)** magnetizing component of current and core loss component of circuit.

   [**Ans. (a)** 0.3125 **(b)** 0.76 A **(c)** 0.25 A]

5. A 230/115 V single phase transformer takes a no-load current of 2 A at a p.f. of 0.2 lagging with low voltage winding kept open. If the low voltage winding is now having a current of 15 A at 0.8 p.f. lagging when loaded, find the current and power factor of primary current now drawn.

   [**Ans.** 9.09 A, 0.7038 lagging]

6. A 4:1 step down transformer takes a no load current of 0.8 A at 0.25 lagging p.f. on h.v. side with l.v. open. If the secondary takes a load current of 100A at **(a)** 0.8 pf lagging and **(b)** 0.8 p.f. leading. Find the primary current and power factor.

   [**Ans. (a)** 25.63, 0.788 lag **(b)** 24.7, 0.818 lead]

7. A 30 KVA, 3000/300 V, single phase 50Hz transformer has a primary resistance and reactance of 3.5 Ω and 4.5 Ω respectively. The secondary resistance and reactance are 0.015 Ω and 0.02 Ω respectively. Find **(a)** Equivalent resistance and reactance referred to h.v. side. **(b)** equivalent resistance and reactance referred to l.v. side. **(c)** full load copper losses.

   [**Ans. (a)** 5 Ω, 6.5 Ω **(b)** 0.05 Ω, 0.065 Ω, **(c)** 500 W]

8. Obtain the approximate equivalent circuit referred to l.v. side of a given 200/2000 V, 30 KVA, 1-phase transformer having following test results.

O.C. test (on l.v. side) : 200 V, 6 A, 360 W

S.C. test (on h.v. side) : 75 V, 18 A, 600 W.

[**Ans.** 111.11 Ω, 34.96 Ω, 0.0185 Ω, 0.0374 Ω]

9. A 4 KVA, 400 / 200 V, 50 Hz, 1-phase transformer has the following test results.

O.C. test (l.v. side) : 200 V, 1 A, 64 W

S.C. test (h.v. side) : 15 V, 10 A, 80 W

Find **(a)** Equivalent circuit referred to h.v. side

(b) Iron losses and full load copper losses

(c) Efficiency and regulation at full load 0.8 pf lagging.

[**Ans. (a)** 2500 Ω, 842.12 Ω, 0.8 Ω, 1.27 Ω **(b)** 64 W, 80 W **(c)** 95.69%, 3.5%]

10. The primary and secondary winding resistances of a 30 KVA, 6600/300 V single phase transformer are 8 Ω and 0.02 Ω respectively. The equivalent leakage reactance referred to primary winding is 30 Ω. Find the full load regulation for load power factor of **(a)** unity **(b)** 0.8 lagging **(c)** 0.8 leading.

[**Ans. (a)** 1.2% **(b)** 2.2% **(c)** –0.28%]

11. A 250/500 V, 1-phase transformer gave the following test results:

O.C. test (l.v. side) : 250 V, 1 A, 80 W

S.C. test (h.v. side) : 20V, 12 A, 100 W

Find **(a)** The circuit constants referred to h.v. side.

(b) Efficiency when 10 A flows through 500 V winding at 0.8 pf lagging.

[**Ans.** 3125 Ω, 1052.64 Ω, 0.69 Ω, 1.52 Ω, 96.41%]

12. Open circuit and short circuit test were conducted on a 50 KVA, 6360/240 V, 50 Hz, 1 phase transformer.

O.C. test : Voltage across primary 6360 V, primary current 1A power input 2 kW.

S.C. test : Voltage across primary 100 V, current in secondary 175 A, power input 0.2 kW.

Draw equivalent circuit referred to secondary side and also find regulation at full load 0.8 pf leading.

[**Ans.** 6.5×10^{-3} Ω, 28.72 Ω, 9.38 Ω, –0.59%]

13. A 15 KVA, 2000/200 V transformer has an iron loss of 250 W and full load copper loss of 400 W. During the days it is loaded as follows :

No. of hrs	Load	Power factor
9	1/4th load	0.6
7	Full load	0.8
6	3/4th load	1.0
2	No load	—

Calculate all days efficiency.

[Ans. 94.3%**]**

14. A 40 KVA transformer has a maximum efficiency of 98% at 80% of full load at upf. During the day it is loaded as follows:

No. of hrs	Load	Power factor
8	6 kW	0.6 lag
6	24 kW	0.8 lag
7	30 kW	0.9 lag
3	No load	—

Calculate all day efficiency.

[Ans. 97.22%**]**

15. A 230 V, 2.5 KVA, 1-phase transformer has an iron loss of 100 W at 40 Hz and 70 W at 30 Hz. Find the hysterias and eddy current losses at 50 Hz.

[Ans. 91.5 W, 40 W**]**

CHAPTER

7 ROTATING ELECTRICAL MACHINE

Rotating electrical machines are widely used for the purpose of converting energy from one form to another. The two most frequently used types of such machines are ***generators*** *and* ***motors****.*

Generators convert mechanical energy to electrical energy i.e. wind generator, hydel power generators, thermal power generators etc. Generator action takes place when a ***conductor*** *is* ***moved*** *in a* ***field****. (Refer art 3.2)*

Motors convert electrical energy to mechanical energy, e.g. fan motors, lifts, mixers etc. Motor action i.e. torque is produced, when a ***current carrying conductor*** *is placed in a* ***field****.*

The motors which are supplied with d.c. supply are called d.c. motors. The motors connected to 3 phase supply line are called 3 phase a.c. motors another ones which work on 1 phase a.c. supply are called ***single phase induction motors****.*

This chapter deals with all the above said motors, to the basic level.

7.1 D.C. Machines

The d.c. machines i.e. generators and motors are dealt here one after the other. The advantages of d.c. motors are

(i) A wide range of speed control, both above and below the rated speed, is easily done without sacrificing its efficiency.

(ii) They can provide high starting torque.

(iii) Reversal of rotation is easily achieved. Though the disadvantages are

- **(a)** High initial cost
- **(b)** High maintenance cost
- **(c)** Have inherent sparking problem at brushes and hence cannot be used in hazardous environment.

This chapter deals with d.c. generators and motors, emf equation, the types of d.c machines.

7.1.1 D.C. Generator Principle

A generator converts mechanical energy to electrical energy. When a conductor is moved in a field emf is induced in it and if a closed path is provided current flows.

Refer to the a.c. dynamo of Fig. 3.2 we have seen that the emf induced in the coil is sinusoidal or alternating. The current in the external resistance (*xy*) is alternating. The two rings R_1 and R_2 are called the *slip rings* which are connected to conductors *AB* and *CD* respectively.

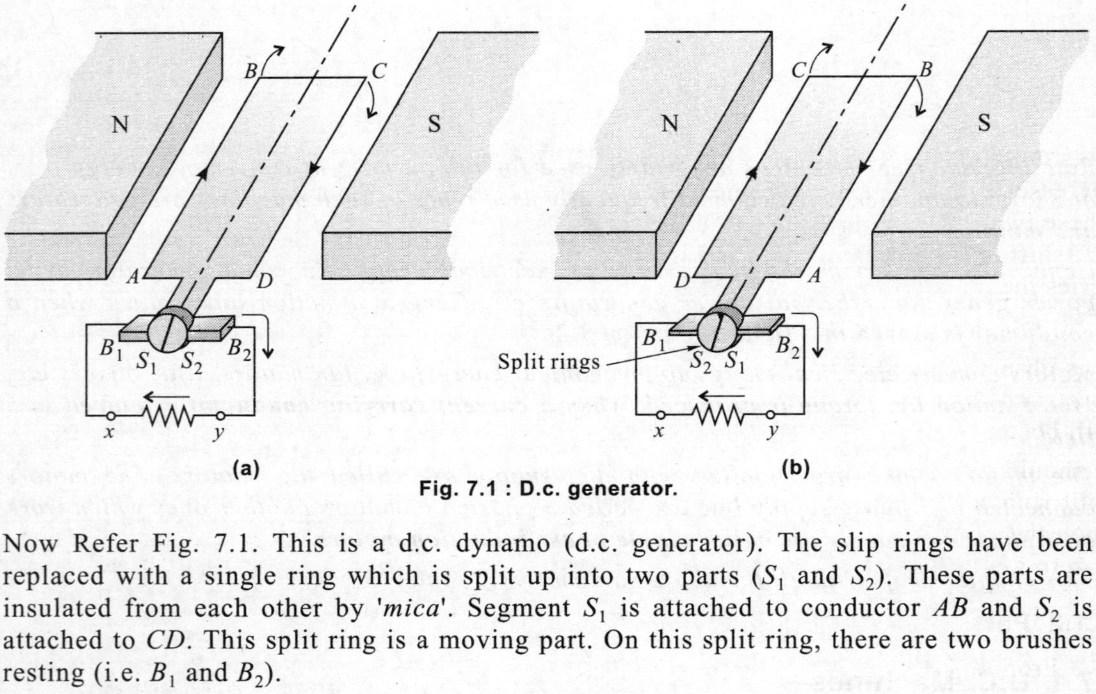

Fig. 7.1 : D.c. generator.

Now Refer Fig. 7.1. This is a d.c. dynamo (d.c. generator). The slip rings have been replaced with a single ring which is split up into two parts (S_1 and S_2). These parts are insulated from each other by '*mica*'. Segment S_1 is attached to conductor *AB* and S_2 is attached to *CD*. This split ring is a moving part. On this split ring, there are two brushes resting (i.e. B_1 and B_2).

Fig. 7.1(a) shows position where maximum emf is induced in *AB* and *CD*. The current in the coil and the outer circuit is as shown. Now, the coil rotates further and reaches position as in Fig. 7.1(b). Conductor *AB* is now under the south pole. The *emf* induced is, therefore, negative maximum the current in *AB* reverses w.r.t. its previous position [Fig. 7.1(a)]. The position of S_1 and S_2 also changes but the brushes remain in the same place. The current in the external circuit remains in the same direction i.e. the bidirectional current of a.c. dynamo is now converted to unidirectional current in d.c. dynamo. The output voltage waveform is as shown in Fig. 7.2.

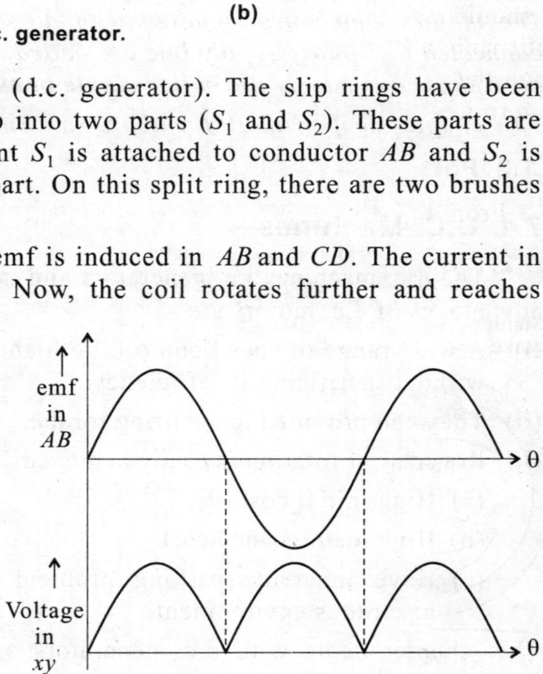

Fig. 7.2 : Output of a.c. dynamo for 1 coil.

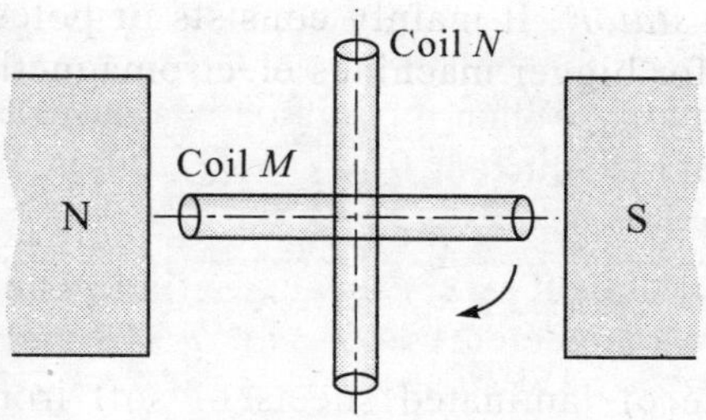

Fig. 7.3(a) : Two coils.

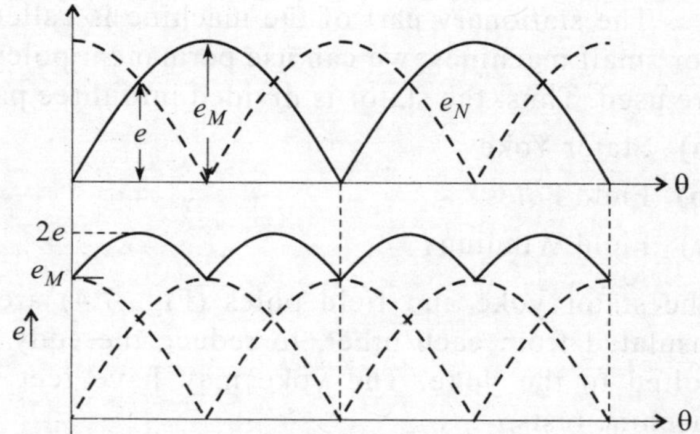

Fig. 7.3(b)

This output current and hence the voltage is unidirectional but not steady d.c. So, let us increase the coils in the dynamo to 2 as in Fig. 7.3(a). Coil M is kept at 90° to coil N. These two coils are now rotated in the field of magnets. The emfs in the two coils will be 90° shifted from each other as in Fig. 7.3(b). If the two coils are connected effectively in series the output voltage e, will be give by

$$e = e_M + e_N$$

It is observed that e has lesser variations in the output (between e_M and $2e$) as compared to e_M and e_N (between 0 to e_M). So if the number of coils is further increased, the output will become smoother and finally constant d.c. will be obtained.

It should be noted that as the number of coils increase, the number of segments on the split rings also increases. It is then called commutator. The number of brushes depends upon the type of winding. The position of brushes is arranged in the axis where coil *emf* is zero i.e. interpolar axis.

7.1.2 Parts of D.C. Machines

From the above discussion the various parts of a d.c. machine are

7.1.2.1 Stator

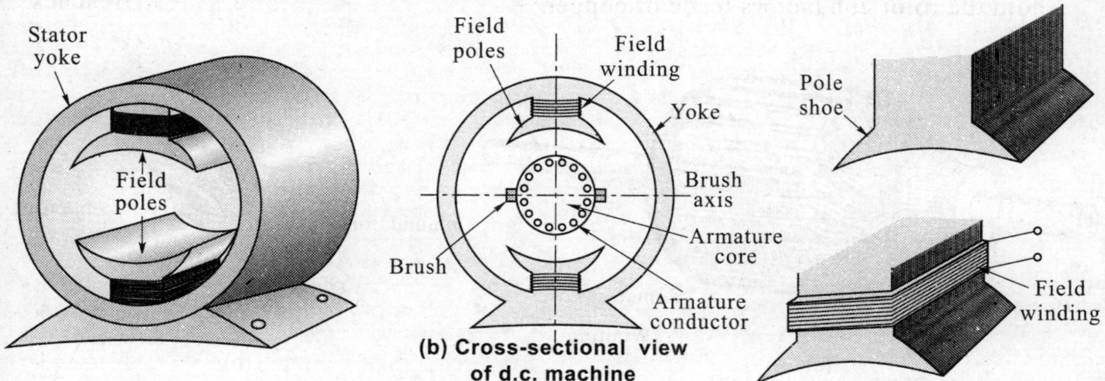

(a)

(b) Cross-sectional view of d.c. machine

(c) Field pole.

Fig. 7.4 : Stator parts.

The stationary part of the machine is called '*the stator*'. It mainly consists of poles. For small machines, we can use permanent poles but for bigger machines electromagnetic are used. Thus, the stator is divided into three parts.

(a) Stator Yoke

(b) Field Poles

(c) Field Windings

The stator yoke and field poles (Fig. 7.4) are made of laminated sheets of soft iron, insulated from each other, to reduce the eddy current loss. The field poles are usually bolted to the yoke. The yoke may have feet or a supporting bracket upon which the machine rests.

The pole core, where the field winding is placed is usually of smaller cross-section than the pole shoes due to the following reasons:-

(i) Reduced cross-section requires less copper for the field winding.

(ii) The large pole shoe area increases the flux per pole entering the armature due to reduction in air gap reluctance.

(iii) Pole shoe provides mechanical strength and support to the field winding.

The concentric field windings, when excited with d.c. produces North and South poles.

7.1.2.2 Rotor

The rotating parts of the machine are called *the rotor parts*. So the rotor should have conductor, large in number. These rotor conductors are placed over a solid core. The rotor conductor are connected to split rings. These split rings have large number of segments according to the number of conductors on the rotor. The split rings are called *commutator*. This entire rotor assembly is called *armature*. The various parts of armature are discussed one by one.

(a) Armature Core

Like the field core, the armature core is a stack of steel laminations (Fig. 7.5). It is cylindrical in shape. The circumferential edge is slotted to a convenient depth to hold the rotor conductors made of copper.

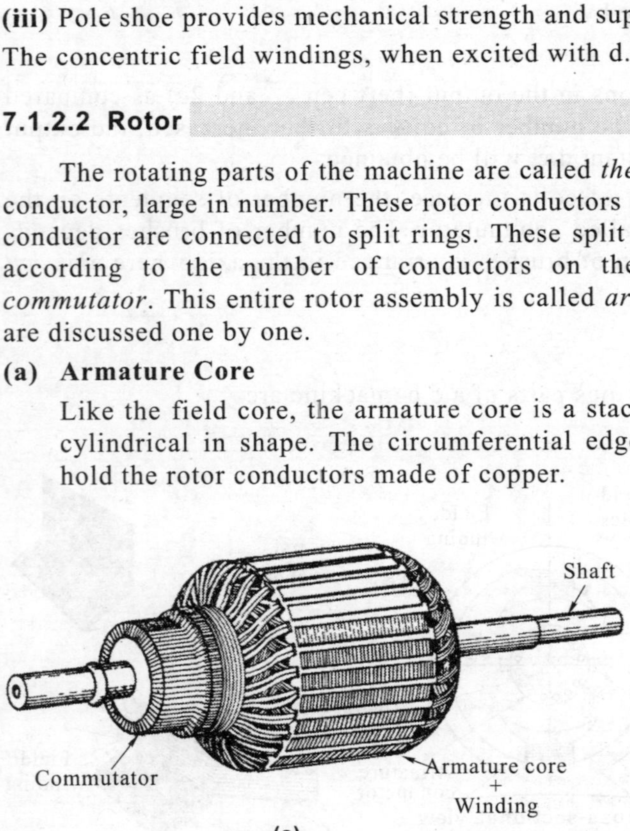

(a)

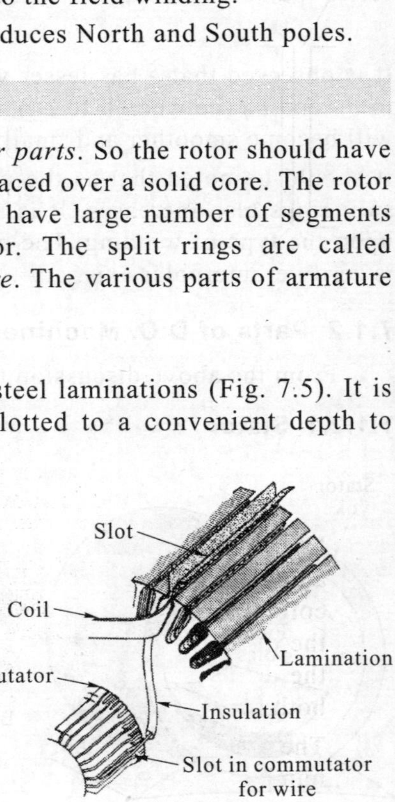

(b)

Fig. 7.5 : Armature core.

One such coil is shown placed in the slots in Fig. 7.5. The commutator shown in Fig. 7.5, which is made of copper segments insulated from each other by mica is also placed on the shaft. The function of the commutator (split rings) is to convert the alternating emf inside the armature to the direct emf at the brush terminals.

The brushes are made of carbon which are placed in the interpolar axis over the commutator. The number of brushes depends upon the type of windings in the armature.

(b) Types of Armature Winding

There are two general types of armature winding i.e. *lap winding* and *wave winding*. They differ from each other in several ways, but from the stand point of construction, they differ from each other in the manner in which the coil ends are connected to the commutator segments. Only simplex lap and wave windings are discussed here.

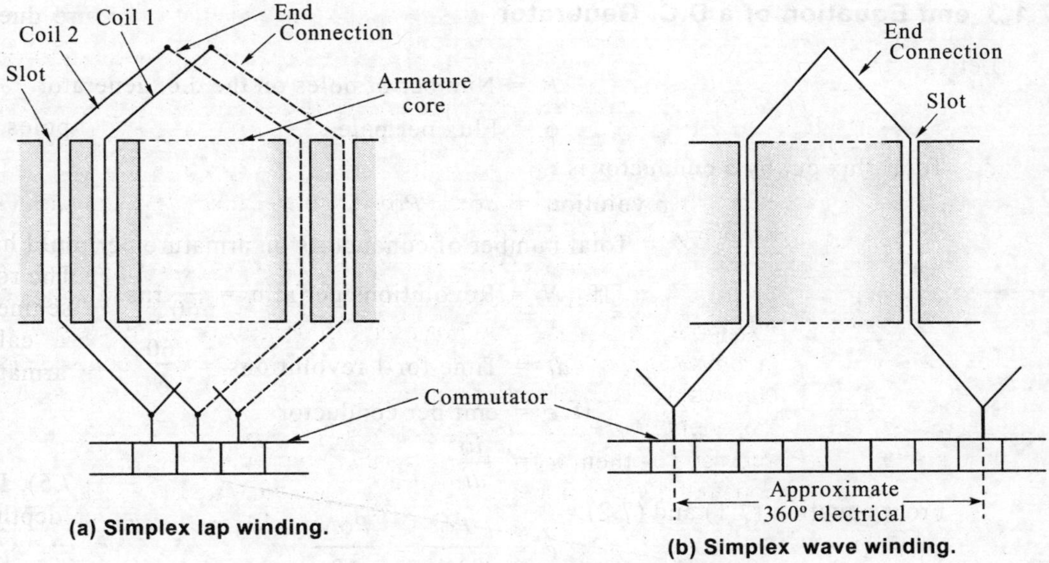

Fig. 7.6 : Types of armature winding.

In the lap winding [Fig. 7.6(a)], the conductors of the same coil are connected to adjacent commutator segments, while in wave winding the conductors of the same coil are connected to commutator segments very nearly, but never exactly, equal to the distance between the poles of same polarity. It should be noted clearly here that the distance between the conductors of the same coil is always same for all coils in both the windings for a particular machine.

The number of brushes for lap winding is equal to number of poles, whereas the number of brushes is always two for wave winding. The number of parallel paths of current inside the armature is always equal to the number of brushes. Fig. 7.7 shows the actual picture of a d.c. machine.

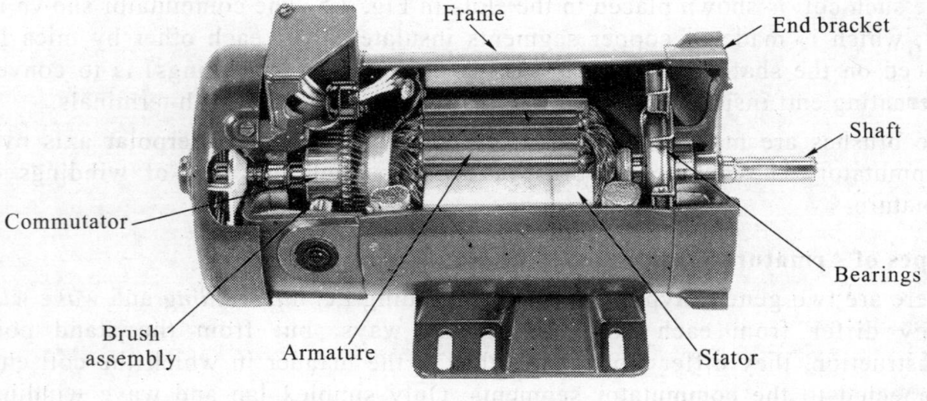

Fig. 7.7 : Picture of actual d.c. machine.

7.1.3 emf Equation of a D.C. Generator

Let,

P = Number of poles on the d.c. generator

ϕ = Flux per pole

∴ Total flux cut by a conductor is

$$1 \text{ revolution} = d\phi = P\phi \quad \text{..... (7.1)}$$

Z = Total number of conductors on armature periphery

If N = Revolutions per min $= \dfrac{N}{60}$ rps

$$dt = \text{Time for 1 revolutions} = \frac{60}{N} \quad \text{..... (7.2)}$$

If e = emf per conductor

then, $e = \dfrac{d\phi}{dt}$

∴ From equation (7.1) and (7.2)

$$e = \frac{P\phi}{60/N} = \frac{P\phi N}{60} \quad \text{..... (7.3)}$$

If Z = Total number of conductors on armature

A = Number of parallel path

= P for lap winding

= 2 for wave winding

$$\therefore \text{ Number of conductors per path} = \frac{Z}{A} \quad \text{..... (7.4)}$$

$$\therefore \quad \text{Total emf generated, } E = e\,\frac{Z}{A}$$

$$\text{or} \quad \boxed{E = \frac{PN\phi Z}{60A}} \quad \text{..... (7.5)}$$

Ex. 7.1 : A 6 pole, 1200 rpm, lap wound d.c. generator has 760 conductors. If the flux per pole is 0.02 wb. Calculate the emf of the generator.

Solution : Given : $P = 6, N = 1200$ rpm, $A = 6$ [$\because A = P$ for lap winding]
$Z = 6, \phi = 0.02$ wb

$$\therefore \quad E = \frac{PN\phi Z}{60A} = \frac{6 \times 1200 \times 0.02 \times 760}{60 \times 6}$$

$$E = \boxed{304 \text{ volts}}$$

Ex. 7.2 : A 8 pole d.c. generator armature has 960 conductors, a flux of 40 mwb/pole and a speed of 400 rpm. Calculate the emf generated on open circuit. If the same armature is wave wound, at what speed must it be driven to generate 400 V.

Solution : Given : $P = 8, Z = 960, \phi = 0.04$ wb, $N_1 = 400$ rpm,
$A = 8$ [as initially lap winding]

$$\therefore \quad E_1 = \frac{PN\phi Z}{60A}$$

$$= \frac{8 \times 400 \times 0.04 \times 960}{60 \times 8}$$

$$E_1 = \boxed{256 \text{ V}}$$

For wound machine $A = 2$, given $E = 400$ V

$$\therefore \quad E_1 = \frac{P\phi NZ}{60A}$$

$$400 = \frac{8 \times N \times 0.04 \times 960}{60 \times 2}$$

$$N = \boxed{156.25 \text{ rpm}}$$

7.1.4 Representation of a D.C. Machine

A d.c. machine (Generator or motor) with one field winding is represented as shown in Fig. 7.8.

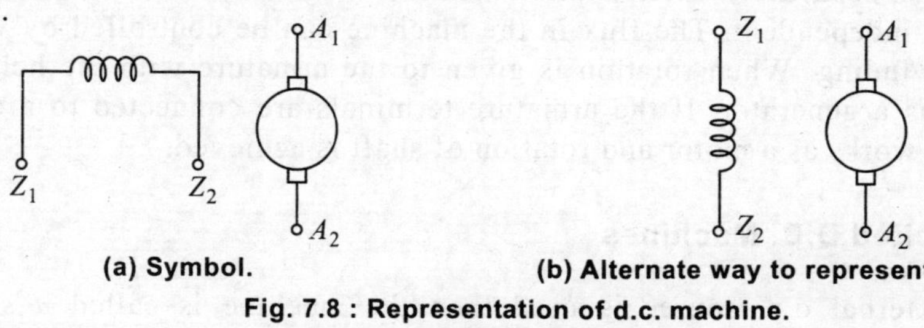

(a) Symbol. **(b) Alternate way to represent d.c. machine.**

Fig. 7.8 : Representation of d.c. machine.

The field winding is shown by a coil, as it produces flux in the air gap. The armature winding is represented by a circle. Two small rectangles touching this circle represent the carbon brushes on commutator.

The field winding in strict electrical sense, should be shown perpendicular to brush axis. However, symbol as shown in Fig. 7.8(b) is also permitted.

7.1.5 Types of D.C. Machines

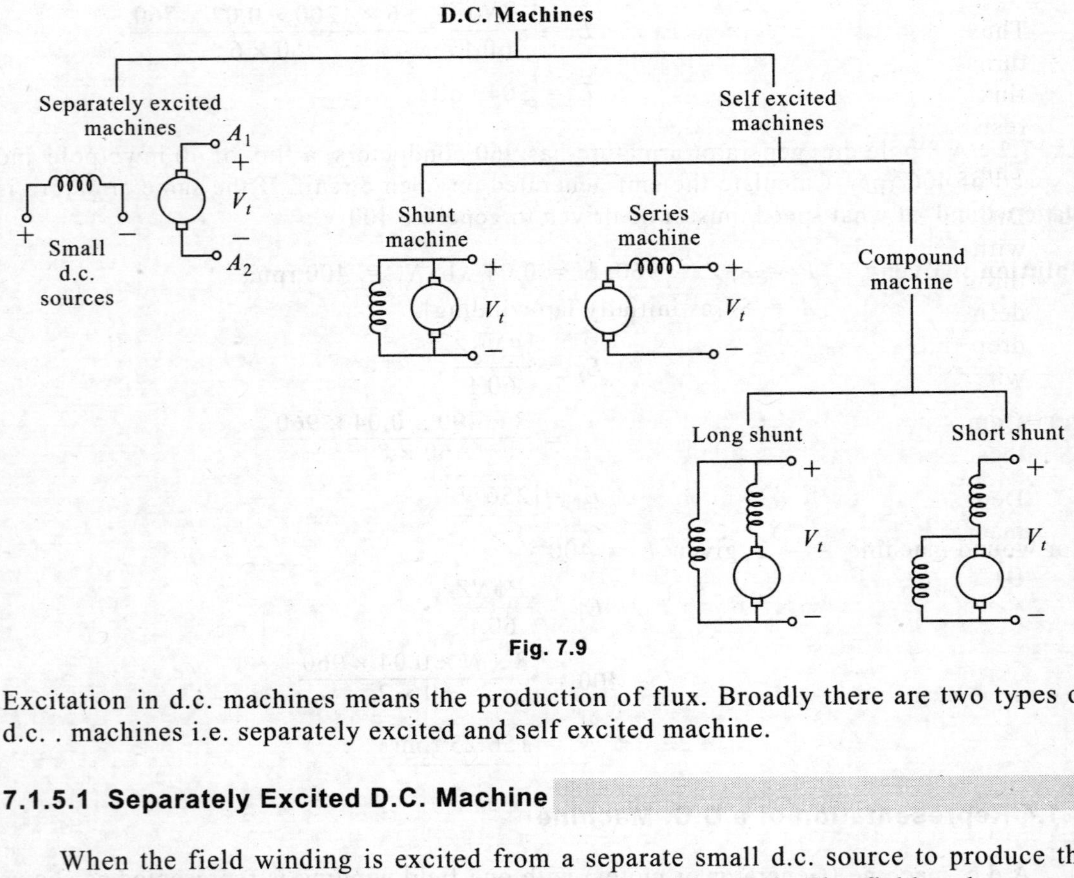

Fig. 7.9

Excitation in d.c. machines means the production of flux. Broadly there are two types of d.c. . machines i.e. separately excited and self excited machine.

7.1.5.1 Separately Excited D.C. Machine

When the field winding is excited from a separate small d.c. source to produce the flux it is called as *separately excited d.c. machine*. (Fig. 7.9). The field and armature circuits are quite independent. The flux in the machine can be controlled by varying the current in field winding. When rotation is given to the armature with the help of prime mover it works as a generator. If the armature terminals are connected to a d.c. supply then the machine works as a motor and rotation of shaft is achieved.

7.1.5.2 Self Excited D.C. Machines

When no external d.c. source is used then the machine is called *a self excited machine*. Here the armature and field winding are excited from the same source. Depending upon how supply is connected to the field and armature winding a further classification of self excited machines is as given below.

(a) D.C. Shunt Machine : When the field winding is connected in parallel to the armature winding, the machine so obtained is a shunt machine. The function of field winding is to produce flux which is proportional to the product of current in the winding and number of turns in the winding i.e.

$$\phi \propto \text{Ampere-turns.}$$

Thus to obtain a predefined flux either we can have high current or large number of turns. In shunt machine as terminal voltage V_t is high, in order to have the required flux large number of turns with less current is preferred. Thus field winding resistance is large ($I = V/R$).

Thus, shunt winding is made of thin wire with large number of turns.

(b) D.C. Series Machine : When the field winding and armature winding are in series with each other the machine is called a *d.c. series machine*. Here as the current through the series field winding is the armature current also the load current, a pre-defined flux as ampers is high, this winding should have less turns. Secondly, the drop in the resistance should be less thus series field winding is made from a thick wire with less number of turns.

(c) Compound Machines : As the name suggest this motor has two field windings. Both these windings are placed on the same pole but carry different currents.

Depending upon the connection (Fig. 7.9) there are two types of compound machines.

(i) Long Shunt Machine : Here, the current through series field winding (*se*) and armature winding is same, where as supply voltage appears across shunt field winding (*sh*) [Fig. 7.10(a)]

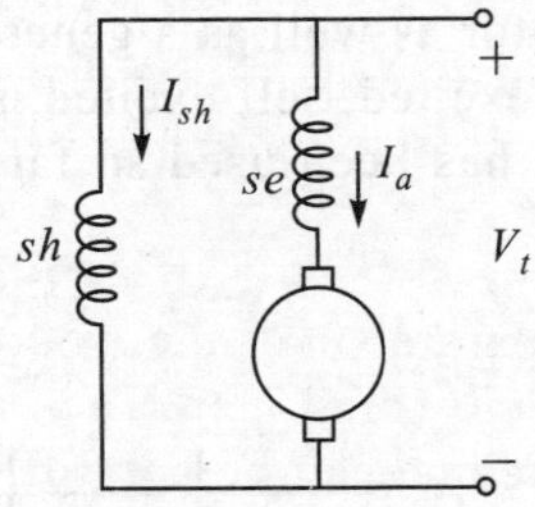

Fig. 7.10(a)

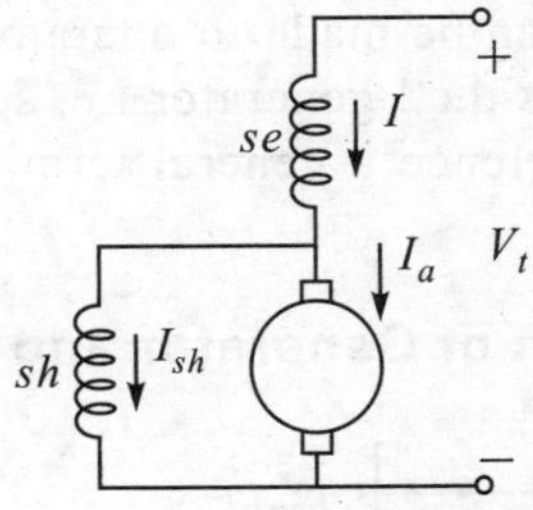

Fig. 7.10(b)

(ii) Short Shunt Machine : The shunt field winding (*sh*) is connected across the armature winding, whereas, the series field winding carries the supply current.

Based on the nature of flux produced by the shunt and series field winding, compound motors can also be classified as

(a) Cumulative compounding

(b) Differential compounding.

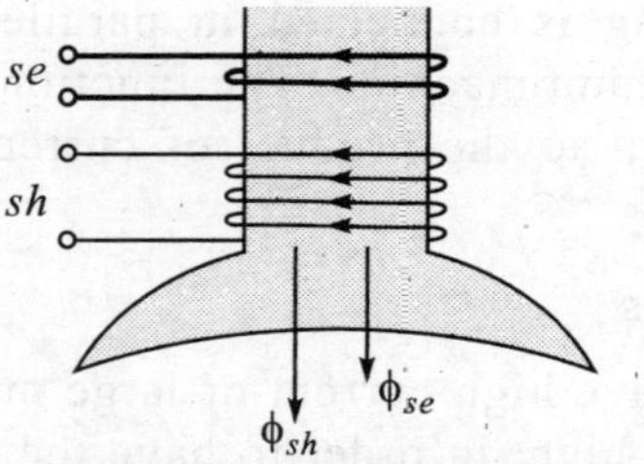

(a) Cumulative compounding.

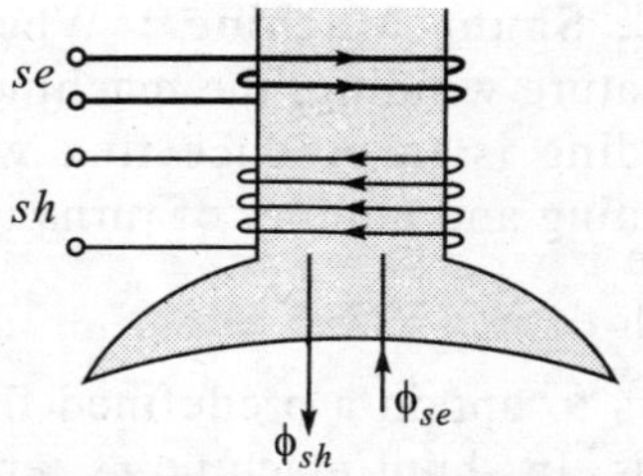

(b) Differential compounding.

Fig. 7.11

Both the field windings i.e. shunt and series field windings are placed on the poles as shown in Fig. 7.11. Both these windings carry currents, and hence both the windings will contribute to the air-gap flux. If the fluxes produced by the shunt field winding and series field winding are in the same direction, it is called *cumulative compounding*.

Whereas, if the fluxes produced by both the windings are in opposite direction than it is called *differential compounding*.

7.1.6 D.C. Motors

When an electric generator is in operation, it is driven mechanically and develops a voltage, which in turn can send a current through the load. Whereas when an electric motor is in operation, it is connected to supply, develops a torque which in turn produces mechanical rotation.

In a generator, when a conductor is moved in a field an emf is induced in the conductor and if a closed path is provided current flows, whereas, in a motor, when a current carrying conductor is placed in a field it experiences a torque. Hence, whether it is a generator as motor, both should have a field, both should have conductors carrying current. This shows that constructionally, both generator and motor are similar. In fact, the same machine can be made to operator as a motor as well as a generator. d.c. motors also are classified as d.c.. generator i.e. separately excited, self excited, shunt, series and compound motors. Hence a general term '*machine*' has been used so far which indicates generator or motor.

7.1.7 Comparison of Generator and Motor

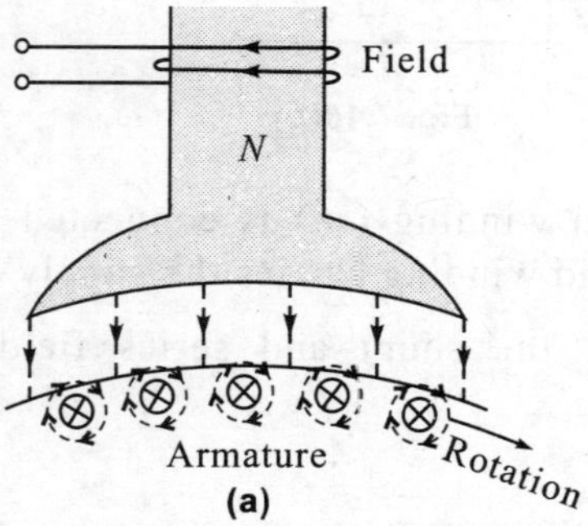

(a)

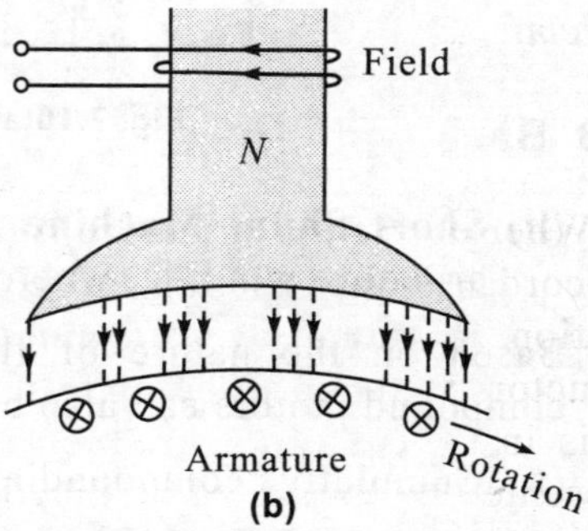

(b)

Fig. 7.12 : D.c. generator section of machine under one pole.

Consider a d.c. machine and study its operation first as a generator and then as a motor.

Consider a section of d.c. generator under the N-pole as in Fig. 7.12(a). The dotted lines from pole to armature indicate *direction of flux*. The armature is rotated in the direction shows (clock-wise). The direction of current as given by "*Flemings right hand rule*" will be as shown in Fig. 7.12(a).

Now each current carrying conductor will have a field around it given by "*right hand thumb rule*" shown by dotted circles around the conductors.

Observe Fig. 7.12(a) carefully, on the left side of a conductor, the field due to N-pole and field due to current in the conductor are in opposite directions, whereas on the right hand side of the conductor, these field are in the same direction. The result of this phenomenon is that the field on left side of the conductor will be weaker as compared to the right side. Thus a crowding of lines of flux is seen on the right edge of the pole Fig. 7.12(b) as compared to the left edge.

This crowding of lines exert a force on the armature in a direction opposite to the direction of rotation [as if there were large number of rubber-bands on the right side of pole and are trying to push the rotar to left hand side]. Thus, there is backward drag on the conductors. It is against this drag action, that prime-mover has to work, the work done in overcoming this opposition is converted into electric energy.

Assume there is no prime-mover attached to the armature. Field is same as previous case and we pass a current in the same direction as in case of the generator (Fig.7.13). There will be crowding of lines on the right hand side of armature. This crowding of lines of flux will push the generator in anti-clockwise direction (opposite to generator rotation). Hence the motor will rotate in anticlockwise direction.

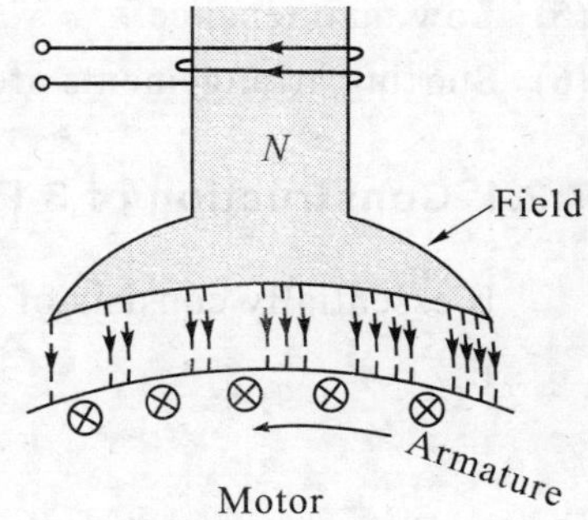

Fig. 7.13

As said, energy conversion is not possible unless there is some opposition, overcoming which provides the necessary means of energy conversion. In case of generator, it was the magnetic drag. In motors it is called *back emf*.

7.1.8 Back emf

When the motor armature rotates, the conductors also rotate and hence cut the flux. In accordance with the laws of electromagnetic induction, emf is induced in them whose direction is found by "*Fleming's Right Hand Rule*". Thus the induced emf in the conductors is found to be opposite of Fig. 7.13, i.e. dots in the conductors. Because this emf is in the opposite direction it is referred to as *back emf or counter emf* (E_b). It is represented as in Fig. 7.14. If R_a is the resistance of armature circuit, the armature current is given by

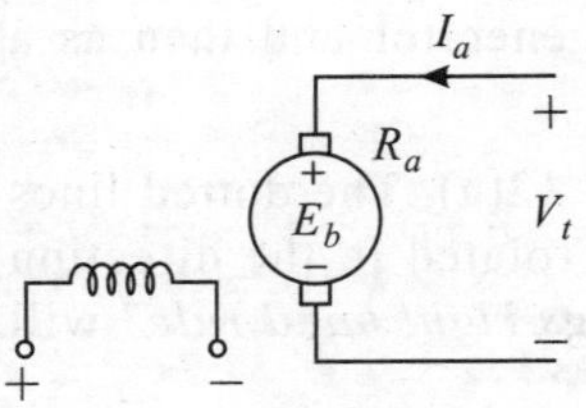

Fig. 7.14

$$I_a = \frac{V_t - E_b}{R_a} \quad \text{..... (7.6)}$$

$$\text{or} \quad V_t = E_b + I_a R_a \quad \text{..... (7.7)}$$

This back emf E_b is the generated emf of the motor and is given by

$$E_b = \frac{p\phi NZ}{60A} \quad \text{..... (7.8)}$$

7.2 3-Phase Induction Motors

With the universal adoption of a.c. system of distribution of electric energy the field of application of ac motors have widened. More than 85% of industrial motors in use are induction motors. It is substantially a constant speed motor with shunt characteristic i.e. a few percent drop in speed from no load to full load.

The advantages of induction motors above other motors are :

(1) Very simple, extremely rugged and almost unbreakable construction.

(2) Low cost and very reliable operation.

(3) Sufficiently high efficiency, no brushes needed hence reduced frictional losses.

(4) Reasonably good power factor.

(5) Low maintenance.

(6) Starting arrangements are simple.

7.2.1 Construction of 3-Phase Induction Motors

It essentially consists of two parts (a) the stator and (b) the rotor.

The stator is made of stampings which are slotted to receive the windings (Fig.7.15). The stator carries a three phase winding and is fed from a three phase supply. It is wound for a definite number of poles, the exact number being determined by the requirement of speed.

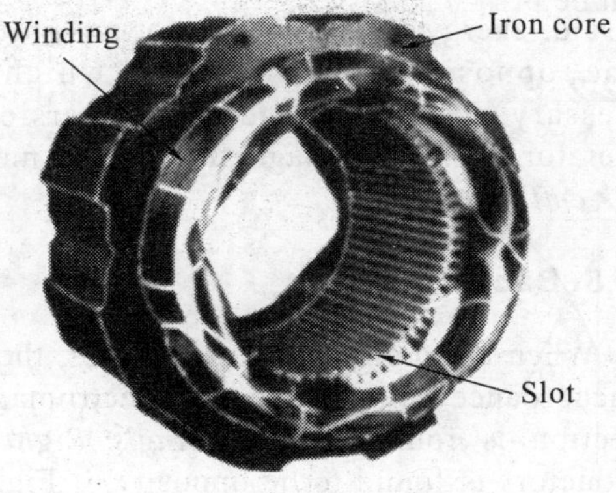

Fig. 7.15 : Stator

The rotor construction is basically of two types (i) squirrel cage, and (ii) phase wound or wound rotor.

The ***squirrel cage construction*** has heavy bars of copper or aluminium or alloy, one in each slot (Fig. 7.16). All these bars are short circuited at the ends so that a closed path of rotor currents is provided. The bars are skewed (twisted) so as to reduce humming and reduce locking tendency i.e. the tendency of rotor teeth to remain under the stator teeth due to direct magnetic attraction between the two.

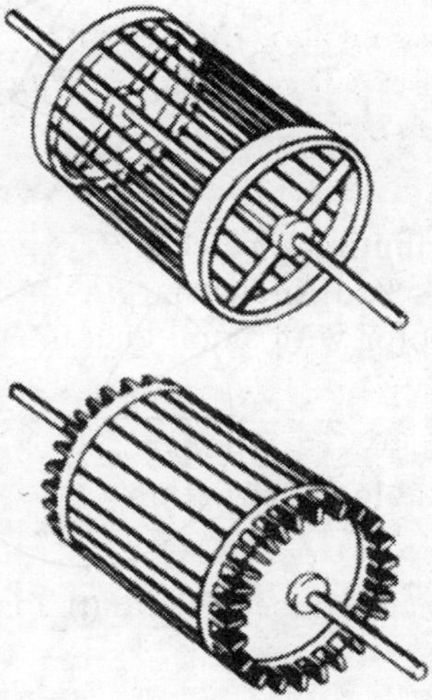

Fig. 7.16 : Squirrel cage rotor

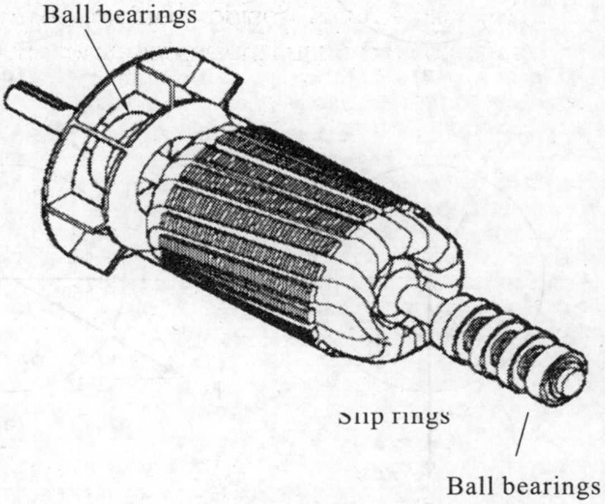

Fig. 7.17 : Wound rotor

The ***wound rotor type construction*** has a three phase, double layer, distributed winding consisting of coils similar to stator (Fig. 7.17). The rotor is wound for as many poles as stator. The three phases are star connected internally. The other three terminals are connected to three insulated slip rings mounted on the shaft with brushes resting on them. The brushes are further connected to star connected rheostats so that high starting torque can be produced.

7.2.2 Production of Rotating Magnetic Field

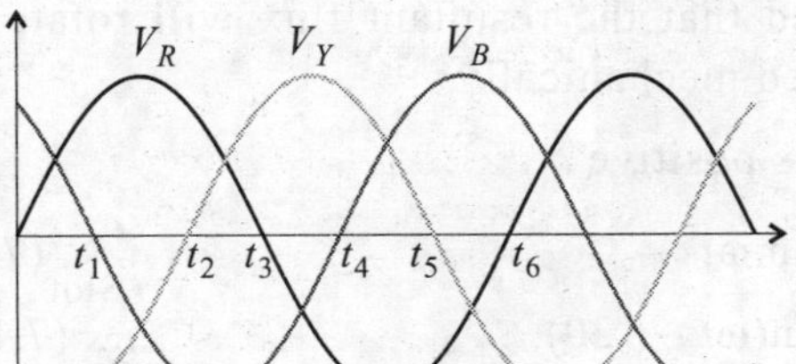

Fig. 7.18

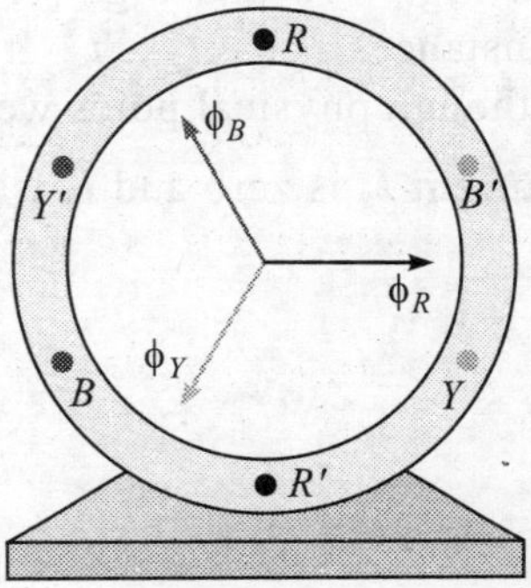

Fig. 7.19

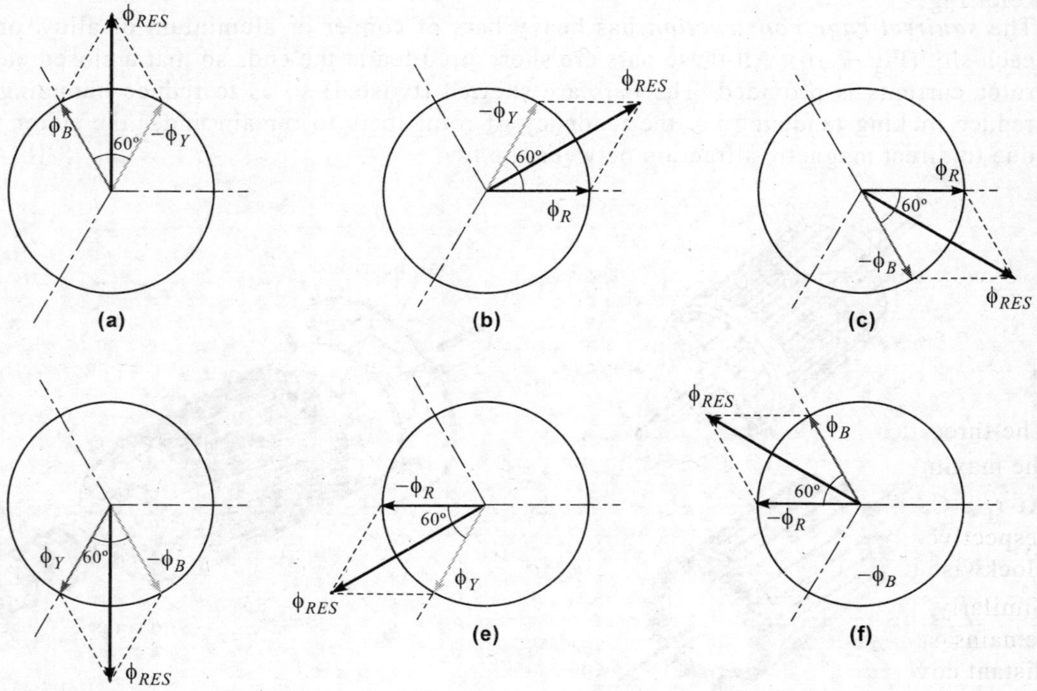

Fig. 7.20

When a three-phase stator winding of an induction motor is connected to a 3-phase source, three independent currents tend to flow, one in each phase. These currents will be displaced from each other by exactly 120° electrical i.e. the currents are as shown Fig. 7.18. The currents are said to be "*displaced in time*" by 120° with phase sequence assumed to be *RYB*. Next consider Fig. 7.19, which schematically represents the three phase windings of a two pole machine. The flux produced by the *R* phase will be along ϕ_R, similarly the fluxes produced by *Y* and *B* phase will be along ϕ_Y and ϕ_B respectively. It can be seen that the three fluxes are at an angle of 120° with respect to each other. With respect to Fig. 7.18 and Fig. 7.19 observe Fig. 7.20, which shows the resultant flux at various instances $t_0, t_1, t_2 \ldots t_6$. It will be observed that the resultant flux will rotate in space as though physical poles were actually rotated mechanically.

At t_0 : Current I_R is zero and I_Y is negative and I_B is positive

$$\text{If} \quad \phi_R = \phi_m \sin \omega t \qquad \text{..... (7.9)}$$

$$\phi_Y = \phi_m \sin(\omega t - 120) \qquad \text{..... (7.10)}$$

$$\phi_B = \phi_m \sin(\omega t - 240) \qquad \text{..... (7.11)}$$

At $\omega t = 0$, we have

$$\phi_R = 0,\ \phi_Y = -\frac{\sqrt{3}}{2}\phi_m,\ \phi_B = \frac{\sqrt{3}}{2}\phi_m$$

Refer Fig.7 6(a), the R phase flux will be zero, Y phase flux will have magnitude of

$\phi_m \frac{\sqrt{3}}{2}$ along $-\phi_y$ axis and $\frac{\sqrt{3}}{2}\phi_m$ along ϕ_B axis.

$$\phi_{RES} = \sqrt{\phi_y^2 + \phi_B^2 + 2\phi_y\phi_B \cos 60} \quad \text{..... (7.12)}$$

$$= \sqrt{\frac{3}{4}\phi_m^2 + \frac{3}{4}\phi_m^2 + 2\left(\frac{\sqrt{3}}{2}\right)\left(\frac{\sqrt{3}}{2}\right)\frac{1}{2}\phi_m^2}$$

$$= \sqrt{\frac{9}{4}\phi_m^2}$$

$$\phi_{RES} = \frac{3}{2}\phi_m \quad \text{..... (7.13)}$$

The three fluxes are added vectorially to get the resultant flux ϕ_{RES} which is (3/2) times the maximum flux in any phase ϕ_m.

At t_1 : Current I_B is zero, I_R is positive and I_Y is negative. The fluxes will have their respective directions and proportionate magnitudes. The resultant flux has shifted in clockwise direction and the magnitude remains same as the previous value.

Similarly, studying time instants t_2, t_3, ...t_6 we observe that magnitude of resultant flux remains same but the direction changes clockwise. Therefore, the field will revolve a distant covered by two poles for each cycle.

If there are P poles, then cycles per revolution will be $P/2$.

If f = frequency of supply in cycles per second, then revolutions of field per second n_s will be

$$n_s = \frac{2f}{P}$$

$$\text{or} \quad N_s = \text{rev per min} = 60 \times \frac{2f}{P} = \frac{120f}{P} \quad \text{..... (7.14)}$$

where, N_s is the speed with which the field revolves, also called the *synchronous speed*.

7.2.3 Principle of Operation

When a 3-phase space distributed winding (120°) (Fig. 7.19) is supplied with a 3-phase time distributed supply (Fig. 7.18), a rotating magnetic field (Fig. 7.20) is produced, as if actual magnetic poles were being rotated mechanically. When this rotating field interacts with stationary rotor conductors an emf is induced in the rotor conductor which causes currents to flow in the short circuited rotor conductor. Due to this a torque is produced and rotor rotates so as to oppose the cause (Lenz law). The cause here is the relative speed between the field and the rotor. Hence the rotor rotates in the direction of the field so that the relative speed between the two becomes zero. But this relative speed can not become zero i.e. the rotor cannot rotate at the speed of stator field (synchronous speed), because the rotor at synchronous speed will not cut any lines of flux and so no emf will be induced in it hence no current and no torque will be developed. The speed of rotor N is always less than the speed of field N_s called the *synchronous speed*.

7.2.4 Slip and Rotor Speed

Although the rotor of an induction motor must rotate in the same direction as the revolving field, it can not do so at synchronous speed and the actual rotor speed is called the *slip speed*. It is generally specified in terms of synchronous speed and as percentage.

$$\% \text{ slip} = \frac{N_s - N}{N_s} \times 100 \qquad \text{..... (7.15)}$$

where, N_s = synchronous speed

N = speed of rotor.

7.3 Single-Phase Induction Motor

A large number of fractional kilowatt a.c. motors are designed to operate from a single phase a.c. supply. Although, 3-phase induction motors can be made in small sizes, but the supply in offices, homes and business premises, where these motors are used, is single-phase.

If a three-phase supply is given to a 3-phase induction motor, a rotating magnetic field is produced starting torque is developed. If a 3-phase induction motor carrying less than half rated load, has its one phase supply disconnected, the motor continues to run, though at reduced speed and increased stator current. The 2 remaining phases constitute in effect a single-phase supply, and therefore a pulsating stator mmf wave is produced. The motor so obtained from a 3-phase motor has poor power factor, low capacity and reduced efficiency. A single-phase induction motor (I.M.) with pulsating magnetic field is not self starting.

7.3.1 Constructional Features of Single-Phase Induction Motors

The rotor of a single-phase I.M. is exactly similar to the squirrel-cage rotor of a 3- phase I.M.

The stator carries two windings namely: main (running) winding and the auxiliary (starting) winding. The main winding is distributed along the stator periphery in about two third of the total slots, because no advantage is achieve if all the slots are wound. The space angle between the main and secondary winding is 90° i.e. the magnetic axis of main and auxiliary windings are in space quadrature.

7.3.2 Double Field Revolving Theory

A single phase I.M. can be represented as in Fig. 7.21. An alternating current in the main winding produces a stator field (mmf) which is stationary in space but pulsating in magnitude. As a result, the stator field ϕ_s produced by the main winding is alternating in polarity but varying sinusoidal with time.

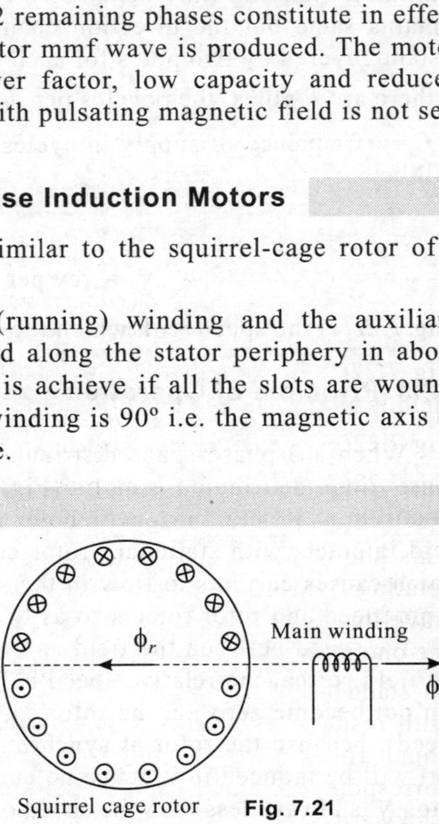

Fig. 7.21

By transformer action, alternating flux ϕ_r induces large currents in the rotor. This rotor current sets up rotor field (mmf) which opposes the stator field at all instants of time. Since the rotor and stator fields are along the same axis, the torque angle between ϕ_s and ϕ_r is zero and no starting torque is developed.

According to '*Revolving Field Theory*' the stationary, pulsating stator field can be resolved into two counter rotating magnetic fields of equal magnitude and moving at synchronous speed. The maximum value of each being $F_s/2$. This is illustrated in Fig. 7.22.

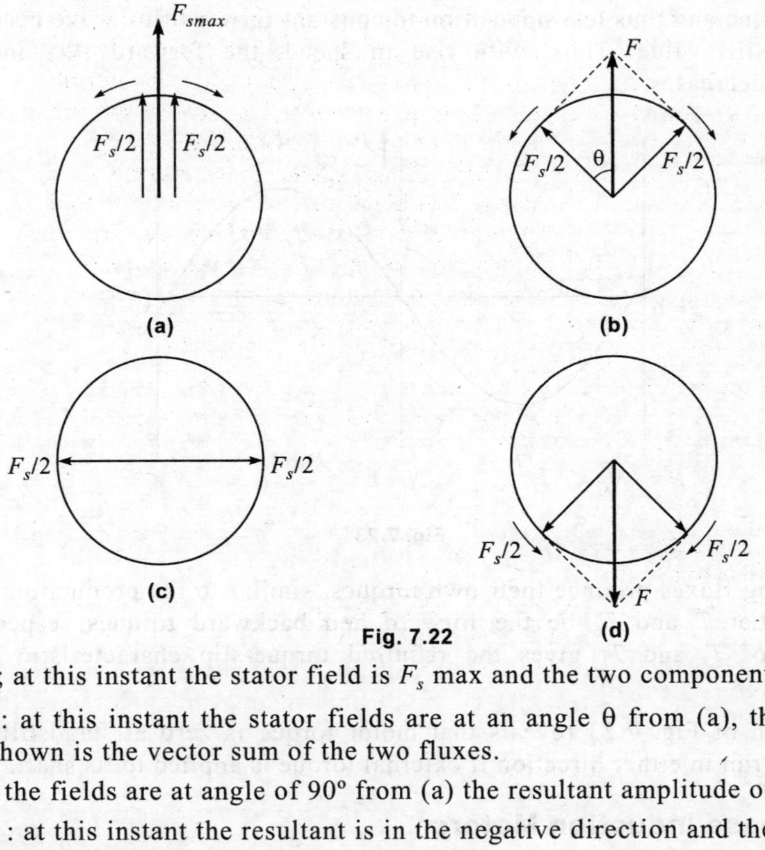

Fig. 7.22

Fig 7.22(a); at this instant the stator field is F_s max and the two component are $F_{smax}/2$.

Fig 7.22(b): at this instant the stator fields are at an angle θ from (a), the amplitude of field is as shown is the vector sum of the two fluxes.

Fig 7.22(c) the fields are at angle of 90° from (a) the resultant amplitude of field is zero.

Fig 7.22(d) : at this instant the resultant is in the negative direction and the resulting field is still along the same axis.

This shows that a stationary, pulsating stator field can be resolved into two counter rotating fields of constant magnitude and moving at synchronous speeds. The stator field travelling in the direction of rotor movement is referred to as forward rotating field and the one in the opposite direction is called *backward rotating field*.

At standstill, both forward and backward rotating fields rotate at synchronous speed N_s with respect to rotor conductors. Both these fields, therefore, induce equal rotor emfs, equal rotor currents and give rise to equal rotor fields. These react with their corresponding equal counter-rotating stator mmfs and, therefore, both forward and backward rotating fields are equal with the rotor at standstill.

When the rotor rotates at a speed N_r, the speed of backward field becomes $N_s + N_r$ with respect to rotor conductors. Hence, backward field induces large rotor emf, large rotor current and thus, large rotor mmf as compared to standstill value. This large mmf opposes its constant rotor backward rotating mmf wave. As a result backward flux wave is reduced considerably from its value at standstill.

The speed of forward flux wave is $N_s - N_r$ with respect to rotor conductors. This relative speed induces small rotor emf, small rotor current and therefore small rotor mmf as compared to their values at standstill. The reduced rotor mmf component as compared to its standstill value and thus less opposition to constant forward flux wave becomes higher than its standstill value. Thus, with rise in speed, the forward flux increases and backward flux decreases.

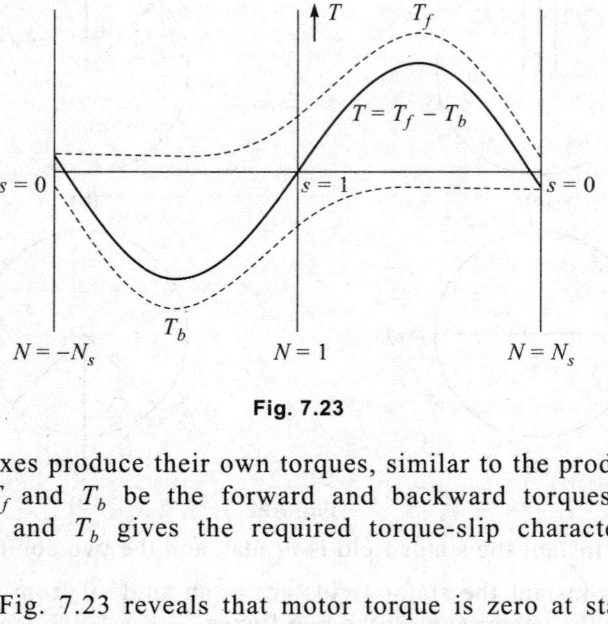

Fig. 7.23

The two rotating fluxes produce their own torques, similar to the production of torque in 3-phase I.M. Let T_f and T_b be the forward and backward torques respectively. The superposition of T_f and T_b gives the required torque-slip characteristic for 1-phase I.M.(Fig.7.23)

An examination of Fig. 7.23 reveals that motor torque is zero at standstill, also the 1 phase I.M. can run in either direction if external torque is applied to its shaft.

7.4 Split-Phase Induction Motors

When a motor is provided with two windings, even though they are excited from the same voltage source, the currents can be made to have a phase difference by having suitable impedance in the auxiliary winding with respect to main winding. As a result $F_{fs} > F_b$ i.e. the forward field is made stronger than the backward rotating field, resulting in a starting in a starting torque. This is how a single phase motor is made self starting.

Two important methods of phase splitting are:

(a) Resistance split-phase motors

(b) Capacitor split-phase motors.

(a) Resistance Split-Phase Motors

The motor employs an auxiliary winding with high resistance (Fig. 7.24). M and A denote main and auxiliary winding respectively. C_s is the centrifugal switch.

The difference in the impedance causes auxiliary winding current I_A to lead the main winding current I_M by angle α (phasor diagram). The fields created by two currents also have a phase difference of α and hence a torque is produced.

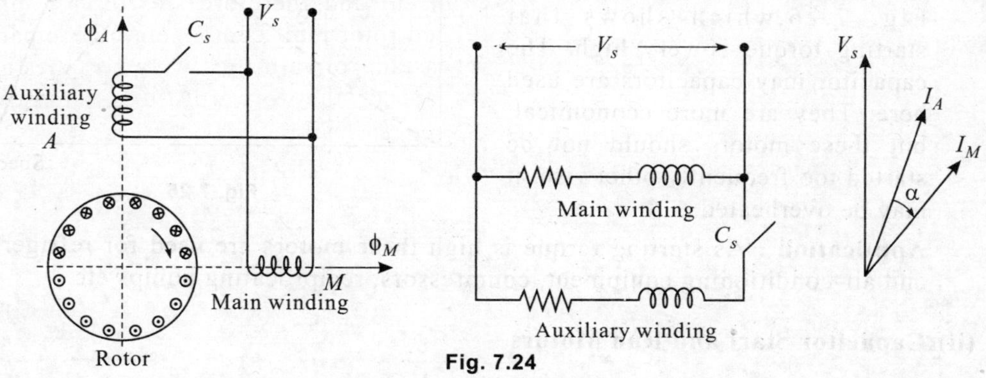

Fig. 7.24

The main winding is made of thick wire hence has a low resistance, and higher leakage reactance, whereas the auxiliary winding is made of higher reactance i.e. thin wire and low leakage reactance.

The starting winding is automatically disconnected by means of centrifugal switch C_s at about 70 - 80% of rated speed.

Applications : Fans, blowers, centrifugal pumps and refrigerators. The economical power ratings are from 10-200 watts.

(b) Capacitor Split-Phase Motors

The problem of poor starting torque in resistance split-phase motor is solved by using a capacitor in series with the auxiliary winding and thereby reaching ideal case $\alpha = 90°$. Auxiliary winding may often be disconnected after starting.

(i) Capacitor Start Motors

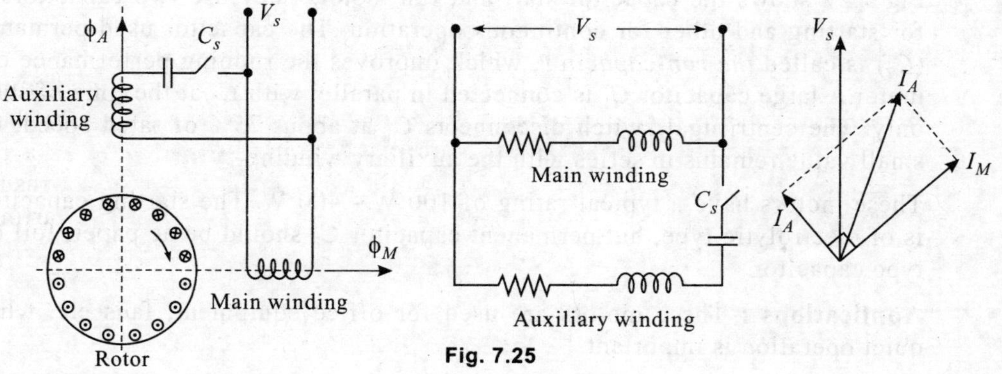

Fig. 7.25

Fig 7.25 shows the schematic diagram of capacitor start motor. The capacitor, here, is used only to start the machine. The value of capacitor is so chosen as to give $\alpha = 90°$ electrical. The torque speed characteristic is as shown in Fig. 7.26, which shows that starting torque is very high. The capacitor may capacitors are used here. They are more economical, but these motors should not be started too frequently otherwise, it may be overheated.

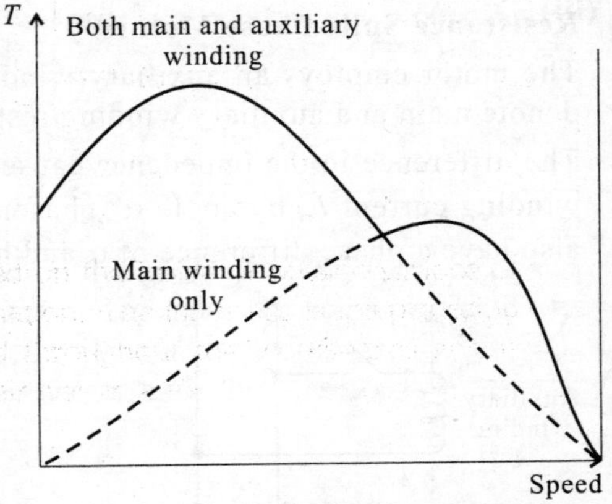

Fig. 7.26

Application : As starting torque is high these motors are used for refrigeration and air-conditioning equipment, compressors, reciprocating pumps etc.

(ii) Capacitor Start and Run Motors

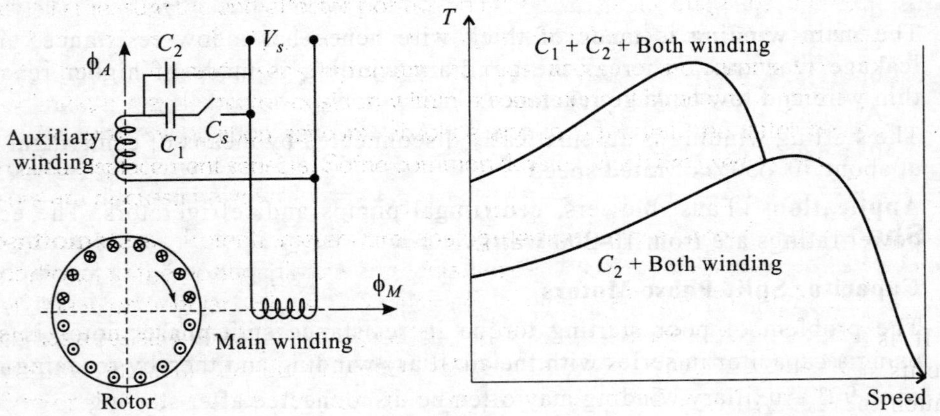

Fig. 7.27

Fig 7.27 shows the capacitor start and run motor. They use two capacitors, one for starting and other for continuous operation. The capacitor used permanently (C_2) is called *the run-capacitor*, which improves the running performance of the motor. A large capacitor C_1 is connected in parallel with C_2 at the time of starting only. The centrifugal switch disconnects C_1 at about 75% of rated speed. C_2 of small value remains in series with the auxiliary winding.

These motors have a typical rating of 100 W - 400 W. The starting capacitor C_1 is of electrolytic type, but permanent capacitor C_2 should be ac paper, foil or oil type capacitor.

Applications : These motors are used for office equipment, fans etc. where a quiet operation is important.

(iii) Capacitor Run Motors

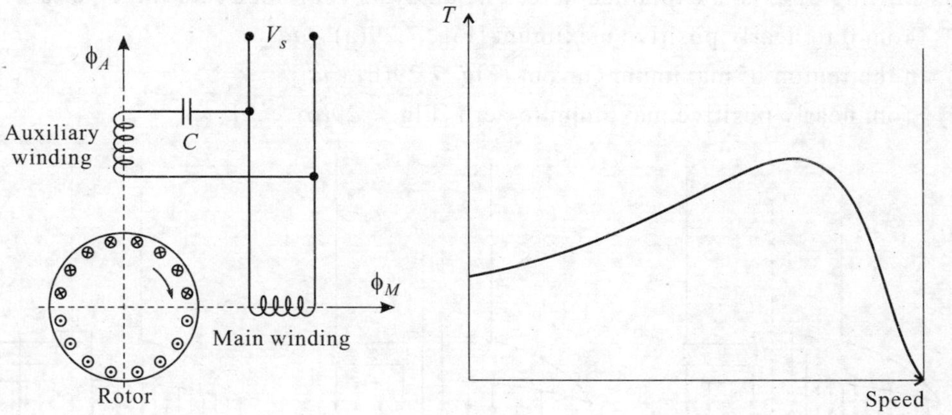

Fig. 7.28

The same capacitor is kept permanently in series with the auxiliary winding both at starting and during running condition. There is no need of centrifugal switch. At a particular designed load the capacitor and auxiliary winding can be so designed as to result in 90° time- phase displacement between the two winding currents. The motor has improved efficiency and better power factor. The motor operation is very quiet.

Applications : Ceiling fans are invariably of capacitor run type in which value of capacitance is 2 - 3μF.

7.5 Shaded Pole Induction Motor

It is essentially an induction motor, since its squirrel cage rotor receives power in much the same way as does the rotor of poly -phase induction motor. The difference between the two is that poly-phase induction motor creates a true revolving field and merely shifts from one side of the pole to other and thus torque is not constant and varies from instant to instant. Fig 7.29 shows a typical shaded pole. A small portion of the pole is covered with a short circuited single turn copper coil called *shading coil*.

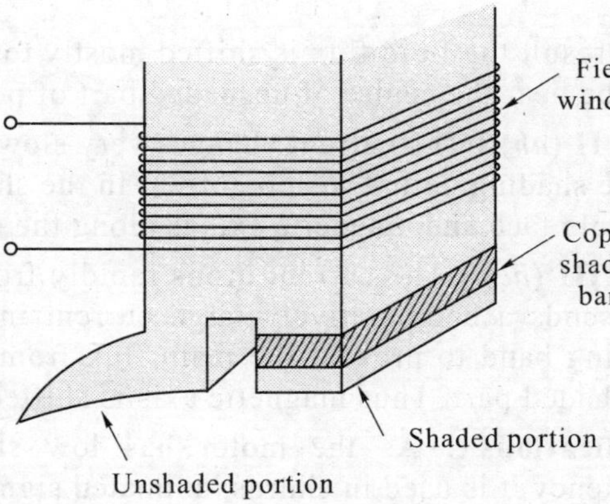

Fig. 7.29

When the field winding is excited by an a.c. source the magnetic axis will shift from unshaded part of the pole to the shaded part of the pole.

This shifting of axis is explained here. The analysis is divided into three parts

(i) From 0 to nearly positive maximum [Fig. 7.29(a) - *oa*]

(ii) In the region of maximum current [Fig. 7.29(b) - *ab*]

(iii) From nearly positive maximum to zero [Fig. 7.29(c) - *bc*]

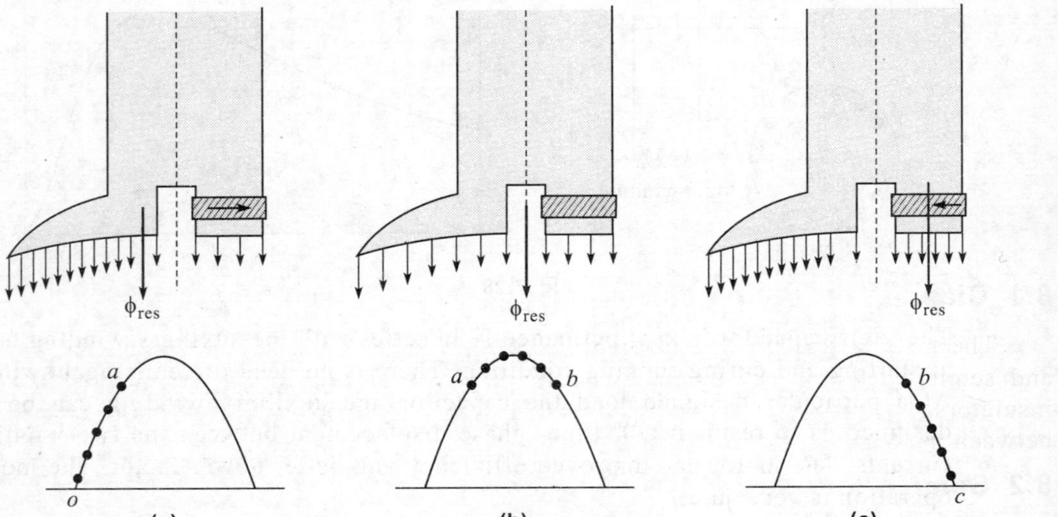

Fig. 7.30

Part I (*oa*) : As shown in Fig.7.30(a), in this part the current rises very sharply from o to a along the sine curve, under this condition, a voltage will be induced in the shading coil by transformer action. The current in the low resistance turn will be comparatively high and will be in such a direction that it

As a result the field flux is shifted mostly to unshaded part of the pole. The magnetic axis will be near the centre of unshaded part of pole.

Part II (*ab*) : The current changes very slowly along ab and practically no emf is induced in the shading coil. Thus no current in the shading coil and flux distribution is even along the pole face and magnetic axis is along the centre of pole face.(Fig. 7.30 b).

Part III (*bc*) : The current drops rapidly from *b* to *c* and emf is induced in shading coil and sends a comparatively large current in such a direction as to create a flux in the shading band to prevent the main flux from dieing out i.e. a strong *N* pole is created in the shaded part. Thus magnetic axis is shifted to centre of shaded part of the pole.

Applications : As the motor has low starting torque, low overload capacity, low efficiency it is used in churns, animated signs and advertising displays.

CHAPTER

8 SEMICONDUCTOR DIODES AND THEIR APPLICATIONS

8.1 Classification of Materials

The materials can be broadly classified into three types viz. conductors, insulators and semiconductors. The conductors allow current to flow easily through them. The insulators do not allow any current through them. Whereas, the semiconductors are in between the conductors and the insulators.

8.2 Semiconductors

Germanium and Silicon are the two most important semiconductor materials used in electronic devices. The crystal structure of these materials consists of regular repetition in three dimensions of a unit cell having the form of a tetrahedron, with an atom at each vertex.(Fig. 8.1)

Germanium (Ge) has 32 electrons (2,8,18,4), and Silicon (Si) has 14 electrons (2,8,4) and each atom contributes four valance electrons. The binding force between neighbouring atoms results from the fact that each valance electron of a germanium atom is shared by one of its four nearest neighbours (Fig. 8.1). This is a co-valent bond. The valence electrons serve to bind one atom to the next. Hence, inspite of the availability of 4 valance electrons the crystal has low conductivity.

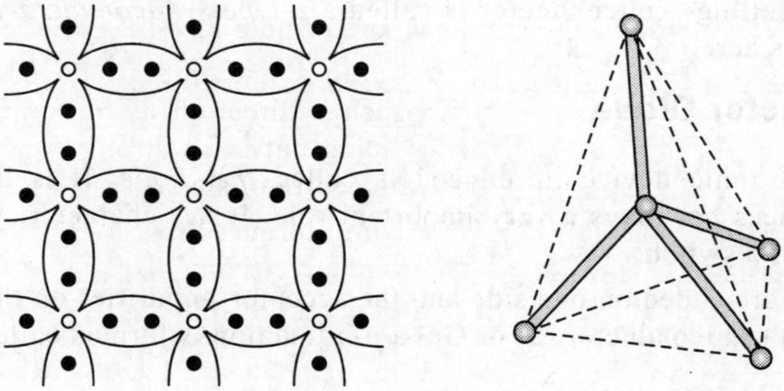

Fig. 8.1

At very low temperatures, the crystal behaves as an insulator, since no free electrons are available. However, at room temperature some bonds are broken because of the thermal energy supplied to the crystal and conduction is made possible

The energy required to break such a co-valent bond is 0.7 eV for Ge and 1.1 eV for Si, thus forming holes (Fig. 8.2). The importance of holes is that it serves as carrier of electricity.

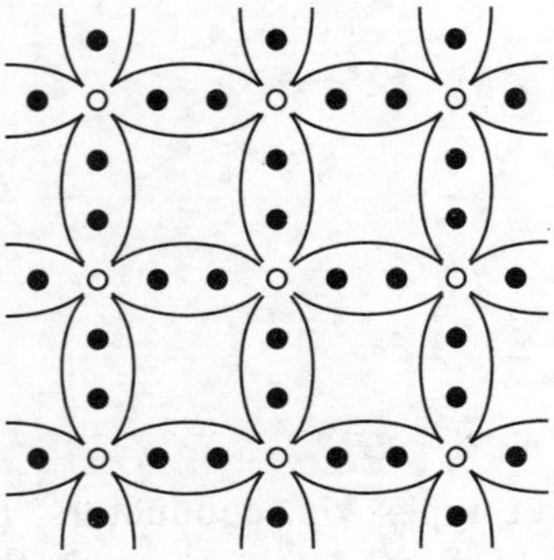

Fig. 8.2

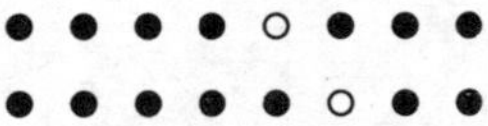

Fig. 8.3 : Flow of hole.

The motion of hole in one direction actually means the transport of negative charge by an equal distance in the opposite direction (Fig. 8.3).

8.3 Donor and Acceptor Impurities

If, to a pure germanium atom, a small impurity is added in the form of a substance with five valance electrons, they displace some of the germanium atoms in the crystal lattice, four of the five valance electrons will occupy co-valent bonds and the fifth will be nominally bound and will be available as a carrier of current. The energy required to detach this fifth electron is 0.0 1 eV for Ge and 0.05 eV for Si.

Suitable pentavalent impurities are Antimony, Phosphorous and arsenic. Such impurities donate excess electron carriers and are referred to as *donor* impurities and the resulting semiconductor is called an *n-type semiconductor*.

If a trivalent impurity like Boron, Gallium or indium, is added to an intrinsic semiconductor, only three co-valent bonds are filled and the vacancy that exists in the fourth bond constitutes a hole. Such an impurity is called an *acceptor* or *p-type* impurities. This resulting semiconductor is called a *p-type semiconductor*. The holes are the majority carriers here.

8.4 Semiconductor Diode

The first electronic device introduced is called *the diode*. It is the simplest of semiconductor devices but plays a very important role. It has characteristic that closely matches with that of a switch.

If donor impurities are added on one side and the acceptor impurities on the other side of a single crystal of a semiconductor (Si or Ge) a *p-n* junction is formed called a *diode*.

(i) **Diode without any Biasing** : Refer Fig. 8.4. The donor ion is indicated by a +ve sign because, after it donates an electron it becomes positive ion. The acceptor ion is indicated by –ve sign because, after this atom accepts an electron it becomes negative ion.

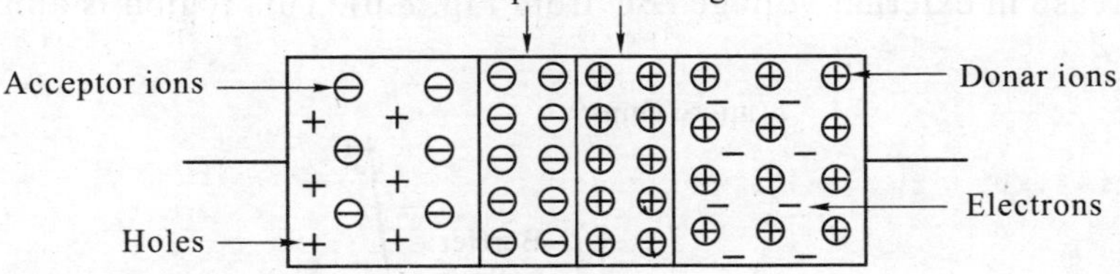

Fig. 8.4

Initially, there are normally only *p*-type carriers to the left of the junction and only *n*-type carriers to the right. But as there is a density gradient across the junction, holes will diffuse to the right across the junction and electrons to the left leaving behind uncompensated negative acceptor ions ⊖ on *p*-side of the junction and positive donor ions ⊕ on *n*-side of the junction (Fig. 8.4) giving rise to a potential barrier at the junction. As a result an electric field will appear across the junction. Equilibrium will be established when the field becomes large enough to restrain the process of diffusion.

Since this region has got depleted of mobile charge carriers, it is called the *Depletion region* or *the space charge region*.

(ii) ***P-N* Junction Diode with Biasing** : The diode allows easy flow of current in one direction but restrains the flow of current in the reverse direction.

(a) Forward Biased Diode : When *p*-type region is connected to positive terminal and *n*-type to the negative terminal of the supply, the potential barrier reduces (Fig. 8.5).

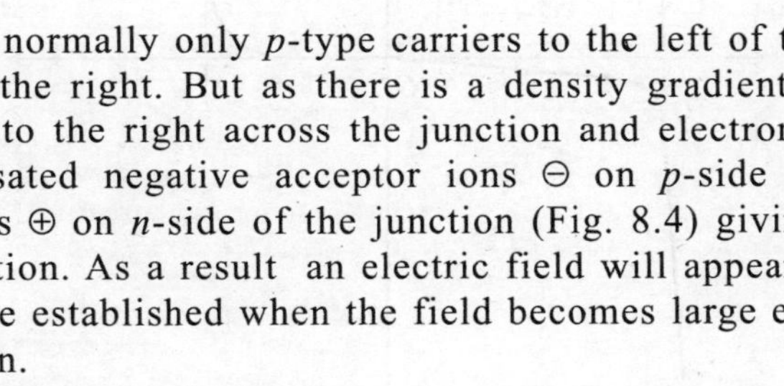

Fig. 8.5

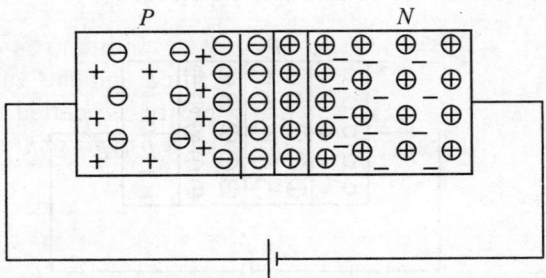

At some forward voltage (0.7 V for Si and 0.3 V for Ge), the potential barrier is completely eliminated and the current starts flowing in the circuit. From now onwards, the current increases with increase in forward voltage. *OC* from Fig. 8.6 is the forward characteristic of diode.

Between *OA* no current flows through the junction and the potential barrier exists.

Between *AB* the current increases very slowly and the curve is non-linear. It is because the external supply voltage is used up in overcoming the barrier potential.

However, once the external voltage exceeds the barrier potential voltage, the *p-n* junction behaves like an ordinary conductor. Therefore, the current rises very sharply with increase in external voltage (*BC* from Fig. 8.6). This region is almost linear.

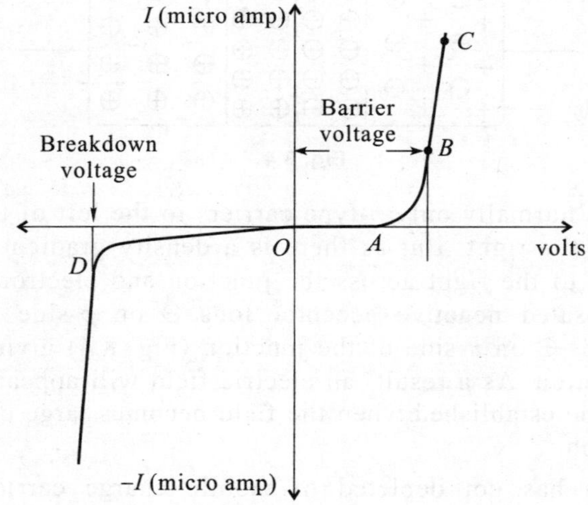

Fig. 8.6

(b) Reverse Biased Diode : The supply is connected with +ve terminal of supply to the *n*-type and –ve to the *p*-type semiconductor (Fig. 8.7). This causes the holes in *p*-region and the electrons in the *n*-region to move away from the junction, and the potential barrier at the junction increases, junction resistance increases and ideally no current flows through the circuit.

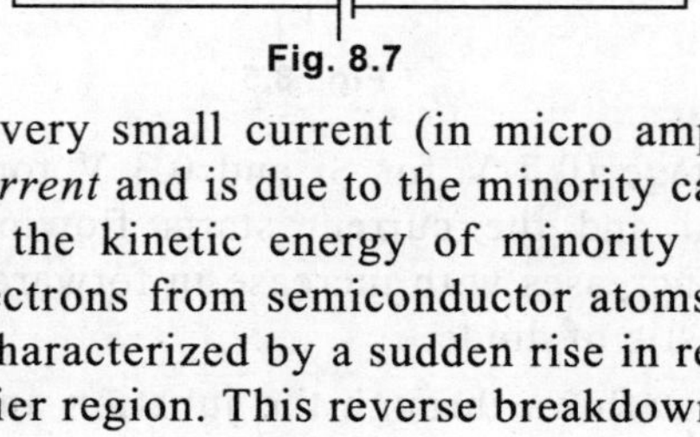

Fig. 8.7

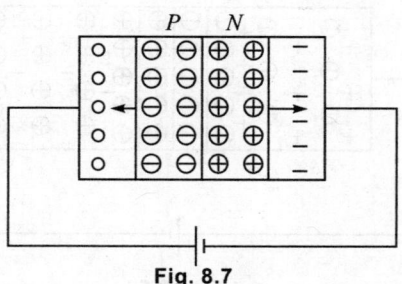

However, in practice a very small current (in micro amperes) flows in the circuit. This is called *reverse current* and is due to the minority carriers. If reverse voltage is increased continuously, the kinetic energy of minority carriers may become high enough to knock out electrons from semiconductor atoms. At this stage break down of the junction occurs, characterized by a sudden rise in reverse current and a sudden fall of resistance of barrier region. This reverse breakdown voltage is very large (it is the peak inverse voltage i.e. PIV rating of diode). This may destroy the junction permanently (beyond point D in Fig.8.6).

Cut-in voltage : The voltage at which the current through the junction starts to increase in the forward direction is called the *cut-in voltage*, Fig. 8.6 (OA). It is 0.2 V for germanium and 0.6 V for silicon.

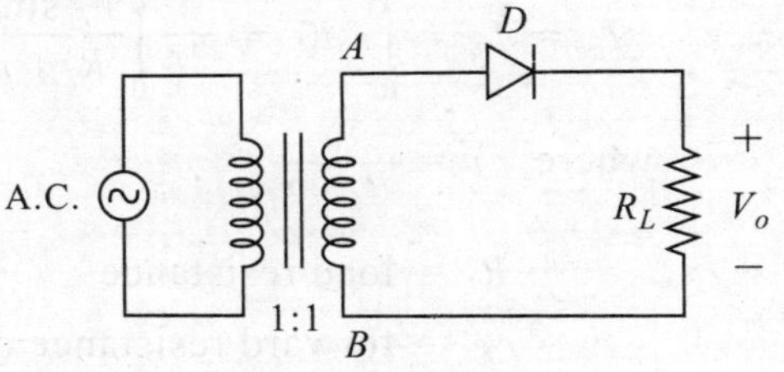

Fig. 8.8

8.5 Half-Wave Rectifier

Fig. 8.8 shows the circuit for a half-wave rectifier. In half-wave rectification, the rectifier conducts only in positive half of the supply cycle. The voltage available across AB (the output terminals of transformer) is as shown in Fig. 8.9.

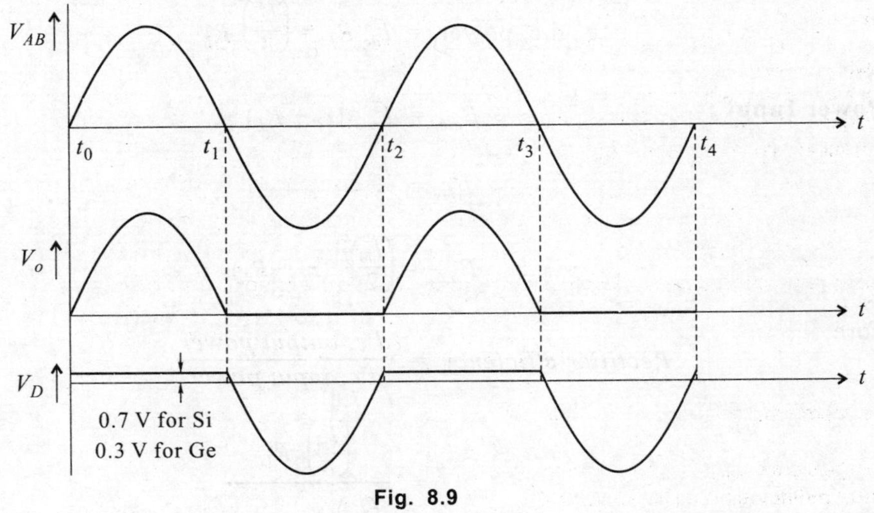

Fig. 8.9

Between t_0 and t_1 : A is at a higher potential as compared to B, therefore diode D is forward biased, and works as a closed switch (i.e. the drop across it is 0.7 for Si and 0.3 for Ge. Under this condition the load voltage will be same as voltage V_{AB}.

Between t_1 and t_2 : V_{AB} is negative or B is more positive with respect to A.

Thus diode D is reversed biased and only the leakage current flows. The output voltage is almost zero, and the voltage across the diode is same as V_{AB}. Observe the output voltage V_O, it contains only the positive half of supply voltage. The output current is always unidirectional. Hence, d.c. output is obtained across R_L, but this output is pulsating. These pulsations can further be smoothened with the help of filter circuits.

$$\textit{Rectifier efficiency} = \frac{\textit{d.c. output power}}{\textit{a.c. input power}} \quad \text{..... (8.1)}$$

D.C. Power Output : The output current is pulsating direct current. To find d.c. power we find I_{av}

$$I_{av} = I_{dc} = \int_0^\pi i\, d\theta = \frac{1}{2\pi}\int_0^\pi \frac{V_m \sin\theta}{R_L + r_f}\, d\theta \quad \text{..... (8.2)}$$

$$\text{where, } i = \frac{v}{R_L + r_f} \quad \text{..... (8.3)}$$

R_L = load resistance

r_f = forward resistance of diode.

$$\text{Therefore, } I_{d.c.} = \frac{V_m}{\pi(r_f + R_L)} = \frac{I_m}{\pi} \quad \text{..... (8.4)}$$

$$\text{where, } I_m = \frac{V_m}{r_f + R_L} \quad \text{..... (8.5)}$$

$$\therefore \quad \text{d.c. power} = I_{dc}^2 R_L = \left(\frac{I_m}{\pi}\right)^2 R_L \quad \text{..... (8.6)}$$

A.C. Power Input :

$$P_{a.c.} = I_{rms}^2 (r_f + R_L) \quad \text{..... (8.7)}$$

$$I_{rms} = \frac{I_m}{2}$$

$$\therefore \quad P_{a.c.} = \left(\frac{I_m}{2}\right)^2 (r_f + R_L) \quad \text{..... (8.8)}$$

Therefore,

$$\textit{Rectifier efficiency} = \frac{\textit{d.c. output power}}{\textit{a.c. input power}}$$

$$= \frac{\left(\frac{I_m}{\pi}\right)^2 R_L}{\left(\frac{I_m}{2}\right)^2 (r_f + R_L)}$$

$$= \frac{0.406\, R_L}{(R_L + r_f)} = \frac{0.406}{1 + \frac{r_f}{R_L}}$$

If r_f is negligible as compared to R_L, then we can get a maximum efficiency of 40.6%.

The use of transformer permits two advantages. Firstly, it allows to step up or step-down the a.c. input voltage. Secondly, the transformer isolates the rectifier circuit from the power circuit and thus reduces the risk of electric shocks.

The main disadvantages of half wave rectifier are :

(a) The a.c. supply delivers power only in half the supply cycle, so the output is low.

(b) Elaborate filtering is required to produce steady direct current.

8.6 Full-Wave Rectifier Circuit (with Centre Tap Transformer)

The circuit employs two diodes D_1 and D_2. The centre tap secondary winding AB is used with the two diodes, so that each half of a.c. input can be utilized (Fig. 8.10).

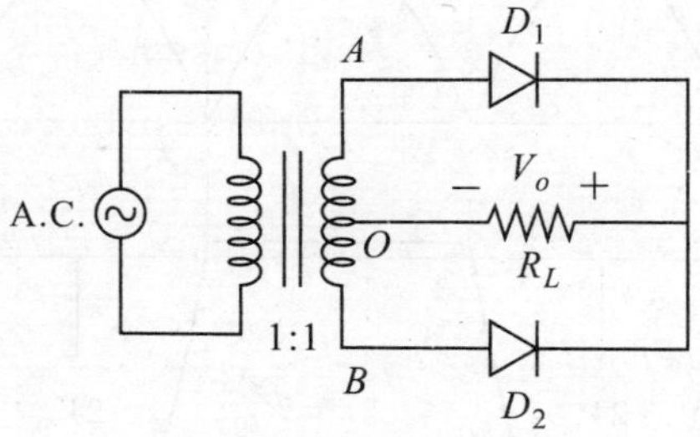

Fig. 8.10

With respect to supply voltage, voltage V_{AO} and V_{BO} are as shown in Fig. 8.11.

Diode D_1 is forward biased till A is at a higher potential than X, and D_2 is forward biased till B is at a higher potential than X. Similarly, D_1 is reversed biased when A is negative w.r.t. X and D_2 is reversed biased when B is negative w.r.t. X.

Between t_0 and t_1 : D_1 is forward biased and D_2 is reversed biased, or D_1 is a closed switch and D_2 open, and the load voltage is V_{AO} [refer Fig. 8.11(a)].

Between t_1 and t_2 interval : D_1 is reversed biased (open switch) and D_2 is forward biased (closed switch). The load voltage is V_{BO} [refer Fig. 8.11(b)].

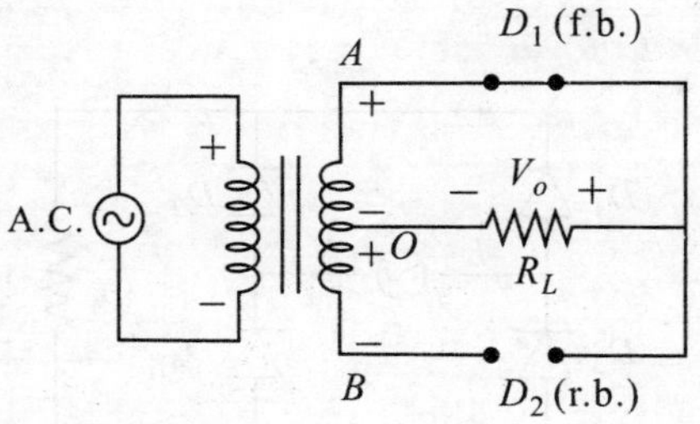

Fig. 8.11(a) : Between t_0 and t_1

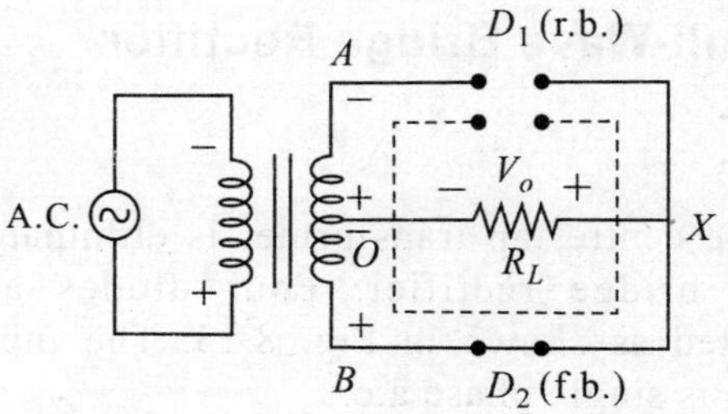

Fig. 8.11(b) : Between t_1 and t_2

Refer Fig. 8.11 and Fig. 8.12, when D_1 is forward biased the voltage across it is 0.7 V and when D_1 is reversed biased between t_1 and t_2 the voltage across D_1 is V_{AB} i.e. $V_{AO} - V_{BO}$.
At t_3 : V_{AO} is V_m and V_{BO} is V_m, thus V_{AB} is $V_m - (-V_m) = 2V_m$.

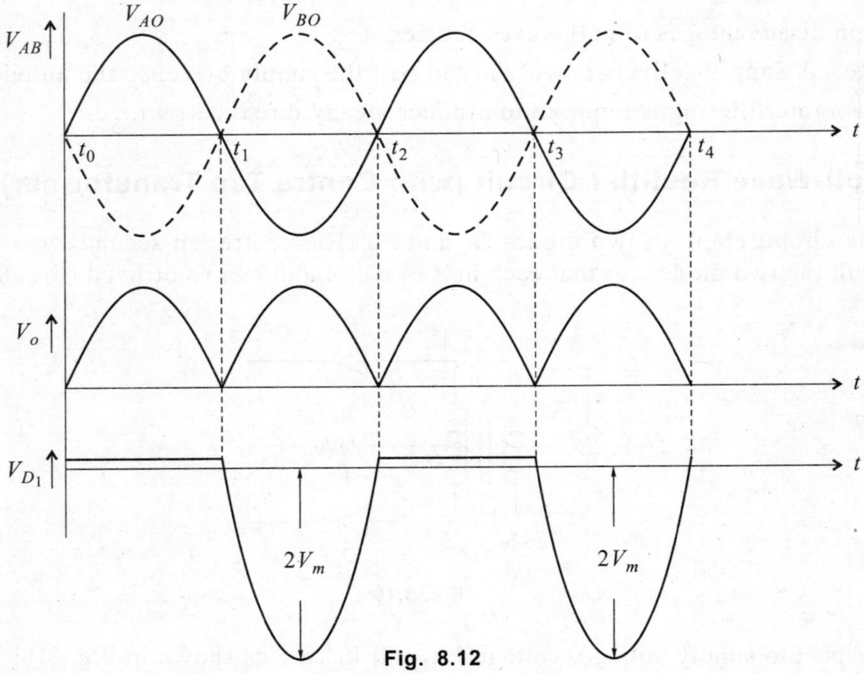

Fig. 8.12

Therefore, peak inverse voltage rating of each diode must be two times the maximum voltage across secondary.

(Derivation of output voltage is done after bridge rectifier).

The disadvantages of this circuit are:

The size of the circuit is big as transformer is used, and

The diodes used should have a higher PIV ($2V_m$) are to be used.

8.7 Full-Wave Bridge Rectifier

The centre tap transformer is eliminated in the bridge rectifier. Four diodes are connected as shown in Fig. 8.13. The input voltage is single phase a.c.

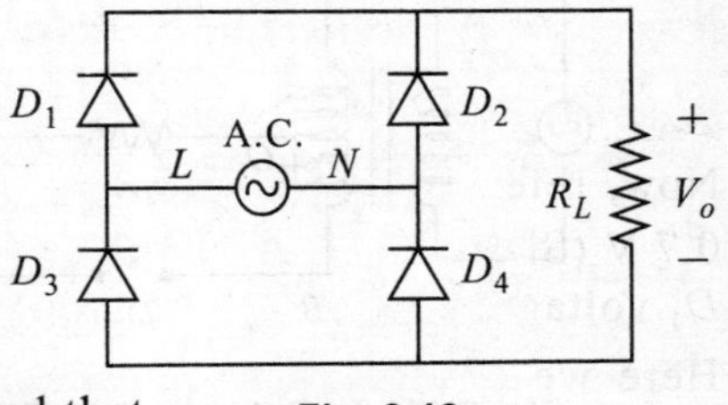

Fig. 8.13

Circuit Operation : Carefully observe the circuit, we find that

(i) D_1 is forward biased (f.b.) till L is +ve w.r.t. any other potential.

(ii) D_2 is f.b. till N is more +ve w.r.t. any other potential.

(iii) D_3 is f.b. till L is more –ve.

(iv) D_4 if f.b. till N is more –ve.

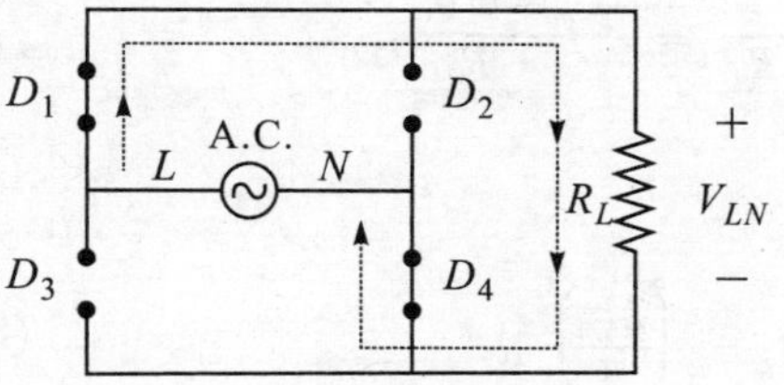

Fig. 8.14(a)

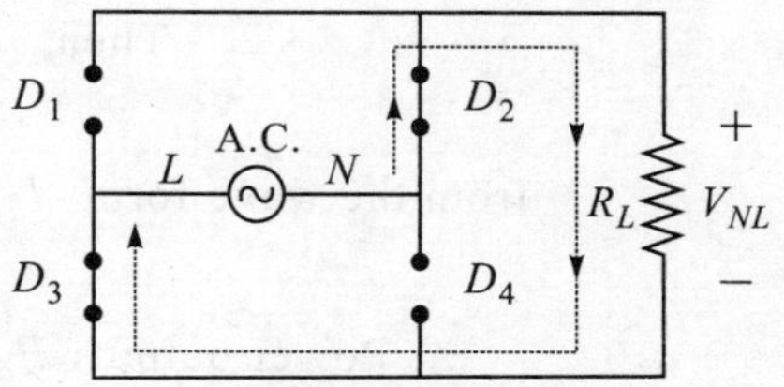

Fig. 8.14(b)

Now, observe Fig. 8.14(a), between interval 0 and π, D_1 and D_4 are f.b. and D_2, are reversed biased (r.b.). Refer Fig. 8.14(a), the output voltage will be equal to V_{LN}.

Now, refer Fig. 8.14(b), between π and 2π, D_2, D_3 are f.b. and D_1, D_4 are r.b., hence, the output voltage is V_{NL}.

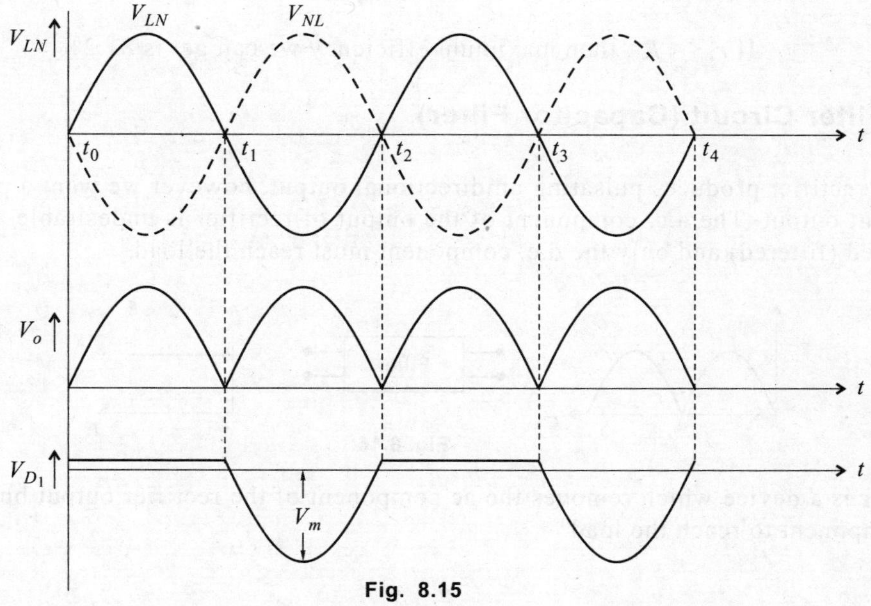

Fig. 8.15

Now, refer Fig. 8.15, between 0 and π, the output voltage is V_{NL} and the D_1 voltage is 0.7 V (Si diodes), between π and 2π the output voltage is the waveform V_{NL} and the diode D_1 voltage is V_{LN}.

Here we observe that output voltage for bridge rectifier is same as that of full wave rectifier with centre tap transformer.

Efficiency of Full-wave Rectifier Circuit :

Let, $v = V_m \sin\theta$

r_f = forward resistance of diode

R_L = load resistance

$$\text{Then,} \quad i = \frac{v}{r_f + R_L} = \frac{V_m \sin\theta}{r_f + R_L} \qquad \text{..... (8.9)}$$

$$\text{from the wave form} \quad I_{d.c.} = \frac{2I_m}{\pi}$$

$$\therefore \text{ Power output } P_{d.c.} = I_{d.c.}^2 \, R_L = \left(\frac{2I_m}{\pi}\right)^2 R_L \qquad \text{..... (8.10)}$$

$$\text{a.c. power input } P_{d.c.} = I_{rms}^2 \, (r_f + R_L) = \left(\frac{I_m}{\sqrt{2}}\right)^2 (r_f + R_L) \qquad \text{..... (8.11)}$$

$$\therefore \quad \text{Efficiency} = \frac{P_{d.c.}}{P_{a.c.}} = \frac{\left(\frac{2I_m}{\pi}\right)^2 R_L}{\left(\frac{I_m}{\sqrt{2}}\right)^2 (r_f + R_L)} = \frac{0.812}{\left(1 + \frac{r_f}{R_L}\right)} \qquad \text{..... (8.12)}$$

If $r_f << R_L$, then maximum efficiency we can get is 81.2%.

8.8 Filter Circuit (Capacitor Filter)

A rectifier produces pulsating unidirectional output, however we want a pure d.c. i.e. constant output. The a.c. component of the output of rectifier is undesirable and must be removed (filtered) and only the d.c. component must reach the load.

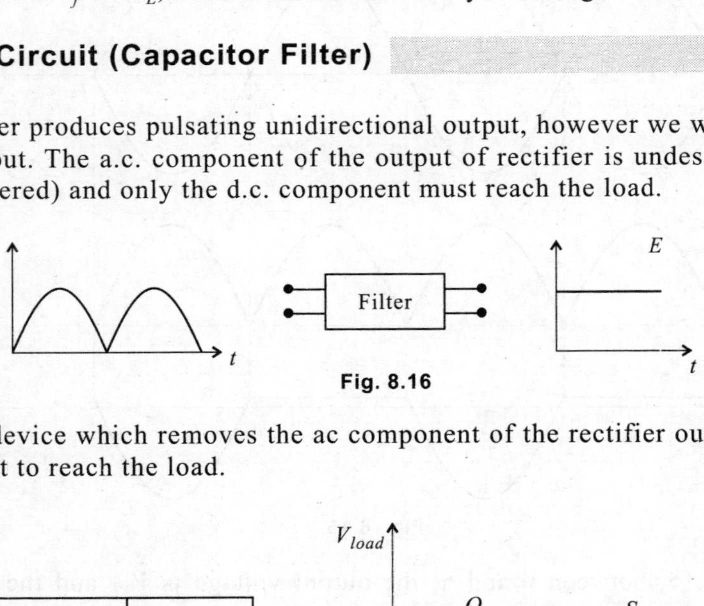

Fig. 8.16

A filter is a device which removes the ac component of the rectifier output but allows the dc component to reach the load.

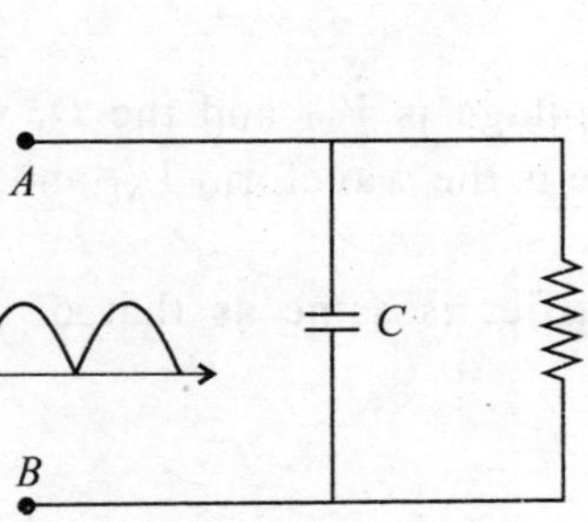

Fig. 8.17(a)

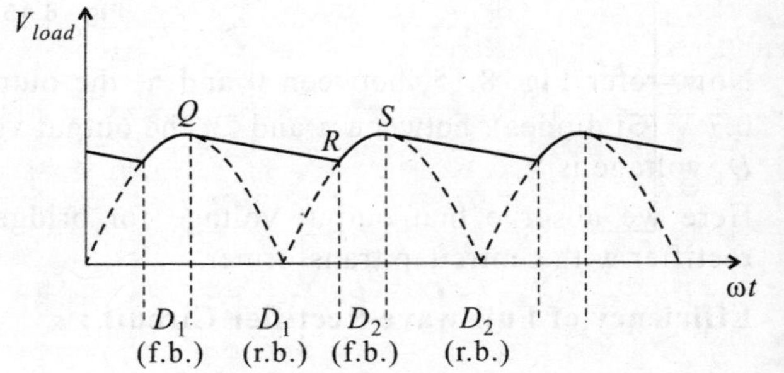

Fig. 8.17(b)

The circuit in Fig. 8.17 shows a capacitor filer. It consists of a capacitor C placed across rectifier output in parallel to the load R_L. The pulsating direct voltage of the rectifier is applied across the capacitor. As the rectifier voltage increases, it charges the capacitor and also supplies current to the load. At Q Fig. 8.17, the capacitor is charged to V_m the peak value of rectifier voltage. Now the rectifier voltage starts decreasing (it follows the sine wave) i.e. potential of X from Fig. 8.18. But due to the basic nature of capacitor (opposes the change in voltage) the capacitor voltage follows the path QR in Fig. 8.17. Thus, Y is at a higher potential as compared to X, Fig. 8.18.

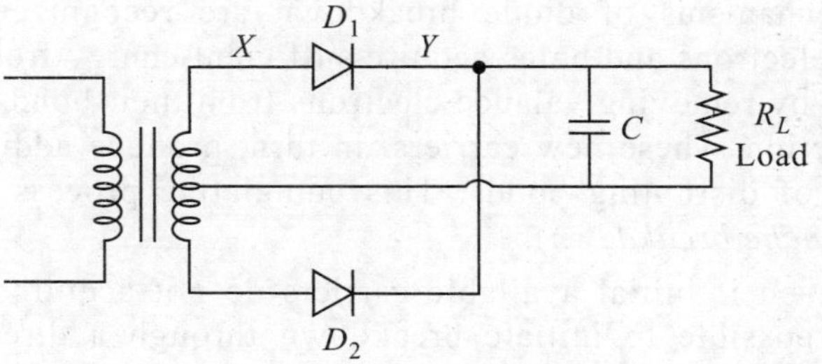

Fig. 8.18

At this instant diode D_1 also becomes reversed biased. At R Fig. 8.17, capacitor voltage and rectifier voltage become equal and between RS diode D_2 becomes forward biased. So, the output voltage with C filter will be the dark line (Fig. 8.17). It can be seen that very little (variation) ripple is left in the output.

8.9 Zener Diode

The reverse-voltage characteristic of semiconductor diode, including the breakdown region is shown in Fig. 8.19(b). Diodes which are designed with adequate power dissipation capabilities to operate in breakdown region are called *zener diodes*.

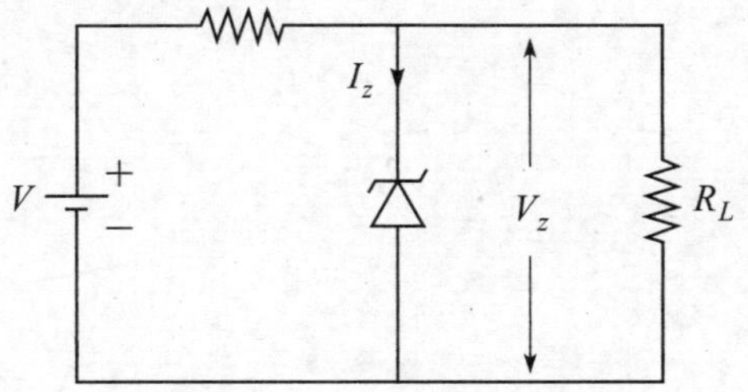

Fig. 8.19(a)

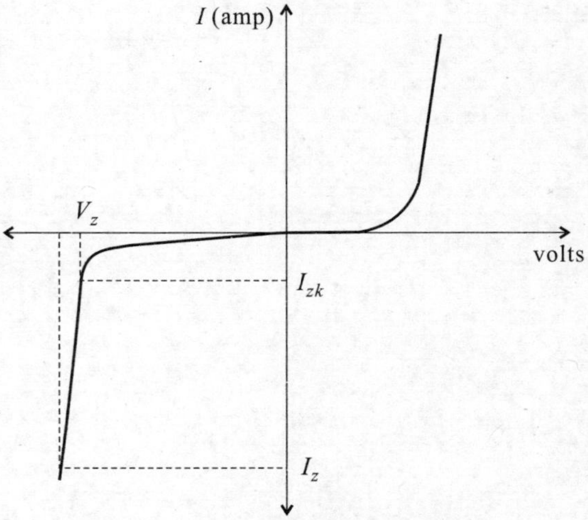

Fig. 8.19(b)

The Zener diodes are typically used as in the circuit of Fig. 8.19(a). The source voltage V and the resistance R are selected so that the diode operates in the breakdown region. Here, the diode voltage, which is also the load voltage, is V_z and the diode current is I_z. The diode regulates the load voltage against the variation in load current and supply voltage, because in the breakdown region large changes in diode current produces small changes in V_z. The upper limit on diode current is determined by the power dissipation rating of the diode.

Working : Two mechanisms of diode breakdown are recognized. In the first one, thermally generated electrons and holes acquire sufficient energy from applied voltage to produce new carriers by removing valance electrons from their bonds in the space charge region of the *pn* junction. These new carriers, in turn, produce additional carriers again through the process of disrupting bonds. This cumulative process is called *avalanche multiplication* (*avalanche breakdown*).

In the second one, even if initial available carriers do not acquire sufficient energy to disrupt bonds, it is possible to initiate breakdown through a direct rupture of bonds because of existence of strong electric field. Under these circumstances the breakdown is referred to as *zener breakdown*.

The zener effect is now known to play an important role in diodes with breakdown voltages below 6 volts. Nevertheless, the term zener is commonly used in more general context even at higher breakdown voltages.

CHAPTER

9 TRANSISTORS

When a third doped element is added to a crystal diode in such a way that two p-n junctions are formed, the resulting device is called a transistor (Fig. 9.1).

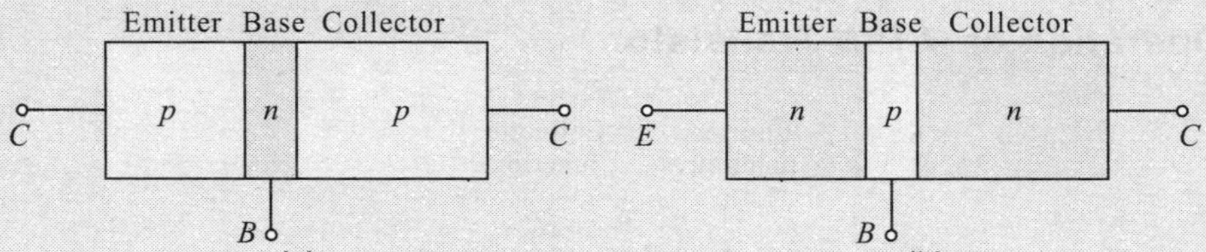

(a) (b)

Fig. 9.1

In both the above types of transistors the following points must be noted.

(1) There are two junctions.

(2) There are three terminals.

(3) The middle layer is thin.

9.1 Naming the Terminals of Transistor

A transistor has three sections of doped semiconductor. The section on one side is the *emitter* and the section on the other side is the *collector*. The middle section is called the *base*.

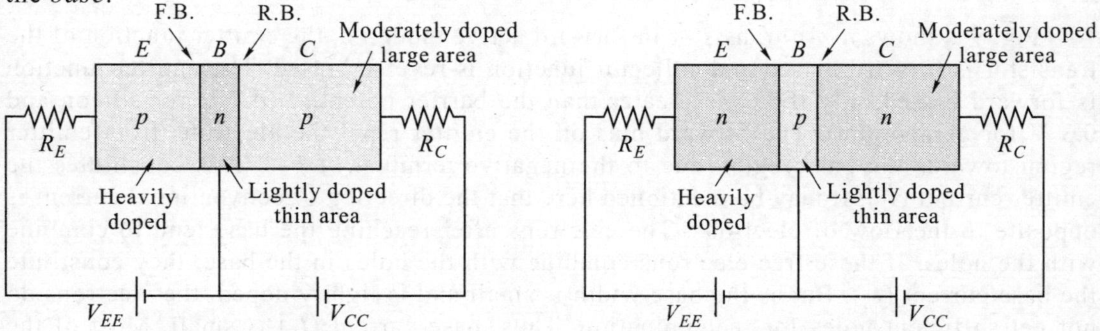

(a) *p-n-p* transistor. **(b) *n-p-n* transistor.**

Fig. 9.2 : Transistor in forward active mode.

Emitter : The section which supplies the charge carriers (holes and electrons) is called the *emitter*. Emitter-base junction is normally forward biased so that it can supply a large number of majority charge carriers. Fig. 9.2(a) shows *p-n-p* transistor. *E-B* junction is forward biased and supplies holes to its base, whereas Fig. 9.2(b) shows transistor with *E-B* junction forward biased and supplies free electrons to its base. Emitter is heavily doped.

Collector : The section on the other side of the base is the *collector* and it collects the charges. For normal operation the collector base junction is reversed biased. Its function is to remove charges from its junction with the base. It is moderately doped and has larger area.

Base : Middle section which forms two junction and is sandwiched between the emitter and the collector is called the *Base*. It is lightly doped region and has a smaller area.

The emitter base junction is forward biased, allowing low resistance for emitter circuit. The base-collector junction is reversed biased and provides high resistance to collector circuit.

9.2 Operation of *N-P-N* Transistor

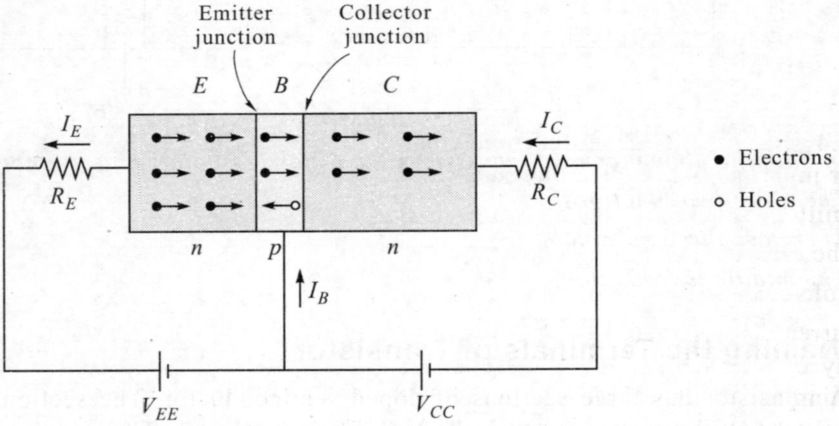

Fig. 9.3 : Operation of *n-p-n* transistor.

Fig. 9.3 shows *n-p-n* transistor in forward active mode i.e. the emitter junction of the transistor is forward biased and collector junction is reverse biased. The emitter junction is forward biased only if V_{EE} is greater than the barrier potential (0.7 V for silicon and 0.3 V for germanium). The forward bias on the emitter repel the electrons from emitter region towards the base region due to the negative terminal of V_{EE}. This constitutes the emitter current (I_E). It may be mentioned here that the direction of conventional current is opposite to the flow of electrons. The electrons after reaching the base tend to combine with the holes. If these free electrons combine with the holes in the base, they constitute the base current (I_B). But as the base width is small and is lightly doped, the electrons do not get sufficient holes for recombination. Thus, base current (I_B) is small. Most of the electrons now diffuse through the collector junction which is reverse biased, and are attracted towards the positive terminal of supply (V_{CC}). These electrons now constitute the collector current (I_C).

The emitter current of the transistor consists of two components namely the base current (I_B) and collector current (I_C). the base current is about 2% of emitter current, while collector current (I_C) is about 98% of I_E.

The resistances R_E and R_C are added to limit the magnitude of current in the transistor.

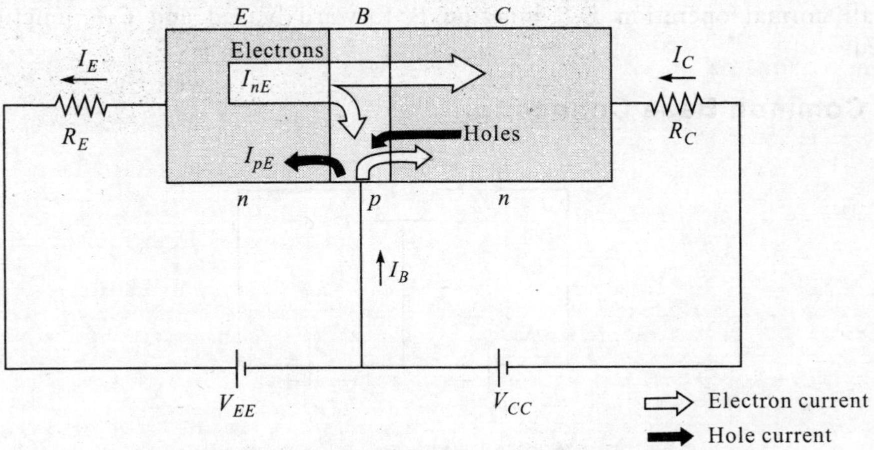

Fig. 9.4 : Current components in a transistor.

Fig. 9.4 shows the various current components which flow across the forward biased emitter junction and reverse biased collector junction of an *N-P-N* transistor.

The emitter current consists of two parts:

(i) The electron current I_{nE} constituted by electrons crossing from emitter into the base.

(ii) Hole current I_{pE} constituted by holes crossing from base to emitter.

The current I_{pE} is negligibly small in comparison to I_{nE}. Thus, the emitter current consists entirely of electrons. a few electrons will recombine with holes in the base region and remaining electrons will diffuse to the collector.

Thus, form Fig. 9.4.

$$I_E = I_B + I_C \qquad \text{..... (9.1)}$$

9.3 Transistor Symbol

Symbol representation of *p-n-p* transistor and *n-p-n* transistor is shown in Fig. 9.5.

Fig. 9.5

9.4 Transistor Connection

The transistor can be connected in a circuit in the following configurations:

(1) Common base connection

(2) Common emitter connection

(3) Common collector connection.

For all normal operation *E-B* junction is forward biased and *C-B* junction is reverse biased.

9.5 Common Base Connection

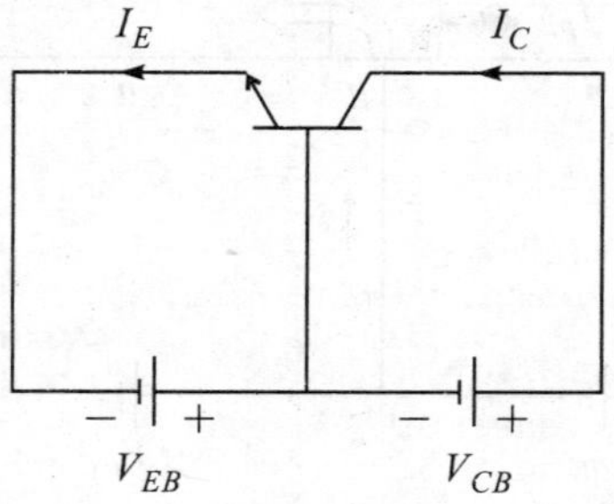

Fig. 9.6

In Fig. 9.6, the potentials are applied on emitter and collector with respect to base, thus, connecting the transistor in common base configuration. The *E-B* junction is forward biased and *C-B* junction is reverse biased. Relating to [Fig. 9.6] and [Fig. 9.4], the conventional currents [Fig. 9.6] are opposite to the electron movement [Fig. 9.4]. Out of the total number of electrons diffusing from emitter into the base, and only 5% of the electrons recombine with the holes in the base consituting the base current I_B, rest 95% electrons are collected by the collector constituting the collector current I_C.

The current amplification factor (α) or the current gain in common base configuration is defined as the ratio of output current (I_C) to input current (I_E).

$$\text{Therefore,} \quad \alpha = \frac{I_C}{I_E} \qquad \text{..... (9.2)}$$

and α is always less than unity. It ranges between 0.9 and 0.998.

There are two components of the collector current, one component is because of the carriers emitted from the emitter and collected by the collector (αI_E) and the other component is because of the minority carriers present in the base and collector regions (I_{CBO}).

$$\text{Therefore,} \quad I_C = \alpha I_E + I_{CBO} \qquad \text{..... (9.3)}$$

I_{CBO} is the reverse saturation current flowing across *C-B* junction with open *E-B* junction. It is very small (in micro amperes).

(a) Input Characteristic :

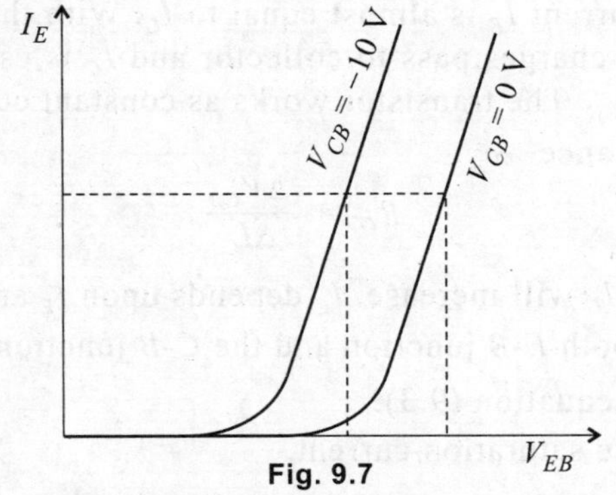

Fig. 9.7

The input characteristic is plotted between the emitter current I_E and the base emitter voltage V_{EB} while the collector base voltage V_{CB} is kept constant.

The emitter- base junction behaves as a forward bias diode, hence the characteristic (Fig. 9.7) is identical to the forward characteristic of a diode. For a fixed value of V_{CB} (reverse biased voltage) few electrons from base are drifted to the collector region, resulting in an increase in concentration gradient for electrons across the emitter base junction. This leads to an increase in diffusion current across the E-B junction.

Thus, the same emitter current I_E (Fig. 9.7) can be obtained at a lower value of V_{BE}.

(b) Output Characteristic :

It is the relation between collector current I_C and V_{CB}. The characteristic is as shown in Fig. 9.8. It consists of three regions, namely

(a) Active region

(b) Cut-off region, and

(c) The saturation region.

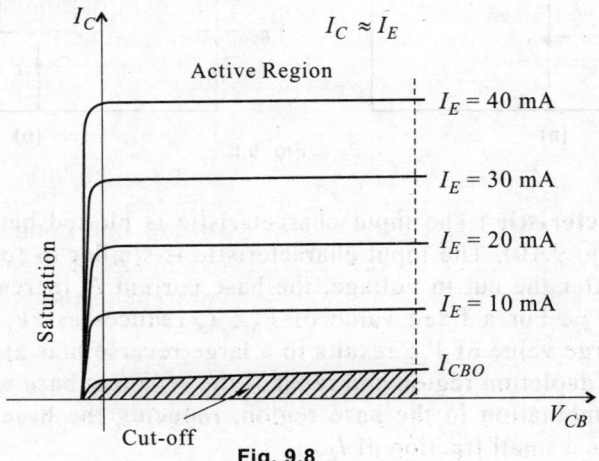

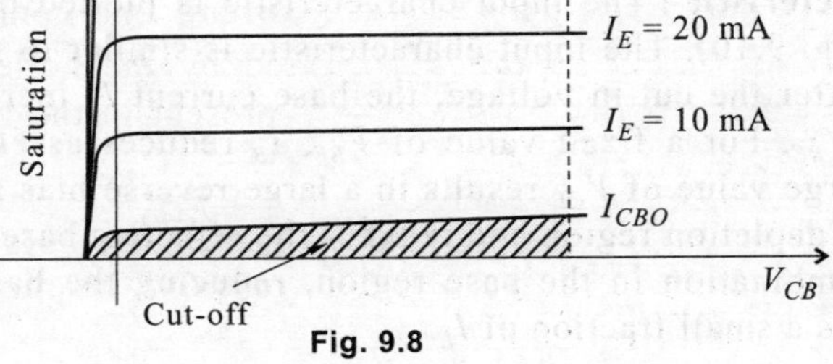

Fig. 9.8

In the active region the *E-B* junction is forward bias and *C-B* junction is reverse biased. The emitter current I_E is almost equal to I_C. With the potential applied at V_{CB} almost all the emitter charges pass to collector and I_C is essentially almost constant. It is independent of V_{CB}. The transistor works as constant current source.

Output dynamic resistance

$$R_O = \frac{\Delta V_{CB}}{\Delta I_C} \qquad \text{..... (9.4)}$$

Here, as I_E increases, I_C will increase. I_C depends upon I_E and not on V_{CB}.

In the cut-off region both *E-B* junction and the *C-B* junction are reverse biased.

If $I_E = 0$, then from equation (9.3).

$I_C = I_{CBO}$, the reverse saturation current.

In the saturation region both junctions are forward biased. In order to make $I_C = 0$, we have to reverse the voltage V_{CB}.

9.6 Common Emitter Configuration

In this configuration the input is applied between base and emitter and output is taken between collector and emitter. Thus, emitter is common to both input and output circuit.

Fig. 9.9 shows common emitter configuration for *n-p-n* transistor. V_{BB} forward biases the *E-B* junction and V_{CC} reverse biases the *C-B* junction.

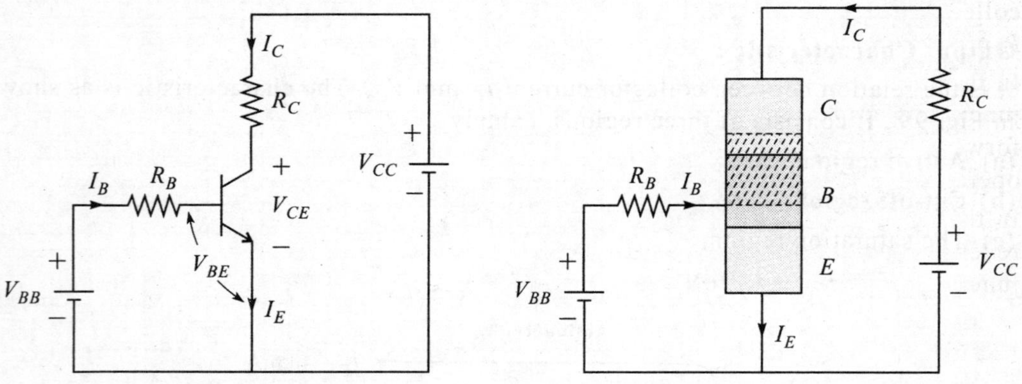

Fig. 9.9

(a) **Input Characteristic :** The input characteristic is plotted between V_{BE} and I_B for a fixed V_{CE} (Fig. 9.10). The input characteristic is similar to forward characteristic of *p-n* diode. After the cut-in voltage, the base current I_B increases rapidly with small increase in V_{BE}. For a fixed value of V_{BE}, I_B reduces as V_{CE} is increased. This is because, a large value of V_{CE} results in a large reverse bias at the *C-B* junction. This increases the depletion region and reduces the effective base width. Hence, There are a fewer recombination in the base region, reducing the base current I_B. In case of transistor I_B is a small fraction of I_E.

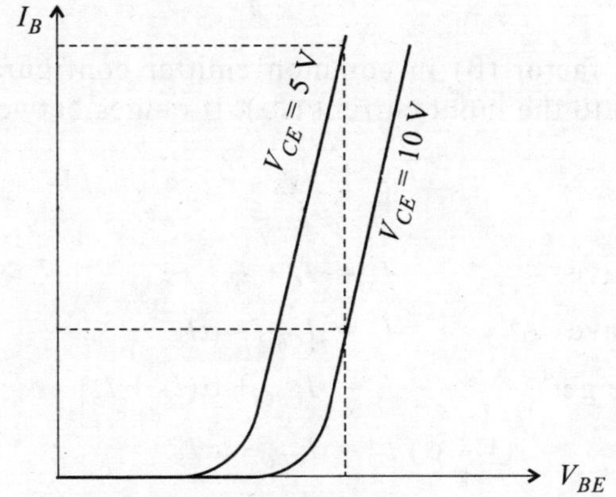

Fig. 9.10

(b) **Output Characteristic :** This characteristic is plotted between collector current I_C and V_{CE}, keeping the base current I_B constant. The characteristic is as shown in Fig. 9.11. It has three regions viz. Active, cut-off and the saturation regions.

In the *active region* the curve is approximately horizontal. The *E-B* junction is forward biased and the *C-B* junction is reverse biased. As V_{CE} is increased, the reverse bias increases which causes the depletion region to spread more in the base than the collector, reducing the chances of recombination. This early effect causes collector current to rise with increase in V_{CE}. Also, a small change in the base current I_B produces large change in output current I_C.

In the *saturation region* if V_{CE} is reduced to a small value (e.g. 0.2 volts), then *C-B* junction becomes forward biased, the emitter junction base junction is already forward biased by 0.7 volts. When both junctions are forward biased the transistor operates saturation.

In the *cut-off region* the input base current I_B is made zero. The collector current is reverse leakage current I_{CEO}. The region below $I_B = 0$ is the cut-off region. Both junctions are reverse biased here.

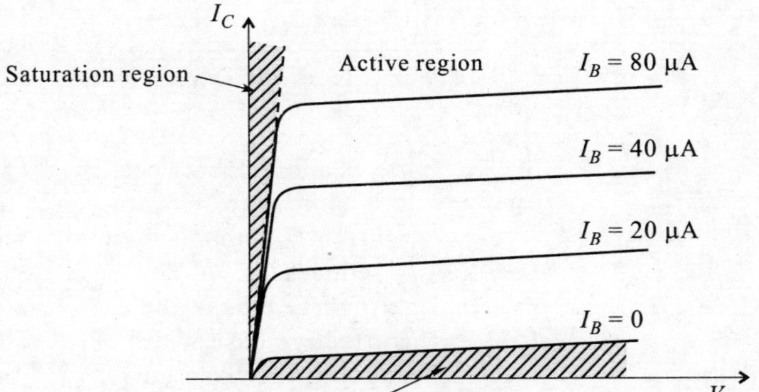

Fig. 9.11

Refer Fig. 9.9(a).

The current amplification factor (β) in common emitter configuration is defined as the ratio of output current (I_C) to the input current (I_B). It ranges between 20 and 300.

$$\beta = \frac{I_C}{I_B} \quad ..... (9.5)$$

From equation (9.1), we have $I_E = I_C + I_B$

From equation (9.3), we have $I_C = I_{CBO} + \alpha I_E$

Using above equations, we get $I_C = I_{CBO} + \alpha(I_C + I_B)$

$$(1-\alpha) I_C = I_{CBO} + \alpha I_B$$

$$I_C = \frac{I_{CBO}}{1-\alpha} + \frac{\alpha}{1-\alpha} I_B \quad ..... (9.6)$$

where $\frac{I_{CBO}}{1-\alpha} = I_{CEO}$

and, $\frac{\alpha}{1-\alpha} = \beta$ ..... (9.7)

therefore, $I_C = I_{CEO} + \beta I_B$ ..... (9.8)

Note : *I_{CEO} is much larger than I_{CBO}.*

APPENDIX

A MULTIPLE CHOICE QUESTIONS

1. What is the equivalent resistance in Fig. M.1.

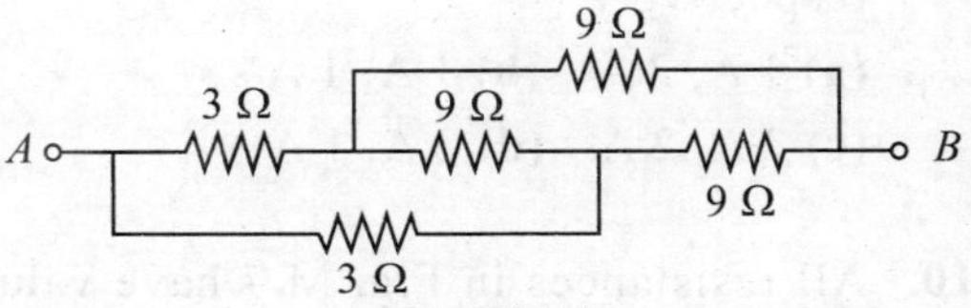

Fig. M.1

(a) 9 Ω (b) 6 Ω (c) 8 Ω (d) 4.5 Ω

2. In the circuit of Fig. M.2 if resistance of voltmeter is 1.2 kΩ find the value of R, if the voltmeter reads 5 V.

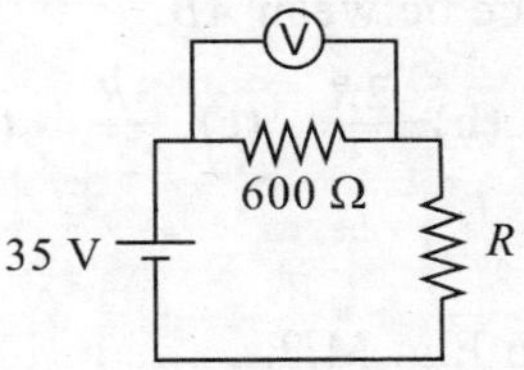

Fig. M.2

(a) 1 kΩ (b) 3.6 kΩ (c) 2.4 kΩ (d) 7.1 kΩ

3. A series R-L-C circuits has $R = 10\ \Omega$, $X_L = 30\ \Omega$, $X_C = 30\ \Omega$. It is connected to a 100 V a.c. supply. The magnitude and phase of voltage across inductance is.

(a) 100 V, 90° (b) 100 V, −90° (c) 20 V, 0° (d) 300 V, 90°

4. Effective inductance of the circuit across terminals AB in Fig. M.3 is

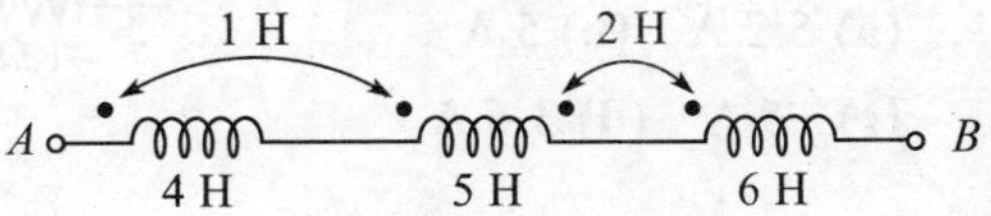

Fig. M.3

(a) 15 H (b) 13 H (c) 18 H (d) 12 H

5. In the circuit of Fig. M.4 find I

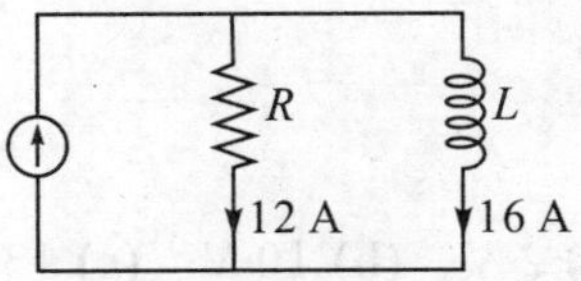

Fig. M.4

(a) 28 A (b) 12 A (c) 20 A (d) 16 A

6. The phasor current through the inductance in Fig. M.5 is

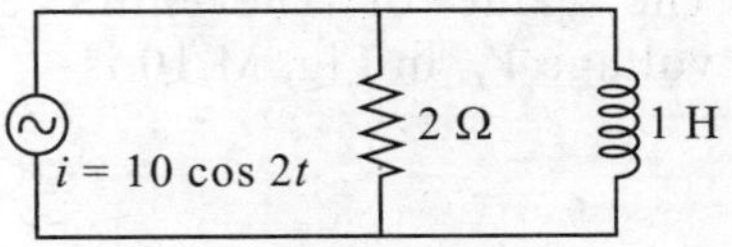

Fig. M.5

(a) $\frac{10}{\sqrt{2}} \angle -45^\circ$ (b) $\frac{10}{\sqrt{2}} \angle 45^\circ$

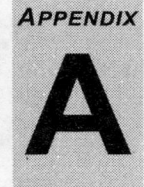

(c) $5 \angle 45^\circ$ (d) $-5 \angle 45^\circ$

7. A series *R-L-C* circuits has $R = 5\ \Omega$, $L = 100\ \mu H$, $C = 1\ \mu f$. The lower half power frequency is

(a) 13.05 kHz **(b)** 11.9 kHz **(c)** 10 kHz **(d)** 715 kHz.

8. The maximum value of mutual inductance of two closely coupled coils with self inductances of 50 mH and 81 mH is

(a) 6.63 mH **(b)** 6363 mH **(c)** 63.63 mH **(d)** 36.36 mH.

9. The value of *I* when switch *S* is open and when *S* is closed in Fig. M.6, is respectively

(a) 1 A, 2 A **(b)** 1 A, 1 A

(c) 2 A, 2 A **(d)** 2 A, 1 A

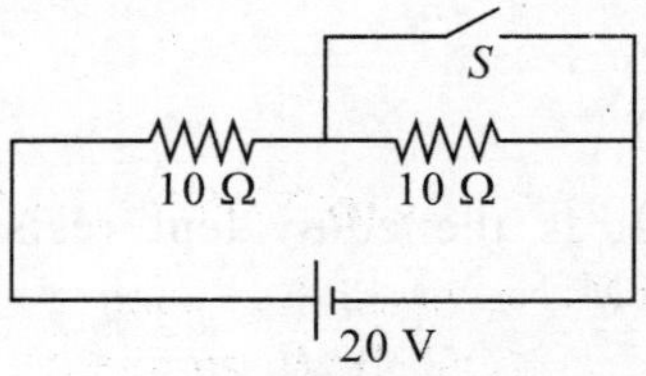

Fig. M.6

10. All resistances in Fig. M.7 have value of *R* ohms, what is the equivalent resistance between *AB*.

(a) $2R$ **(b)** $\frac{2R}{3}$ **(c)** $\frac{3R}{2}$ **(d)** R

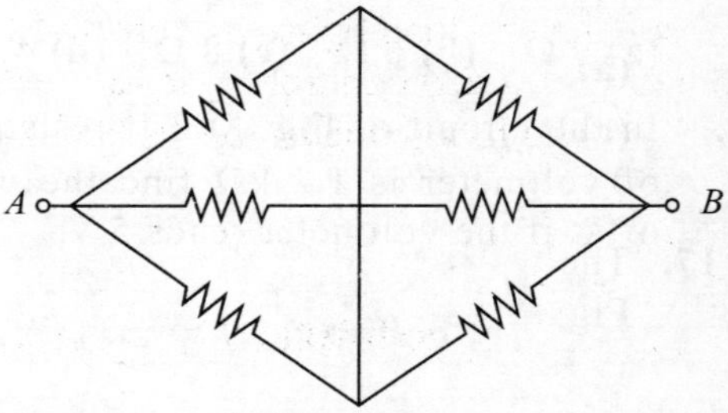

Fig. M.7

11. Find *I* in Fig. M.8.

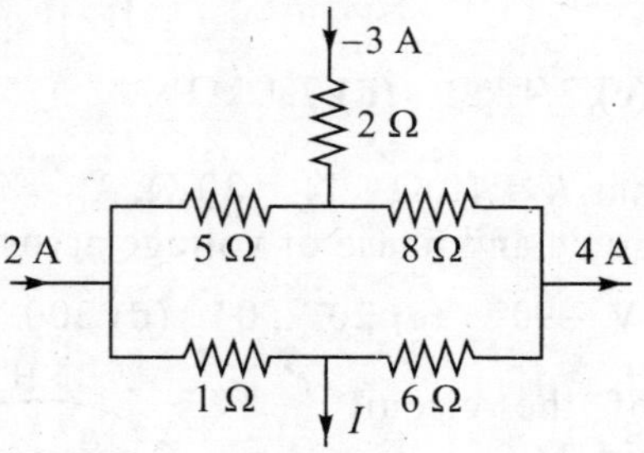

Fig. M.8

(a) 5.2 A **(b)** 5 A

(c) –5 A **(d)** 3.6 A

12. The voltmeter reading in Fig. M.9 is

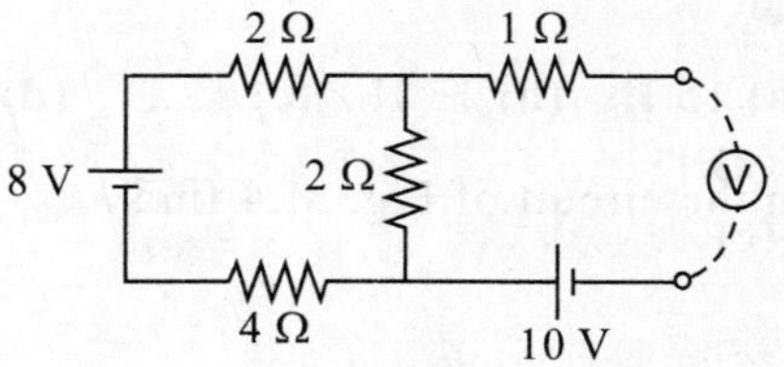

Fig. M.9

(a) 2 V **(b)** 10 V **(c)** 13 V **(d)** 12 V

13. The value of Thevenin's equivalent voltage V_{th} in Fig. M.10 is

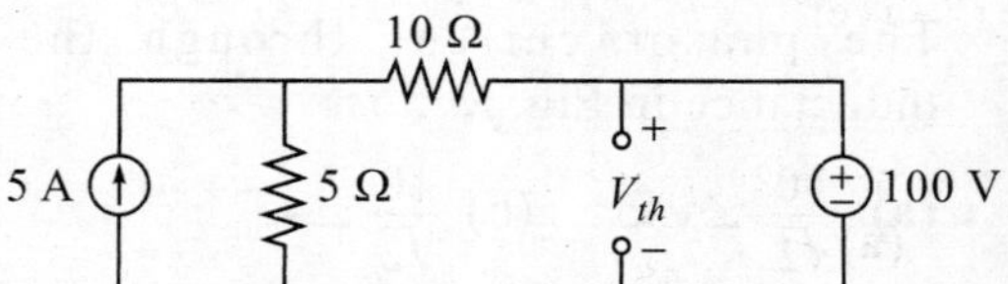

Fig. M.10

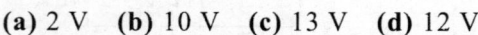

(a) 50 V **(b)** 100 V **(c)** 25 V **(d)** 150 V

14. The value of Thevenin's equivalent resistance for the Fig. M.10

(a) 15 Ω **(b)** 3.3 Ω **(c)** 0 Ω **(d)** 5 Ω

15. The Thevenin's equivalent circuit across 1 Ω resistor in Fig. M.11 is

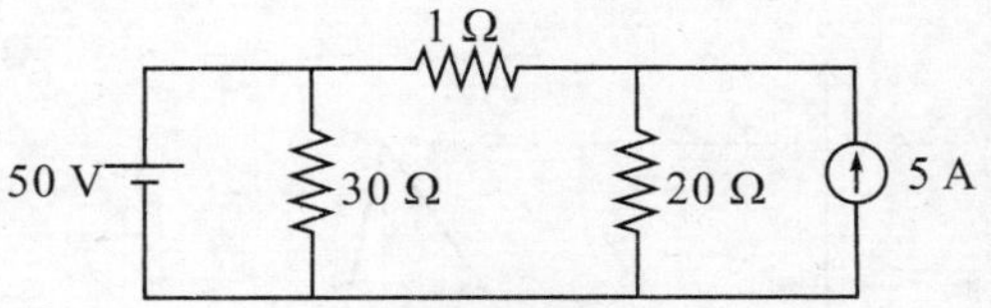

Fig. M.11

(a) V_{th} = 100 V ; R_{th} = 30 Ω **(b)** V_{th} = 100 V ; R_{th} = 50 Ω

(c) V_{th} = 55 V ; R_{th} = 30 Ω **(d)** V_{th} = 50 V ; R_{th} = 20 Ω

16. The current in 3 Ω resistance in Fig. M.12.

(a) 2 A **(b)** 5.143 A

(c) 9 A **(d)** 4.128 A

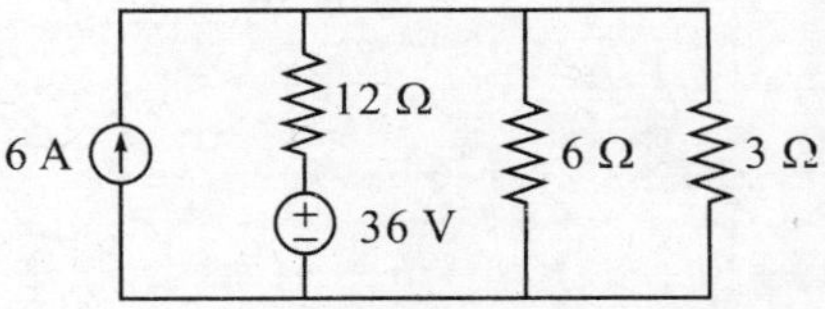

Fig. M.12

17. The current in 3 Ω resistance in Fig. M.13

(a) 0.2 A

(b) 0 A

(c) 0.2162 A

(d) 0.331 A

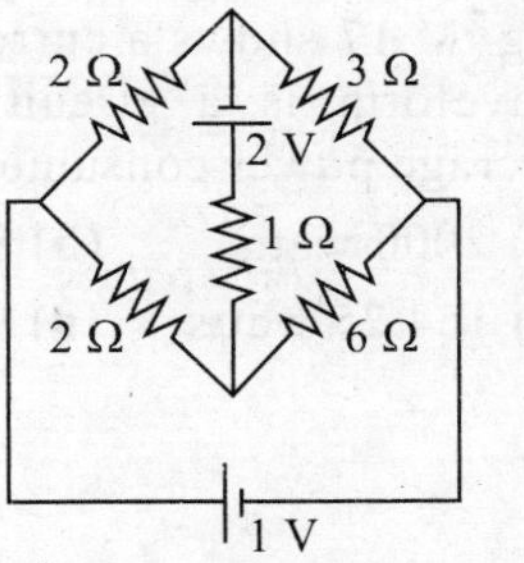

Fig. M.13

18. What is the equivalent capacitance in Fig. M.14.

(a) 14 C **(b)** 1.215 C

(c) 10 C **(d)** 15 C

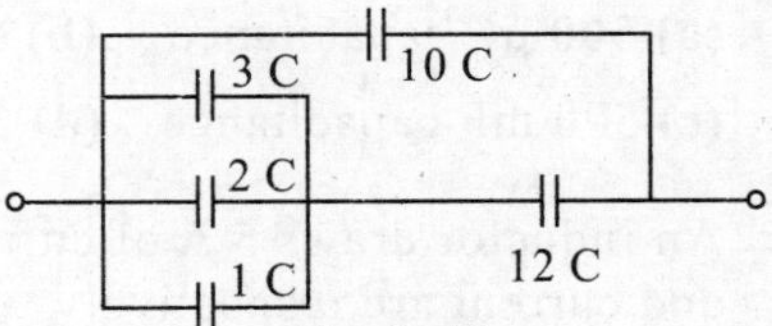

Fig. M.14

19. If the current through a 2 Ω pure resistance is as in Fig. M.15. The average power dissipation is

(a) 18 watts **(b)** 140.5 watts

(c) 162 watts **(d)** 100 watts

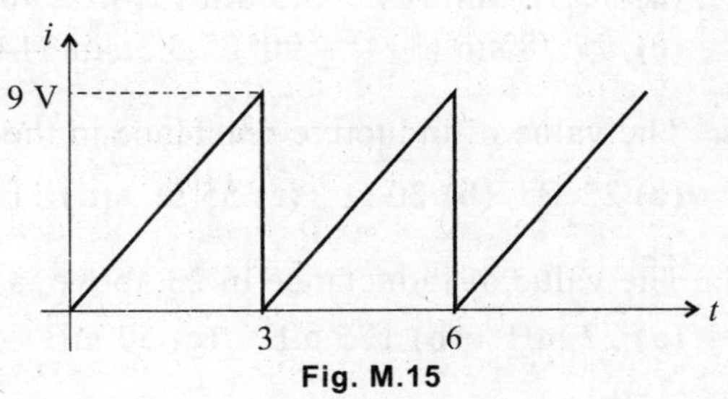

Fig. M.15

20. The current waveform in Fig. M.16 passes through a 2 H inductor. The corresponding voltage waveform is

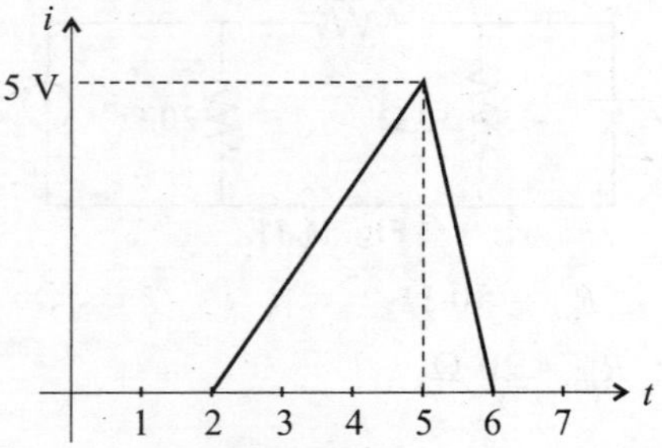

Fig. M.16

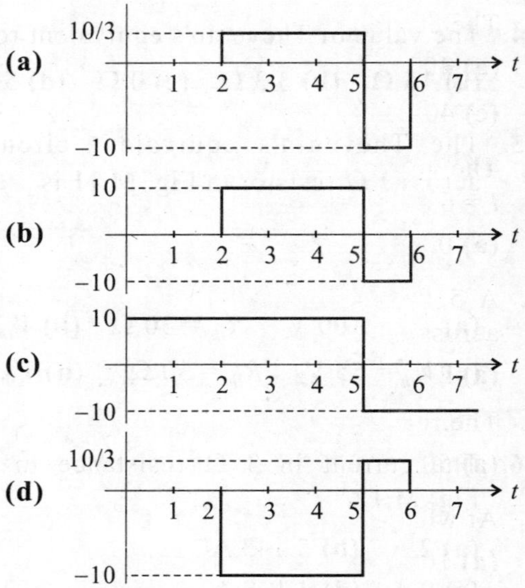

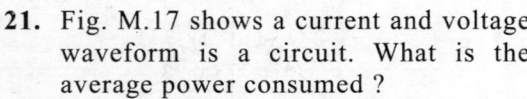

21. Fig. M.17 shows a current and voltage waveform is a circuit. What is the average power consumed ?

(a) 2000 watts **(b)** 866.025 watts

(c) 154.25 watts **(d)** 952.41 watts

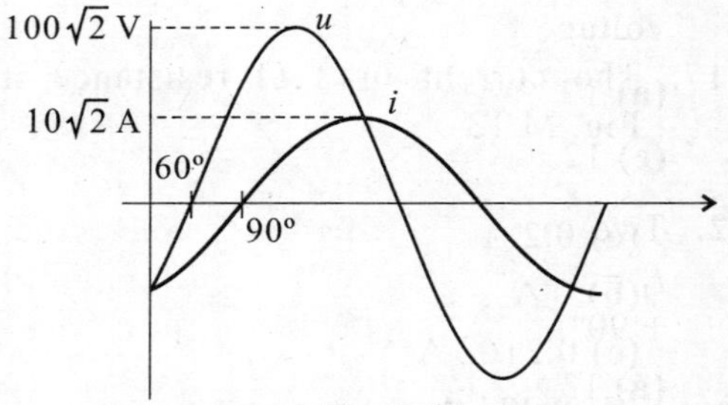

Fig. M.17

22. The voltage and current for a circuit element are $v = 6\cos(1000\,t - 80^\circ)$ volts and $i = 3\cos(1000\,t + 10^\circ)$ A. Identify the element and its value is

(a) 500 μF capacitance **(b)** 500 mH inductance

(c) 500 mF capacitance **(d)** 500 μH Inductance

23. An inductor draws 5 A of current at 110 V, 50 Hz. The instantaneous value of voltage and current are respectively.

(a) $77.78 \sin 314t$, $3.5 \sin(314t - 90^\circ)$ **(b)** $77.78 \cos 314t$, $3.5 \sin(314t - 90^\circ)$

(c) $77.78 \sin(314t - 90^\circ)$, $3.5 \sin 314t$ **(d)** $3.5 \sin 314t$, $77.78 \sin(314t - 90^\circ)$

24. The value of inductive reactance in the problem 23 above is

(a) 22 Ω **(b)** 20 Ω **(c)** 55 Ω **(d)** 11 Ω

25. The value of inductance in 23 above is

(a) 22 mH **(b)** 175 mH **(c)** 50 mH **(d)** 70 mH

26. The current through 50 μF capacitor is $i = 2 \sin 1000t$ A, the instantaneous voltage is
(a) 40 sin (1000t + 90°) **(b)** 40 cos 1000t
(c) 40/2 sin (1000t – 90°) **(d)** 740 cos (1000t + 90°)

27. The voltage and current is a.c. circuit are $v = 100 \sin(314t - 30°)$ volts and $i = 6 \sin(314t + 30°)$ amp. The power factor of the circuit is
(a) 0.866 lagging **(b)** 0.5 lagging **(c)** 0.866 leading **(d)** 0.5 leading

28. A 5 Ω resistor, 100 μf capacitor and 100 mH inductor are connected in parallel across 100 V. 50 Hz supply. The average power drawn by the circuit is
(a) 2 kW **(b)** 3 kW **(c)** 4 kW **(d)** 5 kW

29. The reactance of 50 mH inductor for d.c. supply is
(a) 50 ohms **(b)** infinite ohms **(c)** 0 ohms **(d)** 100 ohms

30. At what frequency will a 100 μF capacitor have a reactance of 100 Ω.
(a) 1000 Hz **(b)** 100 Hz **(c)** 15.9 Hz **(d)** 1 Hz

31. The power factor of a circuit is 0.866 logging. If the input power is 600 W at a voltage of 110 sin (314t + 10°) volts. What is the instantaneous current.
(a) 12.6 sin (314t – 30°) **(b)** 8.9 sin (314t – 30°)
(c) 12.6 sin (314t – 20°) **(d)** 18.9 sin (314t – 20°)

32. Two circuit elements are connected in parallel. The current through one of them is $i_1 = 3 \sin(\omega t - 60°)$ A and the total line current drawn by the circuit is $i = 10 \sin(\omega t + 90°)$. The rms current through the other branch is
(a) 13 A **(b)** 12.687 A **(c)** 7 A **(d)** 8.97 A

33. The instantaneous value of current in problem 32 is
(a) $7\sqrt{2} \sin \omega t$ **(b)** 12.68 sin (ωt + 96.79)
(c) 12.687 cos (ωt + 96.79) **(d)** 12.68 sin (ωt + 92.67)

34. In an a.c. circuit $v = 150 \sin(\omega t + 30°)$ volts and $i = 2 \sin(\omega t - 30°)$ A. The apparent power is
(a) 150 volt-amp **(b)** 150 watts **(c)** 300 volt-amp **(d)** 300 watts

35. What is the reactive power in problem 34.
(a) 692.8 **(b)** 259.8 **(c)** 800 **(d)** 129.9

36. What is the active power in problem 34.
(a) 75 **(b)** 129.9 **(c)** 692.8 **(d)** 800

37. A 20 Ω resistance is connected in series with a parallel combination of capacitor C and a 15 mH pure inductance. At regular frequency ω = 1000 rad/s. Find C such that current is 45° out of phase with line voltage.
(a) 116.7 μF **(b)** 16.67 μF **(c)** 10.5 μF **(d)** both (a) and (b)

38. A inductive coil consumes 500 w of power at 10 A and 110 V at 50 Hz. The resistance and inductance of coil are respectively

(a) 5 Ω, 31.1 mH **(b)** 11 Ω, 9.8 mH **(c)** 11 Ω, 31.1 mH **(d)** 5 Ω, 9.8 mH

39. The series equivalent impedance of the circuit of Fig. M.18 is

(a) $1.44 - 1.8j$ **(b)** $1.44 - 1.92j$

(c) $2.7 - 1.8j$ **(d)** $2.7 - 1.92j$

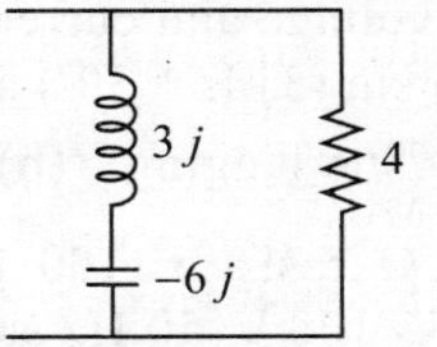

Fig. M.18

40. If the power delivered by source is 400 W in Fig. M.19. Find L if supply frequency is 15.91 Hz.

(a) 100 mH **(b)** 29 H

(c) 10 H **(d)** 29 mH

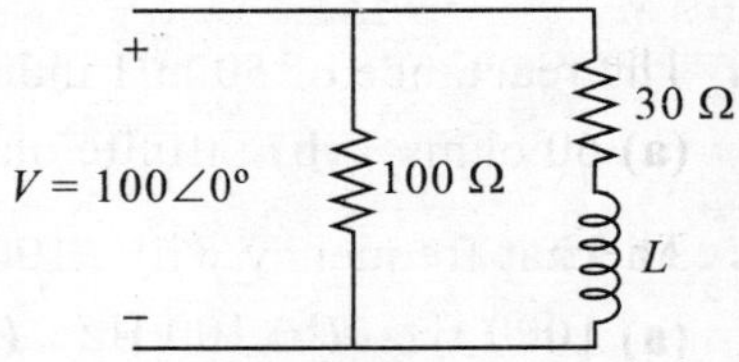

Fig. M.19

41. In the circuit of Fig. M.20, if the voltmeter reads 32 V when connected across 8 Ω resistance and 104 V when across the coil. The values of R and L are respectively

(a) 10 Ω, 10 Ω **(b)** 24 Ω, 10 Ω

(c) 10 Ω, 24 Ω **(d)** 24 Ω, 24 Ω

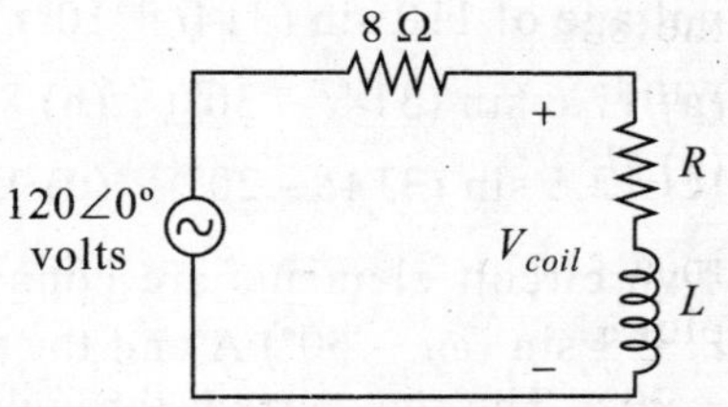

Fig. M.20

42. The condition for circuit of Fig. M.21 to be purely resistive at all frequencies is

(a) $R^2 = \dfrac{4L}{C}$ **(b)** $R^2 < \dfrac{L}{C}$

(c) $R^2 > \dfrac{L}{C}$ **(d)** $R^2 = \dfrac{L}{C}$

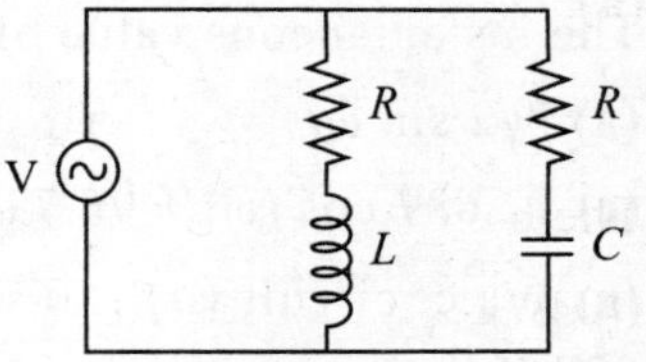

Fig. M.21

43. The current (I) in circuit of Fig. M.22 is

(a) 37.74 ∠–32° **(b)** 5.3 ∠32°

(c) 5.3 ∠– 32° **(d)** 37.74 ∠32°

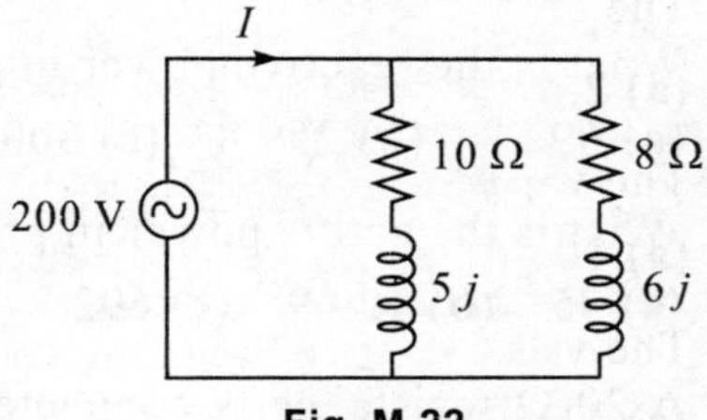

Fig. M.22

44. The power factor of problem 43 is

(a) 0.848 lagging **(b)** 0.848 leading **(c)** 0.886 leading **(d)** 0.886 lagging

45. The value of C such that input voltage and current are in phase in Fig. M.23 is

(a) 1200 μF **(b)** 753.98 μF

(c) 1105 μF **(d)** 1326.3 μF

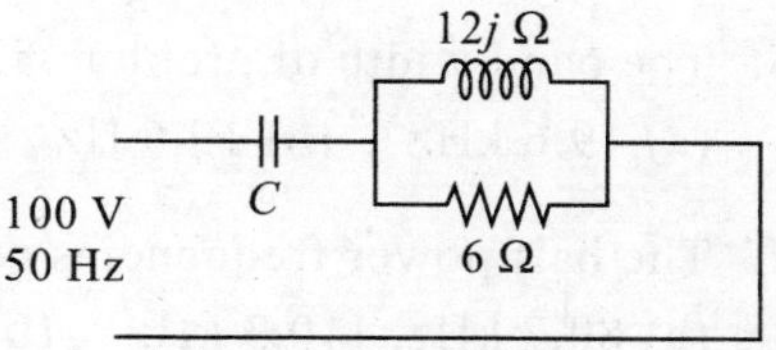

Fig. M.23

46. The mutual inductance for circuit of Fig. M.24 is

(a) 158.17 H **(b)** 19.8 H

(c) 1.98 H **(d)** 15.817 H

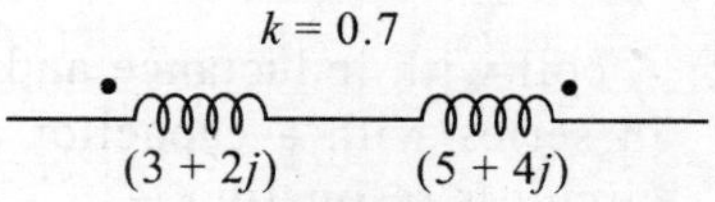

Fig. M.24

47. The equivalent reactance of Fig. M.24 is

(a) 6 Ω **(b)** 2.04 Ω **(c)** 9.96 Ω **(d)** 7.98 Ω

48. The impedance of Fig. M.24 is

(a) 10 ∠36.86° **(b)** 21.35 ∠68° **(c)** 11.4 ∠32.8° **(d)** 8.24 ∠13.9°

49. The primary and secondary turns of a transformer are 200 and 600 respectively. If the source voltage is 50 sin 300t, the rms voltage of the open circuit secondary winding is

(a) $75\sqrt{2}$ **(b)** $25\sqrt{2}$ **(c)** 150 **(d)** 50/3

50. In a series R-L-C circuit, as the supply frequency varies from zero to infinity, the plot of variation of power factor with respect to frequency is

(a)
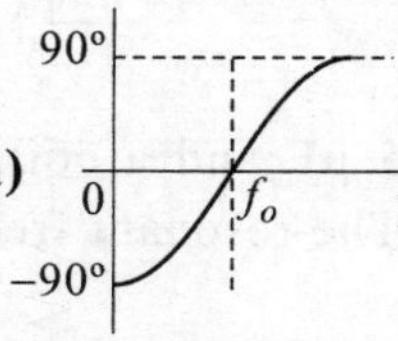

(b)
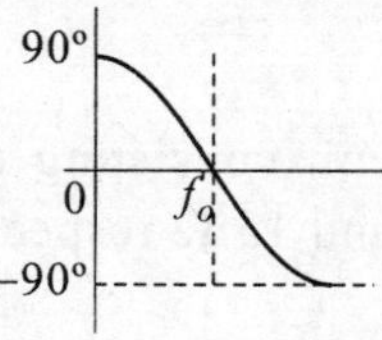

(c)
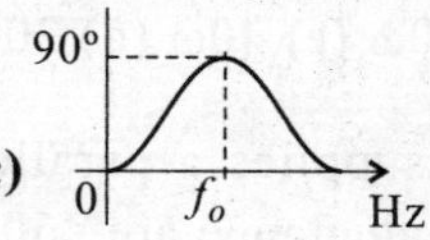

(d)
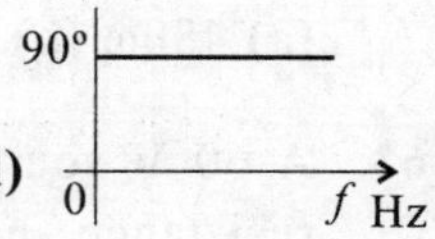

51. The band-width of a series R-L-C circuit is terms of its parameters is

(a) $R/2\pi L$ **(b)** $R/2L$ **(c)** $1/2\pi\sqrt{LC}$ **(d)** $1/\sqrt{LC}$

52. A series R-L-C circuit has resonant frequency of 10 kHz and a band-width of 1 kHz. The circuit draws 15.3 watts from a 200 V source. The resistance is the circuit is

(a) 2.6 Ω **(b)** 2.61 kΩ **(c)** 26.1 Ω **(d)** 261 Ω

53. The value of Q-factor is problem 52 is

(a) 100 **(b)** 10 **(c)** 1 **(d)** 0.1

54. The value of inductance in problem 52 is

(a) 416 mH **(b)** 41.6 mH **(c)** 4.16 mH **(d)** 0.416 mH

55. The value of capacitance in problem 52 is

(a) 61pF **(b)** 610 μF **(c)** 61 μF **(d)** 610 pF

56. The band width of problem 52 is
(a) 19.6 kHz (b) 19.6 Hz (c) 1.96 kHz (d) 196 Hz

57. The half power frequencies of problem 52 are
(a) 80.7 kHz, 110.3 kHz (b) 90.7 kHz, 110.3 kHz
(c) 9.07 Hz, 110.3 Hz (d) 9.07 kHz, 11.03 kHz

58. A coil with inductance and resistance of 30 mH and 20 Ω respectively, is connected in series with a capacitor and a 12 V, 5 kHz source. The circuit current when the circuit is resonating is
(a) 1.6 A (b) 0.6 A (c) 0.32 A (d) 0,8 A

59. The capacitance for circuit in problem 58 is
(a) 338 nF (b) 33.8 nF (c) 338 μF (d) 33.8 μF

60. A series resonant circuit has a resistance of 1 kΩ and half power frequencies are 20 kHz and 100 kHz. The resonant frequency is
(a) 44.72 kHz (b) 80 kHz (c) 40 kHz (d) 50 kHz

61. The band width of problem 60 is
(a) 44.72 kHz (b) 80 kHz (c) 40 kHz (d) 50 kHz

62. A series resonant circuit has R = 5 Ω and operates from 20 V source. The power at half power frequency is
(a) 480ω (b) 100ω (c) 40ω (d) 20ω

63. A 60 V source supplies a parallel circuit consisting of a 2.5 μF and a coil whose resistance and inductance are 260 mH and 15 Ω respectively. The resonant frequency of the circuit is
(a) 19.74 Hz (b) 197.4 Hz (c) 197 Hz (d) 197 kHz

64. In a 3 phase a.c. circuit with balanced star connected load and balanced supply
(a) line and phase currents are in phase
(b) line and phase voltage are in phase
(c) line current is 3 times phase current
(d) phase voltage is 3 times line voltage

65. In a 3-phase a.c. circuit with balanced delta connected load
(a) line and phase currents are in phase
(b) line and phase voltage are in phase
(c) line current phase current equal
(d) phase current is 3 times line current

66. A 3 phase load consists of a 4 Ω resistance in series with 3 Ω capacitive reactance in each phases. This load is connected in star across a 220 V, 3-phase supply, the line currents are

(a) 55 A **(b)** 144 A **(c)** 25.4 A **(d)** 73.3 A

67. The phase current in a 3-phase delta connected load of 3∠20° ohms per phase connected to 240 V. 3-phase supply are

(a) 56.18 **(b)** 46.18 **(c)** 40 A **(d)** 80 A

68 . The total power consumed in problem 67 is

(a) 54.12 kW **(b)** 31.24 kW **(c)** 720 watts **(d)** 2.02 kW

69. The power factor of the load in problem 67 is

(a) 0.94 lead **(b)** 0.94 lag **(c)** upf **(d)** 0.866 lagging

70. A 220 V, 3-phase motor takes 21437 watts at 0.71 lagging power factor. The line current is

(a) 79.2 A **(b)** 29.7 A **(c)** 7.92 A **(d)** 2.97 A

71. If the motor in problem 70 is star connected and balanced. Determine the readings of the two wattmeters connected to measure power

(a) 4.5 W, 16.8 kW **(b)** 4.5 kW, 16.8 W **(c)** 4.5 W, 16.8 W **(d)** 4.5 kW, 16.8 kW

72. Two wattmeters, connected to measure the power in 3 phase circuit, read 60 kW and 40 kw respectively. The total power consumed in the circuit is

(a) 20 kW **(b)** 100 kW **(c)** 80 kW **(d)** 60 kW

73. The power factor of problem 72 is

(a) 0.945 lagging **(b)** 0.945 leading **(c)** 19.1° **(d)** −19.1°

74. A three phase load draws a line current of 30 A when supplied from 450 V three phase a.c. supply. The motor efficiency is 90% and power factor is 0.75. The active power drawn by the load is

(a) 15.88 kW **(b)** 23.5 kW **(c)** 17.537 kW **(d)** 15.783 kW

75. The motor output power in problem 74 is

(a) 15.88 kW **(b)** 23.5 kW **(c)** 17.537 kW **(d)** 15.783 kW

76. Number of diodes in a half wave rectifier is

(a) 1 **(b)** 2 **(c)** 3 **(d)** 4

77. The maximum efficiency of half wave diodes rectifier is

(a) 40.6% **(b)** 81.2% **(c)** 8.12% **(d)** 50%

78. The form factor of a half wave diodes rectifier is

(a) 1.11 **(b)** **1.57** **(c)** 1.21 **(d)** 0.481

79. The transformer utilization factor of a half wave diodes rectifier is
(a) 0.287 **(b)** 0.693 **(c)** 0.81 **(d)** 0.99

80. The maximum efficiency of a full wave bridge rectifier is
(a) 40.6% **(b)** 81.2% **(c)** 28.7% **(d)** 90%

81. The peak inverse voltage appearing across a diode in full wave rectifier using center-top transformer is
(a) zero **(b)** V_m **(c)** $2V_m$ **(d)** 2 V

82. The peak inverse voltage appearing across a diode in full wave bridge rectifier is
(a) zero **(b)** V_m **(c)** $2V_m$ **(d)** 2 V

83. The ripple factor of a half wave diode rectifier is
(a) 1.57 **(b)** 0.481 **(c)** 1.21 **(d)** 1.11

84. The ripple factor of a full wave diode rectifier is
(a) 1.57 **(b)** 0.481 **(c)** 1.21 **(d)** 1.11

85. The basic function of a transformer is to change
(a) power level **(b)** voltage level **(c)** the frequency **(d)** all the above

86. For an ideal transformer windings should have
(a) maximum resistance on primary side and least resistance on secondary side
(b) maximum resistance on secondary side and least resistance on primary side
(c) equal resistance on both sides
(d) no ohmic resistance on both sides

87. The transformer steps up the voltage by a factor of 100. The ratio of current in primary to secondary is
(a) 1 **(b)** 100 **(c)** 0.01 **(d)** 0.1

88. The flux created by the current flowing through the primary winding induces emf in
(a) primary winding only **(b)** secondary winding only
(c) transformer care only **(d)** both primary and secondary windings

89. An ideal transformer does not change
(a) voltage **(b)** current **(c)** power **(d)** all the above

90. The power factor of a power transformer on no load will be above
(a) unity **(b)** 0.75 **(c)** 0.5 **(d)** 0.35

91. The inductive reactance of a transformer depends on
(a) emf **(b)** mmf **(c)** flux **(d)** leakage flux

92. Open circuit test in a transformer is performed with
(a) rated transformer voltage **(b)** rated transformer current
(c) direct current **(d)** high frequency supply

93. The open circuit test on a transformer gives
(a) equivalent resistance and reactance **(b)** magnetizing current and core loss at rated voltage **(c)** copper loss at rated voltage **(d)** both a and b above

94. The short circuit test is performed at
(a) rated current **(b)** rated voltage **(c)** short circuit the secondary at rated primary voltage **(d)** short circuiting the primary winding

95. 1kVA, 200/100 V, 50 Hz single phase transformer gave the following test results
O.C (L.V.side) : 100 V, 20 watts
S.C (h.v. side) : 5 A, 25 watts
The core losses at rated voltage are
(a) 20 W **(b)** 25 W **(c)** 45 W **(d)** 5 W

96. The copper losses at rated load in problem 95 are
(a) 20 W **(b)** 25 W **(c)** 45 W **(d)** 5 W

97. The copper losses at half the rated load in problem 95 are
(a) 20 W **(b)** 6.25 W **(c)** 12.5 W **(d)** 10 W

98. The core loss at half the rated load in problem 95 are
(a) 20 W **(b)** 25 W **(c)** 10 W **(d)** 5 W

99. During the short circuit test on a transformer, the core losses are negligible because
(a) The current on the h.v. side is very small
(b) The power factor is improved
(c) iron becomes saturated
(d) the core loss is proportional to applied voltage, which is small.

100. The transformer will work at maximum efficiency when
(a) hyteresis loss = eddy current loss **(b)** eddy current loss = copper loss
(c) iron loss = copper loss **(d)** hysteresis loss = copper loss

101. To reduce the eddy current loss in a transformer
(a) The core should be made up of wood **(b)** core is made from special steel
(c) core is laminated **(d)** it should be a step-up transformer

102. Grain oriented steel used for transformer core reduces
(a) eddy current loss **(b)** hyteresis loss **(c)** both a and b **(d)** copper loss

103. Transformer core laminations are coated with an enamel layer in order to
(a) reduce humming **(b)** attain adhesion between laminations **(c)** insulate laminations from each other **(d)** prevent corrosion of laminations

104. An induction motor works with
(a) d.c. only **(b)** a.c. only **(c)** both a.c. and d.c. **(d)** non of these

105. In a 3 phase induction motor, the resultant flux is of constant magnitude and is
(a) equal to maximum flux due to any phase
(b) 1.5 times the max-flux due to any phase
(c) $\sqrt{3}/2$ times the max-flux due to any phase
(d) 3 times the max-flux due to any phase

106. 4 pole, 3 phase induction motor is running at 1440 rpm when supply frequency is 50 Hz. The speed of rotation of flux with respect to stator is
(a) 1440 rpm **(b)** 1500 rpm **(c)** 60 rpm **(d)** 0 rpm

107. The speed of rotor conductors with respect to stator conductors in problem 106 is
(a) 1440 rpm **(b)** 1500 rpm **(c)** 60 rpm **(d)** 0 rpm

108. The speed of rotor conductors with respect to stator field in problem 106 is
(a) 1440 rpm **(b)** 1500 rpm **(c)** 60 rpm **(d)** 0 rpm

109. The slip of problem 106 per unit is
(a) 0.04 **(b)** 0.01 **(c)** 4 **(d)** 0.041

110. The frequency of rotor currents in problem 106 is
(a) 20 Hz **(b)** 2 Hz **(c)** 4 Hz **(d)** 50 Hz

111. If any two leads from supply are interchange in a 3-phase induction motor during reconnection after maintenance, then
(a) no change is observed **(b)** motor runs in the reverse direction
(c) motor will not run **(d)** motor will get damaged

112. If any two leads from slip rings are interchange in a 3-phase induction motor, the motor will
(a) continue to run in the same direction **(b)** run in opposite direction
(c) motor will not run **(d)** motor will get damaged

113. The rotor of induction motor runs
(a) in the direction of the stator field **(b)** opposite to the direction of stator field
(c) neither of the two **(d)** either a or be above

114. A single phase induction motor is

(a) self starting **(b)** not self starting

(c) self starting with the help of auxiliary winding **(d)** non of the above

115. Double field revolving theory is based on the idea that pulsating field produced in single phase motors can be resolved into two components of ________ its magnitude and rotating in ________ direction with synchronous speed.

(a) half, same **(b)** half, opposite **(c)** $\sqrt{2}$ time, same **(d)** $\sqrt{2}$ times opposite

116. Single phase induction motors are made self starting by

(a) increasing rotor resistance **(b)** using an external starting device

(c) providing additional winding on the stator

(d) providing additional winding on the rotor

117. Centrifugal switch fitted on the single phase induction motor will operate when

(a) rotor speed is equal to rated speed **(b)** rotor speed exceeds 70% of rated speed

(c) rotor speed exceeds synchronous speed **(d)** as soon as rotor starts running

118. The capacitor in a capacitor-run a.c. motor is connected in series with

(a) main winding **(b)** auxiliary winding

(c) squirrel cage winding **(d)** compensating winding

Answers

1 - (b), **2** - (c), **3** - (d), **4** - (b), **5** - (c), **6** - (c), **7** - (b), **8** - (c), **9** - (a), **10** - (b),

11 - (c), **12** - (d), **13** - (b), **14** - (c), **15** - (d), **16** - (b), **17** - (b), **18** - (a), **19** - (a), **20** - (a),

21 - (b), **22** - (a), **23** - (a), **24** - (a), **25** - (d), **26** - (b), **27** - (d), **28** - (a), **29** - (c), **30** - (c),

31 - (c), **32** - (d), **33** - (b), **34** - (a), **35** - (d), **36** - (a), **37** - (d), **38** - (a), **39** - (b), **40** - (a),

41 - (c), **42** - (d), **43** - (a), **44** - (a), **45** - (d), **46** - (c), **47** - (b), **48** - (d), **49** - (a), **50** - (b),

51 - (a), **52** - (b), **53** - (b), **54** - (a), **55** - (d), **56** - (a), **57** - (b), **58** - (b), **59** - (a), **60** - (a),

61 - (b), **62** - (c), **63** - (c), **64** - (a), **65** - (b), **66** - (c), **67** - (d), **68** - (a), **69** - (b), **70** - (a),

71 - (d), **72** - (b), **73** - (a), **74** - (c), **75** - (d), **76** - (a), **77** - (a), **78** - (b), **79** - (a), **80** - (b),

81 - (c), **82** - (b), **83** - (c), **84** - (b), **85** - (b), **86** - (d), **87** - (b), **88** - (d), **89** - (c), **90** - (d),

91 - (d), **92** - (a), **93** - (b), **94** - (a), **95** - (a), **96** - (b), **97** - (b), **98** - (a), **99** - (d), **100** - (c),

101 - (c), **102** - (b), **103** - (c), **104** - (b), **105** - (b), **106** - (b), **107** - (a), **108** - (c), **109** - (a),

110 - (b), **111** - (b), **112** - (a), **113** - (a), **114** - (c), **115** - (b), **116** - (c), **117** - (b), **118** - (b).

APPENDIX **B**

SOLUTION TO UNSOLVED EXAMPLES

Chapter 1 : D.C. CIRCUITS

Solution to Unsolved Examples

1. Find R_{AB}.

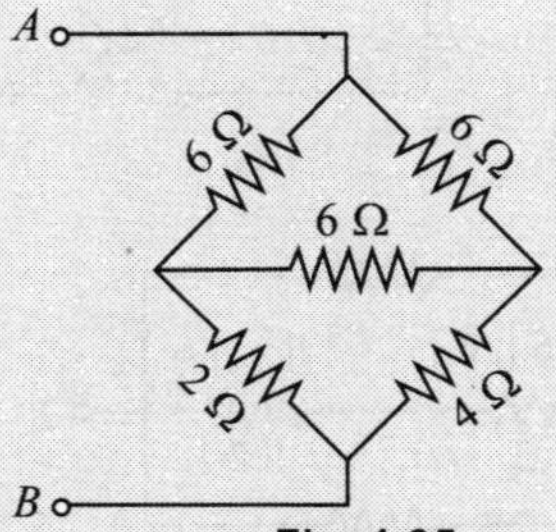

Fig. 1.95

Solution :

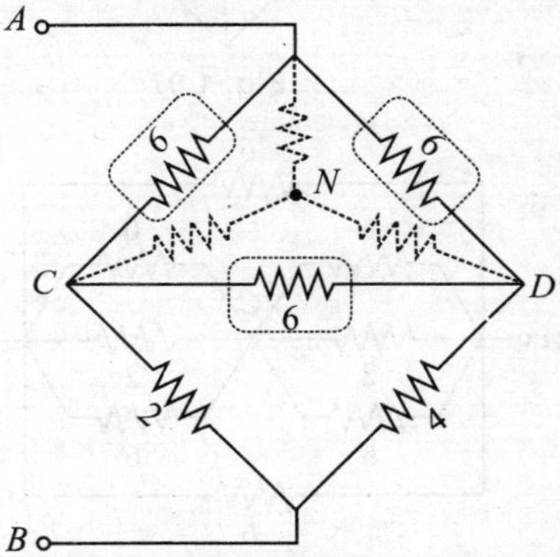

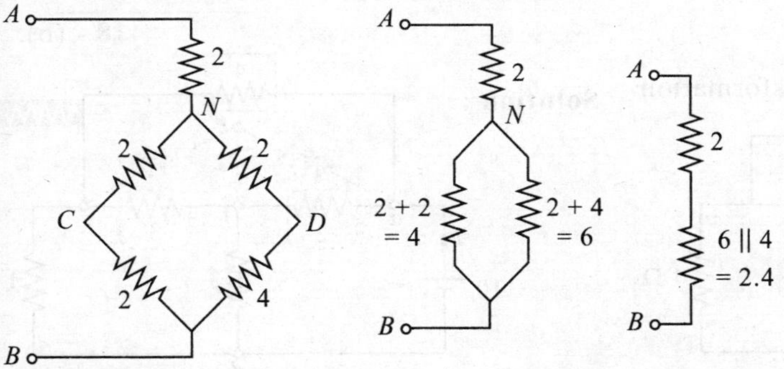

Formula for converting to star from delta is

$$R_1 = \frac{R_{12}\,R_{13}}{R_{12} + R_{23} + R_{13}}$$

$$\therefore\; R_{ab} = 2 + 2.4 = 4.4\ \Omega$$

$$\boxed{R_{ab} = 4.4\ \Omega}$$

2. Find R_{AB}.

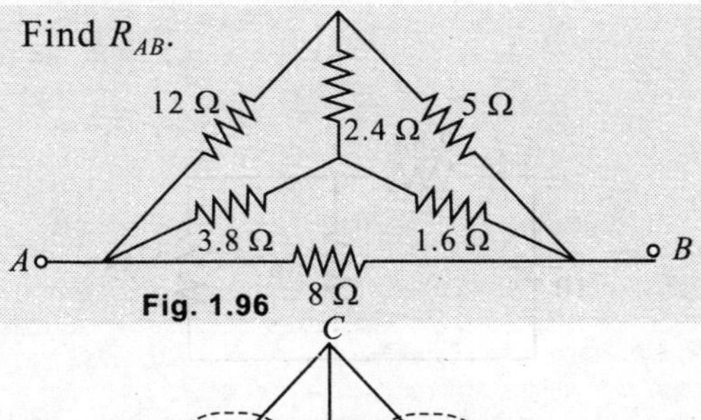

Fig. 1.96

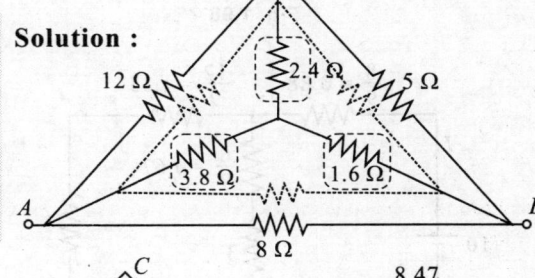

Solution :

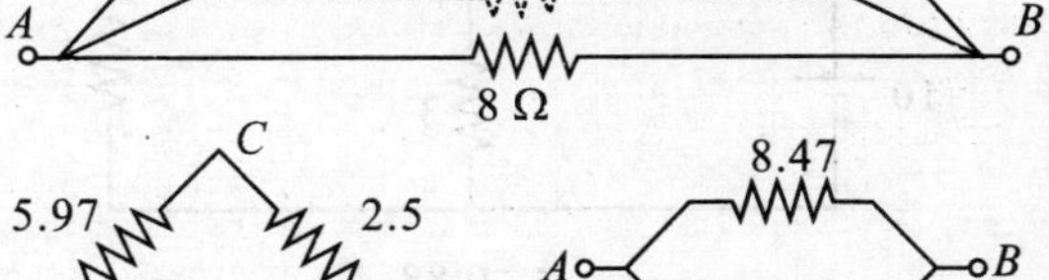

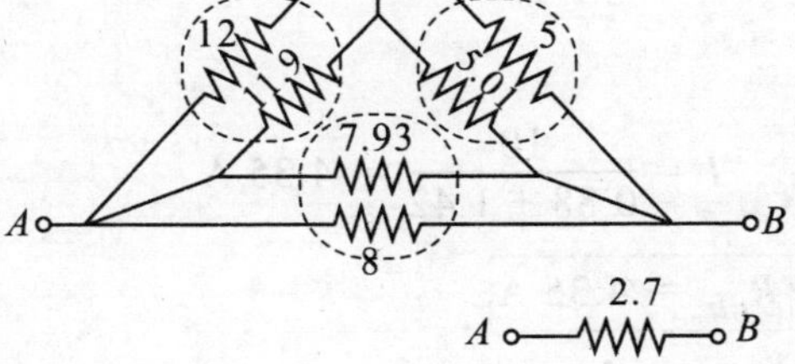

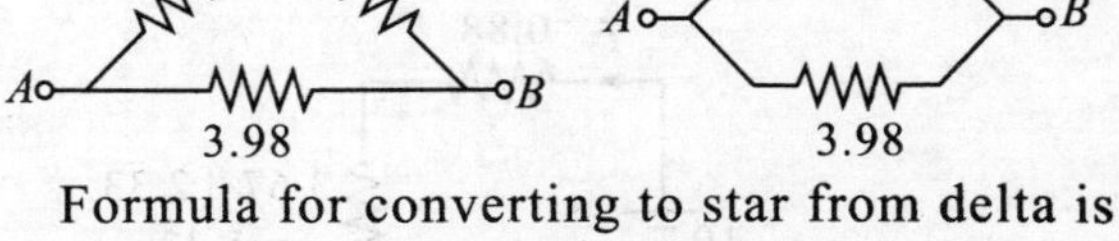

Formula for converting to star from delta is

$$R_{12} = \frac{R_1 R_2 + R_2 R_3 + R_3 R_1}{R_3} \qquad \therefore\; \boxed{R_{AB} = 2.7\ \Omega}$$

3. Find R_{AB}.

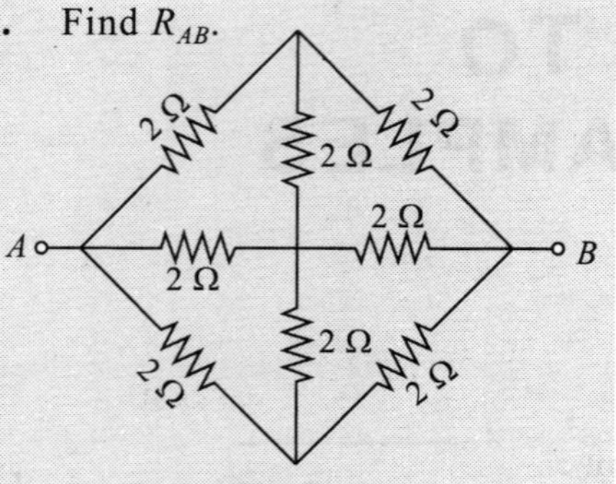

Fig. 1.97

Solution :

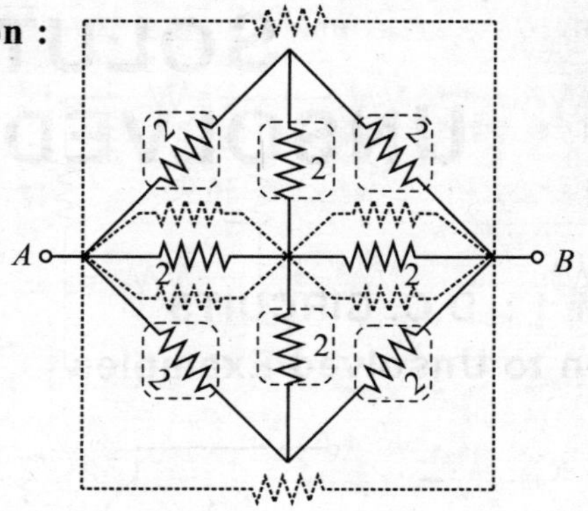

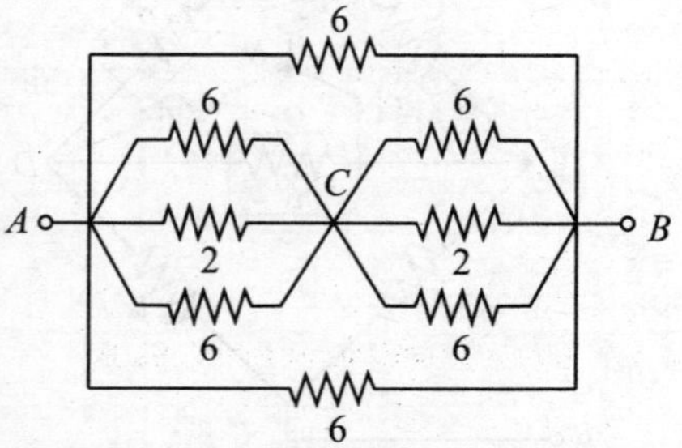

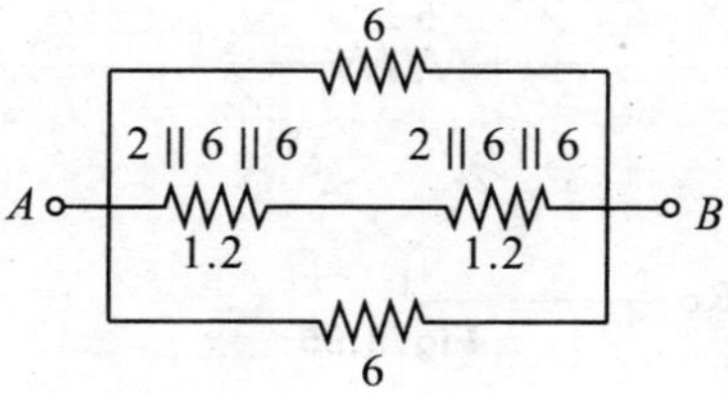

R_{ab} = 1.33 Ω

4. Find I using Star-Delta transformation.

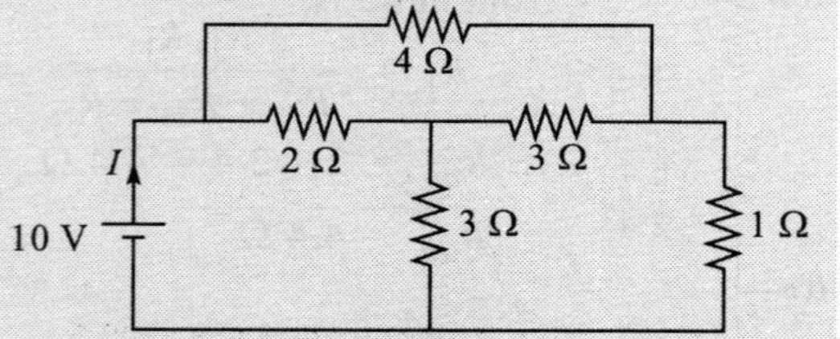

Fig. 1.98

Solution :

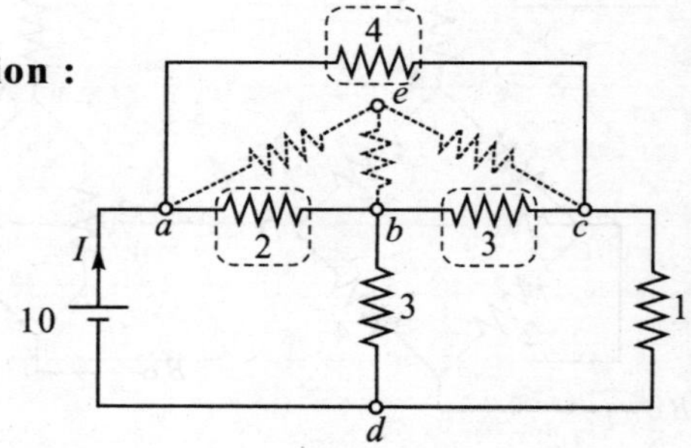

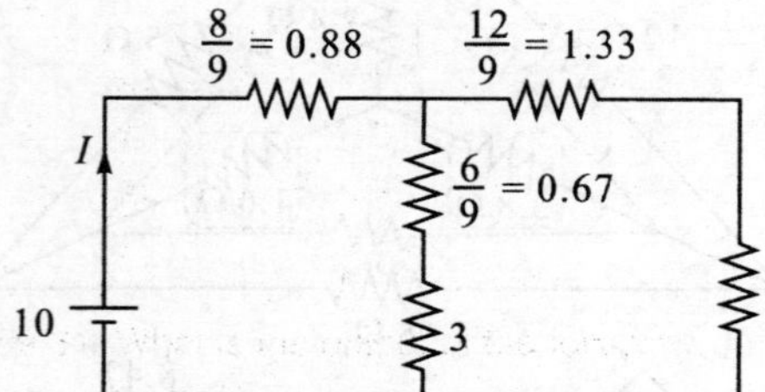

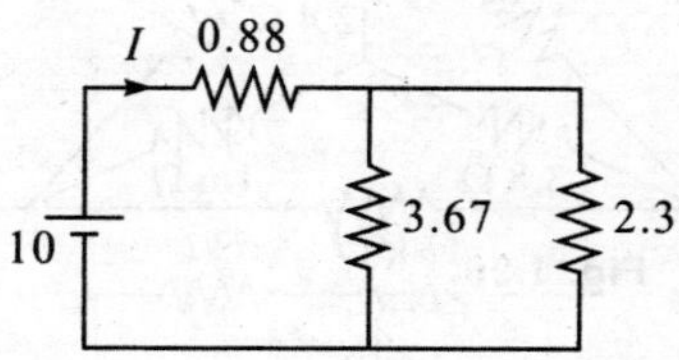

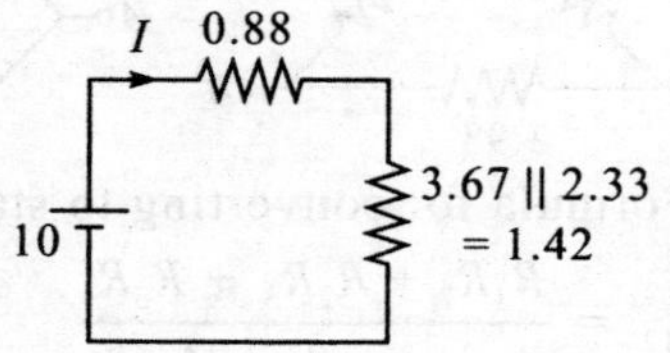

$$\therefore\ I = \frac{10}{0.88 + 1.42} = 4.35 \text{ A}$$

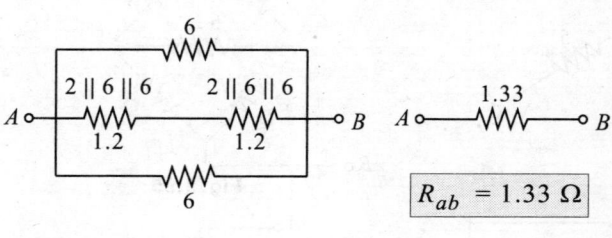

R_{ab} = 4.35 A

5. Using star-delta transformation find I.

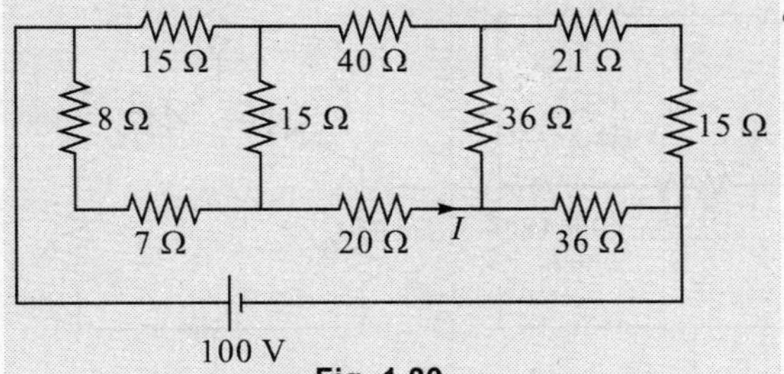

Fig. 1.99

Solution :

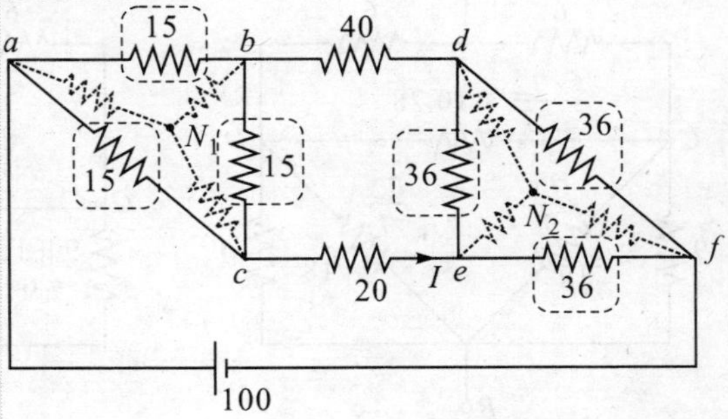

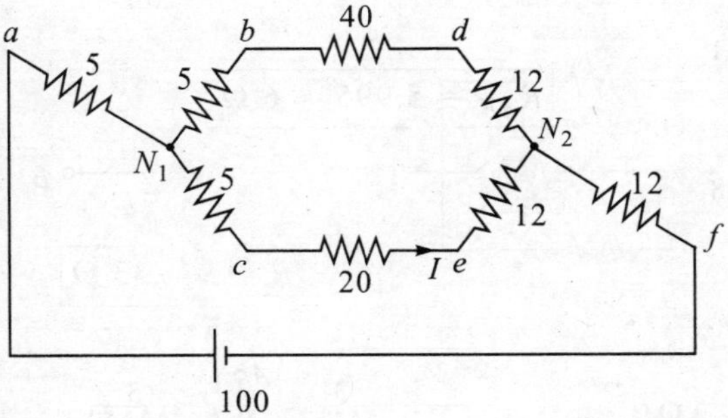

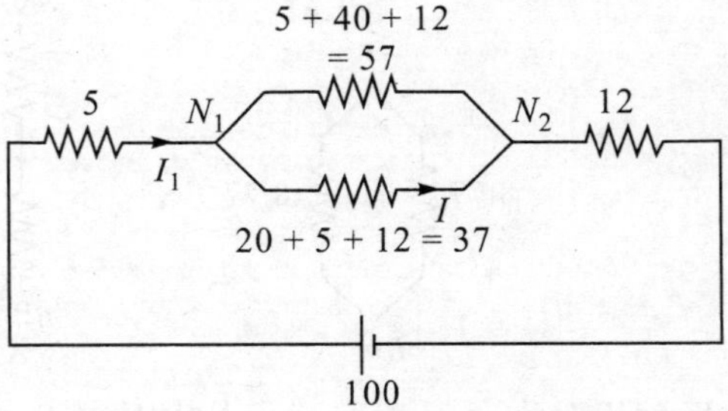

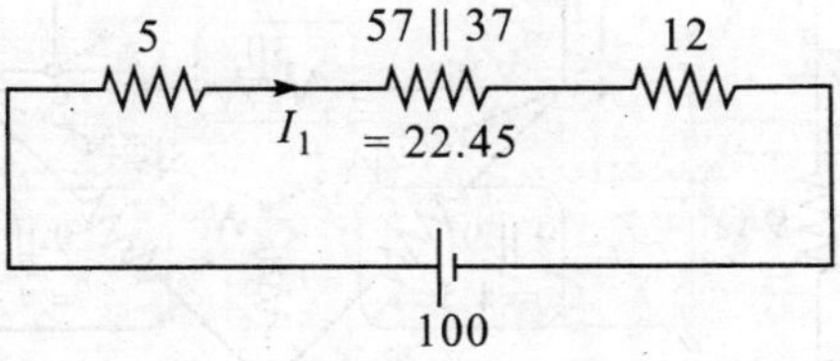

By current division rule

$$I = I_1 \times \frac{57}{57+37} \quad \text{.... (i)}$$

$$\therefore \ I_1 = \frac{100}{5 + 22.45 + 12}$$

$$\therefore \ I_1 = 2.74 \text{ A}$$

from (i) I_1 = **1.66 A**

6. Find R_{AB}.

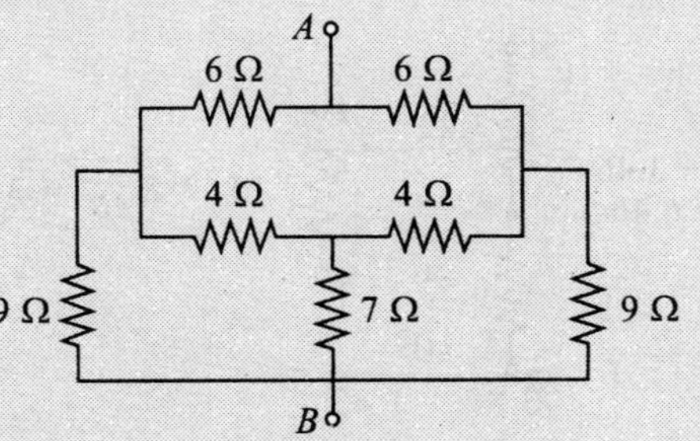

Fig. 1.100

Solution :

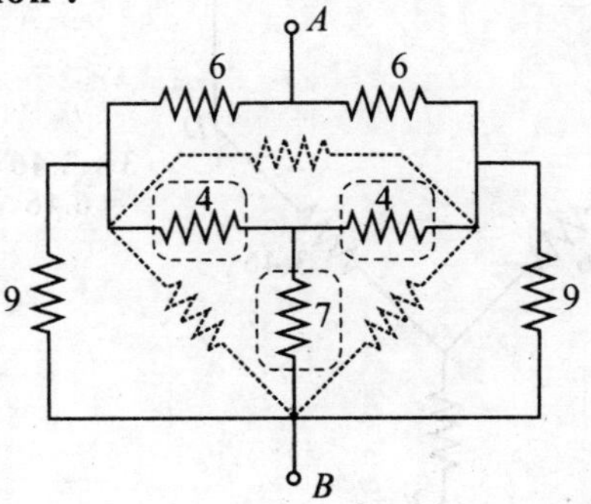

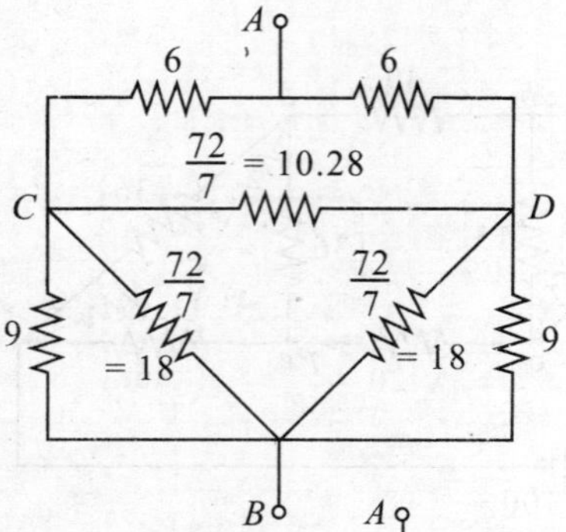

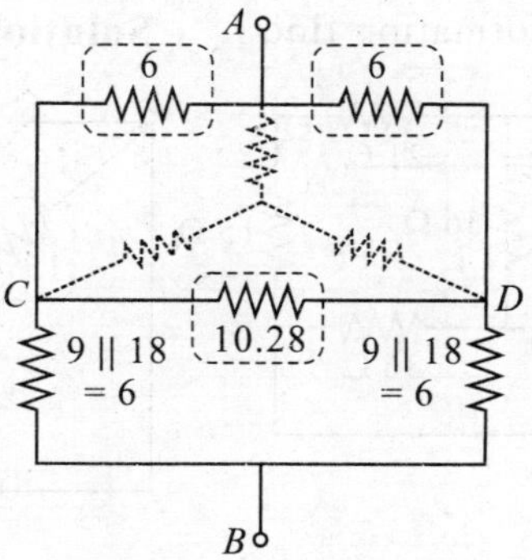

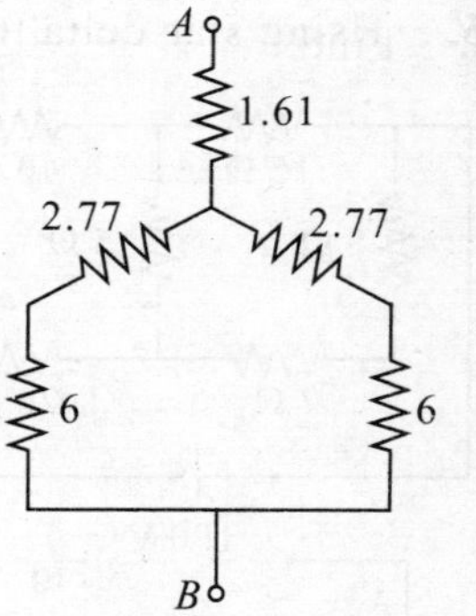

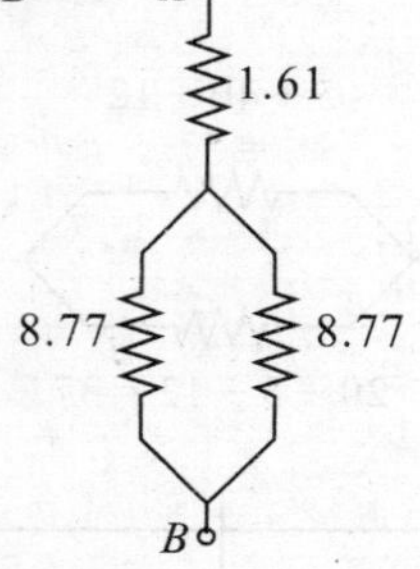

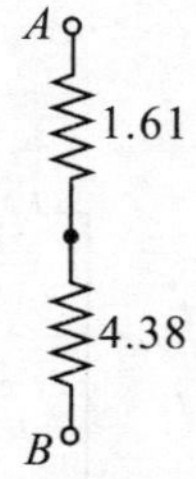

R_{AB} = 5.995 ≈ 6 Ω

7. Find R_{AB}.

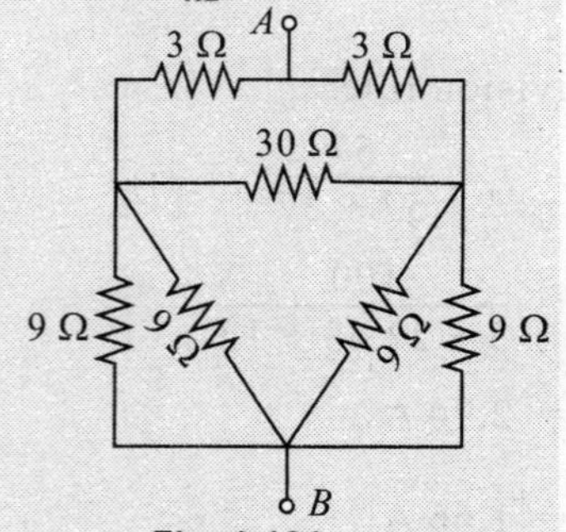

Fig. 1.101

Solution :

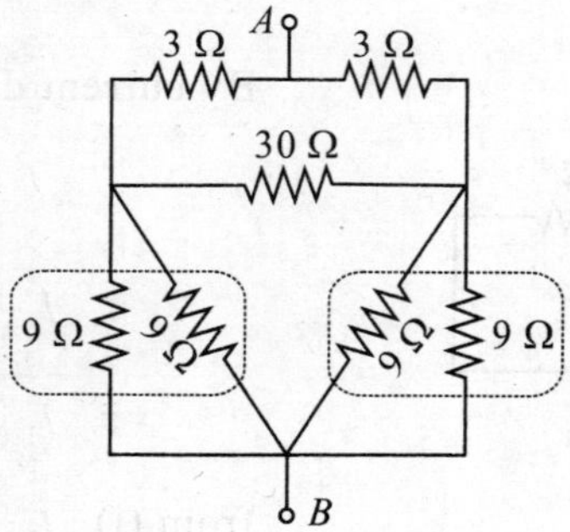

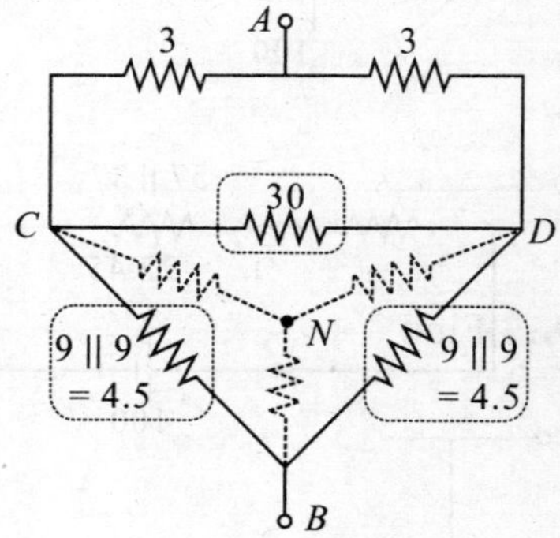

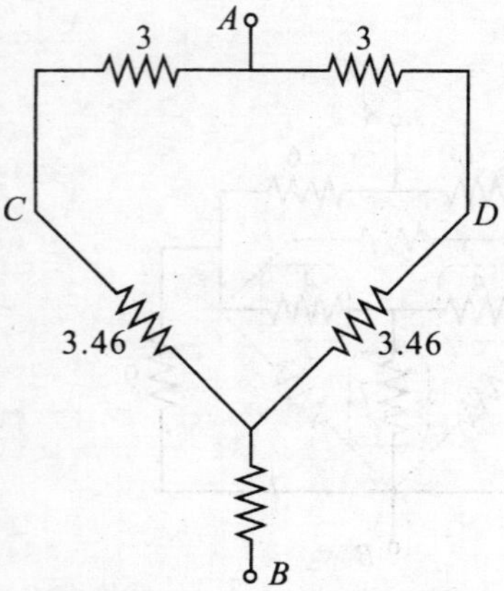

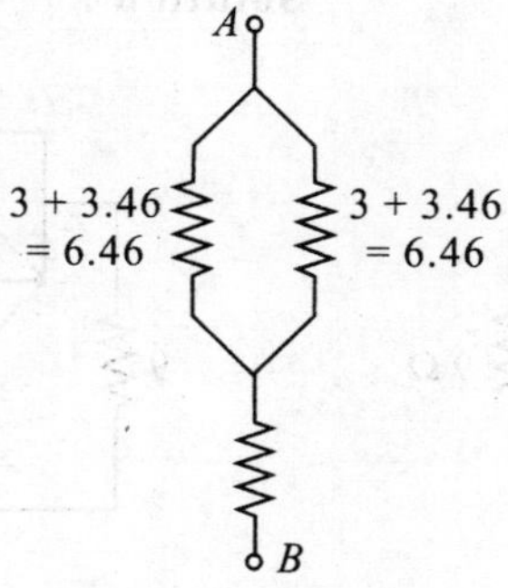

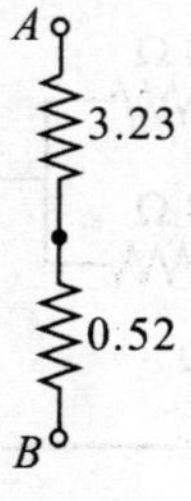

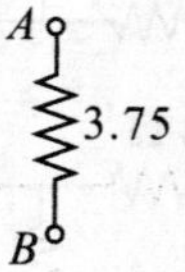

R_{AB} = 3.75 Ω

8. Find R_{xy}.

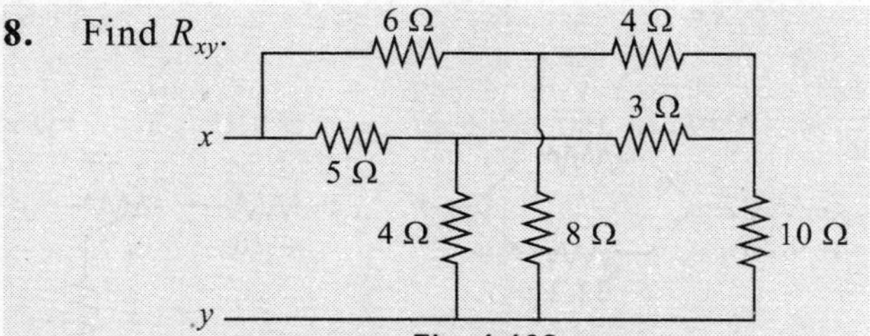

Fig. 1.102

Solution : There are two star connection between *xyz*, one with 5, 3, 4 Ω connected at N_2 and 6, 4, 8 Ω connected at N_1. Converting them to delta we get

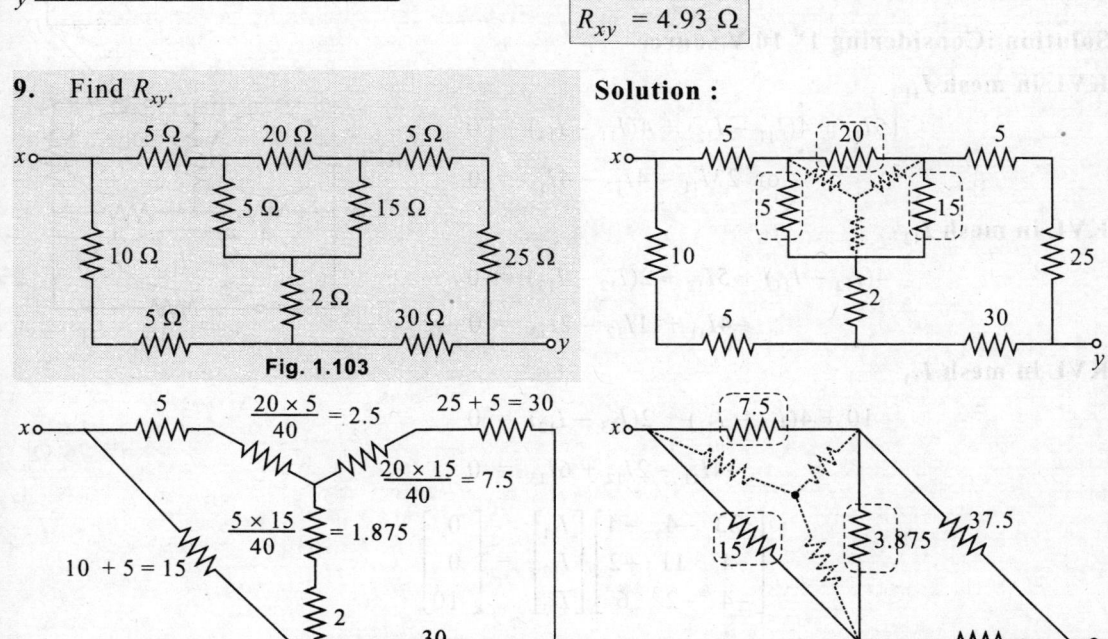

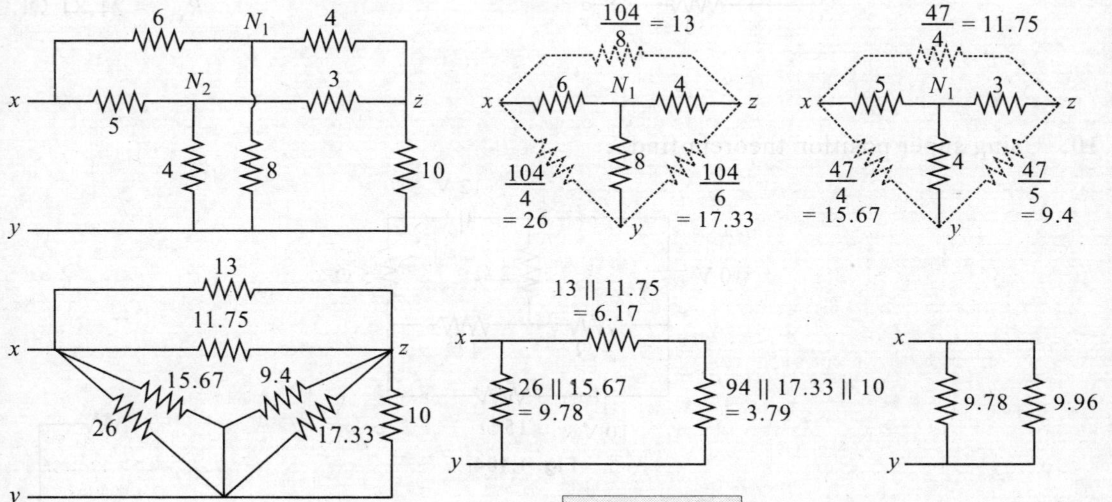

$R_{xy} = 4.93\ \Omega$

9. Find R_{xy}.

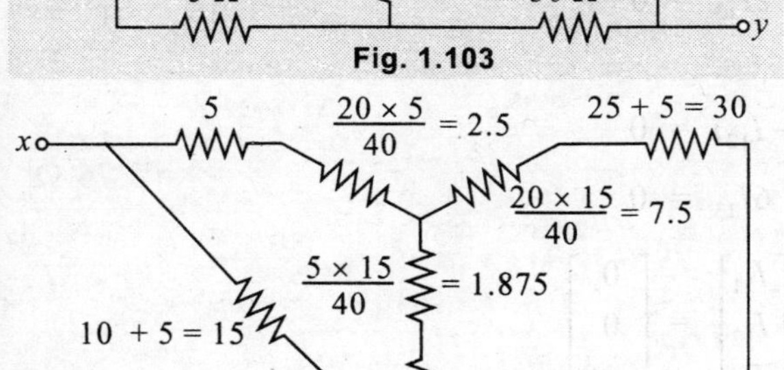

Fig. 1.103

Solution :

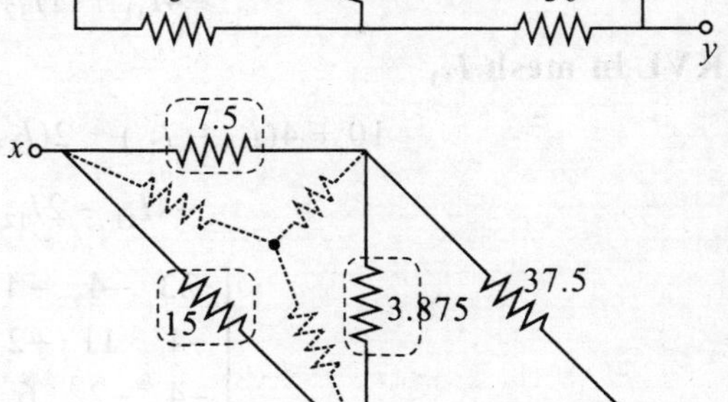

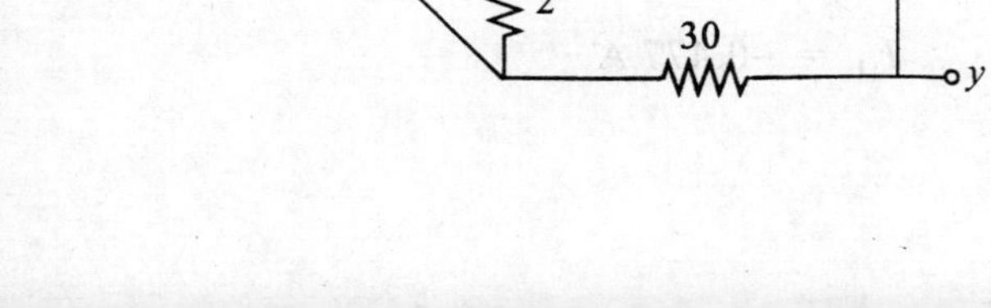

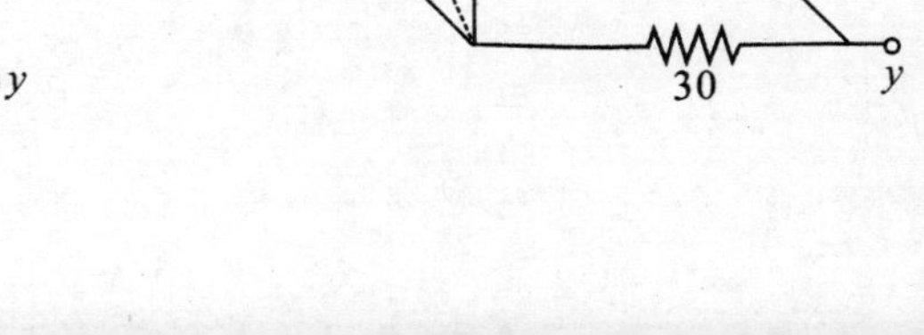

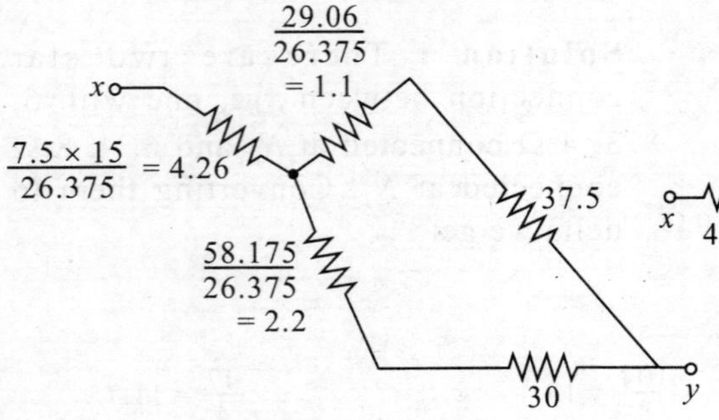

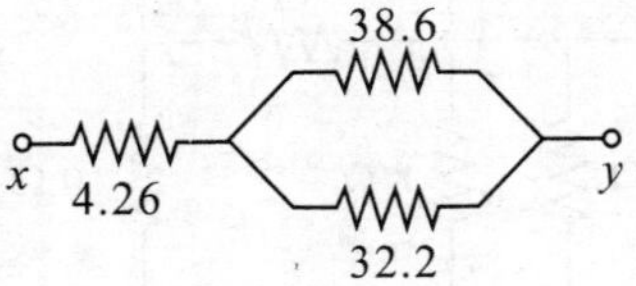

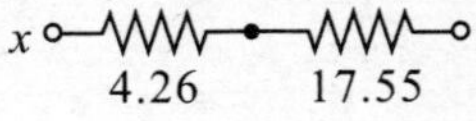

$$R_{xy} = 21.81\ \Omega$$

10. Using super position theorem find I.

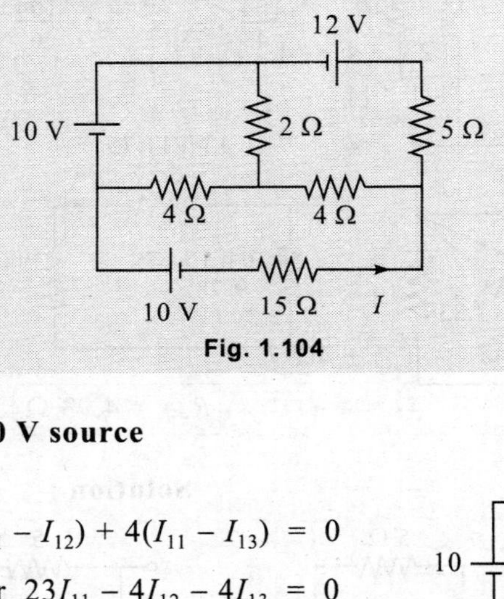

Fig. 1.104

Solution :Considering 1st 10 V source

KVL in mesh I_{11}

$$15I_{11} + 4(I_{11} - I_{12}) + 4(I_{11} - I_{13}) = 0$$

$$\text{or } 23I_{11} - 4I_{12} - 4I_{13} = 0$$

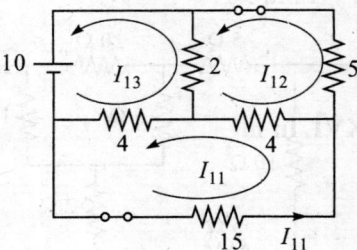

KVL in mesh I_{12}

$$4(I_{12} - I_{11}) + 5I_{12} + 2(I_{12} - I_{13}) = 0$$

$$\therefore\ -4I_{11} + 11I_{12} - 2I_{13} = 0$$

KVL in mesh I_{13}

$$10 + 4(I_{13} - I_{11}) + 2(I_{13} - I_{12}) = 0$$

$$-4I_{11} - 2I_{12} + 6I_{13} = 0$$

$$\begin{bmatrix} 23 & -4 & -4 \\ -4 & 11 & -2 \\ -4 & -2 & 6 \end{bmatrix} \begin{bmatrix} I_{11} \\ I_{12} \\ I_{13} \end{bmatrix} = \begin{bmatrix} 0 \\ 0 \\ -10 \end{bmatrix}$$

$$\therefore I_{11} = -0.477 \text{ A}$$

Considering 2nd 10 V source

KVL in mesh I_{21}

$$+10 + 15(I_{21}) + 4(I_{21} - I_{22}) + 4(I_{21} - I_{23}) = 0$$

$$23 I_{21} - 4I_{22} - 4I_{23} = -10$$

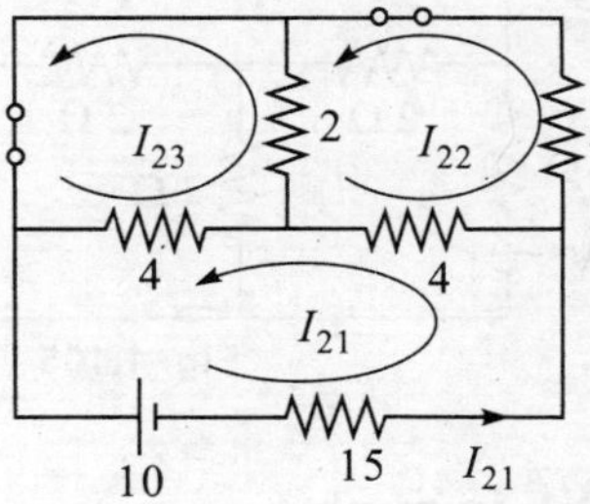

KVL in mesh I_{22}

$$5I_{22} + 2(I_{22} - I_{23}) + 4(I_{22} - I_{21}) = 0$$

$$\therefore -4I_{21} + 11I_{22} - 2I_{23} = 0$$

KVL in mesh I_{23}

$$2(I_{23} - I_{22}) + 4(I_{23} - I_{21}) = 0$$

$$\therefore -4 I_{21} - 2I_{22} + 6I_{23} = 0$$

$$\begin{bmatrix} 23 & -4 & -4 \\ -4 & 11 & -2 \\ -4 & -2 & 6 \end{bmatrix} \begin{bmatrix} I_{21} \\ I_{22} \\ I_{23} \end{bmatrix} = \begin{bmatrix} -10 \\ 0 \\ 0 \end{bmatrix}$$

$$\therefore I_{21} = -0.569 \text{ A}$$

Considering 12 V source

KVL in mesh I_{31}

$$15I_{31} + 4(I_{31} - I_{32}) + 4(I_{31} - I_{33}) = 0$$

$$\therefore 23I_{31} - 4I_{32} - 4I_{33} = 0$$

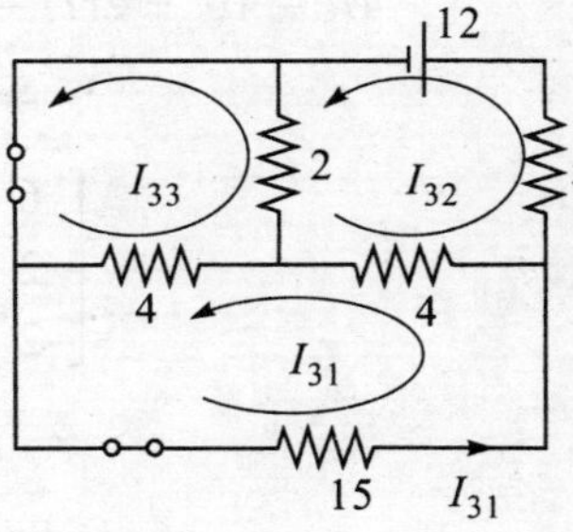

KVL in mesh I_{32}

$$4(I_{32} - I_{31}) + 5I_{32} + 12 + 2(I_{32} - I_{33}) = 0$$

$$\therefore -4 I_{31} + 11I_{32} - 2I_{33} = -12$$

KVL in mesh I_{33}

$$2(I_{33} - I_{32}) + 4(I_{33} - I_{31}) = 0$$

$$\therefore -4I_{31} - 2I_{32} + 11I_{33} = -12$$

$$\begin{bmatrix} 23 & -4 & -4 \\ -4 & 11 & -2 \\ -4 & -2 & 6 \end{bmatrix} \begin{bmatrix} I_{31} \\ I_{32} \\ I_{33} \end{bmatrix} = \begin{bmatrix} 0 \\ -12 \\ 0 \end{bmatrix}$$

$$\therefore I_{31} = -0.352$$

$$\therefore I = I_{11} + I_{21} + I_{31}$$

$$I = -0.477 - 0.569 - 0.352$$

$$I = \boxed{-1.398 \text{ A}}$$

11. Using mesh analysis find I.

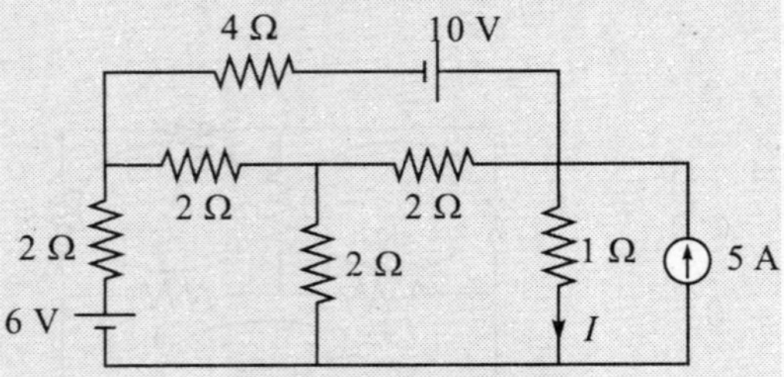

Fig. 1.105

Solution :

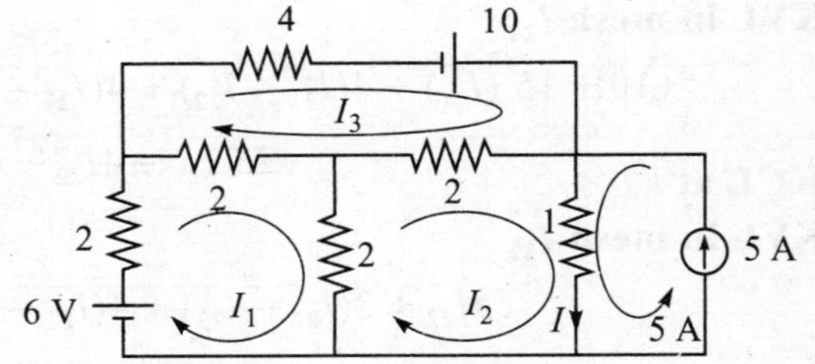

KVL in mesh I_1

$$-6 + 2I_1 + 2(I_1 - I_3) + 2(I_1 - I_2) = 0$$

$$\therefore \; 6I_1 - 2I_2 - 2I_3 = 6 \quad \text{.... (i)}$$

KVL in mesh I_2

$$2(I_2 - I_1) + 2(I_2 - I_3) + 1(I_2 + 5) = 0$$

$$\therefore \; -2I_1 + 5I_2 - 2I_3 = -5 \quad \text{.... (ii)}$$

KVL in mesh I_3

$$4I_3 - 10 + 2(I_3 - I_2) + 2(I_3 - I_2) = 0$$

$$\therefore \; -2I_1 - 2I_2 + 8I_3 = 10 \quad \text{.... (iii)}$$

$$\begin{bmatrix} 6 & -2 & -2 \\ -2 & 5 & -2 \\ -2 & -2 & 8 \end{bmatrix} \begin{bmatrix} I_1 \\ I_2 \\ I_3 \end{bmatrix} = \begin{bmatrix} 6 \\ -5 \\ 10 \end{bmatrix}$$

$$\therefore \; I_1 = 1.73 \text{ A}; \; I_2 = 0.40 \text{ A}; \; I_3 = 1.78 \text{ A};$$

From figure $\quad I = I_2 + 5$

$$I = 0.40 + 5$$

$$I = \boxed{5.40 \text{ A}}$$

12. Using nodal analysis find I.

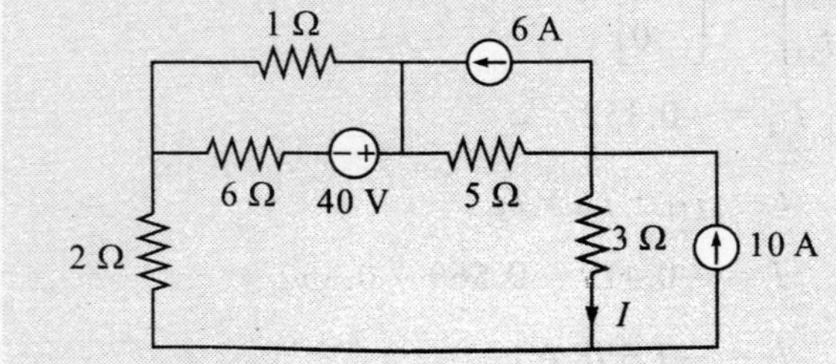

Fig. 1.106

Solution :

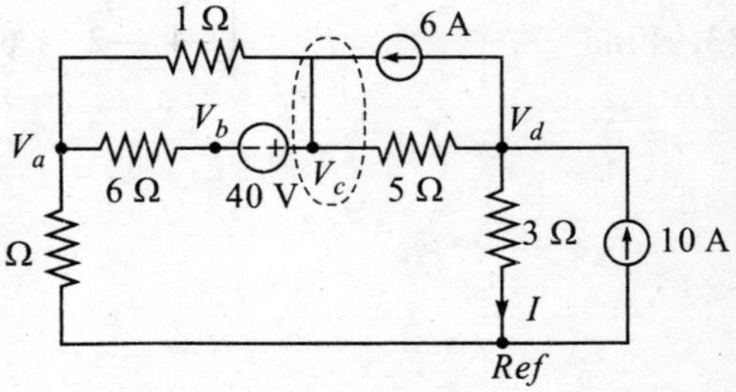

KCL at node *a*

$$\frac{V_a}{2} + \frac{V_a - V_b}{6} + \frac{V_a - V_c}{1} = 0$$

$$\therefore \; 10V_a - V_b - 6V_c = 0 \quad \text{.... (i)}$$

KCL at super node *b, c*

$$\frac{V_b - V_a}{6} + \frac{V_c - V_d}{4} + \frac{V_c - V_a}{1} - 6 = 0$$

$$\therefore \; -14V_a + 2V_b + 15V_c - 3V_d = 72 \quad \text{.... (ii)}$$

$$\text{and} \quad V_c - V_b = 40 \quad \text{.... (iii)}$$

$$\text{or} \quad V_c = V_b + 40 \quad \text{.... (iv)}$$

KCL at node *d*

$$6 + \frac{V_d - V_c}{5} + \frac{V_d}{3} - 10 = 0$$

$$+ 8V_d - 3V_c = 60 \quad \text{.... (v)}$$

Substituting for V_c from (iv) in (i), (ii) and (v), we get

$$10V_a - 7V_b = 240 \quad \text{.... (vi)}$$

$$-14V_a + 17V_b - 3V_d = -528 \quad \text{.... (vii)}$$

$$\text{and} \quad -3V_b + 8V_d = 180 \quad \text{.... (viii)}$$

Solving (vi), (vii) and (viii), we get

$$\begin{bmatrix} 10 & -7 & 0 \\ -14 & 17 & -3 \\ -0 & -3 & 8 \end{bmatrix} \begin{bmatrix} V_a \\ V_b \\ V_c \end{bmatrix} = \begin{bmatrix} 240 \\ -528 \\ 180 \end{bmatrix}$$

$$\therefore \; V_d = 14.81$$

$$I = \frac{V_d}{3} = \frac{14.81}{3}$$

$$I = \boxed{4.94 \text{ A}}$$

13. Find V using super position theorem.

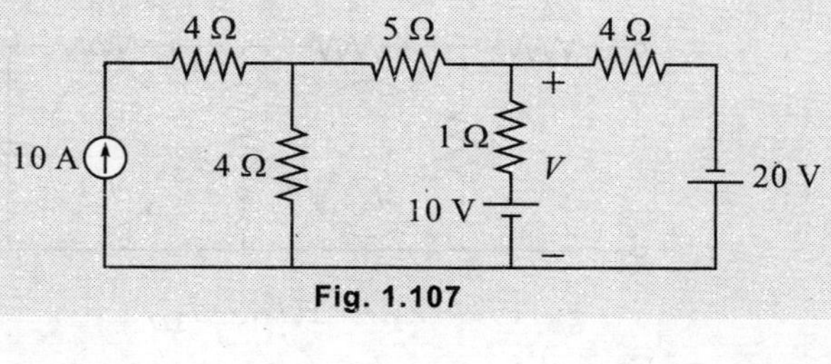

Fig. 1.107

Solution : Considering one 10 A source

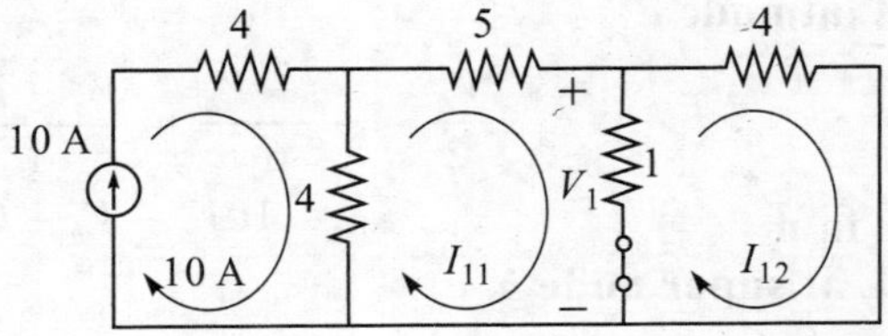

$$V_1 = 1(I_{11} - I_{12})$$

KVL in mesh I_{11}

$$4\,(I_{11} - 10) + 5I_{11} + 1(I_{11} - I_{12}) = 0$$

$$10I_{11} - I_{12} = 40$$

KVL in mesh I_{12}

$$4I_{12} + 1(I_{12} - I_{11}) = 0$$

$$\therefore\ -I_{11} + 5I_{12} = 40$$

$$\therefore \begin{bmatrix} 10 & -1 \\ -1 & 5 \end{bmatrix} \begin{bmatrix} I_{11} \\ I_{12} \end{bmatrix} = \begin{bmatrix} 40 \\ 0 \end{bmatrix}$$

$$\therefore I_{11} = 4.08\text{ A};\ I_{12} = 0.82\text{ A}$$

$$V_1 = 1(I_{11} - I_{12})$$

$$V_1 = \boxed{3.26\text{ V}}$$

Considering 10 V source

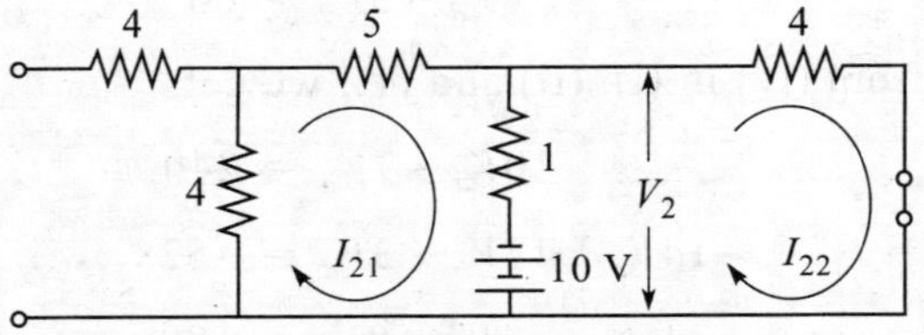

$$V_2 = 1(I_{21} - I_{22}) - 10$$

KVL in mesh I_{21}

$$4I_{21} + 5I_{21} + 1(I_{21} - I_{22}) - 10 = 0$$

$$\therefore\ 10\,I_{21} - I_{22} = 10$$

KVL in mesh I_{22}

$$4I_{22} + 10 + 1(I_{22} - I_{21}) = 0$$

$$\therefore\ -I_{21} + 5I_{22} = -10$$

$$\therefore \begin{bmatrix} 10 & -1 \\ -1 & 5 \end{bmatrix} \begin{bmatrix} I_{21} \\ I_{22} \end{bmatrix} = \begin{bmatrix} 10 \\ -10 \end{bmatrix}$$

$$\therefore I_{21} = 0.82\text{ A};\ I_{22} = -1.84\text{ A}$$

$$V_2 = 1(I_{21} - I_{22}) - 10$$

$$V_2 = -7.34\text{ V}$$

Considering one 20 V source

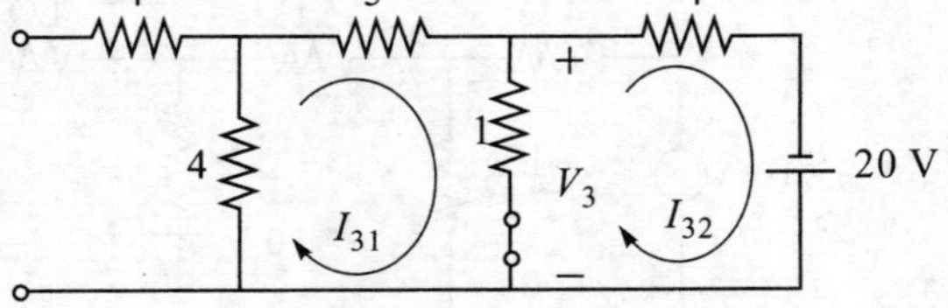

$$V_3 = 1(I_{31} - I_{32})$$

KVL in mesh I_{31}

$$4I_{31} + 5I_{31} + 1(I_{31} - I_{32}) = 0$$

$$10I_{31} - I_{32} = 0$$

KVL in mesh I_{32}

$$4I_{32} - 20 + 1(I_{32} - I_{31}) = 0$$

$$\therefore -I_{31} + 5I_{32} = 20$$

$$\begin{bmatrix} 10 & -1 \\ -1 & 5 \end{bmatrix} \begin{bmatrix} I_{31} \\ I_{32} \end{bmatrix} = \begin{bmatrix} 0 \\ 20 \end{bmatrix}$$

$$\therefore I_{31} = 0.408 \text{ A}; I_{32} = 4.08 \text{ A}$$

$$V_3 = 1(I_{31} - I_{32})$$

$$V_3 = \boxed{-3.672 \text{ V}}$$

Considering all sources together

$$V = V_1 + V_2 + V_3$$

$$V = 3.26 - 7.34 - 3.67$$

$$V = \boxed{-7.75 \text{ V}}$$

14. Using nodal analysis find I.

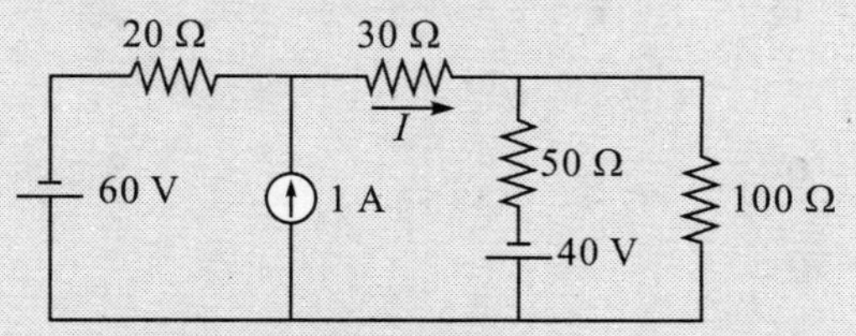

Fig. 1.108

Solution :

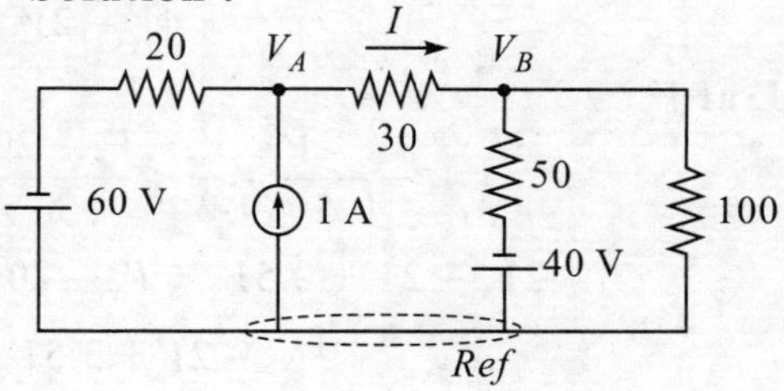

$$I = \frac{V_A - V_B}{30}$$

KCL at super node V_A

$$\frac{V_A + 60}{20} + \frac{V_A - V_B}{30} - 1 = 0$$

Multiplying above equation by 60.

$$\therefore 3V_A + 180 + 2V_A - 2V_B - 60 = 0$$

$$\therefore 5V_A - 2V_B = -120 \quad \text{.... (i)}$$

KCL at V_B

$$\frac{V_B - V_A}{30} + \frac{V_B - (-40)}{50} + \frac{V_B}{100} = 0$$

Multiplying above equation by 150.

$$5V_B - 5V_A + 3V_B + 120 + 1.5V_B = 0$$

$$-5V_A + 9.5V_B = -120 \quad .... \text{(ii)}$$

$$\begin{bmatrix} 5 & -2 \\ -5 & 9.4 \end{bmatrix} \begin{bmatrix} V_A \\ V_B \end{bmatrix} = \begin{bmatrix} -120 \\ -120 \end{bmatrix}$$

$$V_A = -36.97 \text{ V}; \; V_B = -32.43 \text{ V}$$

$$\therefore \; I = \boxed{-0.15 \text{ A}}$$

15. Find V using nodal analysis.

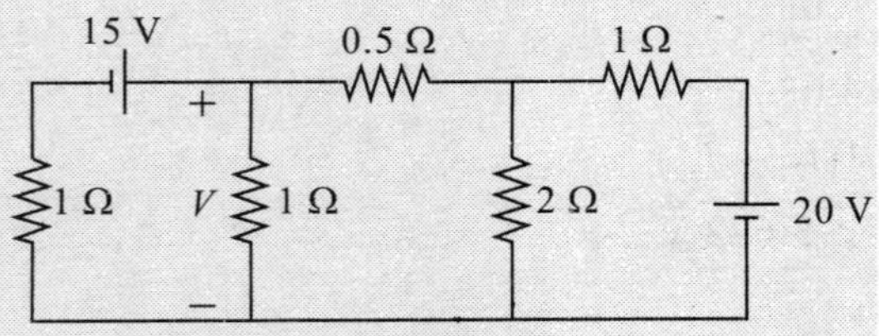

Fig. 1.109

Solution :

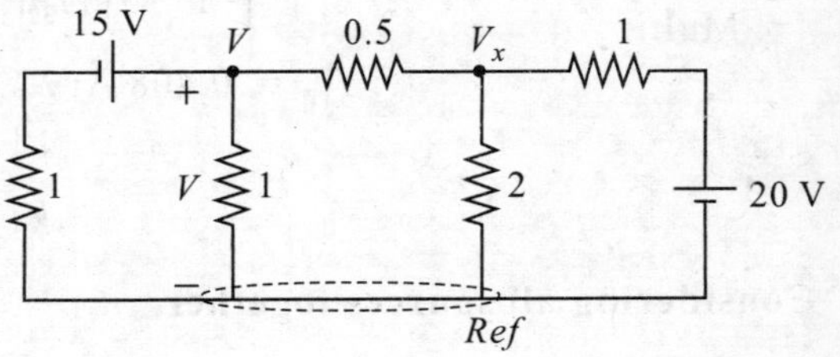

KCL at V

$$\frac{V-15}{1} + \frac{V}{1} + \frac{V-V_x}{0.5} = 0$$

$$V - 15 + V + 2V - 2V_x = 0$$

$$4V - 2V_x = 15 \quad .... \text{(i)}$$

KCL at V_x

$$\frac{V_x - V}{0.5} + \frac{V_x}{2} + \frac{V_x - 20}{1} = 0$$

$$2V_x - 2V + 0.5V_x + V_x - 20 = 0$$

$$-2V + 3.5V_x = 20 \quad .... \text{(ii)}$$

$$\begin{bmatrix} 4 & -2 \\ -2 & 3.5 \end{bmatrix} \begin{bmatrix} V \\ V_x \end{bmatrix} = \begin{bmatrix} 15 \\ 20 \end{bmatrix}$$

$$V = \boxed{9.25 \text{ V}}$$

16. Find I using nodal analysis.

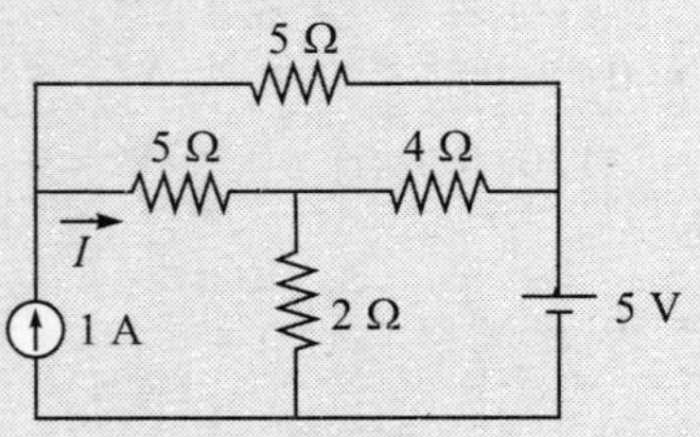

Fig. 1.110

Solution :

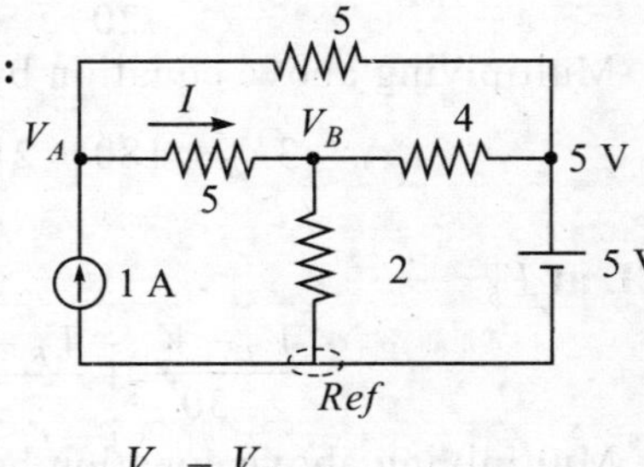

$$I = \frac{V_A - V_B}{5}$$

KCL at node V_A,

$$-1\frac{V_A - V_B}{5} + \frac{V_A - 5}{5} = 0$$

$$\therefore\ -5 + V_A - V_B + V_A - 5 = 0$$

$$2V_A - V_B = 10 \quad .... \text{(i)}$$

KCL at V_B

$$\frac{V_B - V_A}{5} + \frac{V_B}{2} + \frac{V_B - 5}{4} = 0$$

Multiply above equation by 20.

$$4V_B - 4V_A + 10V_B + 5V_B - 25 = 0$$

$$-4V_A + 19V_B = 25 \quad .... \text{(ii)}$$

$$\begin{bmatrix} 2 & -1 \\ -4 & 19 \end{bmatrix} \begin{bmatrix} V_A \\ V_B \end{bmatrix} = \begin{bmatrix} 10 \\ 25 \end{bmatrix}$$

$$V_A = 6.32 \text{ V};\ V_B = 2.65 \text{ V}$$

$$I = \frac{V_A - V_B}{5} = \frac{6.32 - 2.65}{5}$$

$$\therefore\ I = \boxed{0.734 \text{ A}}$$

17. Find I using super position theorem.

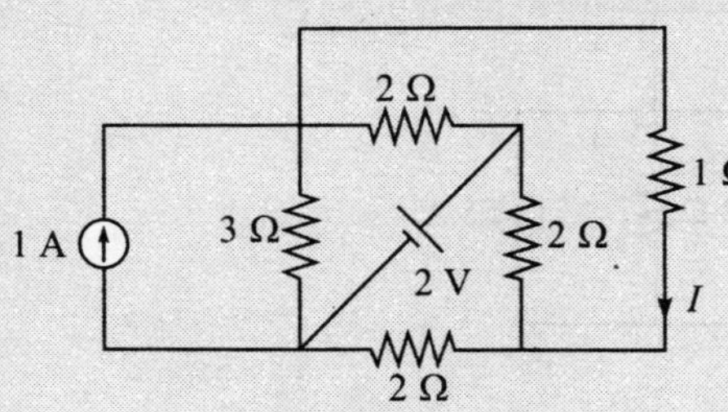

Fig. 1.111

Solution : Considering 1 A source

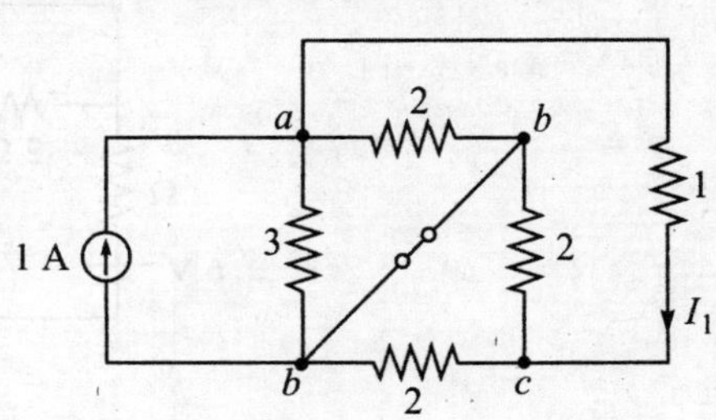

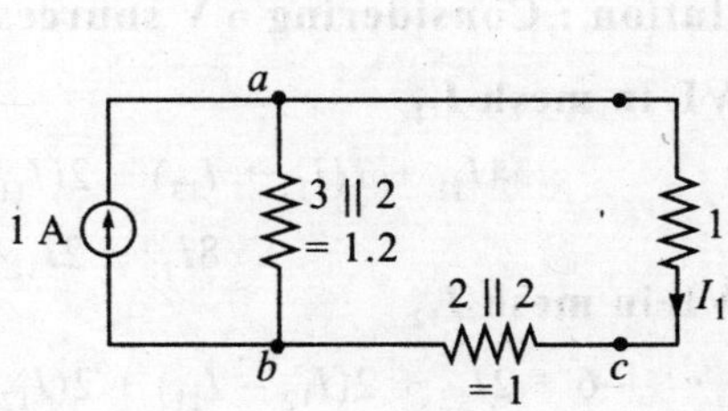

$$\therefore\ I_1 = 1\,\frac{1.2}{1.2 + 1 + 1}$$

$$\therefore\ I_1 = \boxed{0.375 \text{ A}}$$

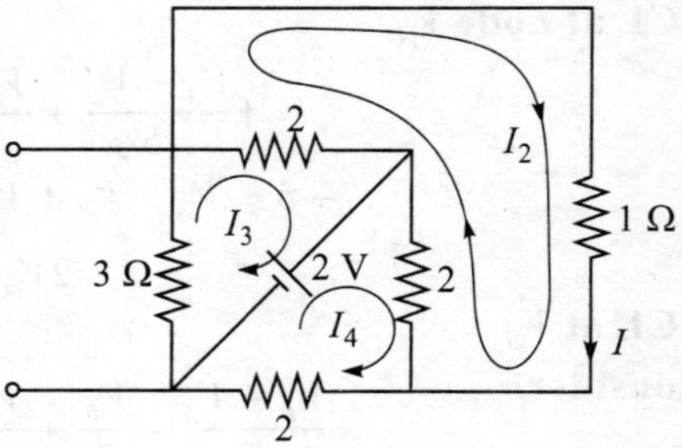

Considering 2 V source

KVL in mesh I_3

$$3I_3 + 2(I_3 - I_2) + 2 = 0$$
$$-2I_2 + 5I_3 = -2$$

KVL in mesh I_4

$$-2 + 2(I_4 - I_2) + 2I_4 = 0$$
$$-2I_2 + 4I_4 = 2$$

KVL in mesh I_2

$$2(I_2 - I_3) + 1.I_2 + 2(I_2 - I_4) = 0$$
$$5I_2 - 2I_3 - 2I_4 = 0$$

$$\begin{bmatrix} -2 & 5 & 0 \\ -2 & 0 & 4 \\ 5 & -2 & -2 \end{bmatrix} \begin{bmatrix} I_2 \\ I_3 \\ I_4 \end{bmatrix} = \begin{bmatrix} -2 \\ 2 \\ 0 \end{bmatrix}$$

$$\therefore I_2 = 0.0625$$

Considering both sources

$$I = I_1 + I_2$$
$$I = 0.375 + 0.0625$$
$$I = \boxed{0.437 \text{ A}}$$

18. Find $I_{4\,\Omega}$ super position theorem.

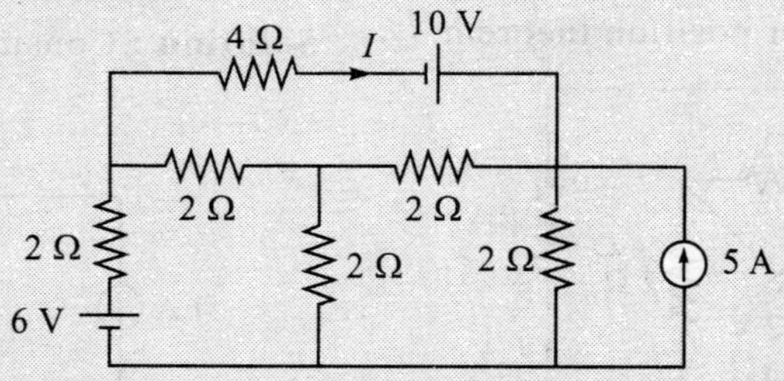

Fig. 1.112

Solution : Considering 6 V sources

KVL in mesh I_{11}

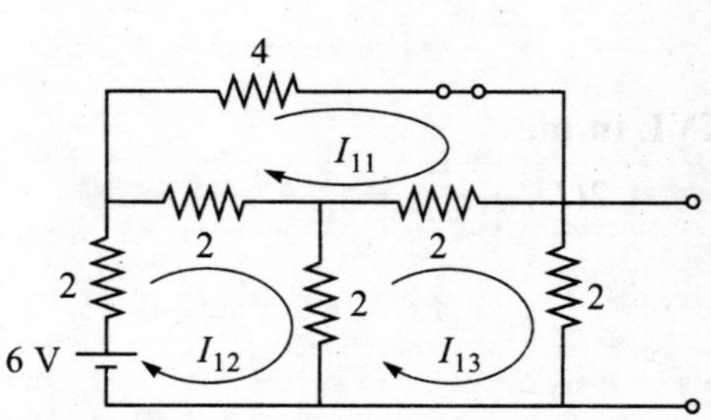

$$4I_{11} + 2(I_{11} + I_{13}) + 2(I_{11} - I_{12}) = 0$$
$$\therefore 8I_{11} - 2I_{12} - 2I_{13} = 0$$

KVL in mesh I_{12}

$$-6 + 2I_{12} + 2(I_{12} - I_{11}) + 2(I_{12} - I_{13}) = 0$$
$$\therefore -2I_{11} + 6I_{12} - 2I_{13} = 6$$

KVL in mesh I_{13}

$$2I_{13} + 2(I_{13} - I_{12}) + 2(I_{13} - I_{11}) = 0$$

$$-2I_{11} - 2I_{12} + 6I_{13} = 0$$

$$\begin{bmatrix} 8 & -2 & -2 \\ -2 & 6 & -2 \\ -2 & -2 & 6 \end{bmatrix} \begin{bmatrix} I_{11} \\ I_{12} \\ I_{13} \end{bmatrix} = \begin{bmatrix} 0 \\ 6 \\ 0 \end{bmatrix}$$

$$\therefore I_{11} = \boxed{0.5 \text{ A}}$$

Considering 10 V source

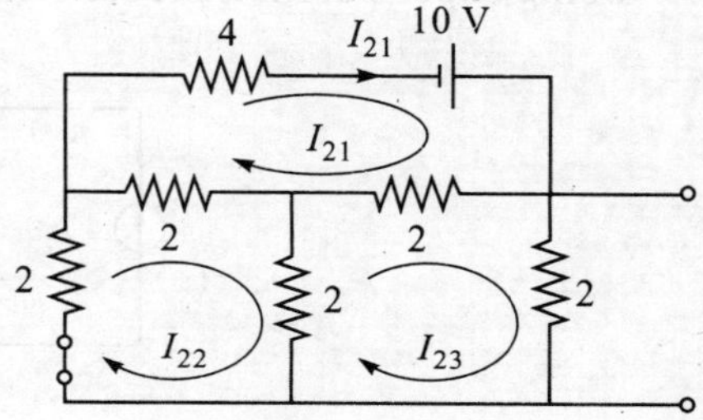

KVL in mesh I_{21}

$$4I_{21} - 10 + 2(I_{21} - I_{23}) + 2(I_{21} - I_{22}) = 0$$

$$\therefore 8\, I_{21} - 2I_{22} - 2I_{23} = 10$$

KVL in mesh I_{22}

$$2(I_{22} - I_{21}) + 2(I_{22} - I_{23}) + 2I_{22} = 0$$

$$\therefore -2I_{21} + 6I_{22} - 2I_{23} = 0$$

KVL in mesh I_{23}

$$2(I_{23} - I_{21}) + 2I_{23} + 2(I_{23} - I_{22}) = 0$$

$$\therefore -2I_{21} - 2I_{22} + 6I_{23} = 0$$

$$\begin{bmatrix} 8 & -2 & -2 \\ -2 & 6 & -2 \\ -2 & -2 & 6 \end{bmatrix} \begin{bmatrix} I_{21} \\ I_{22} \\ I_{23} \end{bmatrix} = \begin{bmatrix} 10 \\ 0 \\ 0 \end{bmatrix}$$

$$\therefore I_{21} = \boxed{1.67 \text{ A}}$$

Considering 5 A source

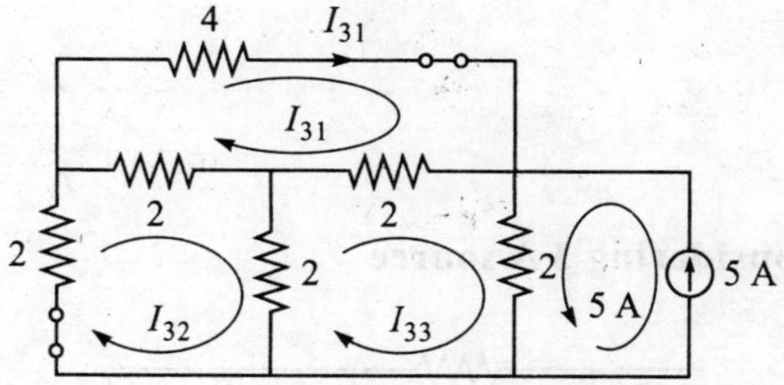

KVL in mesh I_{31}

$$4I_{31} + 2(I_{31} - I_{33}) + 2(I_{31} - I_{32}) = 0$$

$$8I_{31} - 2I_{32} - 2I_{33} = 0$$

KVL in mesh I_{32}

$$2I_{32} + 2(I_{32} - I_{31}) + 2(I_{32} - I_{33}) = 0$$

$$\therefore -2I_{31} + 6I_{32} - 2I_{31} = 0$$

KVL in mesh I_{33}

$$2(I_{33} - I_{31}) + 2(I_{33} + 5) + 2(I_{33} - I_{32}) = 0$$

$$\therefore -2I_{31} - 2I_{32} + 6I_{33} = -10$$

$$\begin{bmatrix} 8 & -2 & -2 \\ -2 & 6 & -2 \\ -2 & -2 & 6 \end{bmatrix} \begin{bmatrix} I_{31} \\ I_{32} \\ I_{33} \end{bmatrix} = \begin{bmatrix} 0 \\ 0 \\ -10 \end{bmatrix}$$

$$\therefore I_{31} = \boxed{-0.83 \text{ A}}$$

$$I = I_{11} + I_{21} + I_{31}$$

$$I = 0.5 + 1.67 - 0.83$$

$$I = \boxed{1.34 \text{ A}}$$

19. Using super position theorem find $I_{6\,\Omega}$.

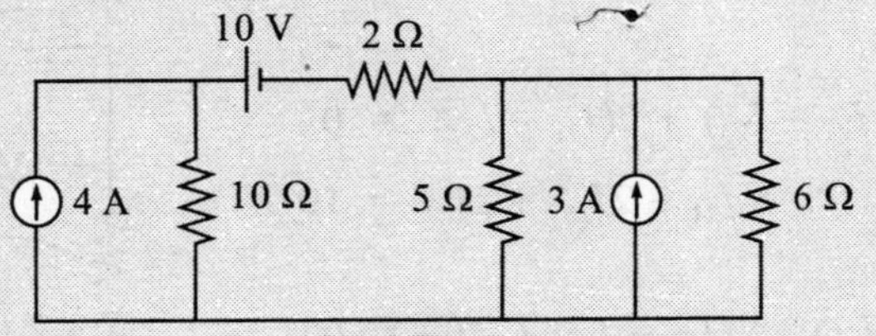

Fig. 1.113

Solution : Considering 4 A source

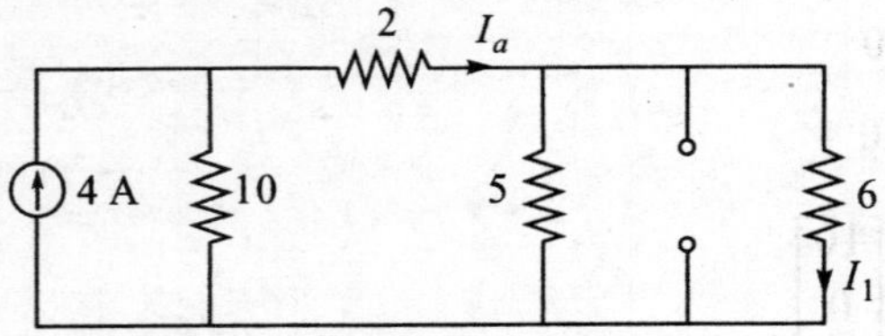

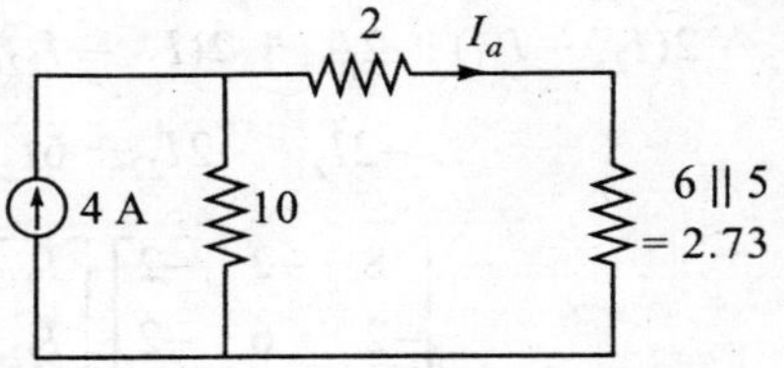

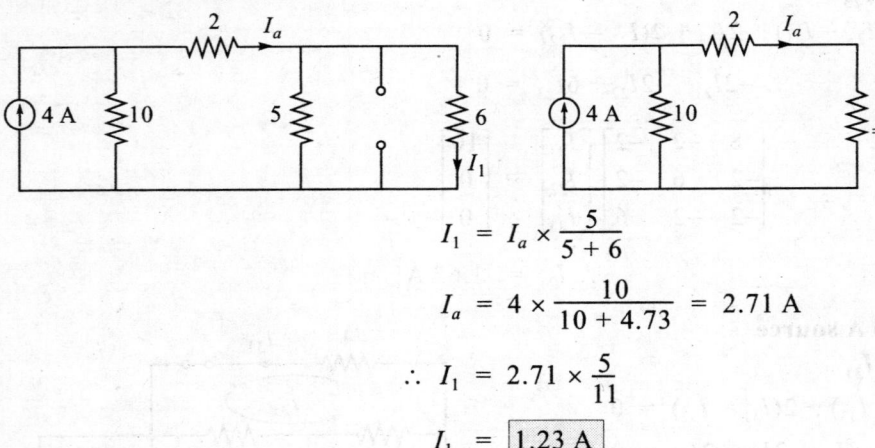

$$I_1 = I_a \times \frac{5}{5+6}$$

$$I_a = 4 \times \frac{10}{10 + 4.73} = 2.71 \text{ A}$$

$$\therefore I_1 = 2.71 \times \frac{5}{11}$$

$$I_1 = \boxed{1.23 \text{ A}}$$

Considering 3 A source

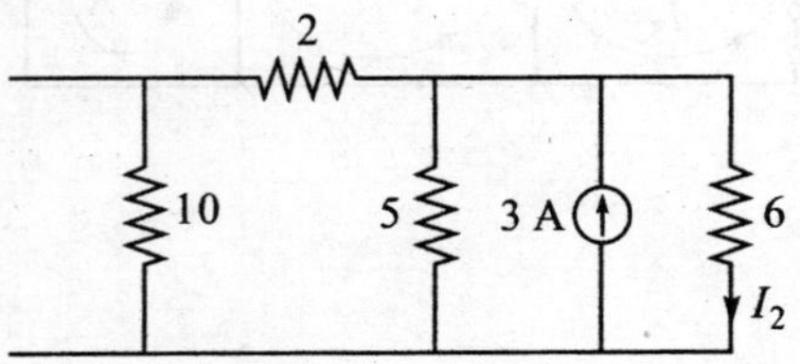

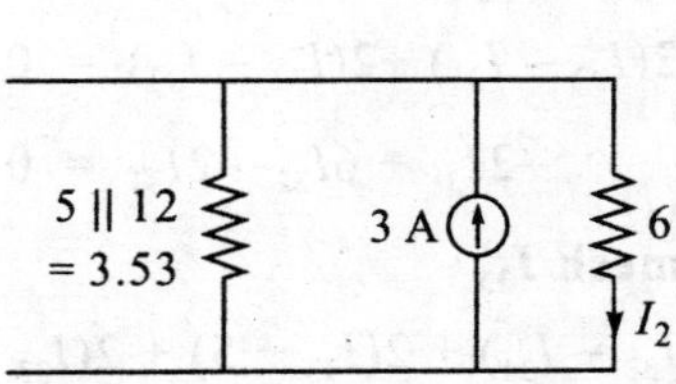

$$I_2 = 3 \times \frac{3.53}{3.53 + 6} = 1.11 \text{ A}$$

$$I_2 = \boxed{1.11 \text{ A}}$$

Considering 10 V source

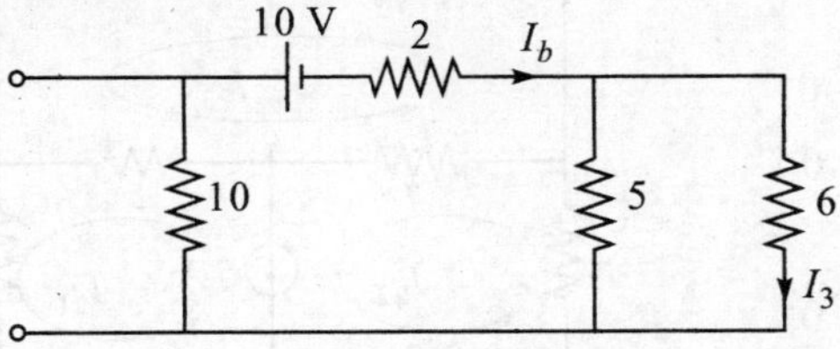

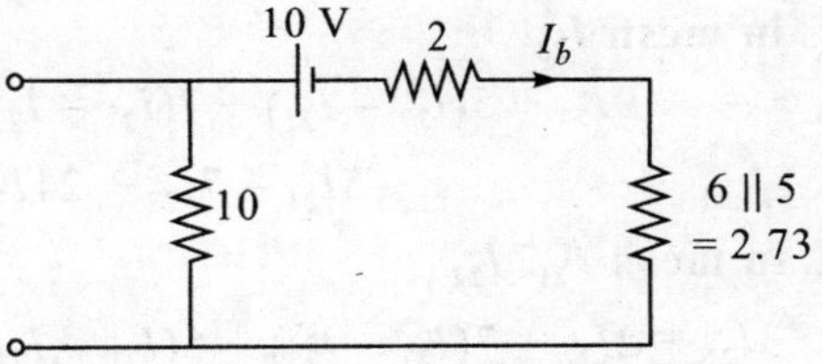

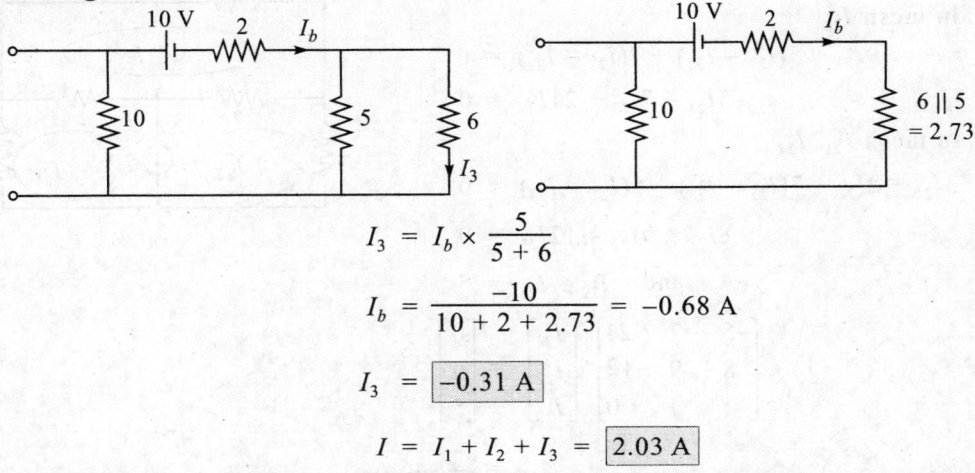

$$I_3 = I_b \times \frac{5}{5+6}$$

$$I_b = \frac{-10}{10+2+2.73} = -0.68 \text{ A}$$

$$I_3 = \boxed{-0.31 \text{ A}}$$

$$I = I_1 + I_2 + I_3 = \boxed{2.03 \text{ A}}$$

20. Using superposition theorem find $I_{3\,\Omega}$.

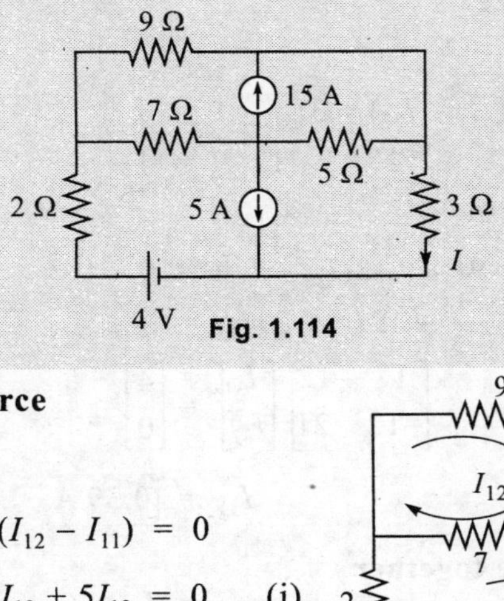

Fig. 1.114

Solution : Considering 15 A source

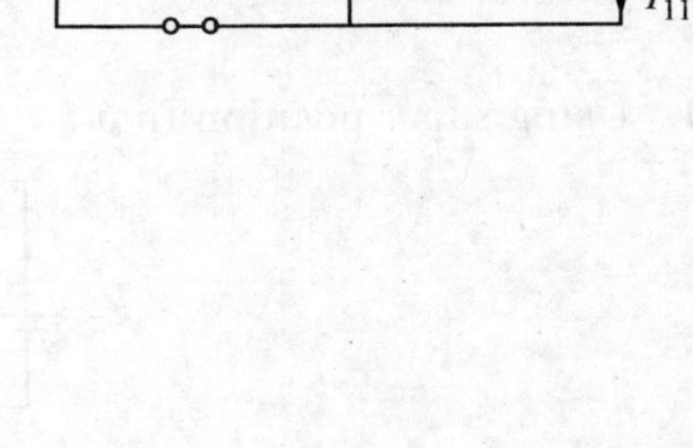

KVL in supermesh I_{12}, I_{13}

$$9I_{12} + 5(I_{13} - I_{11}) + 7(I_{12} - I_{11}) = 0$$

$$\therefore \; -12I_{11} + 16I_{12} + 5I_{13} = 0 \quad \text{...(i)}$$

$$\text{and} \quad I_{13} - I_{12} = 15 \quad \text{...(ii)}$$

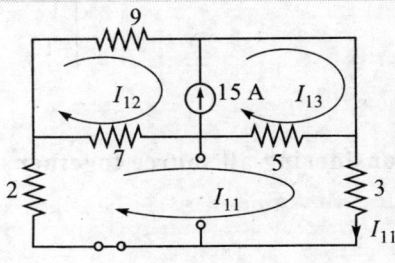

KVL in mesh I_{11}

$$7(I_{11} - I_{12}) + 5(I_{11} - I_{13}) + 3I_{11} + 2I_{11} = 0$$

$$\therefore \; 17I_{11} - 7I_{12} - 5I_{13} = 0$$

$$\begin{bmatrix} -12 & 16 & 5 \\ 0 & -1 & 1 \\ 17 & -7 & -5 \end{bmatrix} \begin{bmatrix} I_{11} \\ I_{12} \\ I_{13} \end{bmatrix} = \begin{bmatrix} 0 \\ 15 \\ 0 \end{bmatrix}$$

$$I_{11} = \boxed{3.17 \text{ A}}$$

Considering 5 A source

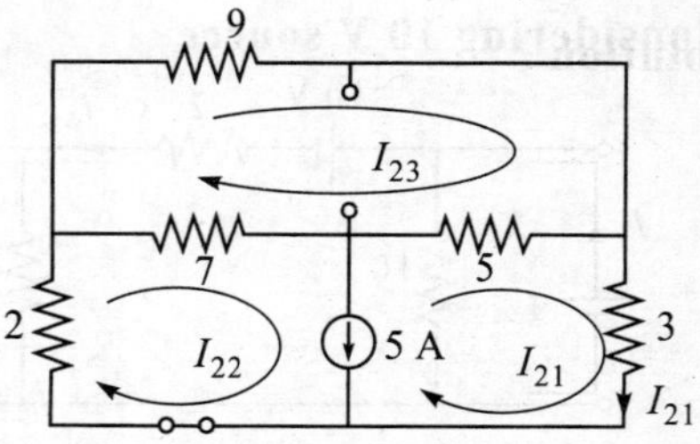

KVL in mesh I_{23}

$$9I_{23} + 5(I_{23} - I_{21}) + 7(I_{23} - I_{22}) = 0$$

$$-5I_{21} - 7I_{22} + 21I_{23} = 0$$

KVL in mesh I_{21}, I_{22}

$$3I_{21} + 2I_{22} + 7(I_{22} - I_{23}) + 5(I_{21} - I_{23}) = 0$$

$$8I_{21} + 9I_{22} - 12I_{23} = 0$$

$$\text{and} \quad I_{22} - I_{21} = 5$$

$$\begin{bmatrix} -5 & -7 & 21 \\ 8 & 9 & -12 \\ -1 & 1 & 0 \end{bmatrix} \begin{bmatrix} I_{21} \\ I_{22} \\ I_{23} \end{bmatrix} = \begin{bmatrix} 0 \\ 0 \\ 5 \end{bmatrix}$$

$$I_{21} = \boxed{-2.46 \text{ A}}$$

Considering 4 V source

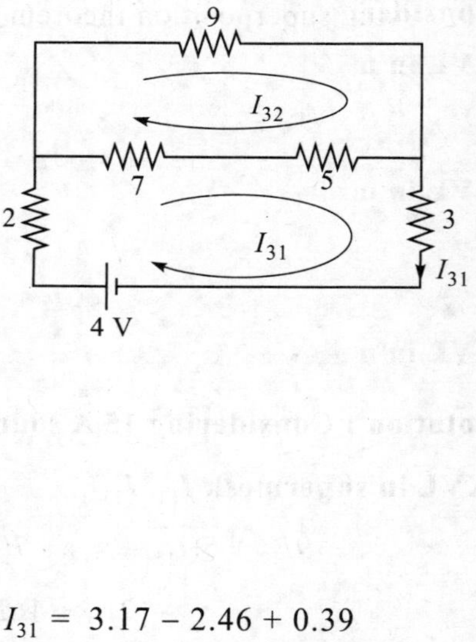

KVL in mesh I_{31}

$$2I_{31} + 12(I_{31} - I_{32}) + 3I_{31} - 4 = 0$$

$$17I_{31} - 12I_{32} = 4$$

KVL in mesh I_{32}

$$9I_{32} + 12(I_{32} - I_{31}) = 0$$

$$-12I_{31} + 21I_{32} = 0$$

$$\begin{bmatrix} 17 & -12 \\ -12 & 21 \end{bmatrix} \begin{bmatrix} I_{31} \\ I_{32} \end{bmatrix} = \begin{bmatrix} 4 \\ 0 \end{bmatrix}$$

$$I_{31} = \boxed{0.39 \text{ A}}$$

Considering all source together

$$I = I_{11} + I_{21} + I_{31} = 3.17 - 2.46 + 0.39$$

$$I = \boxed{1.1 \text{ A}}$$

21. Using super position find I.

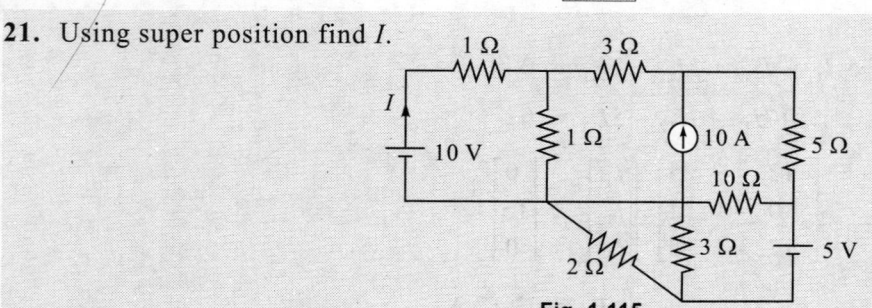

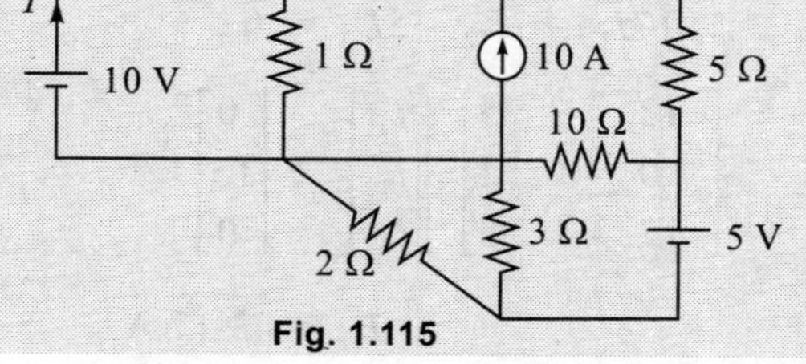

Fig. 1.115

Solution : Considering 10 V source

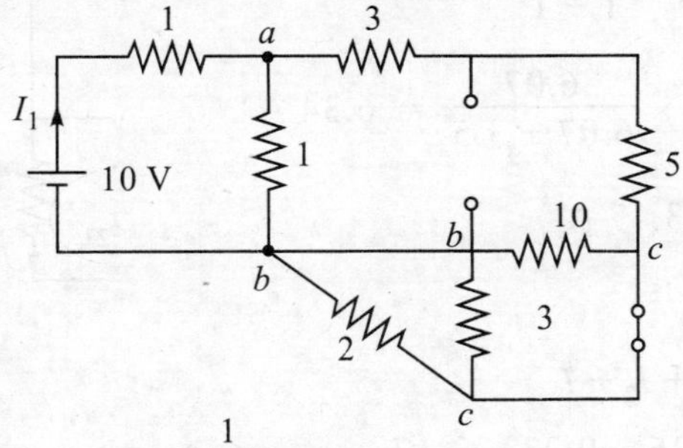

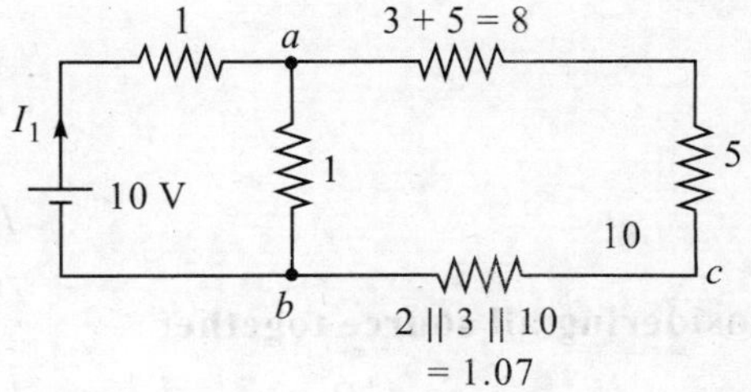

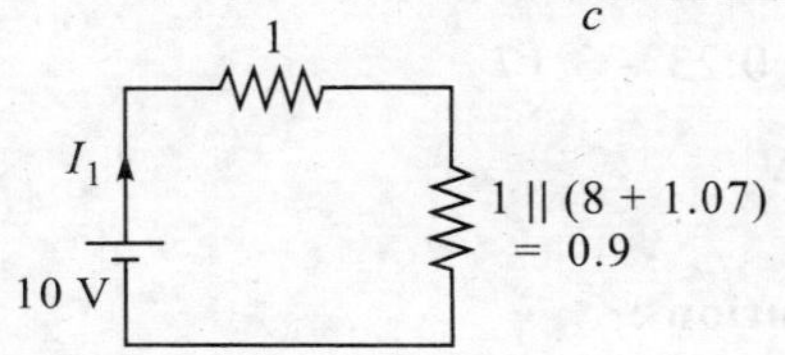

$$I_1 = \frac{10}{1.9}$$

$$I_1 = \boxed{5.26 \text{ A}}$$

Considering 5 V source

KVL in mesh I_a

$$1.2I_a + 10(I_a - I_b) + 5 = 0$$

$$11.2I_a - 10I_b = -5$$

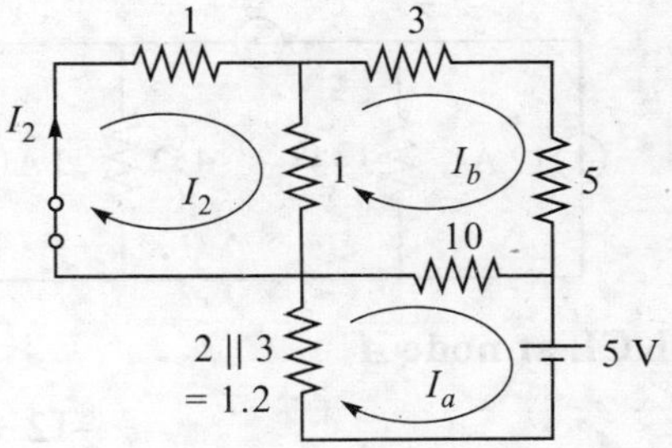

KVL in mesh I_b

$$8I_b + 10(I_b - I_a) + 1(I_b - I_2) = 0$$

$$-10I_a + 19I_b - I_2 = 0$$

KVL in mesh I_2

$$1.I_2 + 1(I_2 - I_b) = 0$$

$$-I_b + 2I_2 = 0$$

$$\begin{bmatrix} 11.2 & -10 & 0 \\ -10 & 19 & -1 \\ 0 & -1 & 2 \end{bmatrix} \begin{bmatrix} I_a \\ I_b \\ I_2 \end{bmatrix} = \begin{bmatrix} -5 \\ 0 \\ 0 \end{bmatrix}$$

$$I_2 = \boxed{-0.23 \text{ A}}$$

Considering 10 A source

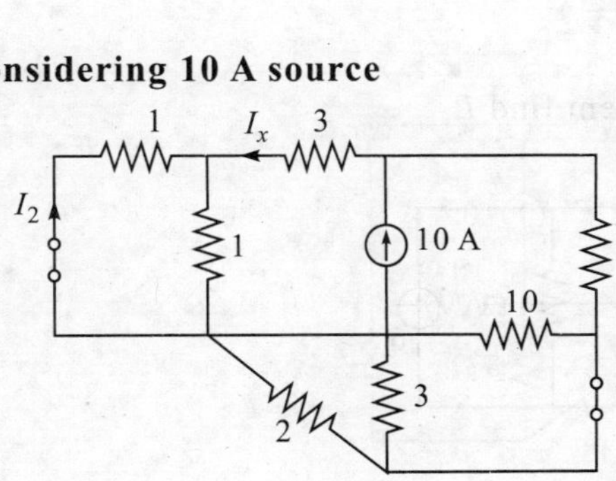

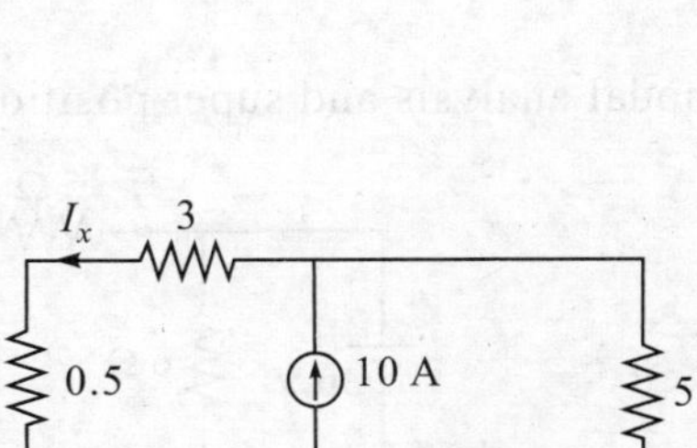

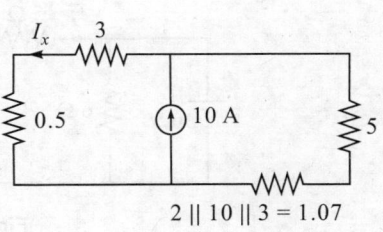

$$I_3 = -I_x \times \frac{1}{1+1} = -\frac{I_x}{2}$$

$$I_x = 10 \times \frac{6.07}{6.07+3.5} = 6.34\text{ A}$$

$$\therefore\ I_3 = \boxed{-3.17\text{ A}}$$

Considering all source together

$$I = I_1 + I_2 + I_3$$

$$I = 5.26 - 0.23 - 3.17$$

$$I = \boxed{1.86\text{ A}}$$

22. Using nodal analysis find *I*.

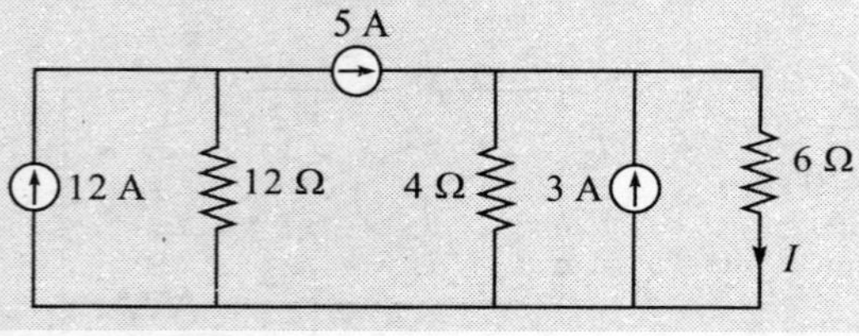

Solution :

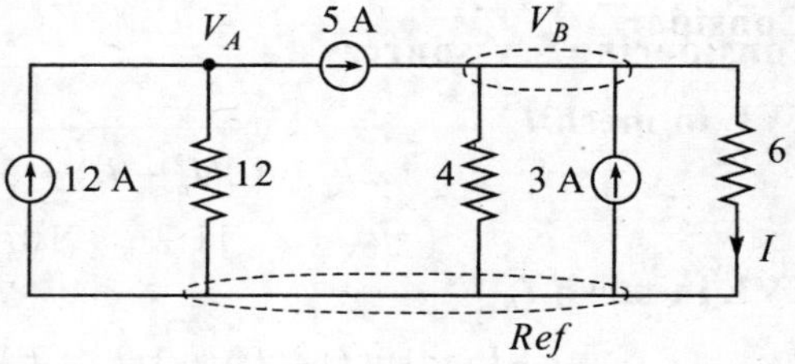

KCL at node *A*

$$-12 + \frac{V_A}{12} + 5 = 0$$

$$\therefore\ V_A = 84\text{ V}$$

KCL at *B*

$$-5 + \frac{V_B}{4} - 3 + \frac{V_B}{6} = 0$$

$$\therefore\ V_B = 19.2$$

$$\therefore\ I = \frac{V_B}{6} = \frac{19.2}{6}$$

$$I = \boxed{3.2\text{ A}}$$

23. Using nodal analysis and super position theorem find *I*.

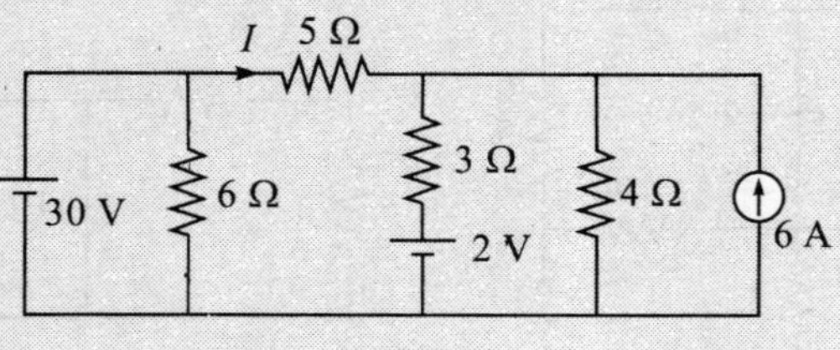

Fig. 1.117

Solution : Nodal Analysis : KCL at V_A

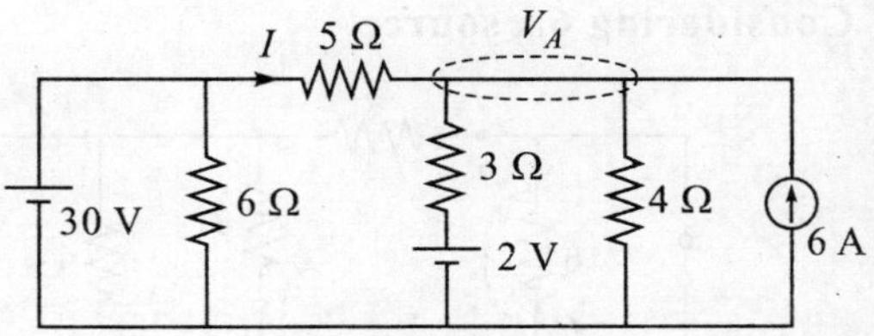

$$\frac{V_A - 30}{5} + \frac{V_A - 2}{3} + \frac{V_A}{4} - 6 = 0$$

$$\therefore \; V_A = 16.17 \text{ V}$$

$$\therefore \; I = \frac{30 - V_A}{5}$$

$$I = \boxed{2.76 \text{ A}}$$

Superposition Theorem

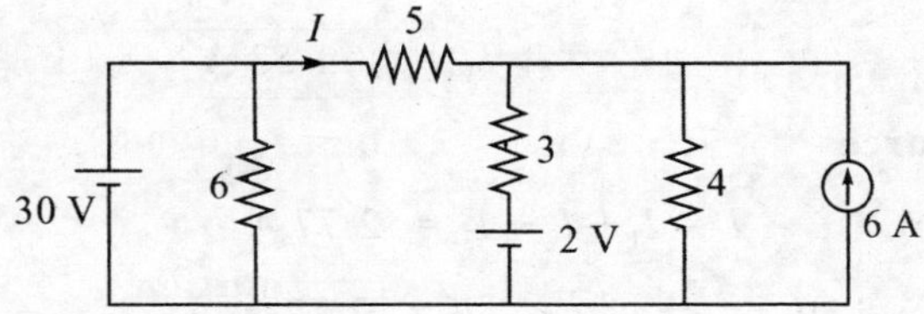

Considering 30 V source

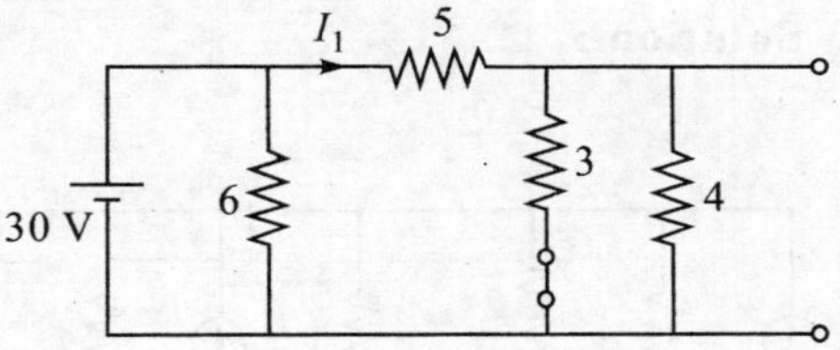

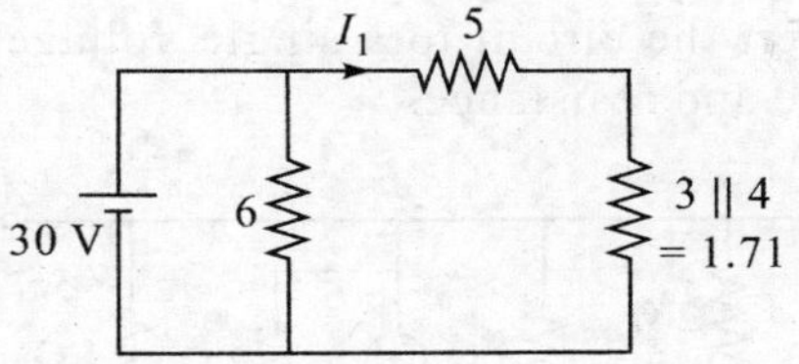

$$I_1 = \frac{30}{6.71}$$

$$I_1 = \boxed{4.47 \text{ A}}$$

Considering 2 V source

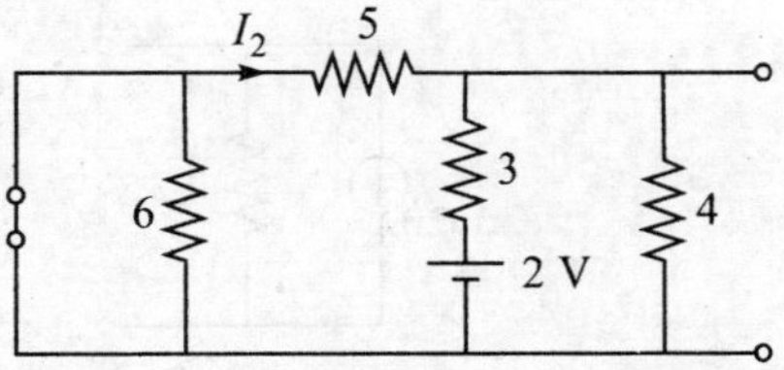

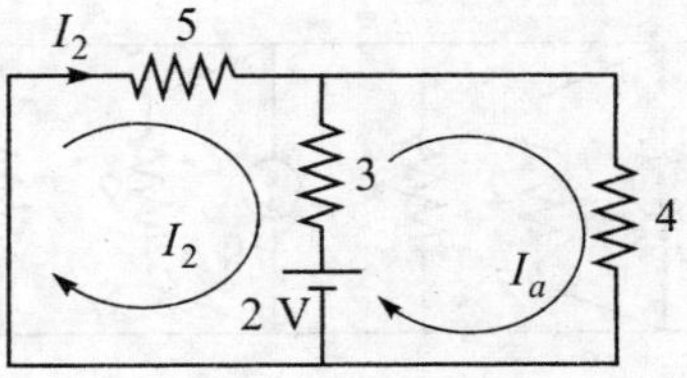

KVL in mesh I_2

$$5I_2 + 3(I_2 - I_a) + 2 = 0$$

$$8I_2 - 3I_a = 0$$

KVL in mesh I_a

$$-2 + 3(I_a - I_2) + 4I_a = 0$$

$$-3I_2 + 7I_a = 2$$

$$\therefore \; I_2 = \boxed{-0.17 \text{ A}}$$

Considering 6A source

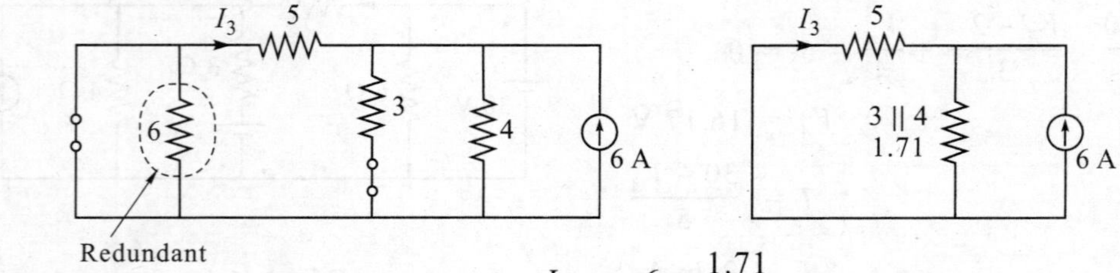

$$I_3 = -6 \times \frac{1.71}{6.71}$$

$$I_3 = \boxed{-1.53\text{ A}}$$

Considering all source

$$I = I_1 + I_2 + I_3 = 2.77\text{ A}$$

$$I = \boxed{2.77\text{ A}}$$

24. Convert the circuit to a single voltage source and resistance.

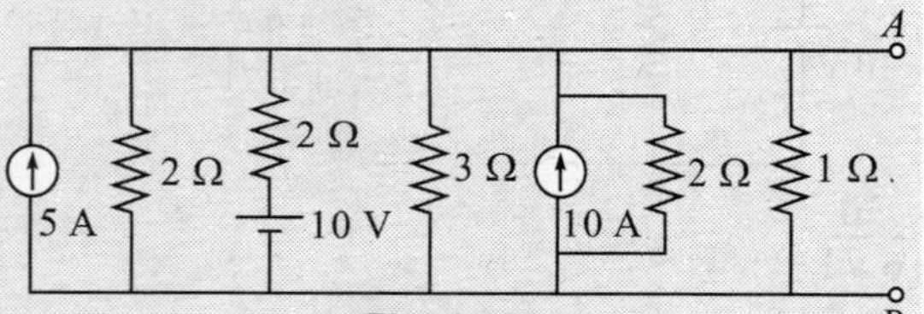

Fig. 1.118

Solution :

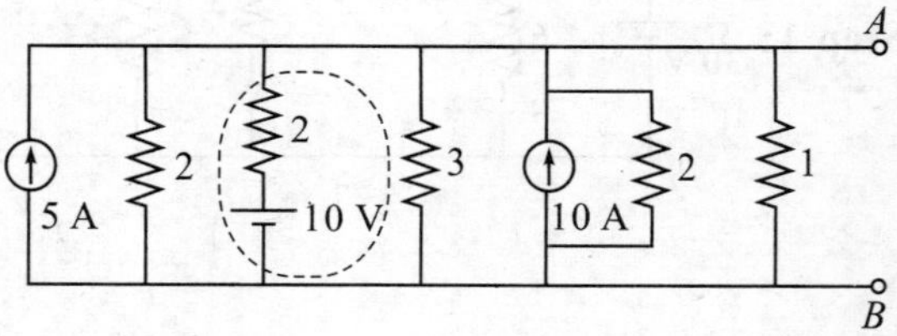

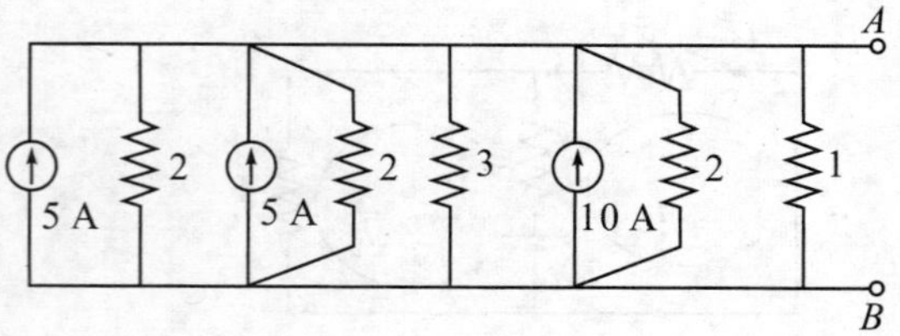

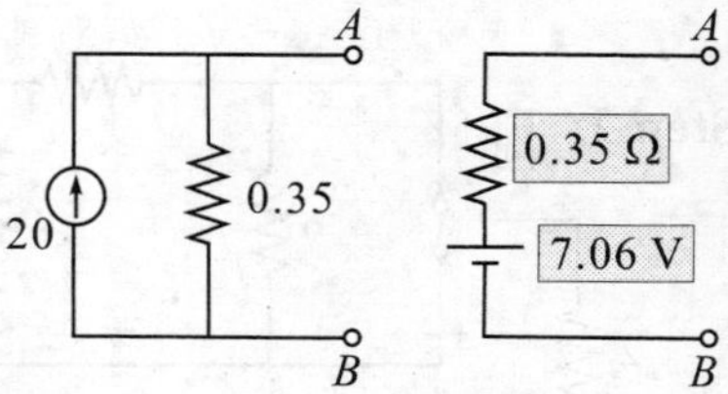

25. Using source transformation and Thevenin's theorem find *I*.

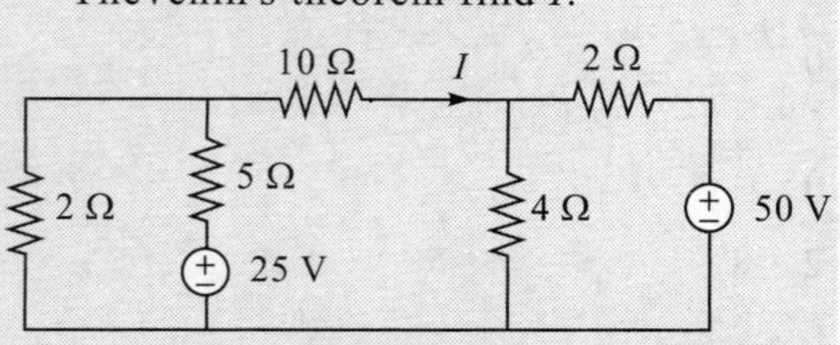

Fig. 1.119

Solution : Source Transformation

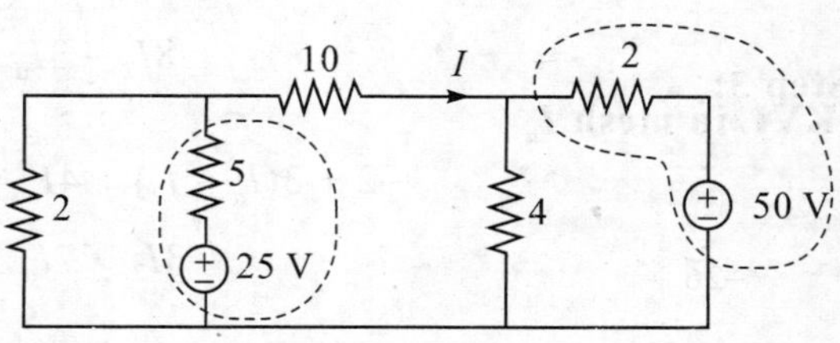

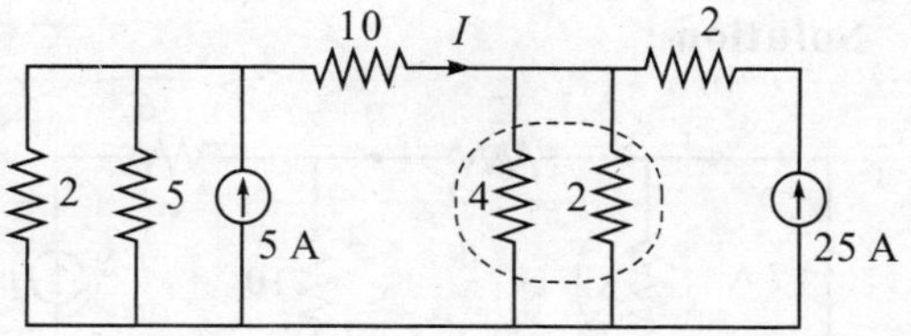

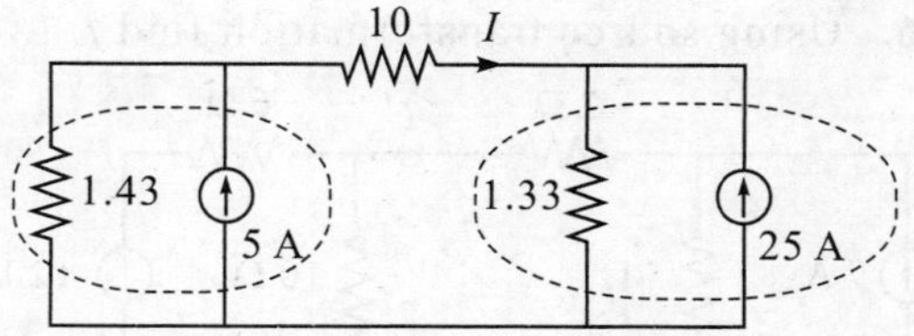

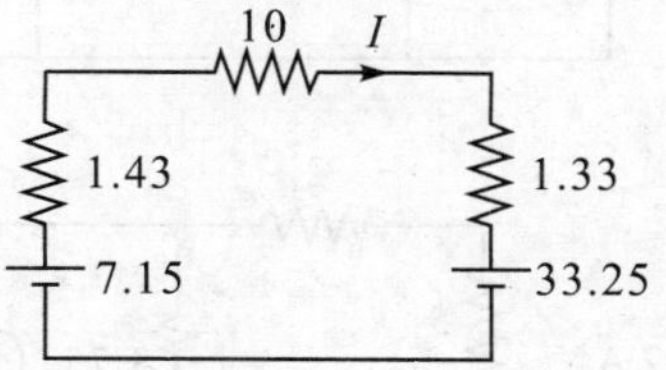

$$\therefore\ I = \frac{7.15 - 633.25}{1.43 + 10 + 1.33}$$

$$I = \boxed{-2.04\text{ A}}$$

Thevenin's Theorem

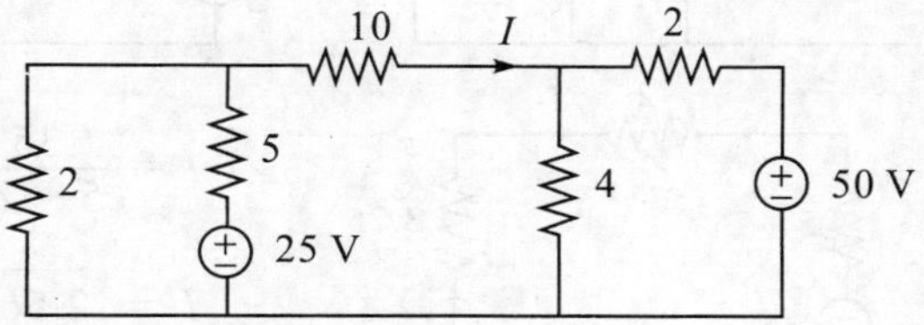

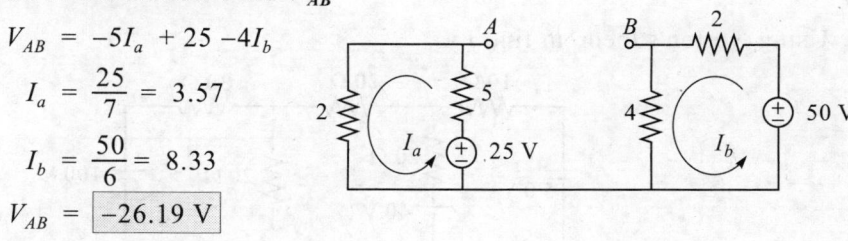

Step 1: Remove 10 Ω resistance. Find V_{AB}

$$V_{AB} = -5I_a + 25 - 4I_b$$

$$I_a = \frac{25}{7} = 3.57$$

$$I_b = \frac{50}{6} = 8.33$$

$$\therefore\ V_{AB} = \boxed{-26.19\text{ V}}$$

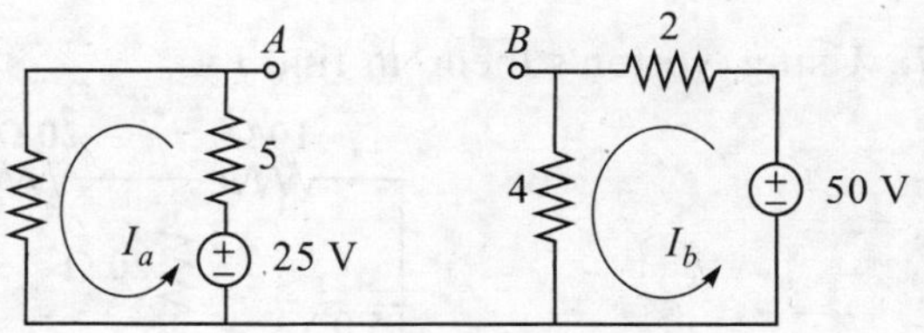

Step 2: Find R_{AB}

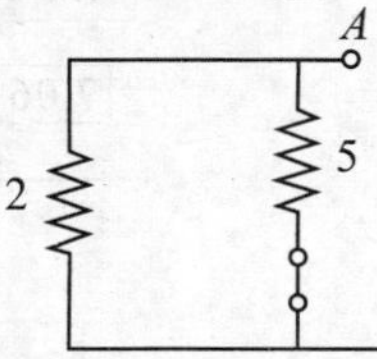

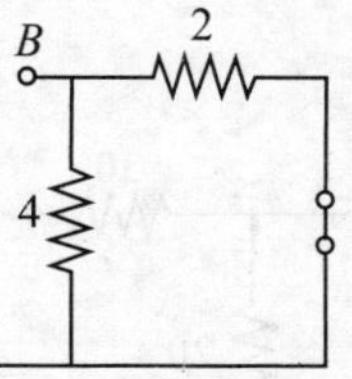

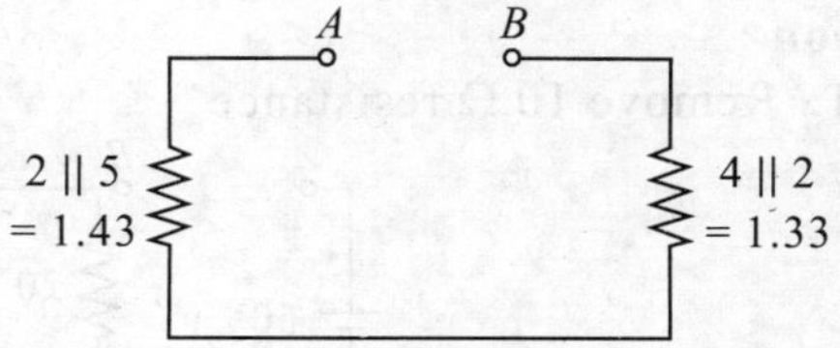

$$\therefore\ R_{AB} = \boxed{2.76\ \Omega}$$

Step 3:

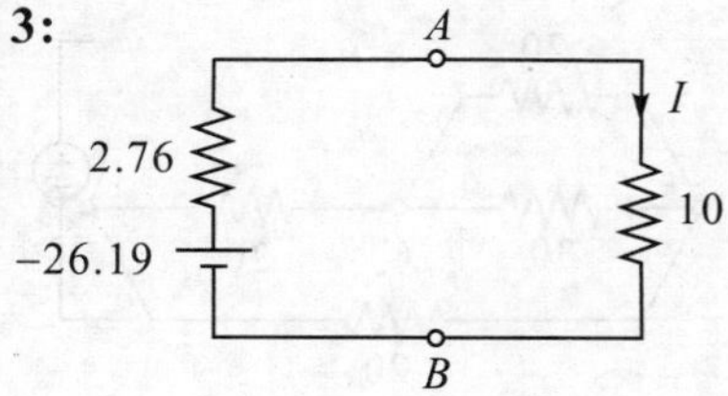

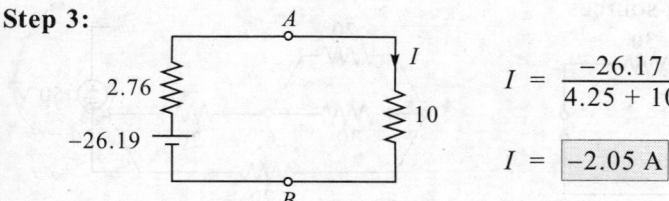

$$I = \frac{-26.17}{4.25 + 10}$$

$$I = \boxed{-2.05\text{ A}}$$

26. Using source transformation find I.

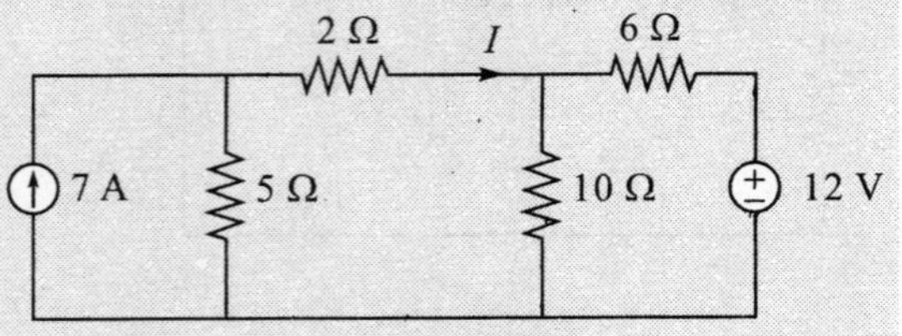

Fig. 1.120

Solution :

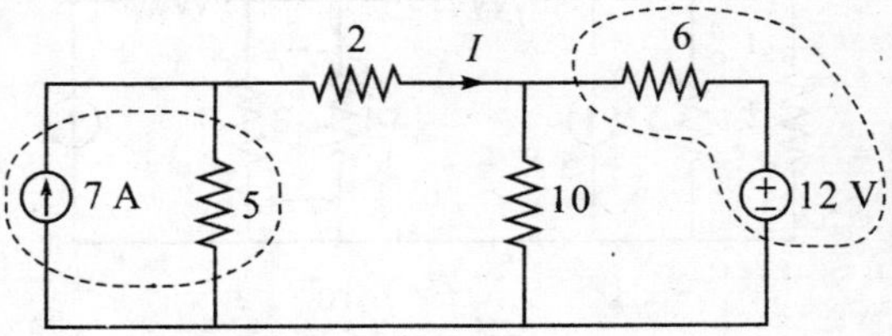

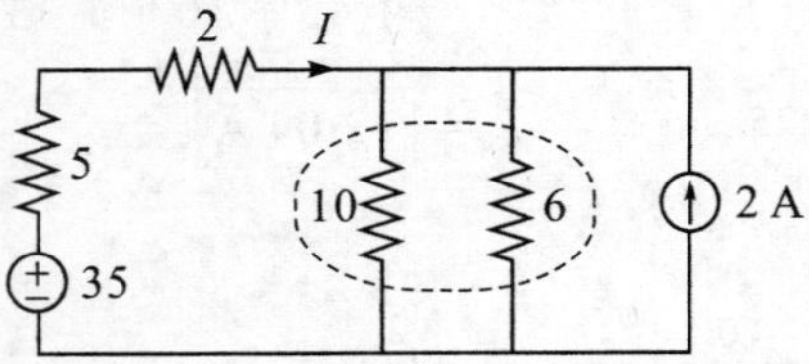

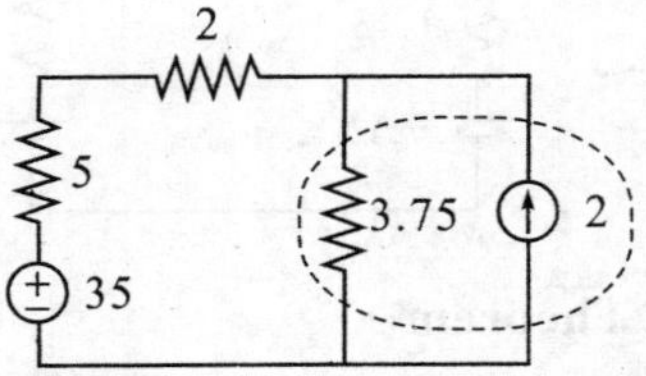

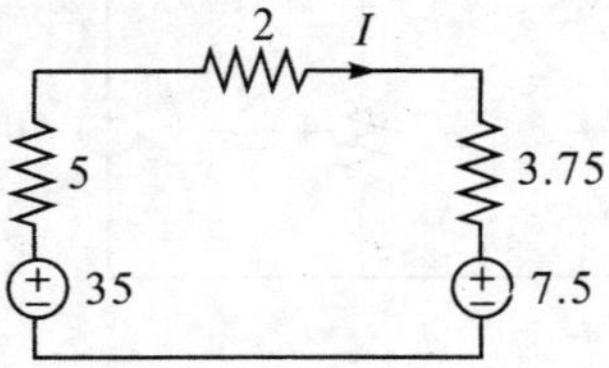

$$I = \frac{35 - 7.5}{5 + 2 + 3.75}$$

$$I = \boxed{2.56 \text{ A}}$$

27. Using Norton's theorem find I.

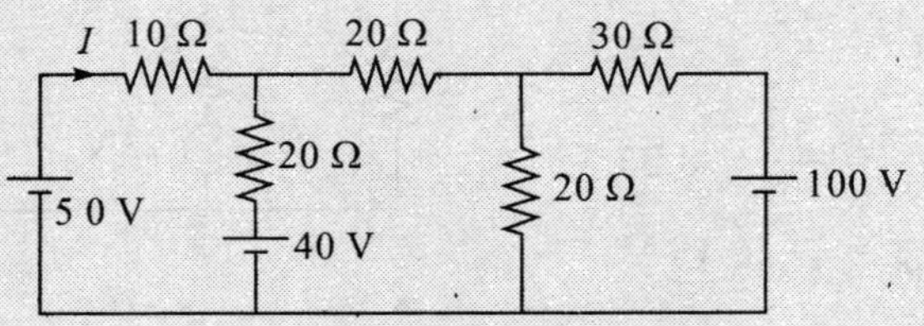

Fig. 1.121

Solution :

Step 1: Remove 10 Ω resistance

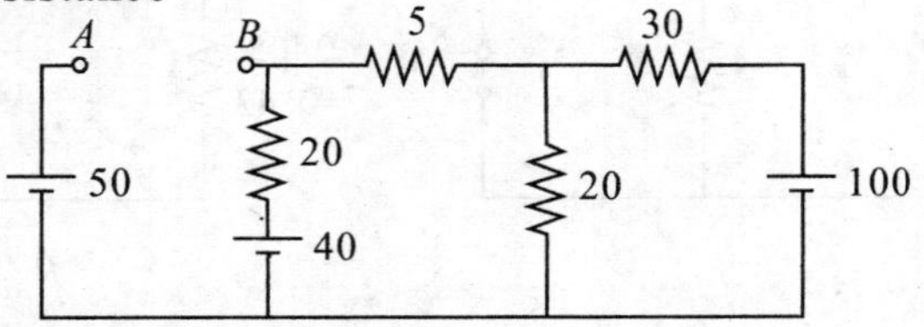

Step 2: Find R_{AB}, after suppressing sources

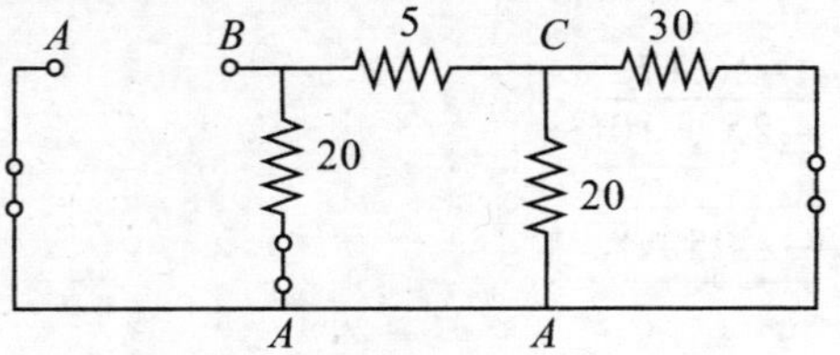

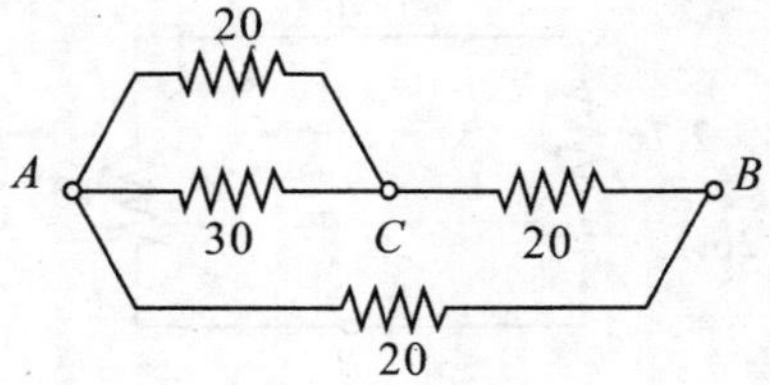

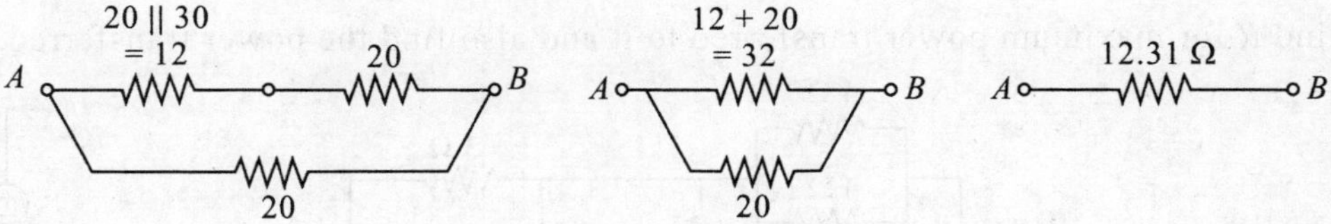

$$R_{AB} = \boxed{12.31\ \Omega}$$

Step 3: Find I_{SC}, i.e. short terminals AB and find I_{AB}

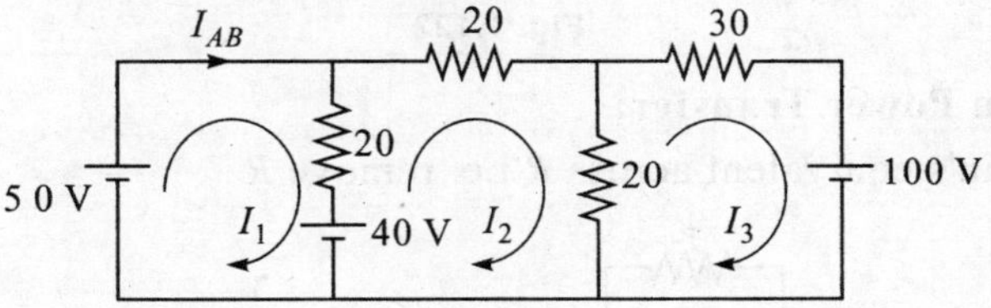

$$I_{AB} = I_1$$

KVL in mesh I_1

$$-50 + 20(I_1 - I_2) + 40 = 0$$

$$\therefore\ 20I_1 - 20I_2 = 10$$

KVL in mesh I_2

$$20I_2 + 20(I_2 - I_3) - 40 + 20(I_2 - I_1) = 0$$

$$\therefore\ -20I_1 + 60I_2 - 20I_3 = 40$$

KVL in mesh I_3

$$30I_3 + 100 + 20(I_3 - I_2) = 0$$

$$\therefore\ -20I_1 + 50I_3 = -100$$

$$\begin{bmatrix} 20 & -20 & 0 \\ -20 & 60 & -20 \\ 0 & -20 & 50 \end{bmatrix} \begin{bmatrix} I_1 \\ I_2 \\ I_3 \end{bmatrix} = \begin{bmatrix} 10 \\ 40 \\ -100 \end{bmatrix}$$

$$\therefore\ I_1 = I_{AB} = \boxed{0.81\ \text{A}}$$

Step 4: Find I from Norton's equivalent circuit

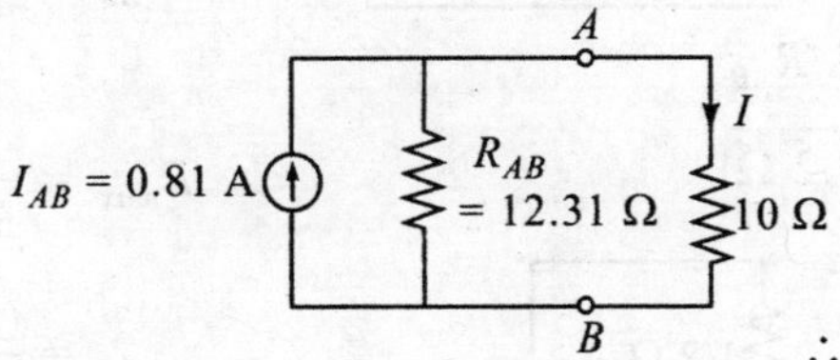

$$\therefore\ I_1 = 0.81 \times \frac{12.31}{12.31 + 10}$$

$$I = \boxed{0.45\ \text{A}}$$

28. Find R for maximum power transferred to it and also find the power transferred.

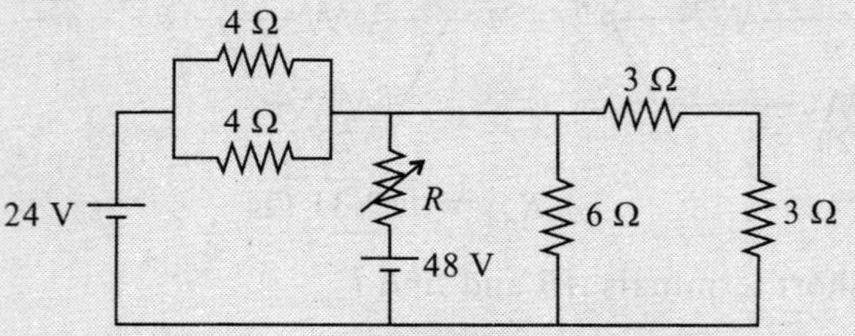

Fig. 1.122

Solution : Maximum Power Transfer:

Step 1: Find Thevenin's equivalent across R i.e. remove R

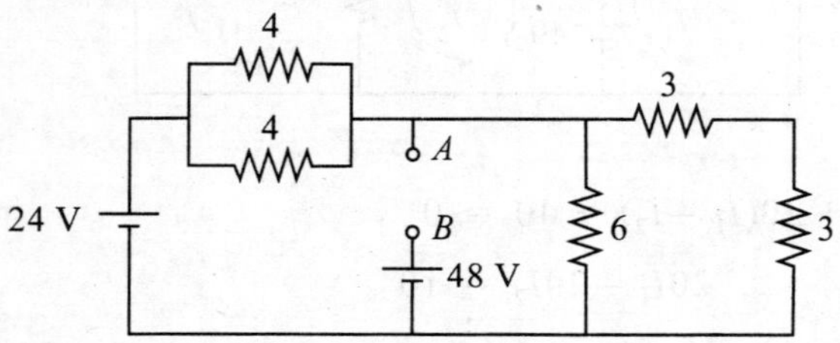

Step 2: Find R_{AB}, by suppressing sources

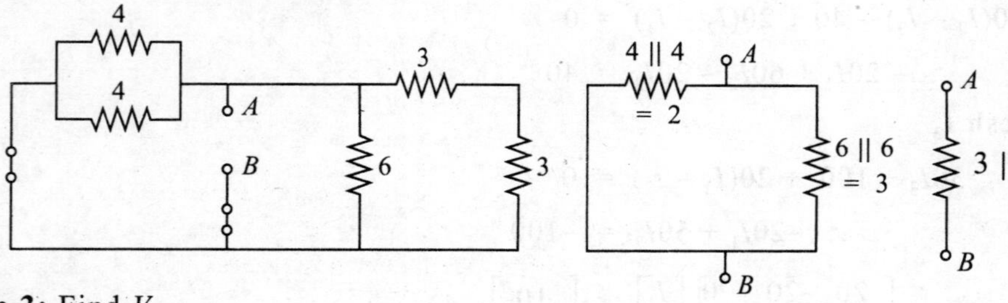

Step 3: Find V_{AB}

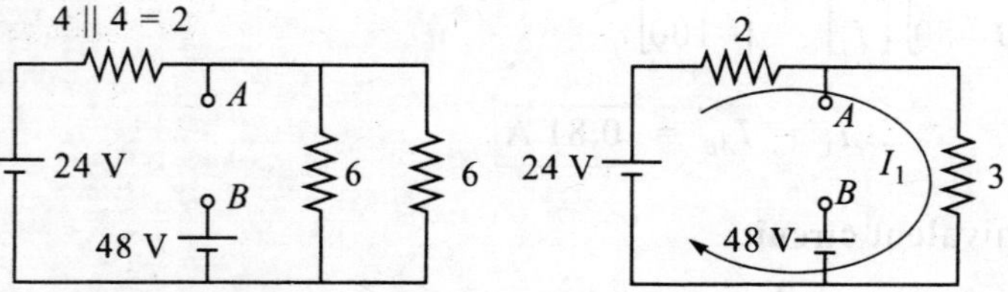

$$V_{AB} = 3I_1 - 48$$

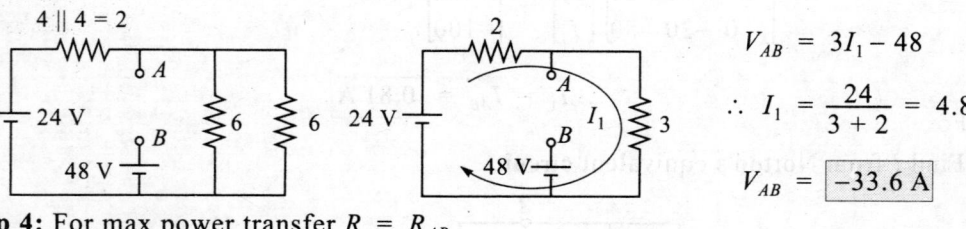

$$\therefore \; I_1 = \frac{24}{3+2} = 4.8$$

$$V_{AB} = \boxed{-33.6 \text{ A}}$$

Step 4: For max power transfer $R = R_{AB}$

$$\therefore \; R = \boxed{1.2 \, \Omega}$$

From Thevenin's equivalent circuit

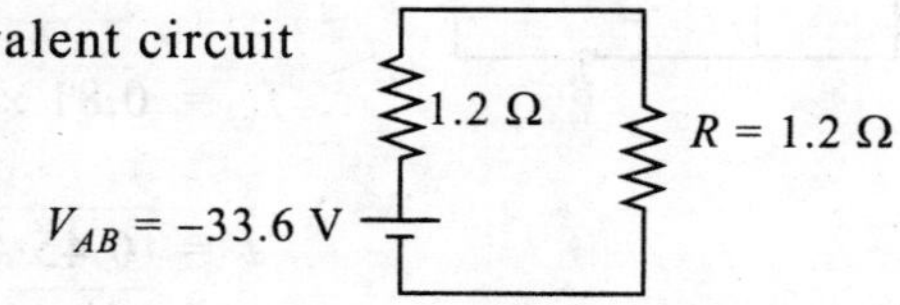

$$\therefore \; P_{max} = \frac{V_{AB}^2}{4R_{th}}$$

$$= \frac{(33.6)^2}{4 \times 1.2}$$

$$\therefore \; P_{max} = \boxed{235.2 \text{ W}}$$

29. Find R for maximum power transferred to it and also find the power transferred.

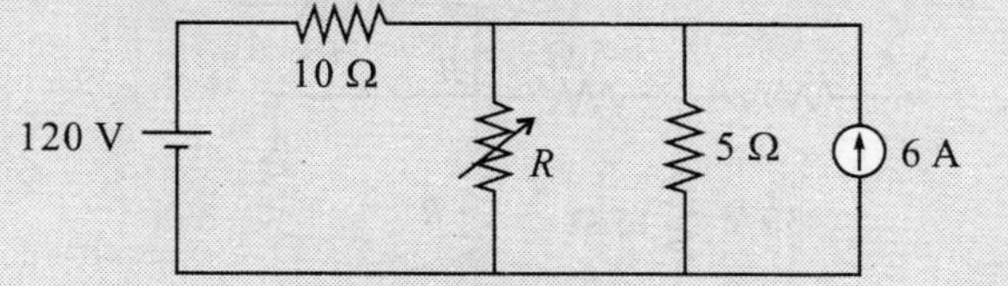

Fig. 1.123

Solution : Maximum Power Transfer:

Step 1: Remove R and find Thevenin's equivalent circuit

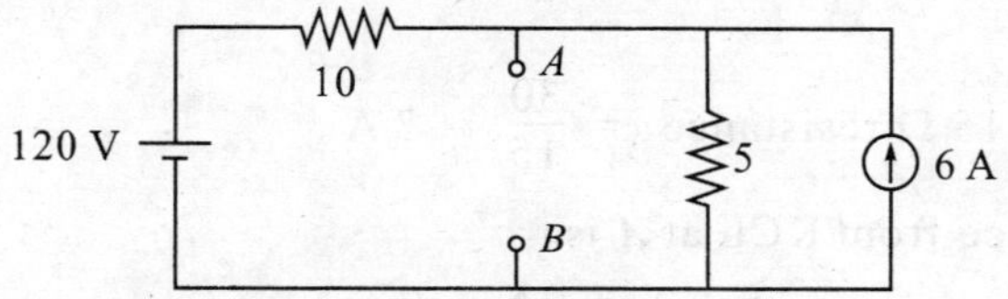

Step 2: Find R_{AB}, after suppressing sources

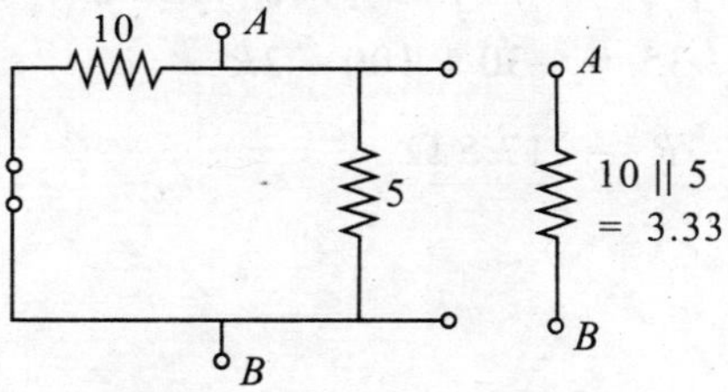

$$R_{AB} = 3.33\ \Omega$$

Step 3: Find V_{AB}, Thevenin's equivalent voltage

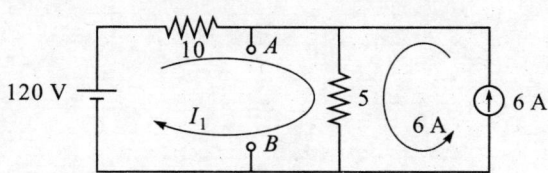

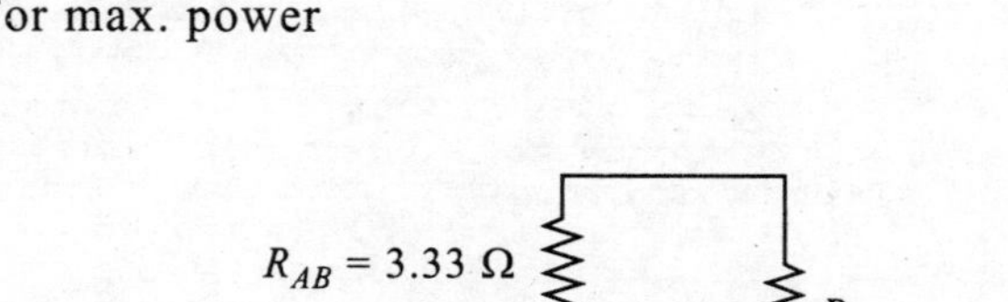

$$V_{AB} = 5(I_1 + 6)$$

$$-120 + 10I_1 + 5(I_1 + 6) = 0$$

$$I_1 = 6\text{A}$$

$$\therefore\ V_{AB} = 60$$

Step 4: For max. power

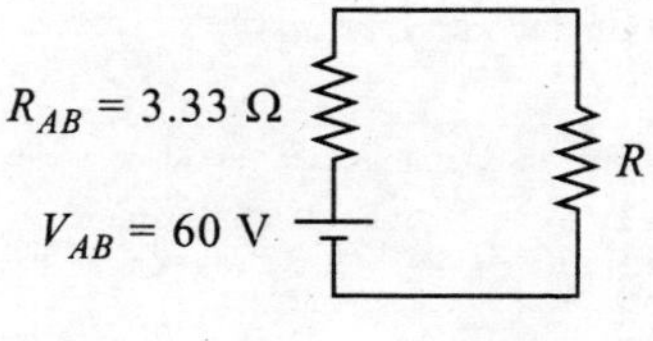

$$R = R_{AB} = \boxed{3.33\ \Omega}$$

$$\therefore\ P_{max} = \frac{V_{AB}^2}{4R_{th}}$$

$$= \frac{(60)^2}{4 \times 3.33}$$

$$\therefore\ P_{max} = \boxed{270.27\ \text{W}}$$

30. Find R.

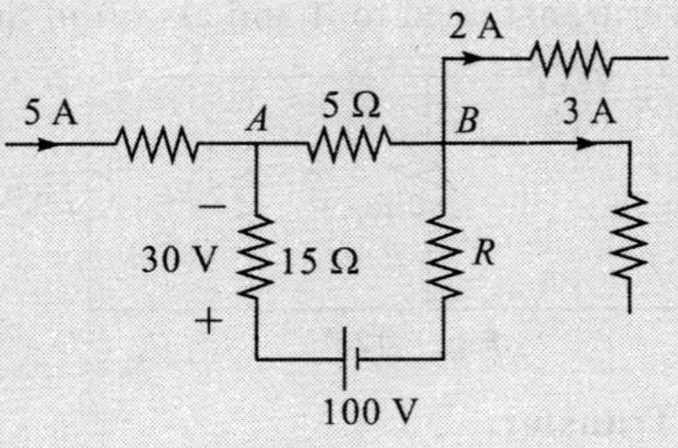

Fig. 1.124

Solution :

$$\text{Current in } 15\ \Omega \text{ resistance } = \frac{30}{15} = 2\text{ A}$$

$\therefore$ Current in 5 Ω resistance from KCL at A is

$$5 + 2 = 7\text{A}$$

$$\therefore\ V_{AB} = 7 \times 5 = -15 \times 2 + 100 - R \times 2$$

$$35 = -30 + 100 - 2R$$

$$R = \boxed{17.5\ \Omega}$$

Chapter 3 : A.C. FUNDAMENTALS

Solution to Unsolved Examples

1. Find rms and average values of the following :

Solutions :

(i)

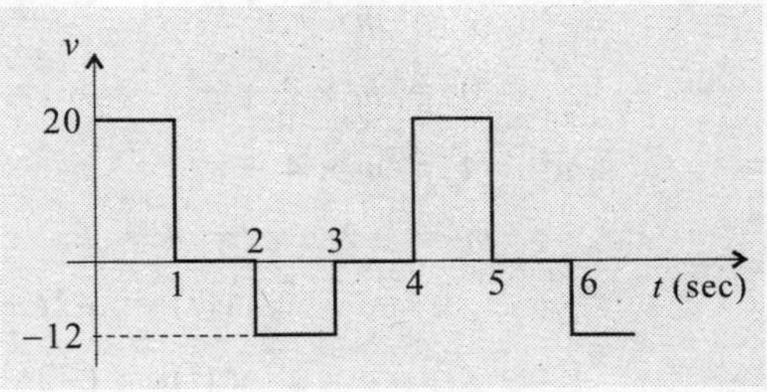

Let us first define the function $v(t)$

$$v(t) = 20 \quad 0 < t < 1$$
$$= 0 \quad 1 < t < 2$$
$$= -12 \quad 2 < t < 3$$
$$= 0 \quad 3 < t < 4$$

$$v^2(t) = 400 \quad 0 < t < 1$$
$$= 0 \quad 1 < t < 2$$
$$= 144 \quad 2 < t < 3$$
$$= 0 \quad 3 < t < 4$$

Interval $T = 4$ sec

$$\therefore \quad V_{av} = \frac{1}{T}\int_0^T v(t)\, dt$$

$$= \frac{1}{4}\left[\int_0^1 20\, dt - \int_2^3 12\, dt\right] = \frac{1}{4}[20(1-0) - 12(3-2)]$$

$$= \frac{1}{4}[20 - 12]$$

$$V_{av} = \boxed{2 \text{ volts}}$$

$$V_{rms} = \sqrt{\frac{1}{T}\int_0^T v^2(t)\, dt}$$

$$= \sqrt{\frac{1}{4}\left[\int_0^1 400\, dt + \int_2^3 144\, dt\right]}$$

$$= \sqrt{\frac{1}{4}[400 + 144]}$$

$$= \sqrt{136}$$

$$V_{rms} = \boxed{11.66 \text{ volts}}$$

(ii)

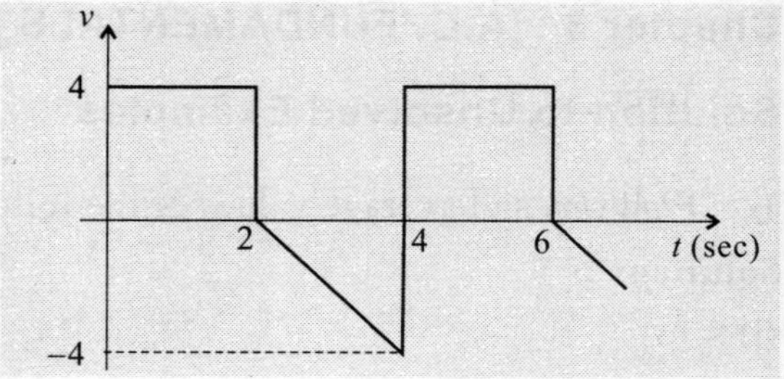

$$v(t) = 4 \qquad 0 < t < 2$$

$$\therefore\ v^2(t) = 16$$

Between 2 sec and 4 sec general equation of line

$$y = mx + c$$

$$\therefore\ 0 = m \times 2 + c$$

$$\text{and}\quad -4 = m \times 4 + c$$

$$\therefore\ m = -2, \quad c = 4$$

$$\therefore\ v(t) = -2t + 4 \qquad 2 < t < 4$$

$$v^2(t) = (-2t + 4)^2 \qquad 2 < t < 4$$

$$= 4t^2 - 16t + 16$$

Here, interval $T = 4$

$$\therefore\ V_{av} = \frac{1}{T}\int_0^T v(t)\, dt$$

$$= \frac{1}{4}\left[\int_0^2 4\, dt + \int_2^4 (-2t + 4)dt\right]$$

$$= \frac{1}{4}\left[4t\Big|_0^2 + \left(\frac{-2t^2}{2} + 4t\right)_2^4\right]$$

$$= \frac{1}{4}\left[4(2 - 0) - (4^2 - 2^2) + 4\,(4 - 2)\right]$$

$$= \frac{1}{4}\left[8 - 12 + 8\right]$$

$$\therefore\ V_{av} = \boxed{1 \text{ volts}}$$

$$V_{rms} = \sqrt{\left[\frac{1}{4}\int_0^2 16\, dt + \int_2^4 (4t^2 - 16t + 16)dt\right]}$$

$$= \sqrt{\left[\frac{1}{4}\, 16t\Big|_0^2 + \frac{4t^3}{3}\Big|_2^4 - \frac{16t^2}{2}\Big|_2^4 + 16t\Big|_2^4\right]}$$

$$= \sqrt{\frac{1}{4}\left[16 \times 2 + \frac{4}{3}(4^3 - 2^3) - 8(4^2 - 2^2) + 16(4 - 2)\right]}$$

$$V_{rms} = \boxed{3.26 \text{ volts}}$$

(iii)

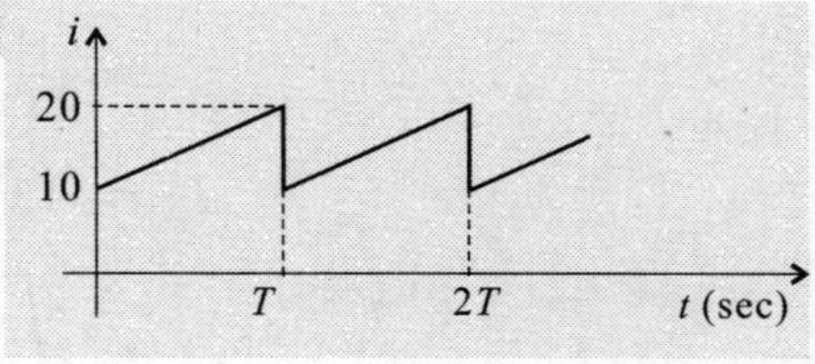

Interval = T

Let, $y = mx + c$ be the general equation of line.

$$10 = m \times 0 + c \quad \therefore \quad c = 10$$

$$20 = mT + 10 \quad \therefore \quad m = \frac{10}{T}$$

$$\therefore \quad i(t) = \frac{10}{T}\,t + 10 \qquad 0 < t < T$$

$$\text{and} \quad i^2(t) = \frac{100}{T^2} \times t^2 + \frac{200}{T}\,t + 100$$

$$I_{av} = \frac{1}{T}\int_0^T \left(\frac{10}{T}\,t + 10\right) dt$$

$$= \frac{1}{T}\left[\frac{10}{T} \times \frac{t^2}{2}\bigg|_0^T + 10t\bigg|_0^T\right] = \frac{1}{T}\left[\frac{10}{2T}\,T^2 + 10t\right]$$

$$I_{av} = \boxed{15 \text{ A}}$$

$$I_{rms} = \sqrt{\frac{1}{T}\int_0^T \left(\frac{100}{T^2}\,t^2 + \frac{200}{T}\,t + 100\right) dt}$$

$$= \sqrt{\frac{1}{T}\left[\frac{100}{T^2} \times \frac{t^3}{3}\bigg|_0^T + \frac{200}{T} + \frac{t^2}{2}\bigg|_0^T + 100\bigg|_0^T\right]}$$

$$= \sqrt{\frac{1}{T}\left[\frac{100}{3T^2} \times T^3 + \frac{100}{T}\,T^2 + 100T\right]} = \sqrt{\frac{700}{3}}$$

$$I_{rms} = \boxed{15.27 \text{ A}}$$

(iv)

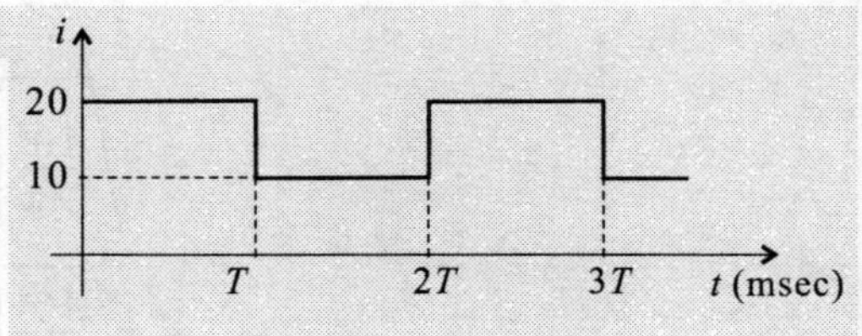

$$i(t) = 20 \qquad 0 < t < T$$
$$= 10 \qquad T < t < 2T$$
$$\therefore \quad i^2(t) = 400 \qquad 0 < t < T$$
$$= 100 \qquad T < t < 2T$$

Interval = $2T$

$$\therefore \quad I_{av} = \frac{1}{2T}\left[\int_0^T 20dt + \int_T^{2T} 10\ dt\right]$$

$$= \frac{1}{2T}\left[20t\Big|_0^T + 10t\Big|_T^{2T}\right] = \frac{1}{2T}[20T + 10T]$$

$$I_{av} = \boxed{15\text{ A}}$$

$$I_{rms} = \sqrt{\frac{1}{2T}\left[\int_0^T 400\,dt + \int_T^{2T} 100\,dt\right]} = \sqrt{\frac{1}{2T}[400T + 100T]} = \sqrt{\frac{500}{2}}$$

$$I_{rms} = \boxed{15.81\text{ A}}$$

(v)

$$v(t) = 200 + 100\sin\omega t \qquad 0 < \omega t < 2\pi$$

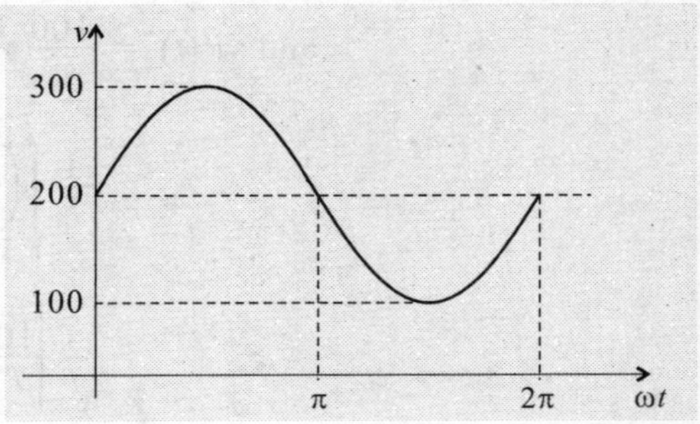

$$\therefore\ V_{av} = \frac{1}{2\pi}\left[\int_0^{2\pi}(200 + 100\sin\omega t)\right]d\omega t$$

$$= \frac{1}{2\pi}\left[200\times\omega t\Big|_0^{2\pi} - 10\cos\omega t\Big|_0^{2\pi}\right]$$

$$= \frac{1}{2\pi}[200\times 2\pi]$$

$$V_{av} = \boxed{200\text{ V}}$$

$$V_{rms} = \sqrt{\frac{1}{2\pi}\left[\int_0^{2\pi}(200 + 100\sin\omega t)^2\,d\omega t\right]}$$

$$= \sqrt{\frac{10^4}{2\pi}\int_0^{2\pi}\left[4 + \sin^2\omega t + 4\sin^2\omega t\right]d\omega t}$$

$$= \sqrt{\frac{10^4}{2\pi}\int_0^{2\pi}\left\{4 + \frac{1}{2}(1 - \cos 2\omega t) + \sin\omega t\right\}d\omega t}$$

$$= \sqrt{\frac{10^4}{2\pi}\left[4\omega t\Big|_0^{2\pi} + \frac{1}{2}\omega t\Big|_0^{2\pi} + \frac{1}{4}\sin 2\omega t\Big|_0^{2\pi} - \cos\omega t\Big|_0^{2\pi}\right.}$$

$$= \sqrt{\frac{10^4}{2\pi}\left[4(2\pi) + \frac{1}{2}(2\pi) - 1 + 1\right]} = \sqrt{\frac{9\times 10}{2}}$$

$$V_{rms} = \boxed{212.13\text{ V}}$$

(vi)

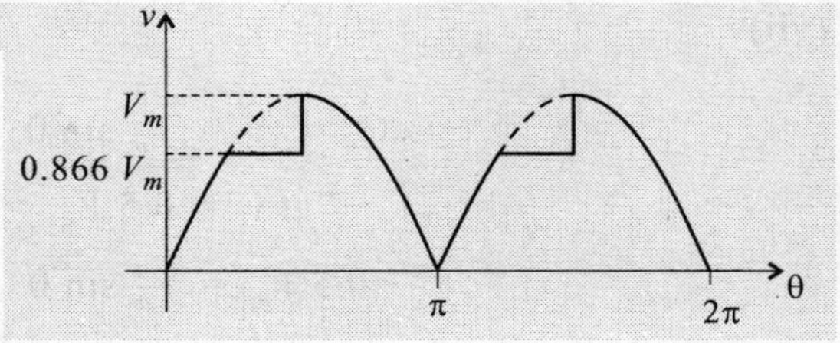

$$v = V_m \sin\theta$$

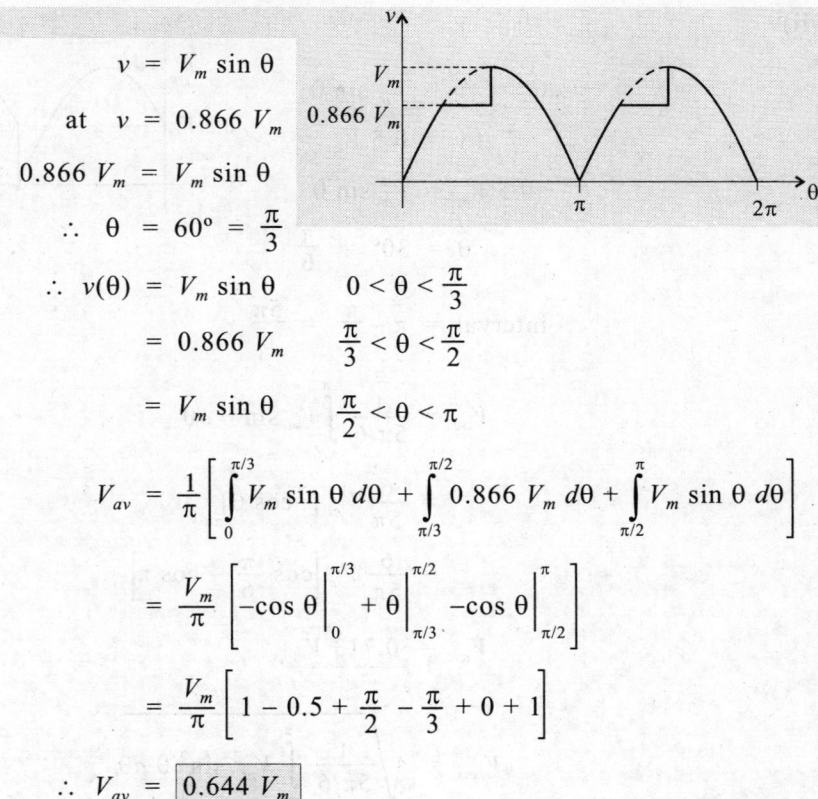

$$\text{at} \quad v = 0.866\, V_m$$

$$0.866\, V_m = V_m \sin\theta$$

$$\therefore \quad \theta = 60^\circ = \frac{\pi}{3}$$

$$\therefore \quad v(\theta) = V_m \sin\theta \qquad 0 < \theta < \frac{\pi}{3}$$

$$= 0.866\, V_m \qquad \frac{\pi}{3} < \theta < \frac{\pi}{2}$$

$$= V_m \sin\theta \qquad \frac{\pi}{2} < \theta < \pi$$

$$V_{av} = \frac{1}{\pi}\left[\int_0^{\pi/3} V_m \sin\theta\, d\theta + \int_{\pi/3}^{\pi/2} 0.866\, V_m\, d\theta + \int_{\pi/2}^{\pi} V_m \sin\theta\, d\theta\right]$$

$$= \frac{V_m}{\pi}\left[-\cos\theta\Big|_0^{\pi/3} + \theta\Big|_{\pi/3}^{\pi/2} - \cos\theta\Big|_{\pi/2}^{\pi}\right]$$

$$= \frac{V_m}{\pi}\left[1 - 0.5 + \frac{\pi}{2} - \frac{\pi}{3} + 0 + 1\right]$$

$$\therefore \quad V_{av} = \boxed{0.644\, V_m}$$

$$V_{rms} = \sqrt{\frac{1}{\pi}\left[\int_0^{\pi/3} V_m^2 \sin^2\theta\, d\theta + \int_{\pi/3}^{\pi/2} 0.75\, V_m^2\, d\theta + \int_{\pi/2}^{\pi} V_m^2 \sin^2\theta\, d\theta\right]}$$

$$= \sqrt{\frac{V_m^2}{\pi}\left[\int_0^{\pi/3} \frac{1 - \cos 2\theta}{2}\, d\theta + 0.75\left(\frac{\pi}{2} - \frac{\pi}{3}\right) + \int_{\pi/2}^{\pi} \frac{1 - \cos 2\theta}{2}\, d\theta\right]}$$

$$= \sqrt{\frac{V_m^2}{\pi}\left\{\frac{1}{2}\left[\theta - \frac{1}{2}\sin 2\theta\right]_0^{\pi/3} + 0.75\,\frac{\pi}{6} + \frac{1}{2}\left[\theta - \frac{1}{2}\sin 2\theta\right]_{\pi/2}^{\pi}\right\}}$$

$$= \sqrt{\frac{V_m^2}{2\pi}\left\{\frac{\pi}{3} - \frac{1}{2}\left[\sin\frac{2\pi}{3} - \sin 0\right] + 0.75\,\frac{\pi}{3} + \pi - \frac{\pi}{2} - \frac{1}{2}\left[\sin 2\pi - \sin\pi\right]\right\}}$$

$$V_{rms} = \boxed{0.6875\, V_m}$$

(vii)

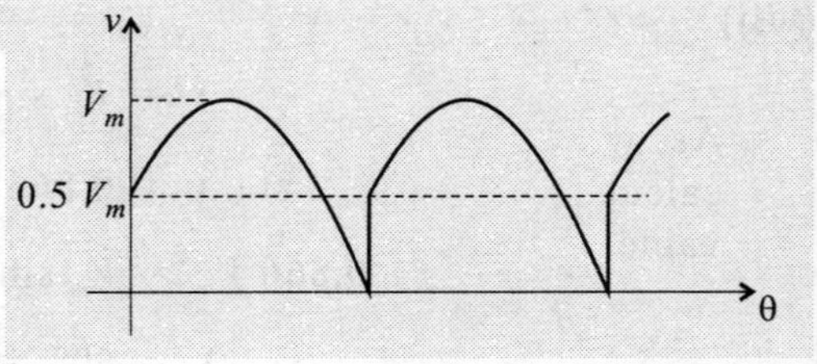

Let, $v = V_m \sin\theta$

at $v = 0.5\ V_m$

$0.5\ V_m = V_m \sin\theta$

$\therefore\ \theta = 30^\circ = \dfrac{\pi}{6}$

$\therefore$ interval $= \pi - \dfrac{\pi}{6} = \dfrac{5\pi}{6}$

$$\therefore\ V_{av} = \frac{1}{5\pi/6}\int_{\pi/6}^{\pi} V_m \sin\theta\, d\theta$$

$$= \frac{6}{5\pi} V_m [-\cos\theta]_{\pi/6}^{\pi}$$

$$= \frac{6}{5\pi} V_m \left[\cos\frac{\pi}{6} - \cos\pi\right]$$

$$V_{av} = \boxed{0.713\ V_m}$$

$$V_{rms} = \sqrt{\frac{1}{5\pi/6}\int_{\pi/6}^{\pi} V_m^{\ 2} \sin^2\theta\, d\theta}$$

$$= \sqrt{\frac{6}{5\pi}\frac{V_m^{\ 2}}{2}\int_{\pi/6}^{\pi}(1-\cos 2\theta)\, d\theta}$$

$$= \sqrt{\frac{3}{5\pi} V_m^{\ 2}\left[\theta\Big|_{\pi/6}^{\pi} - \frac{1}{2}\sin 2\theta\Big|_{\pi/6}^{\pi}\right]}$$

$$= \sqrt{\frac{3}{5\pi} V_m^{\ 2}\left[\pi - \frac{\pi}{6} - \frac{1}{2}\left\{\sin 2\pi - \sin\frac{\pi}{3}\right\}\right]}$$

$$= \sqrt{\frac{3}{5\pi} V_m^{\ 2}\left[\frac{5\pi}{6} + \frac{1}{2}\, 0.866\right]}$$

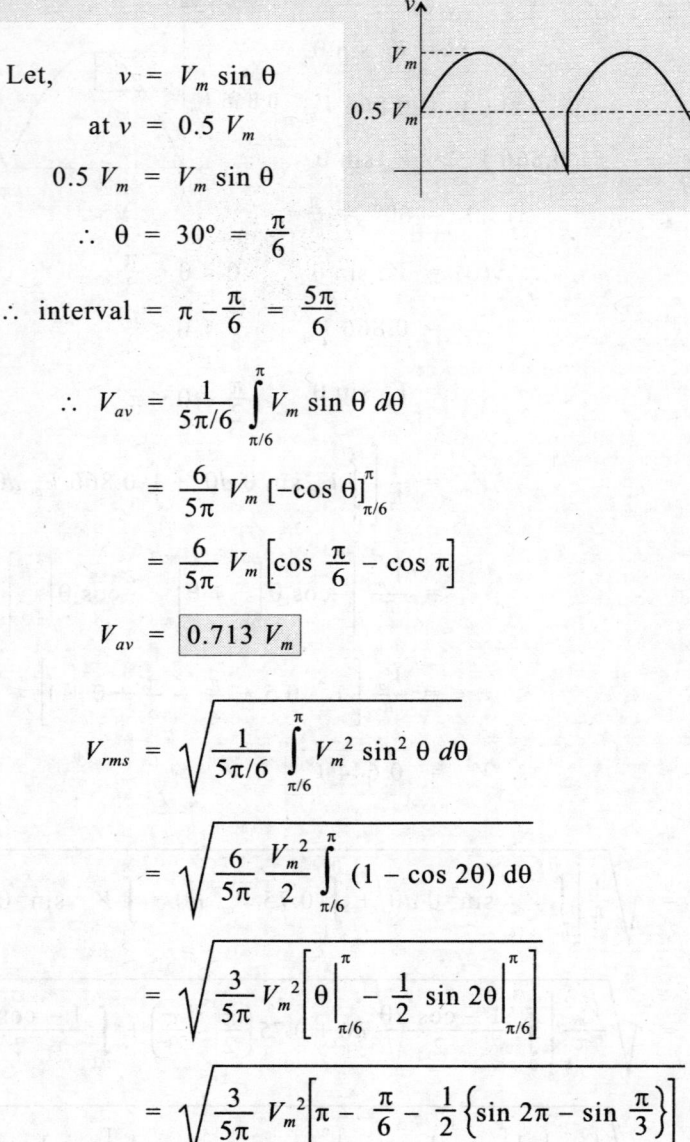

$$V_{rms} = \boxed{0.7633\ V_m}$$

(viii)

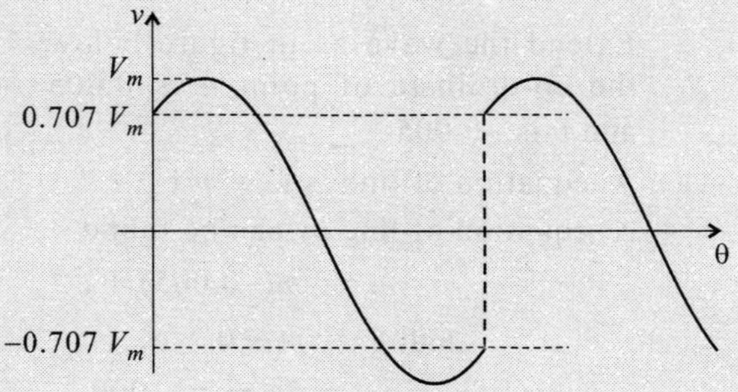

As waveform is symmetrical, we calculate half cycle average and rms value.

$$v = V_m \sin\theta$$

$$\text{at } 0.707\, V_m = V_m \sin\theta$$

$$\therefore \theta = 45^\circ = \frac{\pi}{4}$$

$$\therefore \text{ interval of half cycle} = \pi - \frac{\pi}{4} = \frac{3\pi}{4}$$

$$\therefore V_{av} \text{ half cycle} = \frac{1}{3\pi/4} \int_{\pi/4}^{\pi} V_m \sin\theta \, d\theta$$

$$= \frac{4}{3\pi} V_m [-\cos\theta]_{\pi/4}^{\pi}$$

$$= \frac{4}{3\pi} V_m \left[\cos\frac{\pi}{4} - \cos\pi\right]$$

$$= \frac{4}{3\pi} V_m (1.707)$$

$$V_{av} = \boxed{0.7245\, V_m}$$

$$V_{rms} \text{ half cycle} = \sqrt{\frac{1}{3\pi/4} \int_{\pi/4}^{\pi} V_m^2 \sin^2\theta \, d\theta}$$

$$= \sqrt{\frac{4}{3\pi} V_m^2 \left[\theta\Big|_{\pi/4}^{\pi} - \frac{1}{2} \sin 2\theta\Big|_{\pi/4}^{\pi}\right]}$$

$$= \sqrt{\frac{4}{3\pi} V_m^2 \left[\pi - \frac{\pi}{4} - \frac{1}{2}\left\{\sin 2\pi - \sin\frac{\pi}{2}\right\}\right]}$$

$$= \sqrt{\frac{4}{3\pi} V_m^2 \left[\frac{3\pi}{4} + \frac{1}{2}\right]}$$

$$V_{rms} = \boxed{1.1\, V_m}$$

(ix)

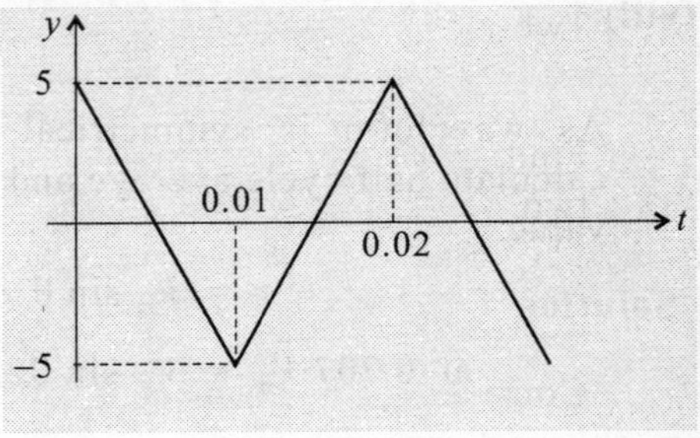

Extend the wave as in figure below the co-ordinate of point a is 0.005 and b is −0.005

$\therefore$ equation of line is $y = mx + c$

$\therefore$ equation of line bx can be found

$$0 = m(-0.005) + c$$

$$\text{and } 5 = m \times 0 + c$$

$$\therefore c = 5, \; m = 1000$$

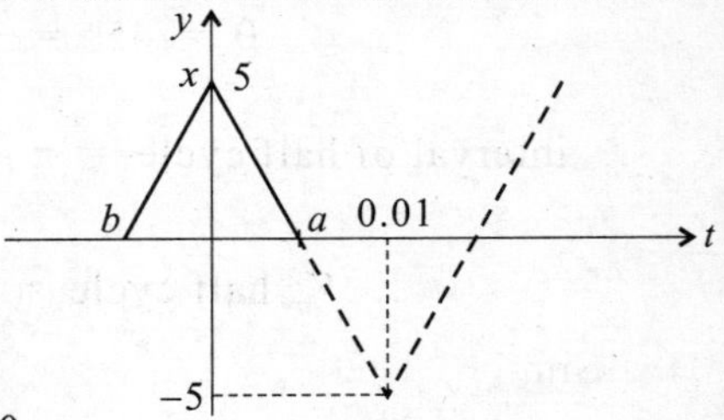

$\therefore$ equation of line bx is

$$y = 1000t + 5$$

Similarly equation of line ax is

$$y = -1000t + 5$$

$$\therefore y(t) = 1000t + 5 \qquad -0.005 < t < 0$$

$$= -1000t + 5 \qquad 0 < t < 0.005$$

This wave is symmetrical about the axis

$$\therefore Y_{av} \text{ half cycle} = \frac{1}{0.01}\left[\int_{-0.005}^{0}(1000t + 5)dt + \int_{0}^{0.005}(-1000t + 5)dt\right]$$

$$= \frac{1}{0.01}\left[\left(1000\frac{t^2}{2} + 5t\right)_{-0.005}^{0} + \left(-1000t\frac{t^2}{2} + 5t\right)_{0}^{0.005}\right]$$

$$= \frac{1}{0.01}\left[-\frac{1000 \times 0.005^2}{2} + 5 \times 0.005 - \frac{1000 \times 0.005^2}{2} + 5 \times 0.005\right]$$

$$Y_{av} = \boxed{2.5}$$

$$Y_{rms} = \sqrt{\frac{1}{0.01}\left[\int_{-0.005}^{0}\left\{10^6t^2 + 10^4t + 25\right\}dt + \int_{0}^{0.005}\left\{10^6t^2 - 10^4t + 25\right\}dt\right]}$$

$$= \sqrt{\frac{1}{0.01}\left[\left\{\frac{10^6}{3}t^3 + \frac{10^4}{2}t^2 + 25t\right\}_{-0.005}^{0} + \left\{\frac{10^6}{3}t^3 - \frac{10^4}{2}t^2 + 25t\right\}_{0}^{0.005}\right]}$$

$$= \sqrt{\frac{1}{0.01}\left[\frac{1}{12}\right]}$$

$$Y_{rms} = \boxed{2.8867}$$

2. Two sine waves are represented by the following expression

$$e = 282 \sin(314t - \pi/6) \quad \text{and} \quad i = 40 \sin(314t + \pi/4).$$

Find maximum and rms value of each. Also, find the phase difference between the two, showing vector diagram.

Solution : Given : $e = 282 \sin\left(\frac{3}{4}t - \frac{\pi}{6}\right)$

Comparing this equation with equation (3.10)

$$E_m = 282$$

$$\therefore \quad E_{rms} = \frac{E_m}{\sqrt{2}} = \frac{282}{\sqrt{2}} = 199.4$$

$$\text{the vector } \bar{E} = \boxed{199.4 \angle -30^\circ} \quad \left[\because \frac{\pi}{6} = 30^\circ\right]$$

Similarly,

$$i = 40 \sin\left(\frac{3}{4}t + \frac{\pi}{4}\right)$$

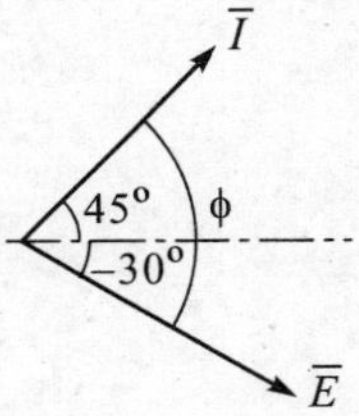

Comparing this equation with equation (3.9)

$$\therefore \quad I_m = 40$$

$$\therefore \quad I_{rms} = \frac{40}{\sqrt{2}} = 28.28 \text{ Amp}$$

$$\text{the vector } \bar{I} = \boxed{28.28 \angle 45^\circ} \quad \left[\because \frac{\pi}{4} = 45^\circ\right]$$

From figure phase difference

$$\phi = 45^\circ + 30^\circ = \boxed{75^\circ}$$

3. $v_1 = 147.3 \cos(\omega t + 98.1^\circ)$

$v_2 = 294 \cos(\omega t - 45^\circ)$

$v_3 = 88 \sin(\omega t + 135^\circ)$

v_1, v_2 and v_3 are the instantaneous voltages in three series connected circuit. Find the resultant voltage. Also show all the vectors on vector diagram.

Solution : Given :

$$v_1 = 147.3 \cos(\omega t + 98.1^\circ)$$

$$v_2 = 294 \cos(\omega t - 45^\circ)$$

$$v_3 = 88 \sin(\omega t + 135^\circ)$$

Writing the above equations in standard form of

$$v = v_m \sin(\omega t \pm \phi)$$

$$v_1 = 147.3 \sin\left(\frac{\pi}{2} + \omega t + 98.1^\circ\right)$$

$$= 147.3 \sin(\omega t + 188.1^\circ)$$

$$v_2 = 294 \cos(\omega t - 45°)$$
$$= 294 \sin(\omega t - 45° + 90°)$$
$$= 294 \sin(\omega t + 45°)$$
$$v_3 = 88 \sin(\omega t + 135°)$$

Now writing vector $\overline{V}_1$, $\overline{V}_2$, and $\overline{V}_3$

$$\overline{V}_1 = \frac{147.3}{\sqrt{2}} \angle 188.1° = 104.16 \angle 188.1°$$

$$\overline{V}_2 = \frac{294}{\sqrt{2}} \angle 45° = 207.9 \angle 45°$$

$$\overline{V}_3 = \frac{88}{\sqrt{2}} \angle 135° = 62.2 \angle 135°$$

For series connected circuit resultant voltage V_R is given by

$$\overline{V}_R = \overline{V}_1 + \overline{V}_2 + \overline{V}_3$$
$$= 104.16 \angle 188.1° + 207.9 \angle 45° + 62.2 \angle 135°$$
$$= \boxed{1176.31 \angle 90°}$$

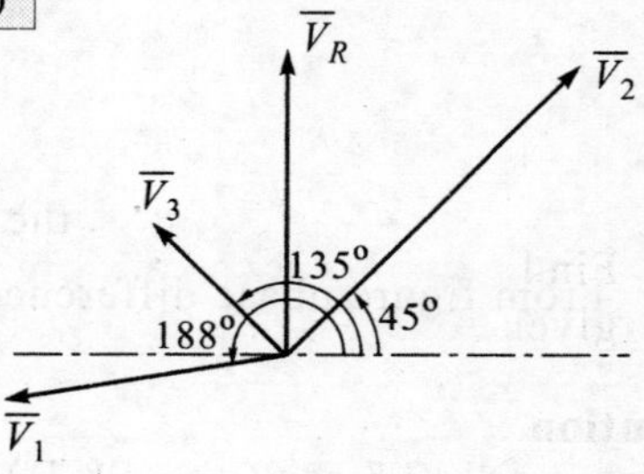

Chapter 4 : A.C. CIRCUITS

Solution to Unsolved Examples

1. Find the impedance of the circuit shown in Fig. 4.58.

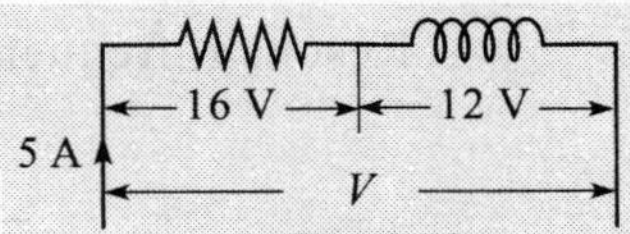

Fig. 4.58

Solution :

$$V^2 = V_R^2 + V_L^2$$

$$\therefore \; V = \sqrt{16^2 + 12^2}$$

$$V = 20$$

$$Z = \frac{V}{I} = \frac{V}{I} = \boxed{4\ \Omega}$$

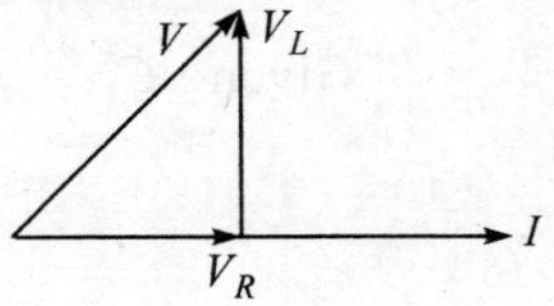

2. Find the applied voltage of the circuit shown in Fig. 4.59.

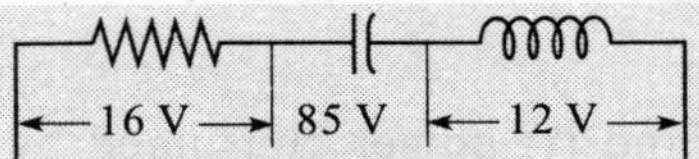

Fig. 4.59

Solution :

$$V = \sqrt{V_R^2 + (V_L - V_C)^2}$$

$$V_L = \sqrt{20^2 + (85 - 100)^2}$$

$$V = \boxed{25\ \text{V}}$$

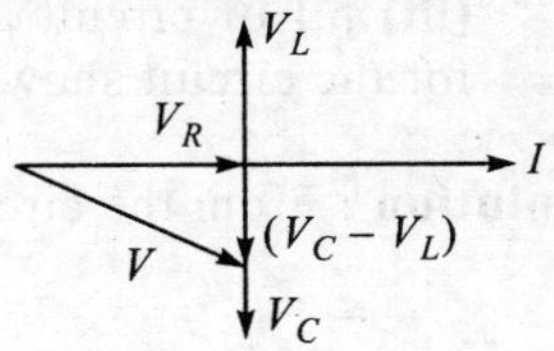

3. Find the power factor of the circuit given in Fig. 4.60.

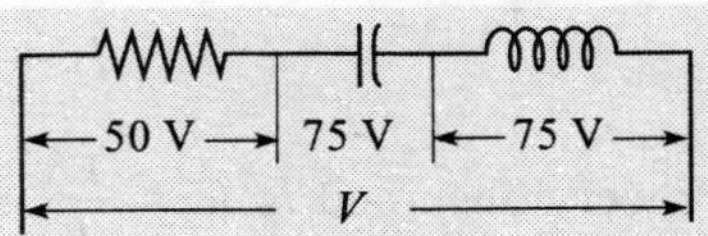

Fig. 4.60

Solution :

$$V = \sqrt{V_R^2 + (V_L - V_C)^2}$$

$$V_L = V_C \text{ (given)}$$

$$\therefore \; V = V_R = 50\ \text{V}$$

as $V = V_R$ the circuit is a resonating circuit hence p.f. $= \cos\phi = \boxed{1}$

4. Find the ammeter and the voltmeter reading in the circuit (Fig. 4.61).

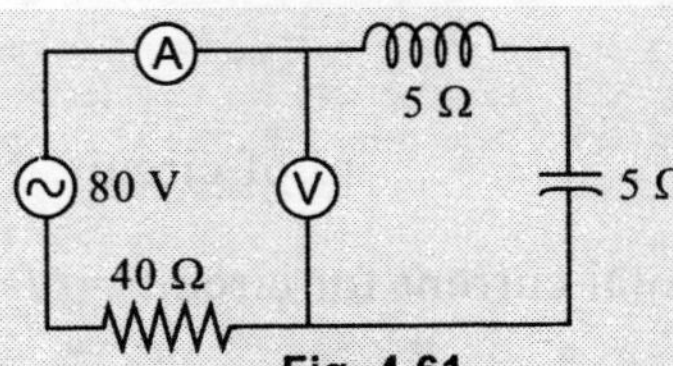

Fig. 4.61

Solution :

$$I = \frac{80}{40 + 5j - 5j} = 2$$

Ammeter reading is $\boxed{2\ \text{A}}$

$$V_1 = V_L + V_C$$

$$= I(5j - 5j) = \boxed{0\ \text{V}}$$

Voltmeter reading is zero.

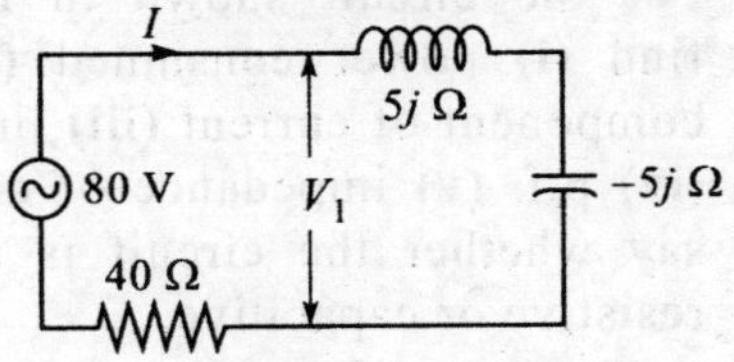

5. In a series R-L-C circuit, the capacitance is changed from C to $4C$. For the same resonating frequency, the inductor should be charged from L to ______.

Solution : Resonant frequency $\omega_o = \sqrt{\frac{1}{LC}}$

$$\therefore \quad \frac{1}{\sqrt{L_1 C_1}} = \frac{1}{\sqrt{L_2 C_2}}$$

Given : $C_1 = C,\ C_2 = 4C$ and $L_1 = L$

$$\therefore \quad \frac{1}{LC} = \frac{1}{4L_2C}$$

$$\text{or } L_2 = \boxed{\frac{L}{4}}$$

6. Find **(i)** power consumed by the circuit **(ii)** active component of line current **(iii)** p.f of circuit and **(iv)** total current for the circuit shown in Fig. 4.62.

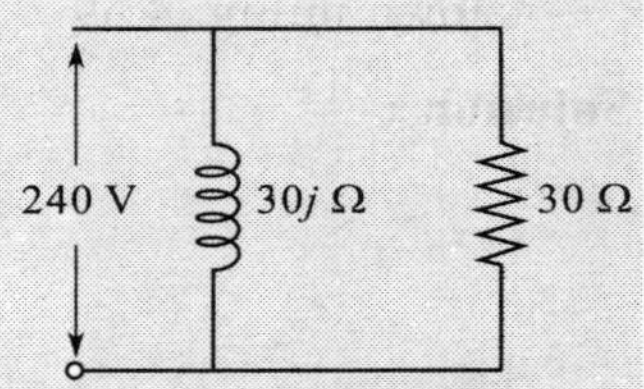

Fig. 4.62

Solution : From the circuit

$$\overline{I_R} = \frac{240}{30} = 8\angle 0^\circ$$

$$\overline{I_L} = \frac{240}{30j} = 8\angle -90^\circ$$

(i) Power consumed $I_R{}^2R = \frac{V^2}{R} = \boxed{1920\text{ W}}$

(ii) Active component of current $I_R = \boxed{8\text{ A}}$

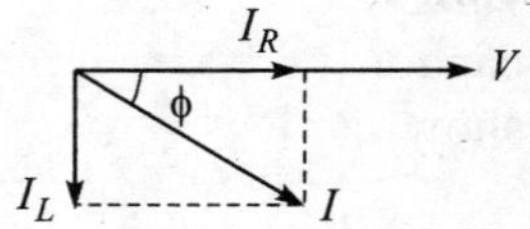

(iii)

$$\overline{I} = \overline{I_R} + \overline{I_L}$$

$$= 8\angle 0 + 8\angle -90^\circ$$

$$= 8\sqrt{2}\angle -45^\circ$$

$$\therefore \text{ pf of circuit} = \cos 45^\circ \text{ (lag)} = \boxed{0.707 \text{ lagging}}$$

(iv) Total current for circuit $= I = \boxed{8\sqrt{2}}$

7. For the circuit shown in Fig. 4.63, find **(i)** power consumed **(ii)** active component of current **(iii)** line current **(iv)** p.f. **(v)** impedance of circuit and say whether the circuit is inductive, resistive or capacitive.

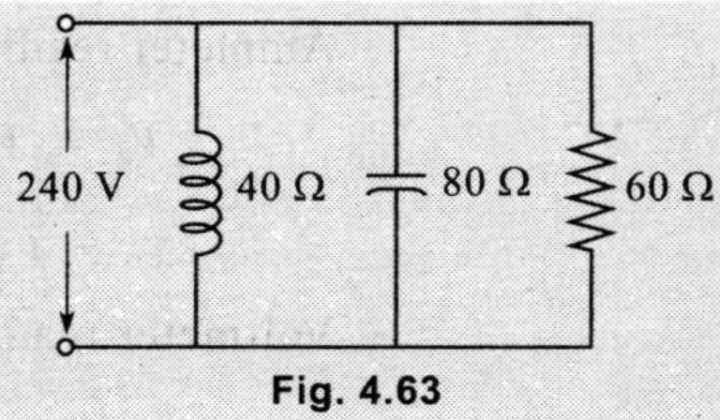

Fig. 4.63

Solution :

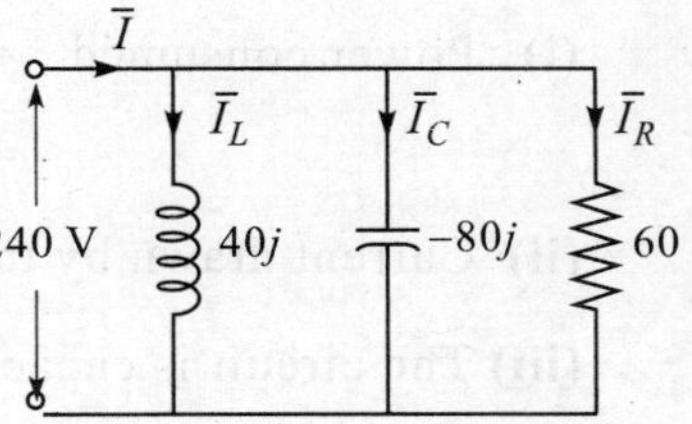

Let $\overline{V} = 240\ \angle 0°$

$$\therefore\ \overline{I}_R = \frac{240\ \angle 0°}{60} = 4\ \angle 0°$$

$$\overline{I}_C = \frac{240\ \angle 0°}{-80j} = 3\ \angle 90°$$

$$\overline{I}_L = \frac{240\ \angle 0°}{40j} = 6\ \angle -90°$$

$$\therefore\ \overline{I} = \overline{I}_R + \overline{I}_L + \overline{I}_C = 4 + 3\ \angle 90° + 6\ \angle -90°$$

$$= 5\ \angle -36.87°$$

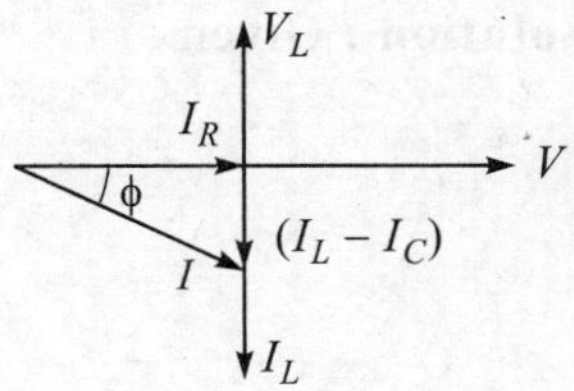

(i) Power consumed $I_R^2 R = 4^2 \times 60 = \boxed{960\ \text{W}}$

(ii) Active component of current $I_R = \boxed{4\ \text{A}}$

(iii) Line current $|I| = \boxed{5\ \text{A}}$

(iv) pf $= \cos(-36.87°) = \boxed{0.8\ \text{lagging}}$

(v) Impedance of circuit $\overline{Z} = \frac{\overline{V}}{\overline{I}} = \frac{240\ \angle 0°}{5\ \angle -36.87°} = 38.4 + 28.8j = 48\ \angle 36.87°$

The circuit is inductive as imaginary part of $\overline{Z}$ is positive and magnitude of impedance $= \boxed{48\ \Omega}$

8. Find **(i)** power consumed **(ii)** current drawn by the circuit and **(iii)** say whether the circuit is inductive or capacitive or resistive for the circuit shown in Fig. 4.64.

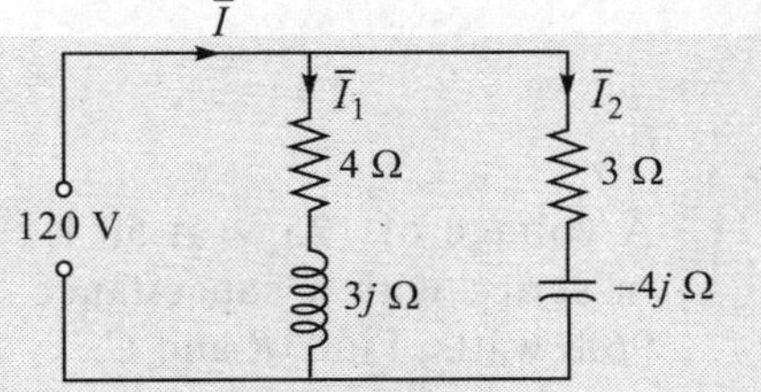

Fig. 4.64

Solution :

Let $\overline{V} = 120\ \angle 0°$

$$\overline{Z}_1 = 4 + 3j$$

$$\overline{Z}_2 = 3 - 4j$$

$$\overline{I}_1 = \frac{\overline{V}}{\overline{Z}_1} = \frac{120\ \angle 0°}{4 + 3j} = 24\ \angle -36.87°$$

$$\overline{I}_2 = \frac{\overline{V}}{\overline{Z}_2} = \frac{120\ \angle 0°}{3 - 4j} = 24\ \angle 53.13°$$

$$\overline{I} = \overline{I}_1 + \overline{I}_2 = 24\ \angle -36.87° + 24\ \angle 53.13°$$

$$= 33.94\ \angle 8.13°$$

(i) Power consumed $= I_1^2 R_1 + I_2^2 R_2 = 24^2 \times 4 + 24^2 \times 3$

$= \boxed{4032 \text{ watts}}$

(ii) Current drawn by the circuit $= \boxed{33.94 \angle 8.13^\circ \text{ amp}}$

(iii) The circuit is capacitive as $\overline{I}$ leads $\overline{V}$ by $\boxed{8.13^\circ}$.

9. A pure inductance of 0.01 H passes a current of 5 cos 2000 t amp. What is the voltage across it ?

Solution : Given :

$$L = 0.01 \text{ H}$$

$$i(t) = 5 \cos 2000t$$

$$v = L\frac{di}{dt} = 0.01 \frac{d}{dt}(5 \cos 2000t)$$

$$= 0.01 \times 5 [-\sin 2000t] \times 2000$$

$$= \boxed{100 \sin (2000t + \pi)}$$

10. A pure capacitance of 30 μf passes a current 12 sin 2000t. Find the voltage.

Solution : Given :

$$i = 12 \sin 2000t$$

$$v = \frac{1}{C}\int i\, dt = \frac{1}{30 \times 10^{-6}} \times \frac{12(-\cos 2000t)}{2000}$$

$$= \boxed{200 \sin\left(2000t - \frac{\pi}{2}\right)}$$

11. A voltage of 125 V at 50 Hz is applied across a non-inductive resistance connected in series with a capacitance. The current is 2.2 A. The power loss in resistance is 96.8 watts. Find R and C.

Solution : Given : $\overline{V} = 125 \angle 0^\circ$, $f = 50$ Hz, $I = 2.2$ A

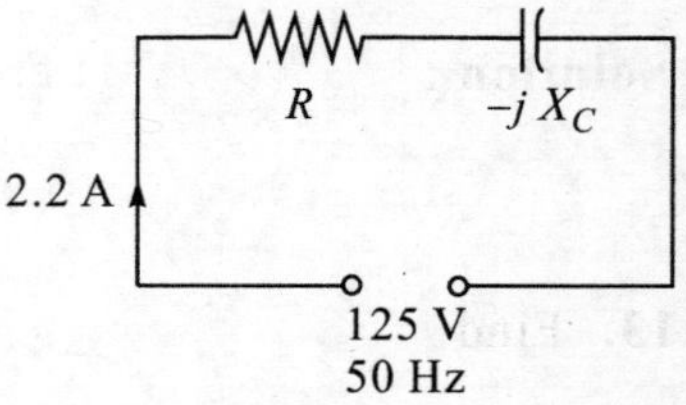

$$P = \text{power loss} = 96.8 \text{ V}$$

$$P = I^2 R$$

$$\therefore \; 96.8 = 2.2^2 \times R$$

$$\therefore \; R = \boxed{20 \; \Omega}$$

$$Z = \frac{V}{I} = \frac{125}{2.2} = 56.82 \; \Omega$$

$$V = \sqrt{R^2 + X_C^2}$$

$$\therefore \; X_C = \sqrt{Z^2 - R^2} = \sqrt{56.82^2 - 20^2}$$

$$= 53.183$$

$$\text{But } X_C = \frac{1}{2\pi f C}$$

$$\therefore C = \frac{1}{2\pi \times 50 \times 53.183} = 59.85 \times 10^{-6}$$

$$= \boxed{59.85 \mu f}$$

12. A coil of pf 0.5 in series with 79.57 µf capacitance is connected across 50 Hz supply. The potential difference across the coil is equal to the potential difference across the capacitance. Find the resistance and inductance of the coil.

Solution :

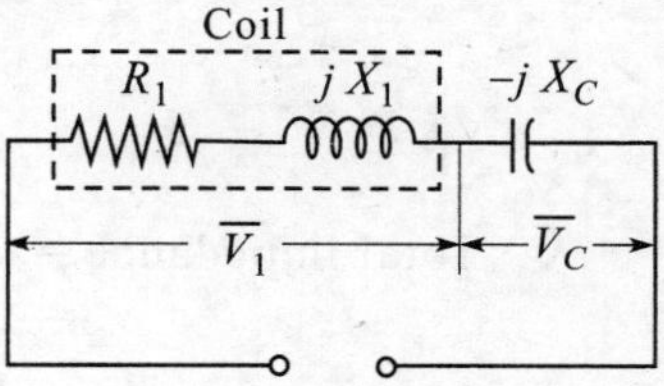

$$\text{pf of coil} = \cos \phi_1 = 0.5$$

$$\phi_1 = 60^\circ$$

$$\therefore C = 79.57 \mu f = 79.57 \times 10^{-6} f$$

$$X_C = \frac{1}{2\pi f C}$$

$$f = 50 \text{ Hz}$$

$$\therefore X_C = 40$$

$$V_1 = V_C \quad \text{...(given)}$$

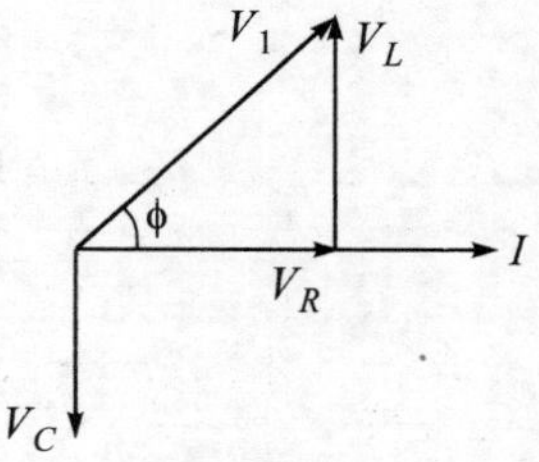

$$\therefore I Z_{coil} = I X_C$$

$$\therefore Z_{coil} = 40$$

$$\therefore R = Z_{coil} \cos \phi_1 = 40 \cos 60^\circ = 20 \ \Omega$$

$$X_L = Z_{coil} \sin \phi_1 = 40 \sin 60^\circ = 34.64 \ \Omega$$

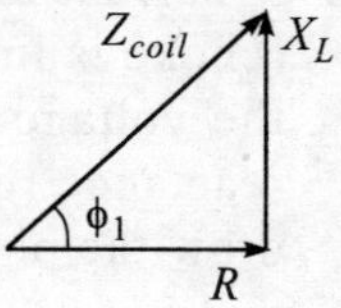

$$\text{but } X_L = \omega L = 2\pi f L$$

$$\therefore L = \frac{34.64}{2\pi \times 50} = 0.11 \text{ H}$$

$$\therefore R = \boxed{20 \ \Omega} \text{ and } L = \boxed{0.11 \text{ H}}$$

13. Find $\overline{I}$, $\overline{V_1}$, $\overline{V_2}$ and power factor of the circuit in Fig. 4.65.

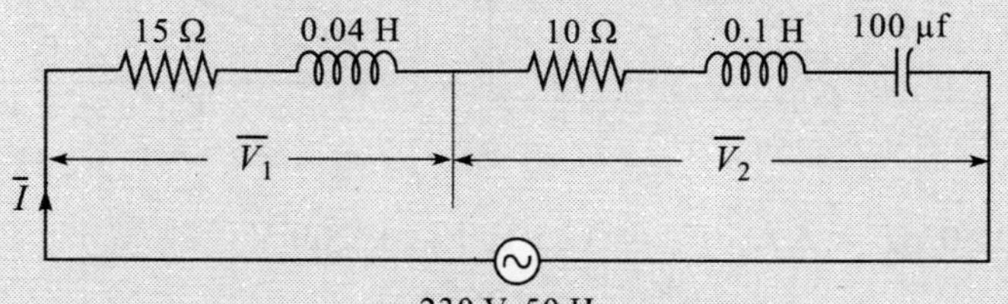

Fig. 4.65

Solution : Given :

$$V = 230 \text{ V} \qquad f = 50 \text{ Hz}$$
$$L_1 = 0.04 \text{ H} \qquad X_{L1} = 2\pi f L_1 = 12.57\ \Omega$$
$$R_1 = 15\ \Omega \qquad R_2 = 10\ \Omega$$
$$L_2 = 0.1 \text{ H} \qquad X_{L2} = 2\pi f L_2 = 31.41\ \Omega$$
$$C = 100\ \mu f \qquad X_C = \frac{1}{2\pi f C} = 31.83\ \Omega$$
$$\overline{Z}_1 = R_1 + jX_{L1} = 15 + 12.57\, j$$
$$\overline{Z}_2 = R_2 + jX_{L2} - jX_C$$
$$= 10 + 31.41j - 31.83j$$
$$= 10 + 0.42j$$

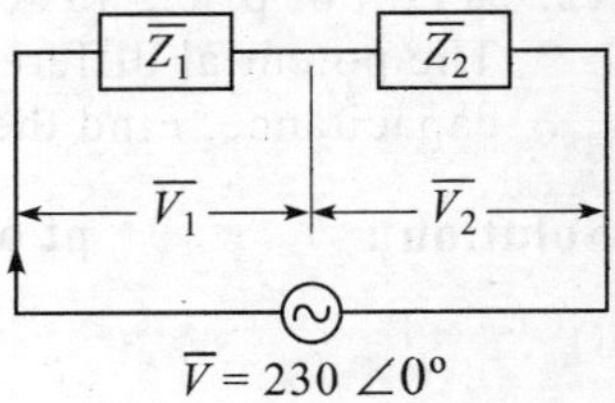

$$\therefore \text{ Total impedance} = \overline{Z} = \overline{Z}_1 + \overline{Z}_2 = 25 + 12.15j$$
$$\overline{I} = \frac{\overline{V}}{\overline{Z}} = \frac{230\ \angle 0°}{25 + 12.15j} = 8.27\ \angle -25.92°$$
$$\overline{I} = \boxed{8.27\ \angle -25.92° \text{ amp}}$$
$$\overline{V}_1 = \overline{I}\,\overline{Z}_1 = (8.27\ \angle -25.92°)\,(15 + 12.57\, j)$$
$$\overline{V}_1 = \boxed{161.94 \angle 14° \text{ volts}}$$
$$\overline{V}_2 = \overline{I}\,\overline{Z}_2 = (8.27\ \angle -25.92°)\,(10 - 0.42j)$$
$$\overline{V}_2 = \boxed{82.77 \angle -28.32 \text{ volts}}$$

14. A current of 5 A flows through a non inductive resistance in series with a choke coil (choke is impure and has some resistance). When supplied by 250 V, 50 Hz supply. If the voltage across resistance is 125 V cross coil is 200 V. Calculate **(i)** Impedence, reactance resistance of coil **(ii)** power absorbed by the coil **(iii)** total power and **(iv)** draw the phasor diagram.

Solution :

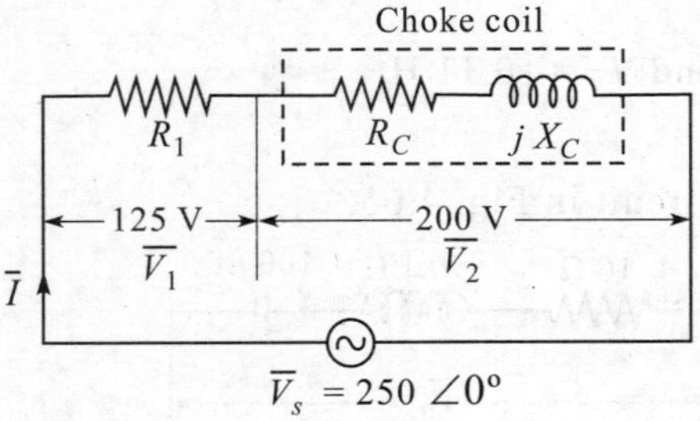

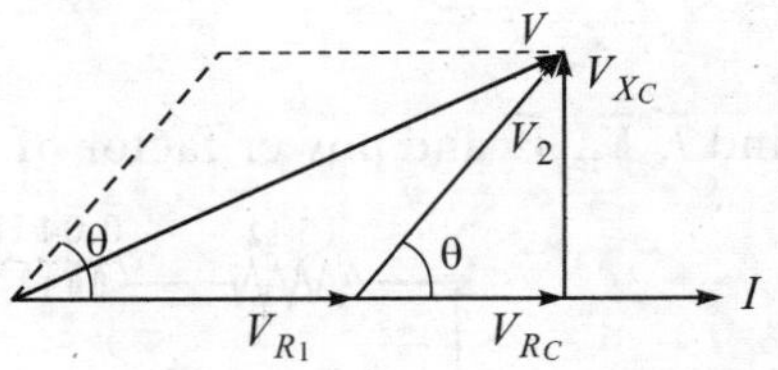

Given : $\overline{V}_s = 250 \angle 0°,\ I = 5 \text{ A},\ V_1 = 125 \text{ V},\ V_2 = 200 \text{ V}$

$$\therefore\ R_1 = \frac{V_1}{I} = \frac{125}{5} = 25\ \Omega$$

From the vector diagram

$$V = \sqrt{V_1^2 + V_2^2 + 2V_1V_2 \cos \phi}$$

$$250 = \sqrt{125^2 + 200^2 + 2 \times 125 \times 200 \cos \phi}$$

$$\therefore \cos \phi_1 = 0.1375$$

$$\therefore \phi_1 = 82.09^\circ$$

(i)
$$Z_{coil} = \frac{V_2}{I} = \frac{200}{5} = \boxed{40}$$

$$\therefore R_C = Z_{coil} \cos \phi = \boxed{5.5\ \Omega}$$

$$X_L = Z_{coil} \sin \phi = \boxed{39.62\ \Omega}$$

(ii) Power absorbed by coil $= I^2 R_C$

$$= 5^2 \times 5.5 = \boxed{137.5 \text{ watts}}$$

(iii) Total power $= I^2 (R_1 + R_C)$

$$= 5^2 (25 + 5.5) = \boxed{762.5 \text{ watts}}$$

15. A resistance in series with a capacitance connected across a 250 V supply draw 5 A current at a frequency of 50 Hz. When the frequency is increased to 60 Hz, it draws 5.8 A. Find R and C and the power drawn by the circuit in the second case.

Solution :

$$V = 250 \text{ V}$$

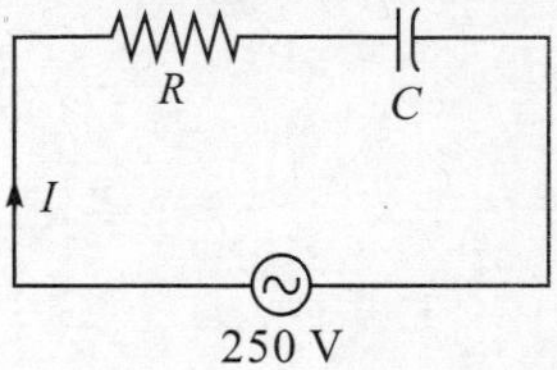

Case I:
$$f_1 = 50 \text{ Hz} \quad \therefore I_1 = 5 \text{ A}$$

$$X_{C_1} = \frac{1}{2\pi f_1 C}$$

Case II:
$$f_2 = 60 \text{ Hz} \quad \therefore I_2 = 5.8 \text{ A}$$

$$X_{C_2} = \frac{1}{2\pi f_2 C}$$

Case I:

$$\frac{V}{I_1} = Z_1 = \sqrt{R^2 + X_{C_1}^2}$$

$$\therefore \frac{250}{5} = 50 = \sqrt{R^2 + X_{C_1}^2}$$

$$\text{or } 2500 = R^2 + X_{C_1}^2$$

$$2500 = R^2 + \frac{1}{(2\pi f_1)^2 C^2} \quad \text{.... (i)}$$

Case II:

$$\frac{V}{I_2} = Z_2 = \sqrt{R^2 + X_{C_2}^2}$$

$$\therefore \frac{250}{5.8} = 43.1 = \sqrt{R^2 + X_{C_1}^2}$$

$$\text{or } 43.1^2 = R^2 + X_{C_1}^2$$

$$1857.61 = R^2 + \frac{1}{(2\pi f_1)^2 C^2} \quad \text{.... (ii)}$$

Solving (i) and (ii)

$$R^2 = 397.63\ \Omega \text{ and } \frac{1}{C^2} = 207 \times 10^6$$

$$\therefore R = \boxed{19.94\ \Omega} \text{ and } C = \boxed{69.4 \times 10^{-6} \text{ f}}$$

16. A voltage of 200 $\angle 25^\circ$ volts is supplied to a circuit composed of two parallel branches. If the branch currents are 10 $\angle 40^\circ$ A and 20 $\angle -30^\circ$ A, determine the KVA, KVAR and KW in each branch. Also the power factor of the combined circuit.

Solution : Given :

$$\overline{V}_s = 200 \angle 25^\circ$$
$$\overline{I}_1 = 10 \angle 40^\circ$$
$$\overline{I}_2 = 20 \angle -30^\circ$$

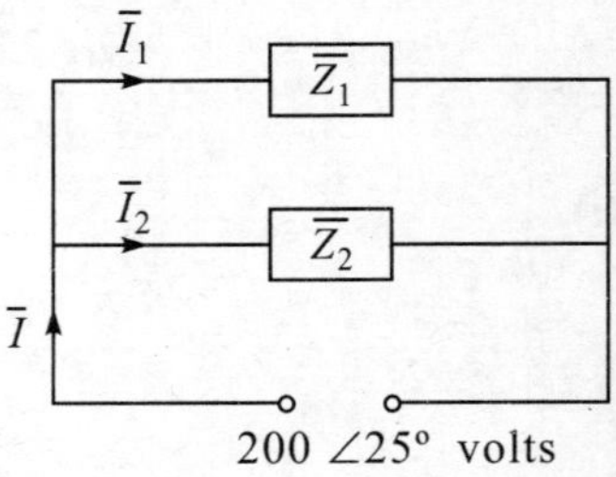

Branch 1

$$\phi_1 = 40^\circ - 25^\circ = 15^\circ$$

$$\therefore \text{KVA}_1 = \frac{V_s \times I_1}{1000} = \frac{200 \times 10}{1000} = \boxed{2}$$

$$\text{KW}_1 = \text{KVA}_1 \cos \phi_1 = 2 \cos 15^\circ$$

$$\text{KW}_1 = \boxed{1.93}$$

$$\text{KVAR}_1 = \text{KVA}_1 \sin \phi_1 = 2 \sin 15^\circ$$

$$\text{KVAR}_1 = \boxed{0.52}$$

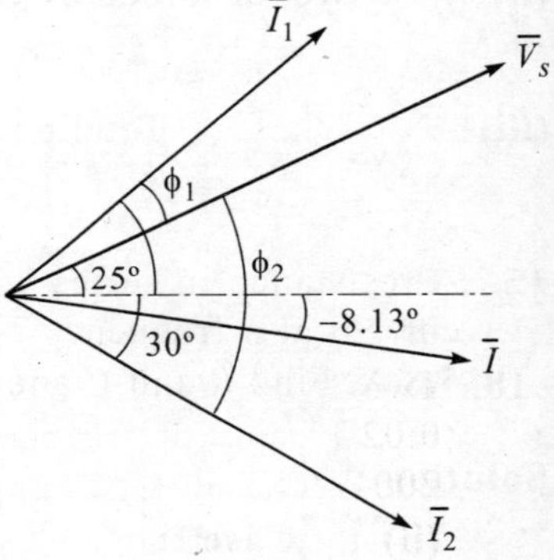

Branch 2

$$\phi_2 = 25^\circ + 30^\circ = 55^\circ$$

$$\therefore \text{KVA}_2 = \frac{V_s \times I_2}{1000} = \frac{200 \times 20}{1000} = \boxed{4}$$

$$\text{KW}_2 = \text{KVA}_2 \cos \phi_2 = 2 \cos 55^\circ$$

$$\text{KW}_2 = \boxed{2.29}$$

$$\text{KVAR}_2 = \text{KVA}_2 \sin \phi_2 = 2 \sin 55^\circ$$

$$\text{KVAR}_2 = \boxed{3.28}$$

Total Current $\overline{I}$

$$\overline{I} = \overline{I}_1 + \overline{I}_2 = 10 \angle 40^\circ + 20 \angle -30^\circ = \boxed{25.23 \angle -8.13^\circ}$$

$$\text{pf angle } \phi = 25^\circ + 8.13^\circ = 33.13^\circ$$

$$\therefore \text{pf} = \cos \phi = \boxed{0.8374 \text{ lagging}}$$

17. In a series circuit of R = 5 and L = 0.06 H, V_L = 15 sin 200 t. Find total voltage, current and the angle by which the current lags the supply voltage and the magnitude of the impedance.

Solution : Given :

$$R = 5\ \Omega$$
$$L = 0.06 \text{ H}$$
$$v_L = 15 \sin 200t$$

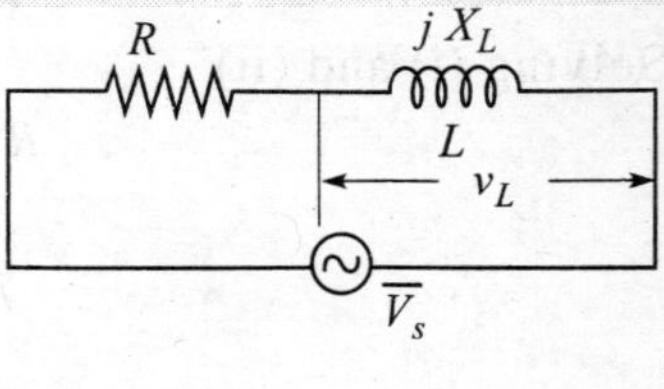

$$\overline{V}_L = \frac{15}{\sqrt{2}} \angle 0° = 10.61 \angle 0°$$

$$\omega = 200$$

$$\therefore X_L = \omega L = 200 \times 0.06 = 12$$

$$\overline{I} = \frac{\overline{V}_L}{X_L j} = \frac{10.61}{12j} = \boxed{0.88 \angle -90°}$$

$$\therefore \overline{V}_R = \overline{I} R = (0.88 \angle -90°) \times 5 = 4.42 \angle -90°$$

$$\overline{V} = \overline{V}_R + \overline{V}_L = 4.42 \angle -90° + 10.61 \angle 0°$$

$$\overline{V} = \boxed{11.49 \angle -22.62°}$$

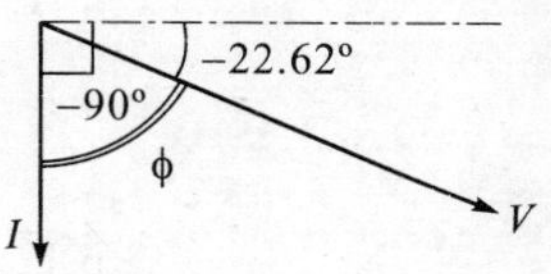

$$\phi = 90° - 22.62° = 15°$$

$$\phi = \boxed{67.38 \text{ lag}}$$

$$Z = \sqrt{R^2 + X_L^{\ 2}} = \sqrt{5^2 + 12^2}$$

$$Z = \boxed{13\ \Omega}$$

18. Two coils A and B have resistances of 12 Ω and 6 Ω respectively and inductance of 0.02 H and 0.03 H respectively. These coil are connected in parallel and a voltage of 200 V and 50 Hz is applied to their common terminals. Find **(i)** current in each coil **(ii)** total current and power factor of combination **(iii)** if a resistance of 15 Ω in series with a condenser of 120 μf is connected in parallel with the above combination. Find the total current and p.f.

Solution : Given : $V_s = 200$ V, $f = 50$ Hz

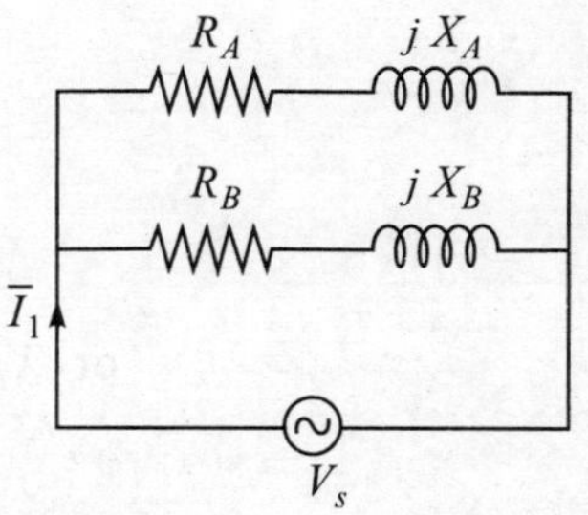

Coil A: $R_A = 12\ \Omega,\ L_A = 0.02$ H

$$X_A = 2\pi f L_A = 6.28\ \Omega$$

Coil B: $R_B = 6\ \Omega,\ L_B = 0.03$ H

$$X_B = 2\pi f L_B = 9.42\ \Omega$$

(i) $$\therefore \overline{I}_A = \frac{V_s}{R_A + X_A j} = \frac{200}{12 + 6.28j} = \boxed{14.77 \angle -27.62°}$$

$$\overline{I}_B = \frac{V_S}{R_B + X_B j} = \frac{200}{6 + 9.42j} = \boxed{17.91 \angle -57.50°}$$

(ii) $$\therefore \overline{I}_1 = \overline{I}_A + \overline{I}_B = 14.77 \angle -27.62° + 17.91 \angle -57.50°$$

$$= \boxed{31.58 \angle -44.03°}$$

$$\therefore \text{pf} = \cos(-44.03°) = \boxed{0.72 \text{ (lagging)}}$$

(iii) Branch *C*: $R_C = 15\ \Omega,\ C = 120\ \mu f$

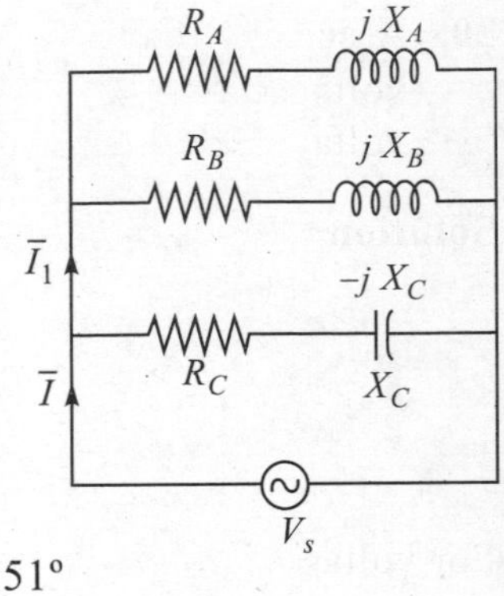

$$X_C = \frac{1}{2\pi f C} = \frac{1}{2\pi \times 50 \times 120 \times 10^{-6}}$$

$$X_C = 26.52\ \Omega$$

$$\therefore\ \overline{I}_C = \frac{V_s}{R_C - X_C j} = \frac{200}{15 - 26.52 j}$$

$$\overline{I}_C = 6.56\ \angle 60.51^\circ$$

$$\therefore\ \overline{I} = \overline{I}_1 + \overline{I}_C = 31.58\ \angle{-44.03^\circ} + 6.56\ \angle 60.51^\circ$$

$$= \boxed{30.6\ \angle{-32.05^\circ}}$$

$$\therefore\ \text{p.f.} = \cos(-32.05^\circ) = \boxed{0.847\ \text{(lagging)}}$$

19. An *R-L-C* series circuit has a current which lags behind the applied voltage by 45°. The voltage across the inductor has maximum value equal to twice the maximum value of voltage across the capacitor. The voltage across the inductance is 300 sin ω*t* and *R* = 20 Ω. Find the value of inductance and capacitance if supply frequency is 50 Hz.

Solution : Given : Angle between $\overline{V}_s$ and $\overline{I}$ is 45 lagging.

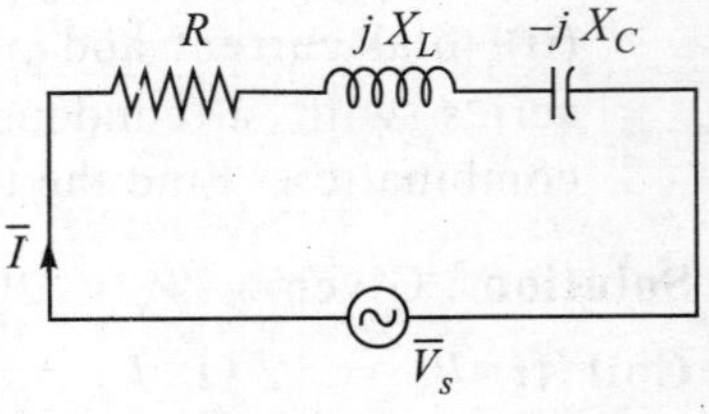

$$V_{L\,max} = 2\ V_{C\,max}$$

$$v_L = 300 \sin \omega t$$

$$R = 20\ \Omega,\ f = 50\ \text{Hz}$$

$$\phi = \tan^{-1}\left(\frac{X_L - X_C}{R}\right)$$

$$\therefore\ R = (X_L - X_C) \qquad [\because\ \phi = 45^\circ]$$

$$\text{or}\ X_L - X_C = 20 \qquad \text{..... (i)}$$

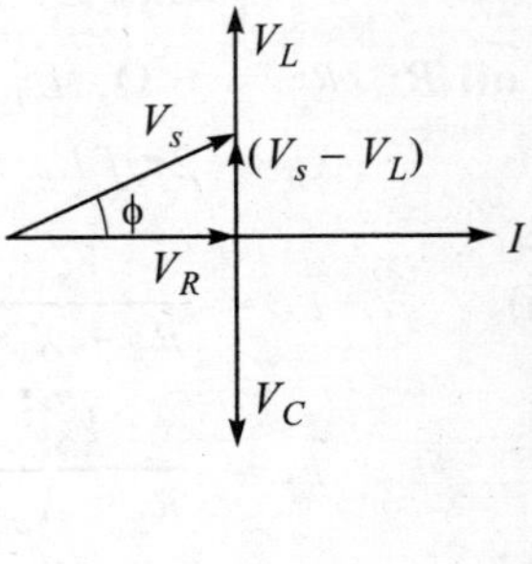

$$V_{L\,max} = 2\ V_{C\,max} \qquad \text{... (given)}$$

$$I_{max} X_L = 2\ I_{max} X_C$$

$$X_L = 2\ X_C \qquad \text{..... (ii)}$$

From (i) and (ii), we get

$$X_C = 20\ \Omega \quad \text{and} \quad X_L = 40\ \Omega$$

$$\frac{1}{2\pi f C} = 20 \quad \text{and} \quad 2\pi f L = 40$$

$$\therefore\ C = \boxed{159.15\ \mu f} \quad \text{and} \quad L = \boxed{127.3\ \text{mH}}$$

20. A series circuit with $R = 5\ \Omega$, C = 20 μf and a variable inductor has an applied voltage of $10 \angle 0°$, with frequency of 1000 rad/s. The inductance is adjusted until the voltage across resistance is maximum. Find the voltage across each element.

Solution : Given : $R = 5\ \Omega,\ \omega = 1000$ rad/s

$C = 20\ \mu f$

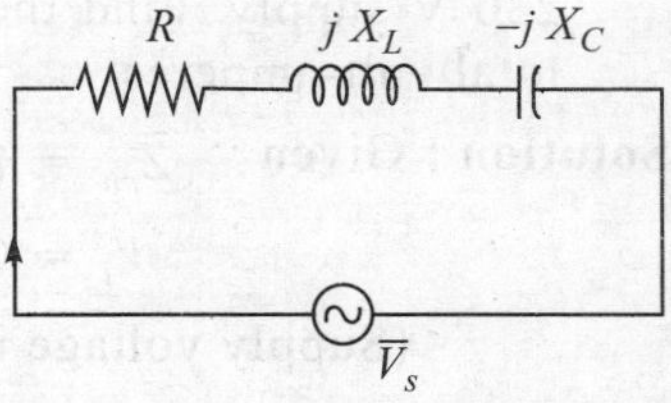

$$X_C = \frac{1}{\omega C} = 50\ \Omega$$

$$\overline{V}_s = 10 \angle 0°$$

For voltage across R to be maximum (resonance)

$$X_L = X_C = 50\ \Omega$$

$$\therefore\ \overline{V}_R = \boxed{10 \angle 0°} \qquad \ldots [\overline{V}_R = \overline{V}_s]$$

At resonance $Z = R$

$$\overline{I} = \frac{\overline{V}_s}{R} = \frac{10 \angle 0°}{5} = 2 \angle 0°$$

$$\therefore\ \overline{V}_L = \overline{I}\,(j X_L)$$

$$\overline{V}_L = \boxed{100 \angle 90°}$$

$$\overline{V}_C = \overline{I}\,(-j X_C)$$

$$\overline{V}_C = \boxed{100 \angle -90°}$$

Chapter 5 : THREE-PHASE CIRCUITS

Solution to Unsolved Examples

(1) A balanced star-connected load of 8 + *j*6 Ω per phase is connected to a 3-phase 230 V supply. Find the line current, power factor, power, reactive volt-ampers and total volt-amperes.

Solution : Given :

$$\overline{Z}_{ph} = 8 + 6j\ \Omega$$

$$V_l = 230 \text{ V}$$

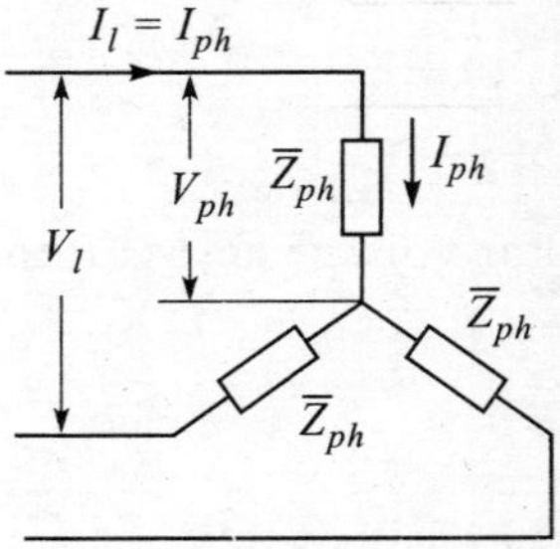

(Supply voltage is always line voltage)

For Star Load :

$$V_{ph} = \frac{V_l}{\sqrt{3}} = \frac{230}{\sqrt{3}} = 132.79 \text{ volts}$$

$$\therefore\ \overline{I}_{ph} = \frac{V_{ph}}{\overline{Z}_{ph}} = \frac{132.79}{8 + 6j} = 13.28\ \angle{-36.87^\circ}$$

$$\therefore\ I_{ph} = \boxed{13.28 \text{ A}} = I_l \quad (\because \text{ star connection})$$

$$\text{Power factor} = \cos(-36.87^\circ)$$

$$\text{p.f.} = \boxed{0.8 \text{ lagging}}$$

$$\text{Power} = 3 V_{ph} I_{ph} \cos\phi$$

$$= 3 \times 132.79 \times 13.28 \times 0.8$$

$$P = \boxed{4232.28 \text{ watts}}$$

$$\text{Reactive volt-ampere } Q = 3 V_{ph} I_{ph} \sin\phi$$

$$P = \boxed{3174.22 \text{ VAR}}$$

$$\text{Total volt-ampere} = 3 V_{ph} I_{ph}$$

$$\text{Total VA} = \boxed{5290.35}$$

(2) A balanced 3-phase, star connected load of 150 kW takes a leading current of 100 A with a line voltage of 1100 V, 50 Hz. Find the circuit constants of the load per phase.

Solution : Given : Star connected load :

$$P = 150 \text{ kW} = 150 \times 10^3 \text{ W}$$

$$I_C = 100 \text{ A} = I_{ph}$$

$$V_L = 1100 \text{ V}$$

$$f = 50 \text{ Hz}$$

$$\text{pf} = \text{leading}$$

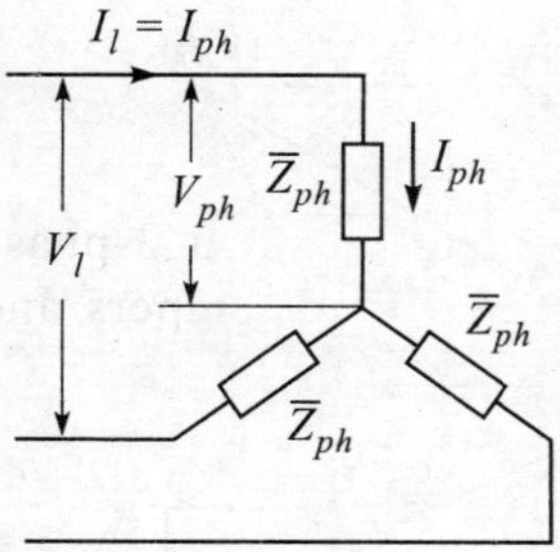

$$P = \sqrt{3}\, V_l\, I_l \cos\phi$$

$$\therefore\ 150 \times 10^3 = \sqrt{3} \times 1100 \times 100 \times \cos\phi$$

$$\therefore\ \cos\phi = 0.7873 \text{ lead}$$

$$\phi = 38.06^\circ$$

$$V_{ph} = \frac{V_l}{\sqrt{3}} = \frac{1100}{\sqrt{3}} = 635.08$$

$$Z_{ph} = \frac{V_{ph}}{I_{ph}} = \frac{635.08}{100}$$

$$\therefore\ Z_{ph} = 6.35\ \Omega$$

$$R = Z_{ph} \cos\phi = 6.35 \cos 38.06^\circ$$

$$\therefore\ R = \boxed{5\ \Omega}$$

$$X_C = Z \sin\phi = 6.35 \sin 38.06^\circ$$

$$\therefore\ X_C = 3.91$$

$$\text{But } X_C = \frac{1}{2\pi f C}$$

$$C = 813.11 \times 10^{-6} \text{ f}$$

$$\therefore\ C = \boxed{813.11\ \mu\text{f}}$$

(3) A balanced star connected load is supplied from a symmetrical 3-phase 400 V system. The current in each phase is 30 A and lags 30° behind the phase voltage. Find **(a)** Phase voltage **(b)** the total power. Draw the vector diagram showing the currents and voltages.

Solution : Given : Star connected load

$$V_l = 400 \text{ V}$$

$$I_{ph} = 30 \text{ A} = I_l$$

$$\phi = 30^\circ \text{ lagging}$$

$$V_{ph} = \frac{V_l}{\sqrt{3}} = \frac{400}{\sqrt{3}}$$

$$\therefore\ V_{ph} = \boxed{230.94 \text{ volts}}$$

$$P = 3 V_{ph}\, I_{ph} \cos\phi$$

$$= 3 \times 230.94 \times 30 \times \cos 30$$

$$P = \boxed{18 \text{ kW}}$$

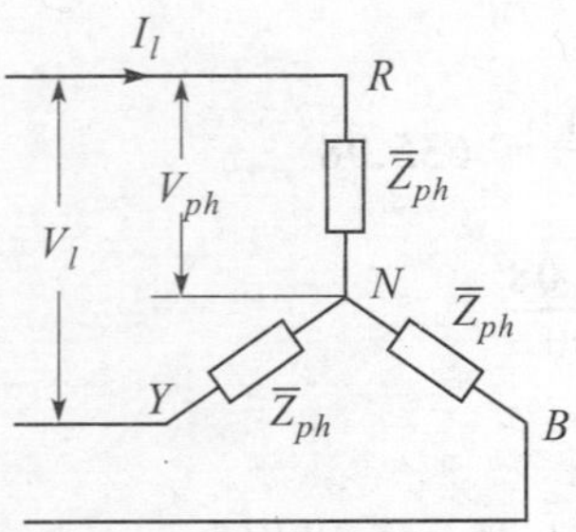

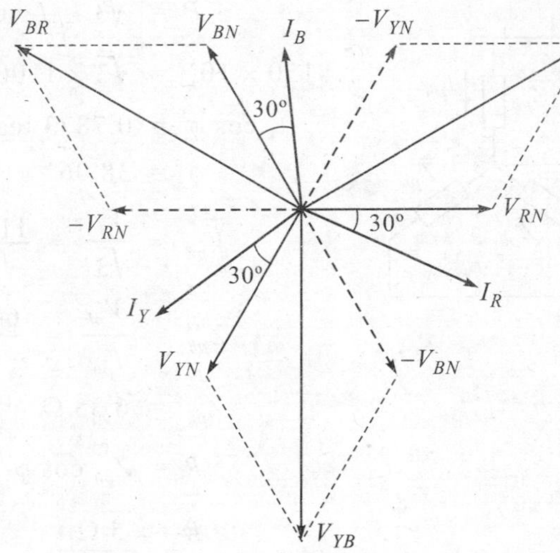

(4) A symmetrical 3-phase 400 V system supplies a balanced delta connected load. The current in each branch circuit is 20 A and phase angle is 40° lagging. Find **(a)** the line current and **(b)** the total power. Draw the vector diagram showing all voltages and currents.

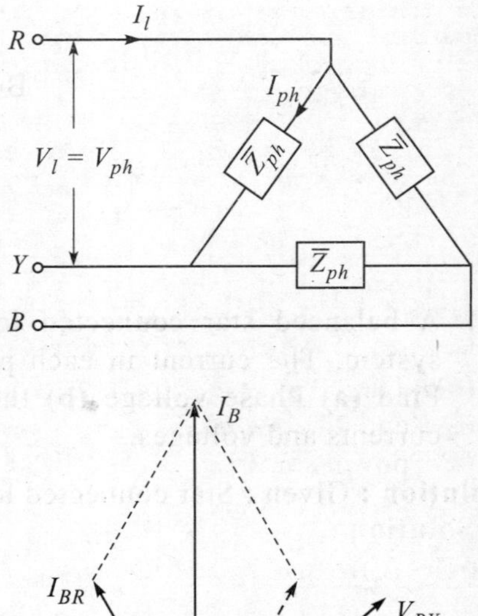

Solution : Given : Delta connected load

$$V_l = 400 \text{ V}$$

$$V_{ph} = 20 \text{ A}$$

$$\phi = 40^\circ \text{ lag}$$

$$I_l = \sqrt{3}\, I_{ph}$$

$$= \sqrt{3} \times 20$$

$$I_l = \boxed{34.64 \text{ A}}$$

$$P = 3 V_{ph}\, I_{ph} \cos\phi$$

$$= 3 \times 400 \times 20 \times \cos 40^\circ$$

$$P = \boxed{18.385 \text{ kW}}$$

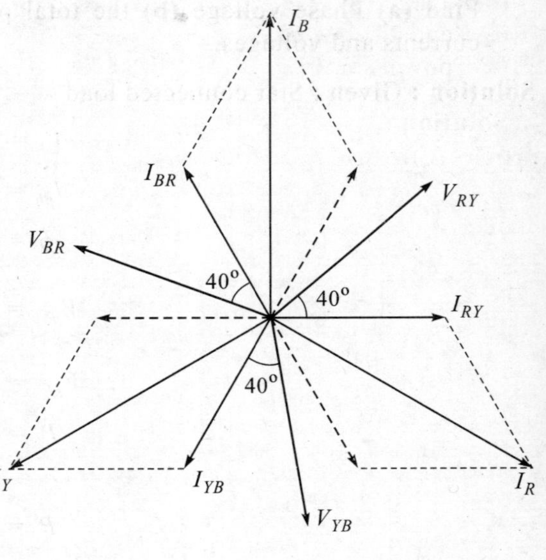

(5) The power input to a 2000 V, 50 Hz, 3-phase motor running on full load at an efficiency of 90% is measured by two wattmeters which indicate 300 kW and 100 kW respectively. Calculate **(a)** input **(b)** power factor **(c)** line current.

Solution : 3-phase motor : $V_l = 2000$ V, $f = 50$ Hz, efficiency $= 90° = \eta$

$$W_2 = 300 \text{ kW}, \; W_1 = 100 \text{ kW}$$

$$\text{Output power} = W_1 + W_2 = 400 \text{ kW}$$

$$\therefore \; \eta = \frac{\text{o/p}}{\text{i/p}}$$

$$\text{Input power} = \boxed{444.44 \text{ kW}}$$

$$\text{Power factor} = \phi = \tan^{-1}\left\{\sqrt{3}\,\frac{W_2 - W_1}{W_1 + W_2}\right\}$$

$$= \tan^{-1}\left\{\sqrt{3}\,\frac{300 - 100}{300 + 100}\right\}$$

$$\phi = 40.89°$$

$$\text{pf} = \boxed{0.7559}$$

$$P = \sqrt{3} V_l I_l \cos\phi$$

$$I_l = \frac{P}{\sqrt{3} V_l \cos\phi} = \frac{400 \times 1000}{\sqrt{3} V_l\, 2000 \times 0.7559}$$

$$I_l = \boxed{152.76 \text{ A}}$$

(6) The power taken by a 3-phase 400 V motor is measured by the two wattmeter method and the readings of the two wattmeters are 460 watts and 780 watts. Estimate the power factor of the motor and the line current.

Solution : Given : $V_L = 400$ V, $W_1 = 460$ W, $W_2 = 780$ W

$$\phi = \tan^{-1}\sqrt{3}\,\frac{W_2 - W_1}{W_2 + W_1} = 24.08°$$

$$\text{pf} = \cos\phi = \boxed{0.9129 \text{ lagging}}$$

$$\text{Power} = W_1 + W_2 = 1240 \text{ W}$$

$$= \sqrt{3}\, V_L I_L \cos\phi$$

$$\therefore \; I_L = \frac{1240}{\sqrt{3} \times 400 \times 0.9129}$$

$$I_L = \boxed{1.96 \text{ A}}$$

(7) Three similar chokes, each having a resistance of 5 Ω and a reactance of 12 W are connected in delta across a 3-phase 440 V supply. Determine **(i)** Total power taken by this load **(ii)** Readings of the two wattmeters connected to measure the total power consumed.

Solution : Given : Delta connection choke : $R = 5\ \Omega, X_L = 12\ \Omega$

$$\therefore\ \bar{Z}_{ph} = 5 + 12j$$

$$V_l = 440 = V_{ph}$$

As the load is inductive, power factor is lagging.

$$\phi = \tan^{-1}\frac{X_L}{R} = \tan^{-1}\frac{12}{5} = 67.38^\circ$$

$$\therefore\ \bar{I}_{ph} = \frac{V_{ph}}{\bar{Z}_{ph}} = \frac{440}{5+12j} = 33.85\angle{-67.38^\circ}$$

$$\therefore\ I_{ph} = 33.85$$

$$\therefore\ I_l = \sqrt{3}\, I_{ph} = 58.63\text{ A}$$

$$P = \sqrt{3}\, V_l\, I_l \cos\phi$$

$$= \sqrt{3} \times 440 \times 58.63 \times \cos 67.38^\circ$$

$$P = \boxed{17.185\text{ kW}}$$

Refer equation (5.52), (5.53), $\phi = -67.38^\circ$ as pf is lagging.

$$\therefore\quad W_1 = V_l I_l \cos(30^\circ + \phi) = 440 \times 58.63 \cos(30^\circ - 67.38^\circ)$$

$$W_2 = V_l I_l \cos(30^\circ - \phi) = 440 \times 58.63 \cos(30^\circ + 67.38^\circ)$$

$$\therefore\ W_1 = \boxed{20.5\text{ kW}}$$

$$W_2 = \boxed{-3.31\text{ kW}}$$

(8) Two wattmeters connected to measure the power input to a 3-phase circuit indicate 8 kW and 0.8 kW, the latter reading obtained after reversing the current coil connections. Find the power and power factor of the load.

Solution : Given : $W_2 = 8$ kW, $W_1 = -0.8$ kW (as reading obtained after reversing current coil connection)

$$P = W_1 + W_2 = 8 - 0.8$$

$$P = \boxed{7.2\text{ kW}}$$

$$\phi = \tan^{-1}\sqrt{3}\,\frac{W_2 - W_1}{W_2 + W_1} = \tan^{-1}\sqrt{3}\,\frac{8+0.8}{8-0.8}$$

$$\therefore\ \phi = 64.71^\circ$$

$$\therefore\ \cos\phi = 0.4271$$

$$\text{p.f.} = \boxed{0.4271}$$

(9) A 7460 watts induction motor runs from 3-phase, 400 V supply. On no-load, the motor takes a line current of 4 A at a power factor of 0.208 lagging. On full load, it operates at a power factor of 0.88 lagging, and an efficiency of 89%. Determine the readings on each of the two wattmeters connected to read total power on **(a)** no load and **(b)** full load.

Solution : Given : 7460 watts, 400 V induction motor.

$$\text{No load current } I_o = 4 \text{ A}$$

$$\text{pf} = \cos \phi_0 = 0.208 \text{ lagging}$$

$$\text{Full load current} = I_{fL}$$

$$\text{Full load efficiency} = \eta = 89\%$$

$$\text{pf} = 0.88 \text{ lagging}$$

Find reading of wattmeters on **(a)** no load **(b)** full load.

(a) No load : $V_L = 400$ V, $I_0 = 4$ A,

$$\cos \phi_0 = 0.208$$

$$\therefore \phi_0 = 78^\circ$$

$$\therefore \quad W_1 = V_l I_l \cos (30^\circ + \phi_0) = 400 \times 4 \times \cos (30^\circ + 78^\circ)$$

$$W_1 = \boxed{-494.43 \text{ watts}}$$

$$W_2 = V_l I_l \cos (30^\circ - \phi_0) = 400 \times 4 \times \cos (30^\circ - 78^\circ)$$

$$W_2 = \boxed{1070.61 \text{ watts}}$$

(b) Full load :

$$\eta = \frac{\text{power o/p}}{\text{power i/p}}$$

$$\text{Power o/p} = \frac{7460}{0.89} = 8382 \text{ watts}$$

$$P = \sqrt{3} V_l I_l \cos \phi$$

$$8382 = \sqrt{3} \times 400 \times I_l \times 0.88$$

$$\therefore I_l = 13.75 \text{ A}$$

$$\phi = \cos^{-1} 0.88 = 28.36^\circ$$

$$\therefore \quad W_1 = V_l I_l \cos (30^\circ + \phi) = 400 \times 13.75 \times \cos (30^\circ + 28.36^\circ)$$

$$W_1 = \boxed{2885.19 \text{ watts}}$$

$$W_2 = V_l I_l \cos (30^\circ - \phi) = 400 \times 13.75 \times \cos (30^\circ - 28.36^\circ)$$

$$W_2 = \boxed{5497.75 \text{ watts}}$$

(10) For a certain balanced 3-phase load, one wattmeter reads 20 kW land the other 5 kW after the voltage circuit of this wattmeter has been reversed. Calculate the power and power factor of the load.

Solution : Given : $W_2 = 20$ kW, $W_1 = -5$ kW (as after reversing voltage circuit).

$$\text{Power} = W = W_1 + W_2 = 20 - 5$$

$$W = \boxed{15 \text{ kW}}$$

$$\phi = \tan^{-1}\sqrt{3}\,\frac{W_2 - W_1}{W_2 + W_1} = \tan^{-1}\sqrt{3}\,\frac{20+5}{20-5}$$

$$\therefore\ \phi = 70.89^\circ$$

$$\text{p.f.} = \cos\phi = \boxed{0.3273}$$

(11) A three-phase three wire 110 V system supplies a delta connected load with equal impedance of 5 ∠45° ohms. Determine the line currents, phase currents and draw the vector diagram.

Solution : Given : Delta connected load

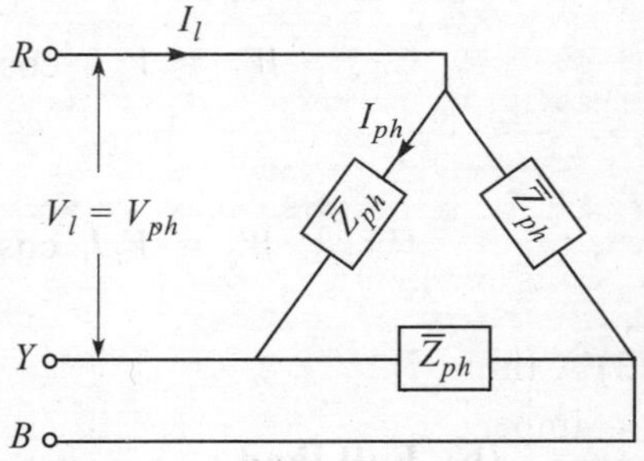

$$V_l = 110 \text{ V} = V_{ph}$$

$$\overline{Z}_{ph} = 5\angle 45^\circ\ \Omega$$

$$\overline{I}_{ph} = \frac{V_{ph}}{\overline{Z}_{ph}}$$

$$= \frac{110}{5\angle 45^\circ}$$

$$= 22\ \angle{-45^\circ}$$

$$I_{ph} = \boxed{22 \text{ A}}$$

$$\phi = -45^\circ$$

$$\text{p.f.} = \cos\phi = \cos(-45^\circ)$$

$$= 0.707$$

$$I_l = \sqrt{3}\,I_{ph} = \sqrt{3} \times 22$$

$$I_l = \boxed{38.1 \text{ A}}$$

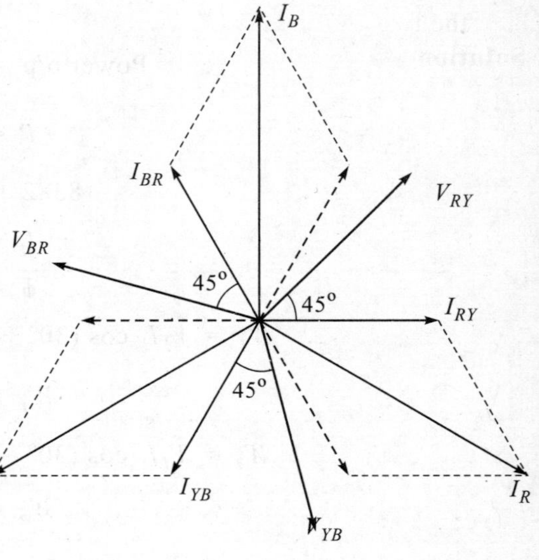

(12) A three 3-phase 208 volt supply is connected to star connected impedances of 20 ∠–30°. Find line and phase currents and voltages. Draw the vector diagram.

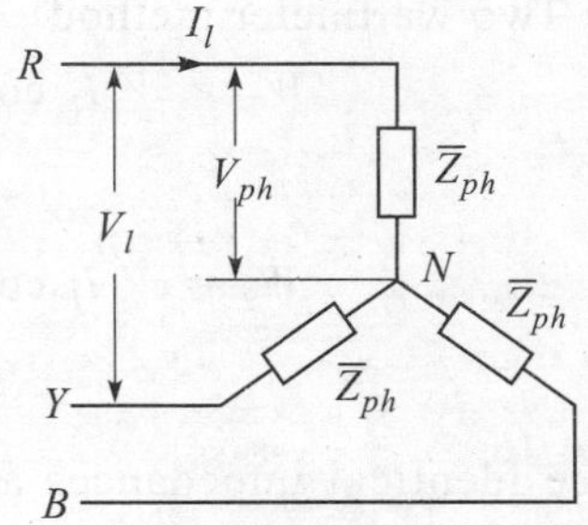

Solution : Given : Star connected load

$$V_l = \boxed{208 \text{ V}} = V_{ph}$$

$$\overline{Z}_{ph} = 20\angle{-30^\circ}$$

$$V_{ph} = \frac{V_l}{\sqrt{3}}$$

$$= \frac{208}{\sqrt{3}} = \boxed{120 \text{ V}}$$

$$\overline{I}_{ph} = \frac{V_{ph}}{\overline{Z}_{ph}}$$

$$= \frac{120}{20\angle{-30^\circ}} = 6\angle 30^\circ$$

$$\therefore I_{ph} = \boxed{6 \text{ A}}$$

$$I_l = I_{ph} = \boxed{6 \text{ A}}$$

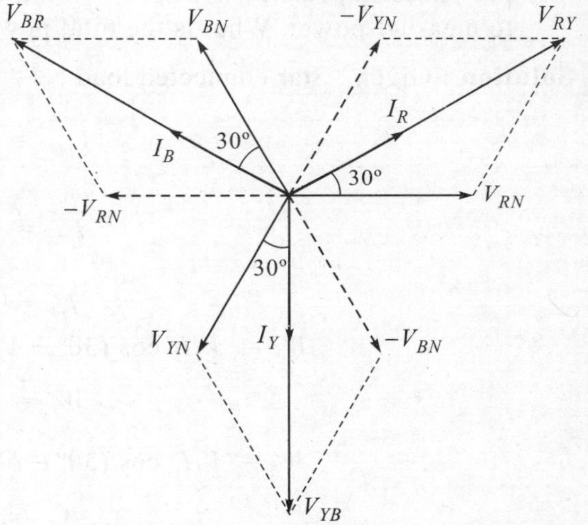

(13) A three-phase, 100 V supplied is connected to a balanced delta connected load with impedance of 20 ∠45°. Determine the line currents and power consumed by the circuit. Also if two wattmeters were used to measure power, indicate the readings of the two wattmeters.

Solution : Given : Delta connected load

$$V_l = 100 \text{ V} = V_{ph}$$

$$\overline{Z}_{ph} = 20\angle 45^\circ \ \Omega$$

$$\therefore \overline{I}_{ph} = \frac{V_{ph}}{\overline{Z}_{ph}} = \frac{100}{20\angle 45^\circ} = 5\angle{-45^\circ}$$

$$\therefore I_{ph} = \boxed{5 \text{ A}}, \ \phi = -45^\circ$$

$$I_l = \sqrt{3}\, I_{ph} = \sqrt{3} \times 5$$

$$I_l = \boxed{8.66 \text{ A}}$$

$$P = \sqrt{3}\, V_l I_l \cos\phi = \sqrt{3} \times 100 \times 8.66 \times \cos 45^\circ$$

$$P = \boxed{1060.63 \text{ W}}$$

Two wattmeter method

$$W_1 = V_l I_l \cos(30° + \phi) = 100 \times 8.66 \times \cos(30° - 45°)$$

$$W_1 = \boxed{836.49 \text{ W}}$$

$$W_2 = V_l I_l \cos(30° - \phi) = 100 \times 8.66 \times \cos(30° + 45°)$$

$$W_2 = \boxed{224.14 \text{ W}}$$

(14) Three identical impedances are connected in star to a 150 V, 3-phase supply. If the per phase impedance is 5 ∠–30°. Find the readings of the two wattmeters connected to measure power. What is the total power consumed.

Solution : Given : Star connected load : $V_l = 150$ V, $\bar{Z}_{ph} = 5\angle -30°\ \Omega$

$$V_{ph} = \frac{V_l}{\sqrt{3}} = \frac{150}{\sqrt{3}} = 86.6 \text{ V}$$

$$\bar{I}_{ph} = \frac{V_{ph}}{\bar{Z}_{ph}} = \frac{86.6}{5\angle -30°} = 17.32\angle 30°$$

$$\therefore I_{ph} = 17.32 = I_l \text{ and } \phi = 30°$$

$$W_1 = V_l I_l \cos(30° + \phi) = 150 \times 17.32 \cos(30° + 30°)$$

$$W_1 = \boxed{1299 \text{ W}}$$

$$W_2 = V_l I_l \cos(30° - \phi) = 150 \times 17.32 \cos(30° - 30°)$$

$$W_2 = \boxed{2598 \text{ W}}$$

$$\text{Total power } W = W_1 + W_2 = 1299 + 2598$$

$$W = \boxed{3897 \text{ W}}$$

(15) The phasor diagram below shows line currents and line voltages of a three phase 346 volt supply. If the magnitudes of line current is 10 A. Find the impedance of star connected load per phase.

Solution : Given : Star connected load : V_l and I_l are in phase.

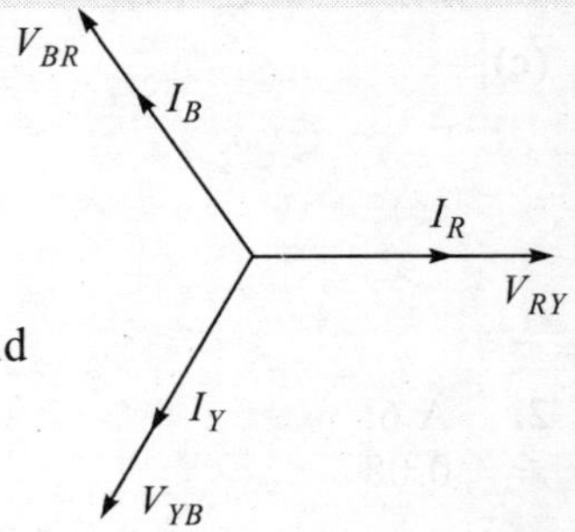

$$V_l = 346 \text{ volts}, I_l = 10 \text{ A} = I_{ph}$$

$$V_{ph} = \frac{V_l}{\sqrt{3}} = 200 \text{ V}$$

For star connected balanced load the angle between phase and line voltages is 30° (line voltage leads)

$\therefore$ Power factor angle = 30° leading $\therefore \phi = 30°$

$$\bar{Z}_{ph} = \frac{V_{ph}}{\bar{I}_{ph}} = \frac{200}{10\angle 30°} = 20\angle -30°$$

$$Z_{ph} = \boxed{20\ \Omega}$$

Chapter 6 : TRANSFORMER

Solution to Unsolved Examples

1. A 300 KVA, single phase transformer has 300 turns on the primary and 100 turns on the secondary. The primary is connected to 1500 V, 50 Hz supply. Determine:

(a) The secondary open circuit voltage

(b) Full load current in both windings

(c) The max. value of flux

Solution : Given : 300 KVA transformers

$$\text{Primary turns} = N_1 = 300$$
$$\text{Secondary turns} = N_2 = 100$$
$$V_1 = 1500 \text{ V}$$
$$f = 50 \text{ Hz}$$

(a) Secondary open circuit voltage $= V_2$

$$\frac{V_2}{V_1} = \frac{N_2}{N_1}$$
$$\therefore\ V_2 = \frac{100}{300} \times 1500$$
$$V_2 = \boxed{500 \text{ V}}$$

(b) Secondary open circuit voltage $= V_2$

$$I_{1fl} = \frac{KVA \times 1000}{V_1} = \frac{300 \times 1000}{1500}$$
$$I_{1fl} = \boxed{200 \text{ A}}$$
$$I_{2fl} = \frac{KVA \times 1000}{V_2} = \frac{300 \times 1000}{500}$$
$$I_{2fl} = \boxed{600 \text{ A}}$$

(c)

$$V_1 = 4.44 f \phi_m N_1$$
$$\therefore\ \phi_m = \frac{1500}{4.44 \times 50 \times 300}$$
$$\phi_m = \boxed{0.0225 \text{ wb}}$$

2. A 6600/600 V, 1-phase, 50 Hz transformer has maximum value of flux in the core as 0.08 wb. Find the number of turns in each winding.

Solution : Given : 6600/600 V, 1-phase, 50 Hz transformer

$$V_1 = 6600,\ V_2 = 600 \text{ V},\ f = 50 \text{ Hz},\ \phi_m = 0.08 \text{ wb.}$$
$$V_1 = 4.44 f \phi_m N_1$$

$$\therefore N_2 = \frac{600}{4.44 \times 50 \times 0.08} = 33.78$$

$$N_2 = \boxed{34 \text{ turns}}$$

$$\frac{N_1}{N_2} = \frac{V_1}{V_2}$$

$$\therefore N_1 = \frac{6600}{600} \times 34$$

$$N_1 = \boxed{374 \text{ turns}}$$

3. A 300 KVA, 3300/300 V single phase transformer has 1100 primary turns. Find **(a)** transformation ratio **(b)** secondary turns **(c)** voltage per turn **(d)** secondary current it supplies a load of 200 kW at 0.8 power factor logging. Assuming primary and secondary winding resistance and leakage reactance to be negligible.

Solution : Given : $V_1 = 3300$ V, $V_2 = 300$ V, $KVA = 300$, $N_1 = 1100$

(a)

$$\text{Turns ratio} = K = \frac{V_2}{V_1} = \frac{300}{3300}$$

$$\text{Turns ratio} = \boxed{\frac{1}{11}}$$

(b)

$$N_2 = \frac{V_2}{V_1} \times N_1 = \frac{300}{3300} \times 1100 = 100$$

$$N_2 = \boxed{100}$$

(c)

$$\text{Voltage per turn} = \frac{V_1}{N_1} = 4.44 f \phi_m$$

$$\text{Voltage per turn} = \frac{3300}{1100} = \boxed{3}$$

(d)

$$P_2 = V_2 I_2 \cos \phi_2$$

$$200 \times 1000 = 300 \times I_2 \times 0.8$$

$$\therefore I_2 = \boxed{833.33 \text{ A}}$$

4. A 4400/1400 V single phase transformer gives 0.8 A and 100 W as ammeter and watt meter readings when supply is given to low voltage windings and high voltage winding is kept open. Find **(a)** Power factor of no-load current **(b)** magnetizing component of current and care loss component of circuit.

Solution : Given : $V_1 = 4400$ V, $V_2 = 400$ V

(a) Current in l.v. winding when h.v. winding is kept open = ?

$$\therefore W_{20} = 100 \text{ W}$$

$$I_{20} = 0.8$$

$$W_{20} = V_2 I_{20} \cos \phi_2$$
$$100 = 400 \times 0.8 \times \cos \phi_2$$
$$\therefore \cos \phi_2 = \boxed{0.3125}$$
$$\phi_2 = 71.79^\circ$$

(b) Magnetizing component of current $= I_m$

$$I_m = I_{20} \sin \phi_0 = 0.8 \sin 71.79^\circ$$
$$I_m = \boxed{0.76 \text{ A}}$$

(c) Core loss component of current $= I_C$

$$I_C = I_{20} \cos \phi_0 = 0.8 \times 0.3125^\circ$$
$$I_C = \boxed{0.25 \text{ A}}$$

5. **A 230/115 V single phase transformer takes a no-load current of 2A at a p.f. of 0.2 lagging with low voltage winding kept open. If the low voltage winding is now having a current of 15 A at 0.8 p.f. lagging when loaded, find the current and power factor of primary current now drawn.**

Solution : Given :

$$V_1 = 230 \text{ V (h.v. winding)}$$
$$V_2 = 115 \text{ V (l.v. winding)}$$
$$I_{10} = 2 \text{ A}$$
$$\cos \phi_0 = 0.2 \text{ lagging}$$
$$\therefore \phi_0 = -78.46$$
$$I_2 = 15 \text{ A}$$
$$\cos \phi_2 = 0.8 \text{ lagging}$$
$$\phi_2 = -36.87$$

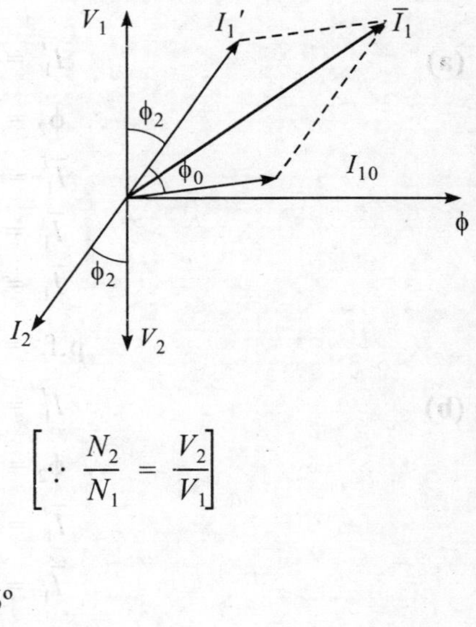

$$N_1 I_1' = N_2 I_2$$
$$\therefore I_1' = \frac{N_2}{N_1} I_2 = \frac{115}{230} \times 15 \qquad \left[\because \frac{N_2}{N_1} = \frac{V_2}{V_1}\right]$$
$$I_1' = 7.5$$
$$\overline{I}_{10} = I_{10} \angle \phi_0 = 2 \angle -78.46^\circ$$
$$\overline{I}_1' = I_1' \angle \phi_2 = 7.5 \angle -36.87^\circ$$
$$\overline{I}_1 = I_1' + I_{10} = 7.5 \angle -36.87^\circ + 2 \angle -78.46^\circ$$
$$\overline{I}_1 = \boxed{9.09 \angle -45.26^\circ}$$
$$\therefore \text{p.f.} = \cos(-45.26)$$
$$\text{p.f.} = \boxed{0.7038 \text{ lagging}}$$

6. A 4:1 step down transformer takes a no load current of 0.8 A at 0.25 lagging p.f. on h.v. side with l.v. open. If the secondary takes a load current of 100 A at **(a)** 0.8 p.f. lagging and **(b)** 0.8 p.f. leading. Find the primary current and power factor.

Solution : Given : 4:1 step down transformer

$$\frac{V_1}{V_2} = \frac{4}{1} = \frac{N_1}{N_2}$$

$$I_{10} = 0.8$$

$$\cos \phi_0 = 0.25 \text{ lagging}$$

$$\text{If } I_2 = 100 \text{ A}$$

(a) 0.8 p.f. lagging **(b)** 0.8 p.f. leading

$$\phi_0 = \cos^{-1} 0.25 = -75.52°$$

$$\bar{I}_{10} = 0.8 \angle -75.52°$$

$$N_1 I_1' = N_2 I_2$$

$$\therefore I_1' = \frac{N_2}{N_1} I_2 = \frac{4}{1} \times 100 = 25 \text{ A}$$

(a)

$$I_1' = 25 \text{ at } 0.8 \text{ p.f. lagging}$$

$$\therefore \phi_2 = -36.87°$$

$$\bar{I}_1' = 25 \angle -36.87°$$

$$\bar{I}_1 = \bar{I}_{10} + \bar{I}_1' = 0.8 \angle -75.52° + 25 \angle -36.87°$$

$$\bar{I}_1 = \boxed{25.63 \angle -37.98°}$$

$$\text{p.f.} = \boxed{0.788 \text{ lagging}}$$

(b)

$$I_1' = 25 \text{ at } 0.8 \text{ pf leading}$$

$$\therefore \phi_2 = 36.87°$$

$$\bar{I}_1' = 25 \angle 36.87° = 0.8 \angle -75.52° + 25 \angle 36.87°$$

$$\bar{I}_1 = \boxed{24.7 \angle 35.15°}$$

$$\text{p.f.} = \boxed{0.818 \text{ leading}}$$

7. A 30 KVA, 3000/300 V, single phase 50Hz transformer has a primary resistance and reactance of 3.5 Ω and 4.5 Ω respectively. The secondary resistance and reactance are 0.015 Ω and 0.02 Ω respectively. Find **(a)** Equivalent resistance and reactance referred to h.v. side. **(b)** equivalent resistance and reactance referred to l.v. side. **(c)** full load copper losses.

Solution : Given : 30 KVA, 3000/300 V, 50 Hz transformer

$r_1 = 3.5\ \Omega\ ;\ x_1 = 4.5\ \Omega$

$r_2 = 0.015\ \Omega\ ;\ x_2 = 0.02\ \Omega$

(a) Referred to h.v. side

$$r_2' = \left(\frac{3000}{300}\right)^2 \times 0.015 = 1.5$$

$$R_1 = r_1 + r_2' = 3.5 + 1.5$$

$$R_1 = \boxed{5\ \Omega}$$

$$X_2' = \left(\frac{3000}{300}\right)^2 \times 0.02 = 2\ \Omega$$

$$X_1 = x_1 + x_2' = 4.5 + 2$$

$$X_1 = \boxed{6.5\ \Omega}$$

(b) Referred to l.v. side

$$r_1' = \left(\frac{300}{3000}\right)^2 \times 3.5 = 0.035$$

$$R_2 = r_1' + r_2 = 0.035 + 0.015$$

$$R_2 = \boxed{0.05\ \Omega}$$

$$X_1' = \left(\frac{300}{3000}\right)^2 \times 04.5 = 0.045$$

$$X_2 = x_1' + x_2 = 0.045 + 0.02$$

$$X_2 = \boxed{0.065\ \Omega}$$

(c) Full load copper loss $= I_{2fl}^2 R_2 = I_{1fl}^2 R_1$

$$I_{2fl} = \frac{\text{KVA} \times 1000}{V_2} = \frac{30{,}000}{300} = 100\text{ A}$$

$$\therefore\ W_{cufl} = 100^2 \times 0.05$$

$$W_{cufl} = \boxed{500\text{ watts}}$$

8. Obtain the approximate equivalent circuit of a given referred to l.v. side. 200/2000 V, 30 KVA, 1-phase transformer having following test results.

O.C. test (on l.v. side) : 200 V, 6 A, 360 W

S.C. test (on h.v. side) : 75 V, 18A, 600 W.

Solution : Given : 200 /2000 V, 30 KVA

(a) O.C. test (on l.v. side)

$V_0 = 200\text{ V}, I_0 = 6\text{ A}$

$W_0 = 360\text{ W}$

$$W_0 = V_0 I_0 \cos \phi_0$$

$$\therefore \cos \phi_0 = \frac{W_0}{V_0 I_0} = \frac{360}{200 \times 6} = 0.3$$

$$\phi_0 = 72.54^\circ$$

$$I_C = I_0 \cos \phi_0 = 1.8 \text{ A}$$

$$R_C = \frac{V_0}{I_C} = \frac{200}{1.8}$$

$$R_C = \boxed{111.11\ \Omega} \quad \text{[Referred to l.v. side]}$$

$$I_m = I_0 \sin \phi_0 = 6 \sin 72.54^\circ = 5.72 \text{ A}$$

$$X_\phi = \frac{V_0}{I_\phi} = \frac{200}{5.72}$$

$$X_\phi = \boxed{34.96\ \Omega} \quad \text{[Referred to l.v. side]}$$

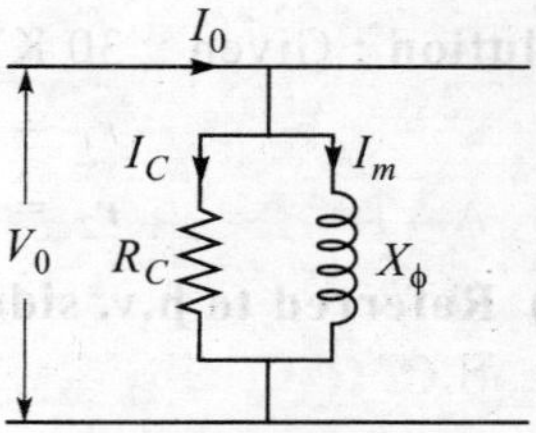

On l.v. side

(b) S.C. test (on h.v. side)

V_{SC} = 75 V; I_{SC} = 18 A; W_{SC} = 600 W

$$Z_{SC} = \frac{V_{SC}}{I_{SC}} = \frac{75}{18} = 4.17\ \Omega$$

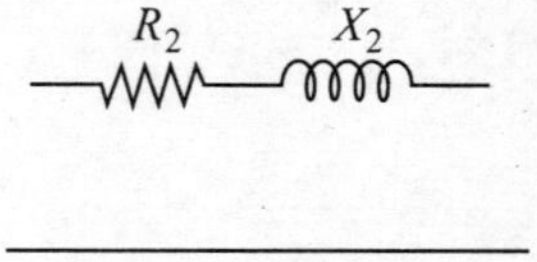

On h.v. side

$$W_{SC} = I_{SC}^2 R_2$$

$$R_2 = \frac{W_{SC}}{I_{SC}^2} = \frac{600}{18^2}$$

$$R_2 = \boxed{1.85\ \Omega}$$

$$Z_2 = \sqrt{R_2^2 + X_2^2}$$

$$X_2 = \sqrt{Z_2^2 - R_2^2} = \sqrt{4.17^2 - 1.85^2}$$

$$X_2 = 3.74\ \Omega$$

$\therefore$ R_1 = resistance referred to l.v. side

$$= \left(\frac{200}{2000}\right)^2 \times 1.85$$

$$R_1 = \boxed{0.0185\ \Omega}$$

$$X_1 = \left(\frac{200}{2000}\right)^2 \times 3.74$$

$$X_1 = \boxed{0.0374\ \Omega}$$

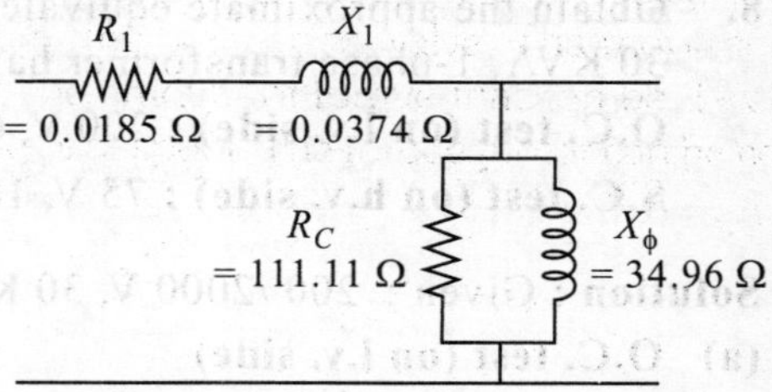

Equivalent circuit referred to l.v. side

9. A 4 KVA, 400 / 200 V, 50 Hz, 1-phase transformer has the following test results.

O.C. test (l.v. side) : 200 V, 1 A, 164 W

S.C. test (h.v. side) : 15 V, 10 A, 80 W

Find **(a)** Equivalent circuit referred to h.v. side

(b) Iron lanes and full load copper lanes

(c) Efficiency and regulation at full load 0.8 p.f. lagging.

Solution : Given : 4 KVA, 400 /200 V, 50 Hz transformer.

(a) O.C. test (on l.v. side)

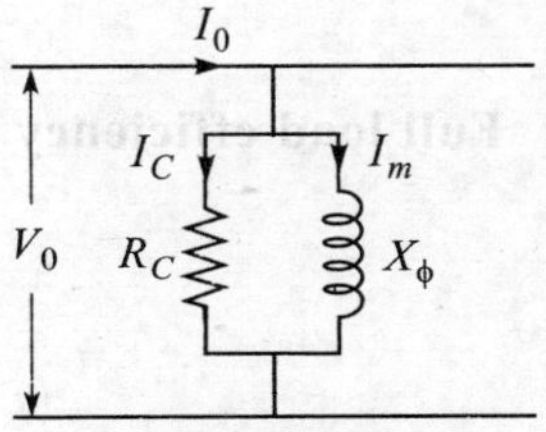

On l.v. side

$V_0 = 200$ V, $I_0 = 1$ A, $W_0 = 64$ W

$$W_0 = V_0 I_0 \cos\phi_0$$

$$\therefore \cos\phi_0 = \frac{64}{200 \times 1} = 0.32$$

$$\phi_0 = 71.33^\circ$$

$$I_C = I_0 \cos\phi_0 = 1 \times 0.32 \text{ A}$$

$$I_m = I_0 \sin\phi_0 = 1 \sin 71.33^\circ = 0.95 \text{ A}$$

$$R_C = \frac{V_0}{I_C} = \frac{200}{0.32} = 625\ \Omega$$

$$X_\phi = \frac{V_0}{I_m} = \frac{200}{0.95} = 210.53\ \Omega$$

Resistance referred to h.v. side

$$R_C' = \left(\frac{400}{200}\right)^2 \times 625 = \boxed{2500\ \Omega}$$

Resistance referred to h.v. side

$$X_C' = \left(\frac{400}{200}\right)^2 \times 210.53 = \boxed{842.12\ \Omega}$$

S.C. test (on h.v. side)

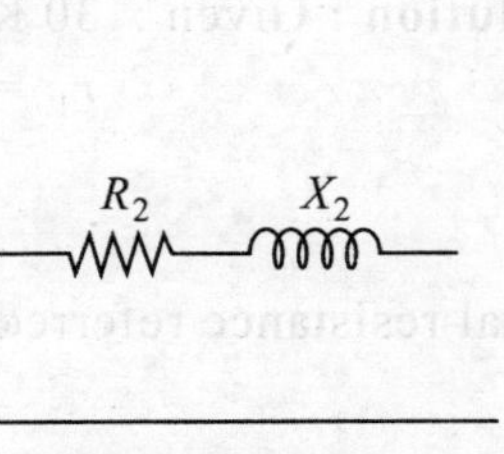

On h.v. side

$V_{SC} = 15$ V, $I_{SC} = 10$ A, $W_{SC} = 80$ W

$$W_{SC} = I_{SC}^2 R_2$$

$$\therefore R_2 = \frac{80}{10^2} = \boxed{0.8\ \Omega}$$

$$Z_2 = \frac{V_{SC}}{I_{SC}} = \frac{15}{10} = 1.5\ \Omega$$

$$X_2 = \sqrt{Z_2^2 - R_2^2} = \sqrt{1.5^2 - 0.8^2}$$

$$X_2 = \boxed{1.27\ \Omega}$$

(b) As O.C. test is performed at rated voltage (200 V)

$$W_o = W_i = \boxed{64 \text{ W}}$$

$$\text{Rated full load current of h.v. winding} = \frac{\text{KVA} \times 1000}{400}$$

$$= \frac{4000}{400} = 10 \text{ A}$$

S.C. test is carried at full load current (10 A)

$$W_{SC} = W_{Cufl} = 80 \text{ W}$$

(c) Full load efficiency $= \eta_{fl}$

$$\eta_{fl} = \frac{\text{KVA} \cos\phi \times 1000}{\text{KVA} \cos\phi \times 1000 + W_i + W_{cufl}} \times 100$$

$$\eta_{fl} = \frac{4 \times 0.8 \times 1000}{4 \times 0.8 \times 1000 + 64 + 80} \times 100$$

$$\eta_{fl} = \boxed{95.69\%}$$

$$\text{Regulation} = \frac{I_2 R_2 \cos\phi_2 + I_2 X_2 \sin\phi_2}{V_2} \times 100$$

$$= \frac{10 \times 0.08 \times 0.8 + 10 \times 1.27 \times 0.6}{400} \times 100$$

$$\text{Regulation} = \boxed{3.5\%}$$

10. The primary and secondary winding resistances of a 30 KVA, 6600/300 V single phase transformer are 8 Ω and 0.02 Ω respectively. The equivalent leakage reactance referred to primary winding is 30 Ω. Find the full load regulation for load power factor of **(a)** unity **(b)** 0.8 lagging **(c)** 0.8 leading.

Solution : Given : 30 KVA, 6600/300 V, transformer

$$r_1 = 8\ \Omega,\ r_2 = 0.02\ \Omega,\ X_1 = 30\ \Omega$$

$$r_1' = \left(\frac{300}{6600}\right)^2 \times 8 = 0.016\ \Omega$$

Total resistance referred to secondary side $= R_2$

$$R_2 = r_1' + r_2 = 0.016 + 0.02$$

$$R_2 = 0.036\ \Omega$$

Total reactance referred to secondary side

$$X_2 = \left(\frac{300}{3000}\right)^2 \times 1 = \left(\frac{1}{22}\right)^2 \times 30$$

$$X_2 = 0.062\ \Omega$$

$$\text{Regulation} = \frac{I_2 R_2 \cos \phi_2 \pm I_2 X_2 \sin \phi_2}{V_2}$$

+ve sign for lagging power factor

–ve sign for leadeing power factor

$$I_2 = \frac{KVA \times 1000}{300} = \frac{30 \times 1000}{300} = 100 \text{ A}$$

(a) Unity p.f. i.e. $\cos \phi = 1, \sin \phi = 0$

$$\% \text{ regulation} = \frac{100 \times 0.036 - 0}{300} \times 100$$

$$\% \text{ regulation} = \boxed{1.2\%}$$

(b) 0.8 lagging power pactor : $\cos \phi = 0.8, \sin \phi = 0.6$

$$= \frac{100 \times 0.036 \times 0.8 + 100 \times 0.062 \times 0.6}{300} \times 100$$

$$\% \text{ regulation} = \boxed{2.2\%}$$

(c) 0.8 leading power pactor : $\cos\phi = 0.8 \ \sin\phi = 0.6$

$$= \frac{100 \times 0.036 \times 0.8 - 100 \times 0.062 \times 0.6}{300} \times 100$$

$$\% \text{ regulation} = \boxed{-0.28\%}$$

11. A 250/500 V 1-phase transformer gave the following test results:

O.C. test (l.v. side) : 250 V, 1 A, 80 W

S.C. test (h.v. side) : 20V, 12 A, 100 W

Find **(a)** The circuit constants referred to h.v. side.

(b) Efficiency when 10 A flows through 500 V winding at 0.8 p.f. lagging.

Solution : Given : 250 /500 V, 1-phase transformer

i.e. $V_1 = 250$ V (l.v.side)

$V_2 = 500$ V (h.v.side)

(a) O.C. test (l.v. side)

$$V_0 = 250 \text{ V}; I_0 = 1 \text{ A}; W_0 = 80 \text{ W}$$

$$W_0 = V_0 I_0 \cos \phi_0$$

$$\therefore \phi_0 = \cos^{-1} \frac{W_0}{V_0 I_0}$$

$$\phi_0 = 71.34$$

$$I_C = I_0 \cos \phi_0 = 0.32 \text{ A}$$

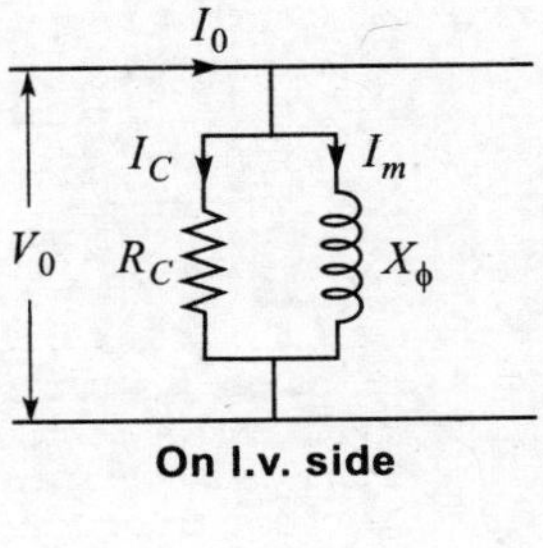

On l.v. side

$$R_C = \frac{V_0}{I_C} = \frac{250}{0.32} = 781.25\ \Omega$$

$$I_\phi = I_0 \sin \phi_0 = 0.95\ \text{A}$$

$$X_\phi = \frac{V_0}{I_\phi} = \frac{250}{0.95} = 263.16\ \Omega$$

$$R_C' = R_C \text{ referred to h.v. side}$$

$$= \left(\frac{500}{250}\right)^2 \times 781.25$$

$$R_C' = \boxed{3125\ \Omega}$$

$$X_\phi' = X_\phi \text{ referred to h.v. side}$$

$$= \left(\frac{500}{250}\right)^2 \times 263.16$$

$$X_\phi' = \boxed{1052.64\ \Omega}$$

S.C. test (on h.v. side)

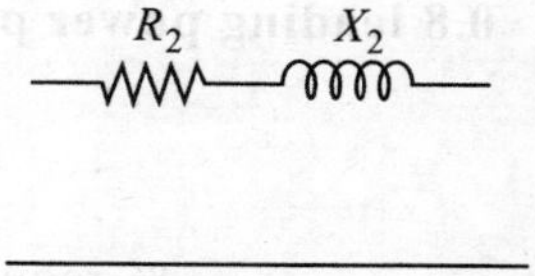

On h.v. side

$$V_{SC} = 20\ \text{V},\ I_{SC} = 12\ \text{A},\ W_{SC} = 100\ \text{W}$$

$$W_{SC} = I_{SC}^2 R_2$$

$$\therefore R_2 = \boxed{0.69\ \Omega}$$

$$Z_2 = \frac{V_{SC}}{I_{SC}} = 1.67\ \Omega$$

$$X_2 = \sqrt{Z_2^2 - R_2^2}$$

$$= \sqrt{1.67^2 - 0.69^2}$$

$$X_2 = \boxed{1.52\ \Omega}$$

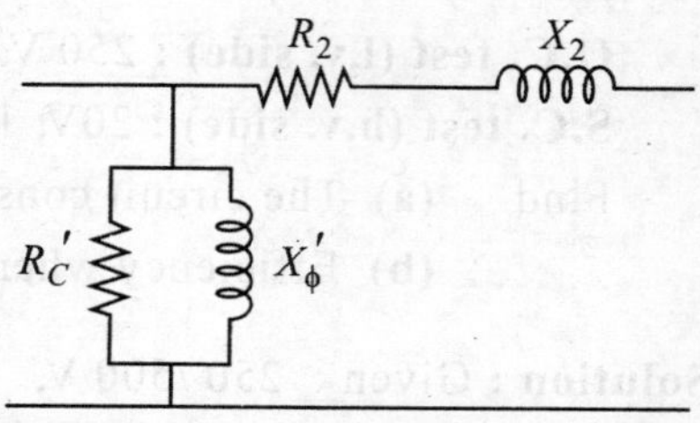

Equivalent circuit referred to h.v. side

(b) Efficiency at 10 A, 0.8 p.f.

$$W_i = W_0 = 80\ \text{W}$$

$$\eta = \frac{V_2 I_2 \cos \phi_2}{V_2 I_2 \cos \phi_2 + W_i + I_2 R_2} \times 100$$

$$\eta = \frac{500 \times 10 \times 0.8}{500 \times 1 \times 0.8 + 80 + 10^2 \times 0.69} \times 100$$

$$\eta = \boxed{96.41\%}$$

12. Open circuit and short circuit test were conducted on a 50 KVA, 6360/240 V, 50 Hz, 1-phase transformer.

O.C. test : Voltage across primary 6360 V, primary current 1A power input 2 kW.

S.C. test : Voltage across primary 100 V, current in secondary 175 A, power input 0.2 kW.

Draw equivalent circuit referred to secondary side and also find regulation at full load 0.8 pf leading.

Solution : Given : 50 KVA, 6360/240 V, 50 Hz, 1-phase transformer

O.C. test (h.v. side)

$$V_0 = 6360 \text{ V}; I_0 = 1 \text{ A}; W_0 = 2 \text{ kW}$$

$$\therefore W_0 = V_0 I_0 \cos\phi_0$$

$$\therefore \phi_0 = 71.67^\circ$$

$$I_C = I_0 \cos\phi_0 = 0.31 \text{ A}$$

$$I_m = I_0 \sin\phi_0 = 0.95 \text{ A}$$

$$R_C = \frac{V_0}{I_C} = 20516\ \Omega$$

$$X_\phi = \frac{V_0}{I_m} = 6700\ \Omega$$

S.C. test (h.v.side)

$$V_{SC} = 100 \text{ V}; W_{SC} = 0.2 \text{ kW}$$

$$I_{2fl} = \frac{\text{KVA} \times 1000}{240} = 208.33 \text{ A}$$

$$I_2 = 175 \text{ A}$$

$$\frac{I_1}{I_2} = \frac{V_2}{V_1}$$

$$I_1 = 175 \times \frac{240}{6360} = 6.6 \text{ A}$$

$$\therefore I_{SC} = 6.6 \text{ A (Primary current)}$$

$$W_{SC} = I_{SC}^2 R_1$$

$$R_1 = 4.59\ \Omega$$

$$Z_1 = \frac{V_{SC}}{I_{SC}} = \frac{100}{6.6} = 15.15\ \Omega$$

$$X_1 = \sqrt{Z_1^2 - R_1^2} = 14.43\ \Omega$$

Equivalent circuit referred to secondary (l.v. side)

$$R_2 = \left(\frac{240}{6360}\right)^2 \times 4.59 = \boxed{6.5 \times 10^{-3}\,\Omega}$$

$$X_2 = \left(\frac{240}{6360}\right)^2 \times 14.43 = 20 \times 10^{-3}\,\Omega$$

$$R_C' = \left(\frac{240}{6360}\right)^2 \times 20516 = \boxed{28.722\,\Omega}$$

$$X_\phi' = \left(\frac{240}{6360}\right)^2 \times 6700 = \boxed{9.38\,\Omega}$$

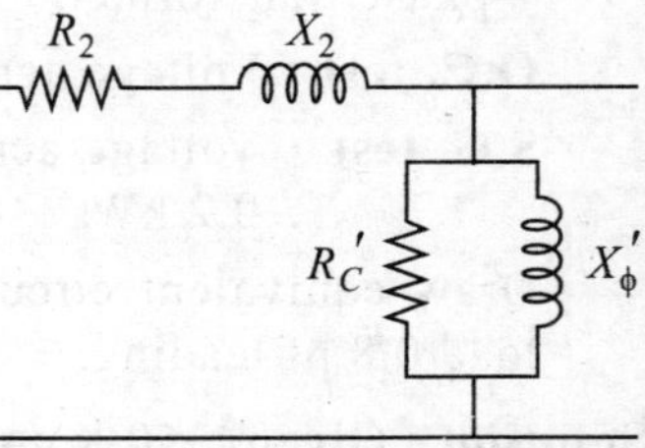

Equivalent circuit referred to l.v. side

Regulation at full load 0.8 p.f. leading

$$= \frac{I_2 R_2 \cos\phi_2 - I_2 X_2 \sin\phi_2}{V_2} \times 100 = \boxed{-0.59\%}$$

13. A 15 KVA, 2000/200 V transformer has an iron loss of 250 W and full load copper loss of 400 W. During the days it is loaded as follows :

No. of hrs	Load	Power factor
9	1/4th load	0.6
7	Full load	0.8
6	3/4th load	1.0
2	No load	—

Calculate all days efficiency.

Solution : Given : 15 KVA, 2000/200 V transformer

$$W_i = 250 \text{ W} = 0.25 \text{ kW}, \; W_{cufl} = 400 \text{ W} = 0.4 \text{ kW}$$

Load α	pf $\cos\phi$	o/p in kW $W = \alpha$ KVA $\cos\phi$	No. of hrs (t)	o/p in kWhr $= Wt$	$W_{cu} = \alpha^2 W_{cufl}$	Copper loss in kWhr $W_{cu} \times t$
0.25	0.6	2.25	9	20.25	0.025	0.225
1	0.8	12	7	84	0.4	2.8
0.75	1	11.25	6	67.5	0.225	1.35
0	---	---	2	---	---	---

Total o/p in kWhr = 20.25 + 84 + 67.5 = 171.75

Total copper loss in 24 hrs = 0.225 + 2.8 + 1.35 = 4.375

$$\therefore \eta_{all\ day} = \frac{\text{o/p in kWhr over 24 hrs}}{\text{o/p in kWhr 24 hrs} + 24\ W_i \text{ over 24 hrs} + W_{cu} \text{ over 24 hrs}} \times 100$$

$$= \frac{171.75}{171.75 + 4.375 + 6} \times 100$$

$$\therefore \eta_{all\ day} = \boxed{94.3\%}$$

14. A 40 KVA transformer has a maximum efficiency of 98% at 80% of full load at 4 pf. During the day it is loaded as follows:

No. of hrs	Load	Power factor
8	6 kW	0.6 lag
6	24 kW	0.8 lag
7	30 kW	0.9 lag
3	No load	—

Calculate all day efficiency.

Solution : Given : 40 KVA transformer, max. efficiency = 98% at α = 0.8 and upf

$$\therefore \eta_{max} = \frac{\alpha \text{ KVA} \times 1000}{\alpha \text{ KVA} \cos\phi + 2Wi} \times 100 \quad \left[\begin{array}{l}\text{as } W_i = W_{cu} \\ \text{for max. efficiency}\end{array}\right]$$

$$98 = \frac{0.8 \times 40 \times 1}{0.8 \times 40 \times 1 + 2Wi} \times 100$$

$$Wi = 0.33 \text{ kW}$$

$$\text{but} \quad Wi = \alpha\, W_{cufl}$$

$$\therefore \quad W_{cufl} = \frac{0.33}{0.8} = 0.41 \text{ kW}$$

Load α	pf $\cos\phi$ *(given)*	o/p in kW $W = \alpha$ KVA $\cos\phi$ *(given)*	No. of hrs (t) *(given)*	o/p in kWhr $= Wt$	$W_{cu} = \alpha^2 W_{cufl}$	Copper loss in kWhr $W_{cu} \times t$
0.25	0.6	6	8	48	0.0256	0.205
0.75	0.8	24	6	144	0.2306	1.38
0.83	0.9	30	7	210	0.282	1.977
0	---	---	3	---	---	---

Total o/p in kWhr = 402

Total copper loss in 24 hrs = 3.562

Iron loss in 24 hrs = 7.92

$$\therefore \eta_{all\ day} = \frac{402}{402 + 7.92 + 3.562} \times 100$$

$$= \boxed{97.22\%}$$

15. A 230 V, 2.5 KVA 1-phase transformer has an iron loss of 100 W at 40 Hz and 70 W at 30 Hz. Find the hysterias and eddy current losses at 50 Hz.

Solution : Given : 230 V, 2.5 KVA transformer

Iron loss at 40 Hz = 100 W

Iron loss at 30 Hz = 70 W

Hysterias loss = $k_1 f$

Eddy current loss = $k_2 f^2$

$$\therefore 100 = k_1 40 + k_2 40^2 \quad ..... (i)$$

$$\text{and} \quad 70 = k_1 30 + k_2 30^2 \quad ..... (ii)$$

Solving (i) and (ii),

$$\therefore k_1 = 1.83 \text{ and } k_2 = 0.016$$

$\therefore$ Hysterias loss at 50 Hz = $k_1 f$

$= 1.83 \times 50$

$W_h = \boxed{91.5 \text{ W}}$

Eddy current loss at 50 Hz = $k_2 f^2$

$= 0.016 \times 50^2$

$W_e = \boxed{40 \text{ W}}$

APPENDIX C

SOME USEFUL FORMULAE

- $\sin(A \pm B) = \sin A \cos B \pm \cos A \sin B$
- $\cos(A \pm B) = \cos A \cos B \mp \sin A \sin B$
- $\sin 2A = 2 \sin A \cos A$
- $\cos 2A = \cos^2 A - \sin^2 A$
- $\sin A + \sin B = 2 \sin\left(\frac{A+B}{2}\right) \cos\left(\frac{A-B}{2}\right)$
- $\sin A - \sin B = 2 \sin\left(\frac{A-B}{2}\right) \cos\left(\frac{A+B}{2}\right)$
- $\cos A + \cos B = 2 \cos\left(\frac{A+B}{2}\right) \cos\left(\frac{A-B}{2}\right)$
- $\cos A - \cos B = 2 \sin\left(\frac{A+B}{2}\right) \sin\left(\frac{B-A}{2}\right)$

	$-\theta$	$90 \pm \theta$	$180 \pm \theta$	$270 \pm \theta$
sin	$-\sin\theta$	$\cos\theta$	$\mp\sin\theta$	$-\cos\theta$
cos	$\cos\theta$	$\mp\sin\theta$	$-\cos\theta$	$\pm\sin\theta$

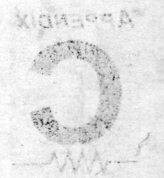